Adult social care law

Stephen Knafler QC is the founder and general editor of the *Community Care Law Reports*. He is based at Landmark Chambers. He practises in every area of public law but has a particular interest in social care.

Available as an ebook at www.lag.org.uk/ebooks

LAG eBook

The purpose of Legal Action Group is to promote equal access to justice for all members of society who are socially, economically or otherwise disadvantaged. To this end, it seeks to improve law and practice, the administration of justice and legal services.

Adult social care law

Stephen Knafler QC

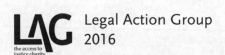

LAG the access to justice charity
Legal Action Group
2016

This edition published in Great Britain 2016
by LAG Education and Service Trust Limited
National Pro Bono Centre, 48 Chancery Lane, London WC2A 1JF
www.lag.org.uk

British Library Cataloguing in Publication Data
a CIP catalogue record for this book is available from the British Library.

FSC
www.fsc.org
MIX
Paper from responsible sources
FSC® C020438

This book has been produced using Forest Stewardship Council (FSC) certified paper. The wood used to produce FSC certified products with a 'Mixed Sources' label comes from FSC certified well-managed forests, controlled sources and/or recycled material.

Print ISBN 978 1 908407 78 8
ebook ISBN 978 1 908407 79 5

Typeset by Regent Typesetting, London
Printed by Hobbs the Printers, Totton, Hampshire

Introduction

The original plan, hatched many years ago, was for a simple, straightforward community care casebook comprising a themed selection of case summaries culled from the *Community Care Law Reports*. If only I had had the time to write that book how much simpler life would have been.

Instead, along came the Care Act 2014, and the native hue of resolution became sicklied o'er with the pale cast of thought.

In the end, after a year or so of sporadic sickly thought, it seemed to me that a simple casebook would not be of much practical use. One needs to know how and why the older cases are relevant now we have the new Act. And in any event, one needs to know the context. In adult social care, cases are only one part of the overall picture so that, to my mind, a simple casebook would afford such an incomplete view of the whole as to be deeply unsatisfactory.

On the other hand, the creation of a full-scale textbook on adult social care struck me as being a task of such monumental proportions, it was best left to writers of genius – such as Professor Luke Clements and the late, greatly missed Pauline Thompson, both colleagues of mine at the *Community Care Law Reports* and authors of the brilliant *Community Care and the Law*, of which I am the proud owner of two copies (at home and chambers), plus one one for luck.

Accordingly, having screwed my courage to the sticking point, I embarked upon the series of compromises, that now form the spine, if it has one, of this book.

I've tried not to compromise on the cases too much because this remains, at its heart, a casebook. I've endeavoured to include all the cases, of any significance, that form part of adult social care and also all the cases that many adult social care practitioners will want to know about from time to time – for example, cases about the NHS, mental health and persons subject to immigration control. I've based my selection on the *Community Care Law Reports* but have often gone beyond them. Where this book differs from other casebooks is that it contains citations and sometimes extensive citations from the judgments and I make no apology for that. On the whole, judgments are the culmination of a lengthy process involving contributions from many different sources and judges think long and hard about how to summarise and adjudicate upon this material. I remain strongly of the view that the words of judges are in general worth a lot of more than the words of textbook writers and repay detailed, careful consideration. So I've included a lot of them. Not everyone has access to all the law reports, or has the time or inclination to read them in the regular, repeated manner they deserve (!), so my hope is that there is enough in the citations in this book to provide for the needs of the average busy practitioner for a lot of the time.

I've taken a similar approach to the legislation and guidance, being of the view that the precise words used are important and useful; a lot of thought has gone into, for example, the *Care and Support Statutory Guidance* which, in many respects, renders superfluous the efforts of the commentator. On the other hand, all the legislation and materials comprise a huge amount of text. So I've tried to strike a balance here, setting out verbatim as much of the legislation, guidance and other material as LAG has allowed me to get away with, whilst summarising the less important passages and, in some cases, simply signposting the reader to documents and websites that will enable him or her to explore particular areas in greater depth. Again, I hope that this method will save the time of busy practitioners and make it possible to use the book as a self-contained resource in some cases and as a starting point, at least, in others.

Finally, at the risk of being shot down in flames, I've tried to introduce each chapter, in particular the chapters with a case-law focus, with a short overarching summary of the legal framework so that readers can get an overview, from the start. I hope readers will find these introductions useful or at least forgive them: I had to write them because I was in blood stepped so far that should I wade no more, returning were as tedious as go o'er.

I intended, initially, to include children's social care but there has been such an explosion of cases and material in this area in recent years, and in areas closely associated with children's social care, in particular relating to children from abroad, that this will have to wait for another book.

I'd like to thank the whole team of editors at the *Community Care Law Reports*: Richard Gordon QC, Stephen Cragg QC, Paul Bowen QC, Simon Bull, Luke Clements, Jean Gould, Nicola Mackintosh QC, Kate Markus QC, Sophy Miles, Camilla Parker, Paul Ridge and Lucy Scott-Moncrieff, and in particular the headnote editors: Christopher Baker, Tim Baldwin, Stephen Broach, Bethan Harris and Stephen Simblet whose case summaries I have relied on a great deal and, in a few cases, verbatim. I would like to recollect, with gratitude and deep respect, the contribution made by Pauline Thompson before her death. I give a special thanks to Roger Pezzani for his guidance on the mental health chapter and to David Lock QC for his assistance on the health chapter; both pre-eminent mental health and health practitioners.

My editor Esther Pilger has been absolutely brilliant. I can't thank her or the team at LAG enough, especially Lesley Exton and Lucy Logan-Green.

I have tried to make the book as up to date as possible, and whilst some of the more recondite of recent materials may have passed me by, I think the law is up to date as at the end of August 2016. I aim to update the book each quarter in its ebook format and I would be very grateful indeed for any corrections, additions and observations that readers send in: please write to SKnafler@landmarkchambers.co.uk.

I count myself as having been extremely fortunate to have practised as a barrister in the social care field for many years and to have had the opportunity to advise and represent across a very broad spectrum from individuals and families needing care and support, to private and social sector operators and to social services, housing and health authorities and regulators. It's been an eye-opening and often an amazing and humbling experience. I hope that this book gives something back that others find useful. That is the purpose of the book. Ultimately, it's the people who need care and support and the families and friends who support them who need help the most and I really hope that in some way this tome will, in the difficult years that lie ahead, provide a sword and shield for those who need its help most and who often achieve incredible things in the face of huge adversity. But it would be churlish and wrong not to acknowledge, also, the sympathetic devotion and hard work of many who toil in the often unloved social and public sector, and private sector operators, who do their very best, but so often get the brickbats and not the compliments. If this book is of some practical use, saves time and helps everyone concerned reach fair and equitable solutions, I will shuffle off my mortal coil just that little bit more happily when the time comes, hopefully after many more editions of this epistle which, despite the best efforts of the drafters of some of the secondary legislation, I have very much enjoyed writing.

Stephen Knafler QC
September 2016

Contents

Table of cases

R v Mayor and Burgesses of the London Borough of Hackney ex p S (No 2) [2001] EWHC 228 (Admin)	8.63, 27.24
R v Mental Health Review Tribunal ex p Hall [2000] 1 WLR 1323, [1999] 4 All ER 883, (1999) 2 CCLR 383, [1999] Lloyd's Rep Med 417, (2000) 51 BMLR 117, [1999] COD 429, (1999) 96(33) LSG 31, (1999) 149 NLJ 1368, CA	12.53, 19.14, 19.126
R v Mental Health Review Tribunal for South Thames Region ex p Smith (1999) 47 BMLR 104, [1999] COD 148, QBD	19.8, 19.12
R v Merseyside Mental Health Review Tribunal ex p K [1990] 1 All ER 694, CA	19.85, 19.88
R v Merton Sutton and Wandsworth HA ex p Perry (2000) 3 CCLR 378, [2001] Lloyd's Rep Med 73, [2001] ACD 9, QBD	4.25, 16.28, 22.14
R v Ministry of Defence ex p Smith [1996] QB 517, [1996] 2 WLR 305, [1996] 1 All ER 257, [1996] ICR 740, [1996] IRLR 100, (1996) 8 Admin LR 29, [1996] COD 237, (1995) 145 NLJ 1689, CA	25.55
R v Monopolies and Mergers Commission ex p Argyll Group Plc [1986] 1 WLR 763, [1986] 2 All ER 257, (1986) 2 BCC 99086, CA	3.30
R v Montila (Steven William) [2004] UKHL 50, [2004] 1 WLR 3141, [2005] 1 All ER 113, [2005] 1 Cr App R 26, [2005] Crim LR 479, (2005) 102(3) LSG 30, (2004) 148 SJLB 1403	7.2, 7.102, 17.9
R v Newcastle-upon-Tyne City Council ex p Dixon, 20 October 1993, unreported	14.19
R v Newham LBC ex p Medical Foundation for the Care of Victims of Torture (1998) 30 HLR 955, (1997–98) 1 CCLR 227, QBD	9.87, 20.37
R v Newham LBC ex p Patrick (2001) 4 CCLR 48, QBD	8.60, 9.85
R v North and East Devon HA ex p Coughlan [2001] QB 213, [2000] 2 WLR 622, [2000] 3 All ER 850, (2000) 2 LGLR 1, [1999] BLGR 703, (1999) 2 CCLR 285, [1999] Lloyd's Rep Med 306, (2000) 51 BMLR 1, [1999] COD 340, (1999) 96(31) LSG 39, (1999) 143 SJLB 213, CA	3.13, 3.31, 3.33, 3.36, 3.37, 3.40, 13.16, 16.5, 16.27, 16.39, 16.49, 18.6, 18.20, 18.50, 18.51, 18.56, 22.14, 25.55
R v North and East Devon HA ex p Pow [1997] EWHC 765 (Admin), (1997–98) 1 CCLR 280	3.12
R v North Derbyshire HA ex p Fisher (1998) 10 Admin LR 27, (1997–98) 1 CCLR 150, [1997] 8 Med LR 327, (1997) 38 BMLR 76, QBD	4.8, 4.11, 4.21, 18.11, 18.28, 25.3
R v North West Lancashire HA ex p A [2000] 1 WLR 977, [2000] 2 FCR 525, (1999) 2 CCLR 419, [1999] Lloyd's Rep Med 399, (2000) 53 BMLR 148, CA	18.11, 18.30, 25.3
R v North West Thames RHA ex p Daniels (Rhys William) [1993] 4 Med LR 364, [1994] COD 44, DC	3.12
R v North Yorkshire CC ex p Hargreaves (1997–98) 1 CCLR 104, QBD	8.56, 8.57, 9.5, 23.24, 27.16
R v North Yorkshire CC ex p Hargreaves (1997–98) 1 CCLR 331, [1997] COD 390, QBD	4.19, 8.3
R v Oxford Regional Mental Health Tribunal ex p Secretary of State for the Home Department [1988] AC 120, [1987] 3 WLR 522, [1987] 3 All ER 8, (1987) 84 LSG 2690, (1987) 137 NLJ 735, (1987) 131 SJ 1086, HL	19.14
R v Powys CC ex p Hambidge (No 2) (1999) 2 CCLR 460, QBD	3.14, 3.15, 11.68

R (HA) v Hampstead School Governors [2016] EWHC 278 (Admin), [2016] ELR 125	3.8, 4.13, 5.13, 27.10
R (Haggerty) v St Helens BC [2003] EWHC 803 (Admin), [2003] HLR 69, (2003) 6 CCLR 352, (2003) 74 BMLR 33, [2003] ACD 73	3.19, 16.36
R (Haringey Consortium of Disabled People and Carers Association) v Haringey LBC (2002) 5 CCLR 422, (2001) 58 BMLR 160, QBD	3.15
R (Harris) v Haringey LBC [2010] EWCA Civ 703, [2011] PTSR 931, [2010] Eq LR 98, [2010] BLGR 713, [2010] JPL 1635, [2010] NPC 72	5.58
R (Harrison) v Secretary of State for Health [2009] EWHC 574 (Admin), (2009) 12 CCLR 355, [2009] LS Law Medical 246, [2009] ACD 61	18.41
R (Hawke) v Secretary of State for Justice [2015] EWHC 3599 (Admin)	3.8, 5.67, 27.10
R (Heather) v Leonard Cheshire Foundation [2002] EWCA Civ 366, [2002] 2 All ER 936, [2002] HRLR 30, [2002] UKHRR 883, [2002] HLR 49, (2002) 5 CCLR 317, (2003) 69 BMLR 22, [2002] ACD 43	15.7
R (Heffernan) v Sheffield City Council [2004] EWHC 1377 (Admin), (2004) 7 CCLR 350	8.62
R (Hillsden) v Epping Forest DC [2015] EWHC 98 (Admin)	4.3
R (Holloway) v Oxfordshire CC [2007] EWHC 776 (Admin), [2007] BLGR 891, (2007) 10 CCLR 264	19.37, 19.49
R (Hooper) v Secretary of State for Work and Pensions [2002] EWHC 191 (Admin), [2002] UKHRR 785	19.97
R (Hooper) v Secretary of State for Work and Pensions [2005] UKHL 29, [2005] 1 WLR 1681, [2006] 1 All ER 487, [2005] 2 FCR 183, [2005] HRLR 21, [2005] UKHRR 717, [2005] Pens LR 337	17.17
R (Hooper) v Secretary of State for Work and Pensions [2003] EWCA Civ 813, [2003] 1 WLR 2623, [2003] 3 All ER 673, [2003] 2 FCR 504, [2003] UKRR 1268, 14 BHRC 626, (2003) 100(29) LSG 35	25.44
R (Howard League for Penal Reform) v Secretary of State for the Home Department (No 2) [2002] EWHC 2497 (Admin), [2003] 1 FLR 484, (2003) 6 CCLR 47, [2003] Prison LR 128, [2003] Fam Law 149, (2003) 100(3) LSG 30, (2003) 147 SJLB 61	25.18
R (Hughes) v Liverpool City Council [2005] EWHC 428 (Admin), [2005] BLGR 531, (2005) 8 CCLR 243	9.91, 25.72
R (Hunt) v North Somerset Council [2013] EWCA Civ 1320, [2014] BLGR 1, (2013) 16 CCLR 502	27.7
R (Hunt) v North Somerset Council [2015] UKSC 51, [2015] 1 WLR 3575, [2016] 1 All ER 95, [2015] BLGR 859, [2015] LLR 516	27.38
R (Hurley) v Secretary of State for Business, Innovation and Skills [2012] EWHC 201 (Admin), [2012] HRLR 13, [2012] Eq LR 447, [2012] ELR 297, [2012] ACD 50	3.30, 5.8, 5.9, 5.11, 5.22, 5.58, 5.62, 5.64, 5.68
R (Ireneschild) v Lambeth LBC [2007] EWCA Civ 234, [2007] HLR 34, [2007] BLGR 619, (2007) 10 CCLR 243, [2007] NPC 31	8.4, 8.64, 9.6, 27.5
R (J) v Caerphilly CBC [2005] EWHC 586 (Admin), [2005] 2 FLR 860, [2005] 2 FCR 153, (2005) 8 CCLR 255, [2005] ACD 80, [2005] Fam Law 611, [2005] Fam Law 528	8.61

R (Mooney) v Southwark LBC [2006] EWHC 1912 (Admin), (2006) 9 CCLR 670, [2006] NPC 94	20.41
R (Morge) v Hampshire CC [2011] UKSC 2, [2011] 1 WLR 268, [2011] 1 All ER 744, [2011] PTSR 337, [2011] Env LR 19, [2011] BLGR 271, [2011] JPL 865, [2011] 4 EG 101 (CS), (2011) 108(5) LSG 20	5.68
R (Morris) v Newham LBC [2002] EWHC 1262 (Admin)	20.38, 25.61
R (Morris) v Rhondda Cynon Taf CBC [2015] EWHC 1403 (Admin), [2015] ELR 559, (2015) 18 CCLR 550	3.44
R (Morris) v Trafford Healthcare NHS Trust [2006] EWHC 2334 (Admin), (2006) 9 CCLR 648, [2006] Lloyd's Rep Med 529, [2007] ACD 11, (2006) 150 SJLB 1290	3.21, 16.40
R (Morris) v Westminster City Council (No 3) [2005] EWCA Civ 1184, [2006] 1 WLR 505, [2005] HRLR 43, [2006] UKHRR 165, [2006] HLR 8, [2006] BLGR 81, [2006] ACD 29	17.17, 20.39, 20.44, 25.44
R (Moseley) v Haringey LBC [2014] UKSC 56, [2014] 1 WLR 3947, [2015] 1 All ER 495, [2014] PTSR 1317, [2014] BLGR 823, [2015] RVR 93	3.2, 3.3, 3.4, 3.5, 3.37, 3.39, 3.40, 3.42, 3.43, 3.44, 3.45
R (MS) v Independent Monitor of the Home Office [2016] EWHC 655 (Admin), [2016] 4 WLR 88	29.69
R (Munjaz) v Mersey Care NHS Trust [2005] UKHL 58, [2006] 2 AC 148, [2005] 3 WLR 793, [2006] 4 All ER 736, [2005] HRLR 42, [2006] Lloyd's Rep Med 1, (2005) 86 BMLR 84, [2005] MHLR 276	4.26, 4.27
R (MVN) v Greenwich LBC (Costs) [2015] EWHC 2663 (Admin)	27.39
R (Mwanza) v Greenwich LBC [2010] EWHC 1462 (Admin), [2011] PTSR 965, [2010] BLGR 868, (2010) 13 CCLR 454, [2010] MHLR 226, [2010] ACD 86	19.110, 19.123, 20.1, 21.20, 21.35
R (N) v Mental Health Review Tribunal (Northern Region) [2005] EWCA Civ 1605, [2006] QB 468, [2006] 2 WLR 850, [2006] 4 All ER 194, (2006) 88 BMLR 59, [2006] MHLR 59	19.78
R (National Association of Health Stores) v Secretary of State for Health [2005] EWCA Civ 154	5.8
R (NM) v Islington LBC [2012] EWHC 414 (Admin), [2012] 2 All ER 1245, [2012] PTSR 1582, [2012] BLGR 435, (2012) 15 CCLR 563	8.50
R (Noble Organisation Ltd) v Thanet DC [2005] EWCA Civ 782, [2006] Env LR 8, [2006] 1 P&CR 13, [2006] JPL 60, [2005] NPC 86	14.4
R (Novartis Pharmaceuticals UK Ltd) v Licensing Authority (C106/01) [2004] ECR I-4403, [2004] 2 CMLR 26, [2005] All ER (EC) 192, (2005) 81 BMLR 200, ECJ	25.9
R (O) v East Riding of Yorkshire CC [2011] EWCA Civ 196, [2011] 3 All ER 137, [2012] PTSR 328, [2011] 2 FLR 207, [2011] 1 FCR 453, [2012] BLGR 171, [2011] ELR 347, (2011) 14 CCLR 256, [2011] Fam Law 586, (2011) 108(11) LSG 18	22.18
R (O) v Haringey LBC [2004] EWCA Civ 535, [2004] 2 FLR 476, [2004] 2 FCR 219, [2004] HLR 44, [2004] BLGR 672, (2004) 7 CCLR 310, [2004] Fam Law 634	21.65
R (OH) v Bexley LBC. *See* OH v Bexley LLP	
R (Otley) v Barking and Dagenham NHS Primary Care Trust [2007] EWHC 1927 (Admin), (2007) 10 CCLR 628, [2007] LS Law Medical 593, (2007) 98 BMLR 182, [2007] ACD 78	18.8, 18.39

R (VC) v Newcastle City Council [2011] EWHC 2673 (Admin), [2012] 2 All ER 227, [2012] PTSR 546, [2012] 1 FLR 944, [2012] 1 FCR 206, (2012) 15 CCLR 194, [2012] Fam Law 280	21.72
R (W) v Birmingham City Council [2011] EWHC 1147 (Admin), [2011] Eq LR 721, [2012] BLGR 1, (2011) 14 CCLR 516, (2011) 120 BMLR 134, [2011] ACD 84	3.29, 5.50, 5.53
R (W) v Croydon LBC [2011] EWHC 696 (Admin), (2011) 14 CCLR 247, [2011] ACD 64	3.26, 10.20
R (W) v Doncaster MBC [2004] EWCA Civ 378, [2004] BLGR 743, [2004] MHLR 201, (2004) 101(22) LSG 32, (2004) 148 SJLB 572	19.111, 19.119
R (W) v Lambeth LBC [2002] EWCA Civ 613, [2002] 2 All ER 901, [2002] 2 FLR 327, [2002] 2 FCR 289, [2002] HLR 41, [2002] BLGR 351, (2002) 5 CCLR 203, [2002] Fam Law 592, (2002) 146 SJLB 125	17.5, 17.13
R (W) v Secretary of State for Home Department [2016] EWCA Civ 82, [2016] 1 WLR 2793, [2016] Imm AR 585	27.42
R (W) v Secretary of State for Justice [2015] EWHC 1952 (Admin), [2015] ACD 139	29.65
R (W, X, Y, Z) v Secretary of State for Health [2015] EWCA Civ 1034, [2016] 1 WLR 698	18.68
R (Wahid) v Tower Hamlets LBC [2002] EWCA Civ 287, [2003] HLR 2, [2002] BLGR 545, (2002) 5 CCLR 239	9.87, 20.8, 20.37
R (Watkins-Singh) v Aberdare Girls' High School Governors [2008] EWHC 1865 (Admin), [2008] 3 FCR 203, [2008] ELR 561, [2008] ACD 88	7.27
R (Watts) v Bedford Primary Care Trust (C-372/04) [2006] QB 667, [2006] 3 WLR 213, [2006] ECR I-4325, [2006] 3 CMLR 5, [2006] All ER (EC) 835, [2006] CEC 884, (2006) 90 BMLR 150, ECJ	18.35
R (WC) v South London & Maudsley NHS Trust [2001] EWHC 1025(Admin), [2001] 1 MHLR 187	19.47
R (Weaver) v London & Quadrant Housing Trust [2009] EWCA Civ 587, [2010] 1 WLR 363, [2009] 4 All ER 865, [2010] PTSR 1, [2009] HRLR 29, [2009] UKHRR 1371, [2009] HLR 40, [2009] BLGR 962, [2009] L&TR 26, [2009] 25 EG 137 (CS), (2009) 153(25) SJLB 30, [2009] NPC 81	15.4, 15.11, 25.28, 25.75
R (West Berkshire DC) v Secretary of State for Communities and Local Government [2016] EWCA Civ 441, [2016] PTSR 982	3.4, 4.6, 4.8, 5.17
R (Westminster City Council) v National Asylum Support Service [2002] UKHL 38, [2002] 1 WLR 2956, [2002] 4 All ER 654, [2002] HLR 58, [2003] BLGR 23, (2002) 5 CCLR 511, (2002) 146 SJLB 241	21.60, 21.71
R (Whapples) v Birmingham Cross City Clinical Commissioning Group [2015] EWCA Civ 435, [2015] PTSR 1398, (2015) 18 CCLR 300	18.47, 18.64
R (Wilkinson) v Broadmoor Hospital [2001] EWCA Civ 1545, [2002] 1 WLR 419, [2002] UKHRR 390, (2002) 5 CCLR 121, [2002] Lloyd's Rep Med. 41, (2002) 65 BMLR 15, [2001] MHLR 224, [2002] ACD 47, (2001) 98(44) LSG 36, (2001) 145 SJLB 247	19.13
R (Wilkinson) v Inland Revenue Commissioners [2005] UKHL 30, [2005] 1 WLR 1718, [2006] 1 All ER 529, [2006] STC 270, [2005] UKHRR 704, 77 TC 78, [2005] STI 904, (2005) 102(25) LSG 33	17.17

W v L [1974] QB 711, [1973] 3 WLR 859, [1973] 3 All ER 884, 72 LGR 36, (1973) 4 Fam Law 134, (1973) 117 SJ 775, CA	19.36
W v United Kingdom, judgment of 8 July 1987, Series A no 121-A, (1988) 10 EHRR 29, ECtHR	25.58, 25.66
Waldron, Re [1986] QB 824, [1985] 3 WLR 1090, [1985] 3 All ER 775, (1986) 83 LSG 199, (1985) 129 SJ 892, CA	19.16
Wandsworth LBC v Winder (No 1) [1985] AC 461, [1984] 3 WLR 1254, [1984] 3 All ER 976, (1985) 17 HLR 196, 83 LGR 143, (1985) 82 LSG 201, (1985) 135 NLJ 381, (1984) 128 SJ 838, HL	20.42
Wasif and Hossain v Secretary of State for the Home Department. *See* R (W) v Secretary of State for the Home Department	
Watts v United Kingdom (Admissibility), Application no 53586/09, [2011] Inquest LR 157, (2010) 51 EHRR SE5, ECtHR	16.18, 16.46, 25.80
WD v Belgium, Application no 73548/13, 6 September 2016	19.24
Welsh Ministers v Care Standards Tribunal [2008] EWHC 49 (Admin), [2008] 1 WLR 2097, (2008) 11 CCLR 234	29.34
Whitbread (Habeas Corpus: Compulsory Admission), Re (1998) 39 BMLR 94, (1997) 94(27) LSG 23, (1997) 141 SJLB 152, CA	19.43, 19.47
Williams v Hackney LBC [2015] EWHC 2629 (QB)	25.89
Wilson v First County Trust Ltd (No 2) [2003] UKHL 40, [2004] 1 AC 816, [2003] 3 WLR 568, [2003] 4 All ER 97, [2003] 2 All ER (Comm) 491, [2003] HRLR 33, [2003] UKHRR 1085, (2003) 100(35) LSG 39, (2003) 147 SJLB 872	29.65
Winterwerp v Netherlands, 24 October 1979, 60, Series A no 33	25.86
Woodland v Swimming Teachers Association [2013] UKSC 66, [2014] AC 537, [2013] 3 WLR 1227, [2014] 1 All ER 482, [2014] ELR 67, (2013) 16 CCLR 532, [2014] PIQR P6, (2013) 163(7582) NLJ 15, (2013) 157(41) SJLB 39	26.9
Wright and others v Secretary of State for Health. *See* R (Wright) v Secretary of State for Health	
X & Y v Netherlands (1985) 8 EHRR 235	25.25, 25.54, 25.67, 25.82
X (Emergency Protection Orders), Re [2006] EWHC 510 (Fam), [2006] 2 FLR 701, [2007] 1 FCR 551, [2006] Fam Law 627	23.27, 24.20
X (Minors) v Bedfordshire CC [1995] 2 AC 633, [1995] 3 WLR 152, [1995] 3 All ER 353, [1995] 2 FLR 276, [1995] 3 FCR 337, 94 LGR 313, (1995) 7 Admin LR 705, [1995] ELR 404, [1995] Fam Law 537, (1996) 160 LG Rev 103, (1996) 160 LG Rev 123, (1995) 145 NLJ 993, HL	19.97, 26.5, 26.14
X Local Authority v B (Emergency Protection Orders) [2004] EWHC 2015 (Fam), [2005] 1 FLR 341, [2007] 1 FCR 512, [2005] Fam Law 13	23.27, 24.20
X v Austria (2013) 57 EHRR 405	25.90
X v Bedfordshire CC	19.116, 26.11
X v Hounslow LBC [2009] EWCA Civ 286, [2009] PTSR 1158, [2009] 2 FLR 262, [2009] 3 FCR 266, [2010] HLR 4, (2009) 12 CCLR 254, [2009] Fam Law 487, (2009) 153(14) SJLB 30, [2009] NPC 63	26.8, 26.25
X v Latvia, Application no 27853/09, [2014] 1 FLR 1135, (2014) 59 EHRR 3, [2014] Fam Law 269, ECtHR	9.101, 10.23, 25.85
X v United Kingdom (1981) 4 EHRR 188	19.16
Yule v South Lanarkshire Council (No 2), 2001 SC 203, 2000 SLT 1249, 2001 SCLR 26, (2001) 4 CCLR 383, 2003 Hous LR 2, 2000 GWD 27-1066, CS IH	11.59

Table of statutes

Table of statutory instruments

Table of treaties and conventions

Abbreviations

ADASS	Association of Directors of Adult Social Care Services
ADR	alternative dispute resolution
AMHP	approved mental health professional
ASW	approved social worker
CCG	clinical commissioning group
CFR	Charter of Fundamental Rights
CJEU	Court of Justice of the European Union
COP	Court of Protection
CPR	Civil Procedure Rules
CQC	Care Quality Commission
CSDPA 1970	Chronically Sick and Disabled Persons Act 1970
CTO	community treatment order
DDA 1995	Disability Discrimination Act 1995
DOLS	Deprivation of Liberty Safeguards
ECHR	European Convention on Human Rights
ECRC	Enhanced Criminal Records Certificate
ECtHR	European Court of Human Rights
EHRC	Equality and Human Rights Commission
EIA	Equality impact assessment
EU	European Union
FTT	First-tier Tribunal
GMC	General Medical Council
GPC	general power of competence
GWP	general well-being power
HCPC	Health and Care Professions Council
HRA 1998	Human Rights Act 1998
ILF	independent living fund
ILR	indefinite leave to remain
IMCA	Independent Mental Capacity Advocate
JSC	Justice of the Supreme Court
LASSA 1970	Local Authority and Social Services Act 1970
LGA 2000	Local Government Act 2000
LGA	Local Government Association
LGO	Local Government Ombudsman
LHB	local health board
LJ	Lord Justice
LTR	leave to remain
MAPPA	multi-agency public protection arrangements
MCA 2005	Mental Capacity Act 2005
MHA 1983	Mental Health Act 1983
MHRT	Mental Health Review Tribunal
NAA 1948	National Assistance Act 1948
NHS	National Health Service
NICE	National Institute for Care and Excellence
PCT	Primary Care Trust
PSED	public sector equality duty

PSIC	person subject to immigration control
PTSD	post traumatic stress disorder
RMO	responsible medical officer
SVGA 2006	Safeguarding Vulnerable Groups Act 2006
TFEU	Treaty on the Functioning of the European Union
UKVI	United Kingdom Visas and Immigration
UNCRC	United Nations Convention on the Rights of the Child
UNCRDP	United Nations Convention on the Rights of Persons with Disabilities

Part I

CHAPTER 1

Introduction: the main statutory provisions in outline

Legislation

1.1 In outline:

- For **adult social care** in England, see the Care Act 2014.[1]
- For **children's social care** in England, see the Chronically Sick and Disabled Persons Act 1970, the Children Act 1989, the Carers and Disabled Children Act 2000, the Children Act 2004, the Childcare Act 2006, sections 58–66 of the Care Act 2014 and the Children and Families Act 2014.
- For **adult and children's social care in Wales**, see the Social Services and Well-being (Wales) Act 2014.
- For **residual local authority powers**, see the Localism Act 2011 in England and the Local Government Act 2000 in Wales.
- For **health care** see the National Health Service Act 2006 in England and the National Health Service (Wales) Act 2006 for Wales.

Regulation

1.2 In outline:

- Most adult social care services in England are regulated by the Care Quality Commission,[2] operating under the Health and Social Care Act 2008, supplemented by Part 2 of the Care Act 2014.
- In England, health services are regulated by Monitor[3] (now part of NHS Improvement) and in Wales by the Healthcare Inspectorate Wales.[4]
- Throughout Great Britain, the Health and Safety Executive[5] operates as an independent regulator for health and safety in the workplace, which includes all private and publicly owned health and social care settings.
- Most children's services in England are regulated by Ofsted (the Office for Standards in Education, Children's Services and Skills)[6] led by Her Majesty's Chief Inspector of Education, Children's Services and Skills, operating under the Care Standards Act 2000, the Children Act 1989 and the Adoption and Children Act 2000.
- In Wales, the Care and Social Services Inspectorate Wales[7] regulates most adults' and children's social services, under the Health and Social Care (Community Health and Standards Act) 2003, the Care Standards Act 2000, the Children Act 1989, the Adoption and Children Act 2002 and the Children and Families (Wales) Measure 2010.

1 The Care Act 2014 replaces earlier adult social care legislation: the National Assistance Act 1948, the Health Services and Public Health Act 1968, the Chronically Sick and Disabled Persons Act 1970 (in relation to adults), the Health and Social Services and Social Security Adjudications Act 1983, the Disabled Persons (Services, Consultation and Representation) Act 1986, parts of the National Health Service and Community Care Act 1990 and parts of the Health and Social Care Act 2001.

2 www.cqc.org.uk.

3 www.gov.uk/government/organisations/monitor.

4 www.hiw.org.uk/home.

5 www.hse.gov.uk/healthservices/arrangements.htm#a1.

6 www.gov.uk/government/organisations/ofsted.

7 www.cssiw.org.uk.

- In England and Wales, regulation of professionals is undertaken by a range of professional bodies, operating under diverse legislation, overseen by the Professional Standards Authority,[8] the Administrative Court and sometimes the tribunal system. This self-regulatory machinery sits alongside the Safeguarding Vulnerable Groups Act 2006, which provides machinery whereby individuals are required to disclose criminal convictions and other relevant information about themselves and may be barred from working with children or adults, by the Disclosure and Barring Service.[9]

8 www.professionalstandards.org.uk.

9 www.gov.uk/government/organisations/disclosure-and-barring-service/.

CHAPTER 2

Strategy, policy and challenges

Introduction

2.1 Social and health care bodies assess individuals and make decisions about whether and how to meet their needs. They also make overarching decisions about strategy and policy: see below, at 'Adult social care strategy and policy materials' (para 2.5) and 'Health care strategy and policy materials' (para 2.13).

2.2 In recent years, due to 'financial austerity', such 'macro' decisions have involved increases in charging and/or reductions in service provision, and have been subject to legal challenge by way of judicial review.

2.3 The usual grounds of challenge have been:

- inadequate consultation (see below, chapter 3);
- failure to act under statutory guidance, or take into account non-statutory guidance (see below, chapter 4);
- breach of what is now the public sector equality duty (PSED) at section 149 of the Equality Act 2010 (see below, chapter 5).

2.4 All these grounds of challenge are also available in the context of decisions about individual needs but have proven particularly suited to macro challenges.

Adult social care strategy and policy materials

England

2.5 The Care Act 2014 contains a number of discrete duties to publish strategies and policies, but for an overarching duty one has to turn to sections 116–116B of the Local Government and Public Involvement in Health Act 2007.

2.6 These provisions, set out below, apply to both local authorities and clinical commissioning groups. They require joint social and health care planning:

- section 116 imposes a duty on local authorities and clinical commissioning groups to assess local social care and health care needs;
- section 116A requires them to prepare and publish a strategy for meeting the needs included in the assessment ('a joint health and wellbeing strategy'), taking account the Secretary of State's Mandate to the National Health Service Commissioning Board, published under section 13A of the National Health Service Act 2006, and any statutory guidance published by the Secretary of State. They are also required to consider increased joint working and closer integration;
- sections 116(8) and 116A(5) require local authorities and clinical commissioning groups to involve the Local Healthwatch organisation and also 'the people who live or work in that area' in the assessment and strategy;
- section 116B requires local authorities and clinical commissioning groups, and the National Health Service Commissioning Board, to have regard to these assessments and strategies when discharging their functions;

- by virtue of section 116A(8) of the 2007 Act and section 195 of the Health and Social Care Act 2012, these provisions apply to all local authority social services functions, as defined in the Local Authority Social Services Act 1970. Thus, for example, children's services under the Children Act 1989 and Children Act 2004 are included.

2.7 Sections 116–116B of the Local Government and Public Involvement in Health Act 2007 are as follows:

Health and social care: joint strategic needs assessments

116(1) An assessment of relevant needs must be prepared in relation to the area of each responsible local authority.

(2) A further assessment of relevant needs in relation to the area of a responsible local authority–
(a) must be prepared if the Secretary of State so directs; and
(b) may be prepared at any time.

(3) A direction under subsection (2)(a) may be revoked.

(4) It is for–
(a) the responsible local authority, and
(b) each of its partner clinical commissioning groups,
to prepare any assessment of relevant needs under this section in relation to the area of the responsible local authority.

(5) The responsible local authority must publish each assessment of relevant needs prepared under this section in relation to its area.

(6) For the purposes of this section, there is a relevant need in relation to so much of the area of a responsible local authority as falls within the area of a partner clinical commissioning group if there appears to the responsible local authority and the partner clinical commissioning group to be a need or to be likely to be a need to which subsection (7) applies.

(7) This subsection applies to a need–
(a) which–
(i) is capable of being met to a significant extent by the exercise by the responsible local authority of any of its functions; and
(ii) could also be met, or could otherwise be affected, to a significant extent by the exercise by the partner clinical commissioning group or the National Health Service Commissioning Board of any of its functions; or
(b) which–
(i) is capable of being met to a significant extent by the exercise by the partner clinical commissioning group or the National Health Service Commissioning Board of any of its functions; and
(ii) could also be met, or could otherwise be affected, to a significant extent by the exercise by the responsible local authority of any of its functions.

(8) In preparing an assessment under this section, the responsible local authority and each of its partner clinical commissioning groups must–
(a) co-operate with one another;
(b) have regard to any guidance issued by the Secretary of State;
(ba) involve the Local Healthwatch organisation for the area of the responsible local authority;
(bb) involve the people who live or work in that area; and
(c) if the responsible local authority is a county council, involve each relevant district council.

(8A) In preparing an assessment under this section, the responsible local authority or a partner clinical commissioning group may consult any person it thinks appropriate.

(9) In this section–

'partner clinical commissioning group', in relation to a responsible local authority, means any clinical commissioning group whose area coincides with or falls wholly or partly within the area of the authority;

'relevant district council' means–

(a) in relation to a responsible local authority, any district council which is a partner authority of it; and

(b) in relation to a partner clinical commissioning group of a responsible local authority, any district council which is a partner authority of the responsible local authority and whose district falls wholly or partly within the area of the clinical commissioning group.

Health and social care: joint health and wellbeing strategies

116A(1) This section applies where an assessment of relevant needs is prepared under section 116 by a responsible local authority and each of its partner clinical commissioning groups.

(2) The responsible local authority and each of its partner clinical commissioning groups must prepare a strategy for meeting the needs included in the assessment by the exercise of functions of the authority, the National Health Service Commissioning Board or the clinical commissioning groups ('a joint health and wellbeing strategy').

(3) In preparing a strategy under this section, the responsible local authority and each of its partner clinical commissioning groups must, in particular, consider the extent to which the needs could be met more effectively by the making of arrangements under section 75 of the National Health Service Act 2006 (rather than in any other way).

(4) In preparing a strategy under this section, the responsible local authority and each of its partner clinical commissioning groups must have regard to–

(a) the mandate published by the Secretary of State under section 13A of the National Health Service Act 2006, and

(b) any guidance issued by the Secretary of State.

(5) In preparing a strategy under this section, the responsible local authority and each of its partner clinical commissioning groups must–

(a) involve the Local Healthwatch organisation for the area of the responsible local authority, and

(b) involve the people who live or work in that area.

(6) The responsible local authority must publish each strategy prepared by it under this section.

(7) The responsible local authority and each of its partner clinical commissioning groups may include in the strategy a statement of their views on how arrangements for the provision of health-related services in the area of the local authority could be more closely integrated with arrangements for the provision of health services and social care services in that area.

(8) In this section and section 116B–

(a) 'partner clinical commissioning group', in relation to a responsible local authority, has the same meaning as in section 116, and

(b) 'health services', 'health-related services' and 'social care services' have the same meaning as in section 195 of the Health and Social Care Act 2012.

Duty to have regard to assessments and strategies

116B(1) A responsible local authority and each of its partner clinical commissioning groups must, in exercising any functions, have regard to–

(a) any assessment of relevant needs prepared by the responsible local authority and each of its partner clinical commissioning groups under section 116 which is relevant to the exercise of the functions, and

(b) any joint health and wellbeing strategy prepared by them under section 116A which is so relevant.

(2) The National Health Service Commissioning Board must, in exercising any functions in arranging for the provision of health services in relation to the area of a responsible local authority, have regard to–

(a) any assessment of relevant needs prepared by the responsible local authority and each of its partner clinical commissioning groups under section 116 which is relevant to the exercise of the functions, and

(b) any joint health and wellbeing strategy prepared by them under section 116A which is so relevant.

2.8 The Mandate published under section 13A of the National Health Service Act 2006 (see section 116A(4)(a)) is published annually.[1]

2.9 The Department of Health has published *Statutory Guidance on Joint Strategic Needs Assessments and Joint Health and Wellbeing Strategies* (2013) (see section 116B(4)(b)).[2]

2.10 Important though the Local Government and Public Involvement in Health Act 2007 is, the Care Act 2014 also imposes strategic and policy obligations. Such obligations arise from the terms of section 2 (the duty to prevent needs for care and support arising), section 4 (the duty to provide information and advice), section 5 (the duty to promote diversity and quality in the provision of services – 'market shaping') and section 6 (the duty to co-operate with 'partners'). The need to devise and publish strategies and policies, arising out of these duties, is explained by the *Care and Support Statutory Guidance* (see chapter 4 below on Guidance).

Wales

2.11 Whereas the duty on English local authorities, to prepare community care plans under section 46 of the National Health Service and Community Care Act 1990, has been a dead letter since the Care Plans (England) Directions 2003, it still applies in Wales. Thus, by virtue of section 46 of the National Health Service and Community Care Act 1990 and, also, section 40 of the National Health Service (Wales) Act 2006, local authorities and Local Health Boards in Wales are to produce Health, Social Care and Well-Being Strategies.[3] The policy objective is to co-ordinate adult social care and health planning, together with Children and Young People's Plans.

1 The current version is at: www.gov.uk/government/uploads/system/uploads/attachment_data/file/383495/2902896_DoH_Mandate_Accessible_v0.2.pdf.

2 At www.gov.uk/government/uploads/system/uploads/attachment_data/file/223842/Statutory-Guidance-on-Joint-Strategic-Needs-Assessments-and-Joint-Health-and-Wellbeing-Strategies-March–2013.pdf.

3 The statutory guidance and associated materials are at http://gov.wales/topics/health/publications/health/strategies/strategies/?lang=en.

2.12 In addition, by virtue of sections 14 and 14A of the Social Services and Well-Being (Wales) Act 2014, Welsh local authorities are required to publish their assessment, and a strategy, addressing local needs for care and support, help for carers and preventative services. This is to be undertaken jointly with Local Health Boards and provision is made for co-ordination with Children and Young People's Plans:

Assessment of needs for care and support, support for carers and preventative services

14(1) A local authority and each Local Health Board any part of whose area lies within the area of the local authority must, in accordance with regulations, jointly assess–

(a) the extent to which there are people in the local authority's area who need care and support;

(b) the extent to which there are carers in the local authority's area who need support;

(c) the extent to which there are people in the local authority's area whose needs for care and support (or, in the case of carers, support) are not being met (by the authority, the Board or otherwise);

(d) the range and level of services required to meet the care and support needs of people in the local authority's area (including the support needs of carers);

(e) the range and level of services required to achieve the purposes in section 15(2) (preventative services) in the local authority's area;

(f) the actions required to provide the range and level of services identified in accordance with paragraphs (d) and (e) through the medium of Welsh.

(2) Regulations under subsection (1) may, for example, provide for the timing and review of assessments.

(3) In section 40 of the National Health Service (Wales) Act 2006 (health and well-being strategies)–

(a) after subsection (2) insert–

'(2A) The responsible bodies must take into account the most recent assessment under section 14 of the Social Services and Well-being (Wales) Act 2014 (assessment of needs for care and support, support for carers and preventative services) in the formulation or review of the strategy.

(2B) The responsible bodies must jointly publish the strategy.

(2C) The Local Health Board (or Boards) responsible for the strategy must submit to the Welsh Ministers any part of the strategy which relates to the health and well-being of carers (and if more than one Board is responsible for the strategy, they must do so jointly).';

(b) in subsection (6), after paragraph (g) insert–

'(h) the submission of the strategy or a part of the strategy, to the Welsh Ministers (including, for example, the form in which and the time by which the strategy or part is to be submitted).';

(c) in subsection (9), insert in the appropriate place–

'"carer" has the same meaning as in the Social Services and Well-being (Wales) Act 2014,'

(4) In section 26 of the Children Act 2004 (children and young people's plans), after subsection (1A) insert–

'(1AA) A local authority in Wales must take into account the most recent assessment under section 14 of the Social Services and Well-being (Wales) Act 2014 (assessment of needs for care and support, support for carers and preventative services) in the preparation and review of the plan.'

Plans following assessments of needs under section 14

14A(1) In this section, 'relevant body' means a local authority or Local Health Board which has carried out a joint assessment under section 14(1).

(2) Each relevant body must prepare and publish a plan setting out–

(a) the range and level of services the body proposes to provide, or arrange to be provided, in response to the assessment of needs under paragraphs (a) to (c) of section 14(1);

(b) in the case of a local authority, the range and level of services the authority proposes to provide, or arrange to be provided, in seeking to achieve the purposes in section 15(2) (preventative services);

(c) in the case of a Local Health Board, anything the Board proposes to do in connection with its duty under section 15(5) (Local Health Boards to have regard to the importance of preventative action when exercising functions);

(d) how the services set out in the plan are to be provided, including the actions the body proposes to take to provide, or arrange to provide, the services through the medium of Welsh;

(e) any other action the body proposes to take in response to the assessment under section 14(1);

(f) the details of anything the body proposes to do in response to the assessment jointly with another relevant body;

(g) the resources to be deployed in doing the things set out in the plan.

(3) A relevant body's plan may be published by including it within a local well-being plan published under section 39 or 44(5) of the Well-being of Future Generations (Wales) Act 2015 (the '2015 Act') by a public services board of which the body is a member.

(4) A local authority and a Local Health Board who have carried out a joint assessment together under section 14(1) may jointly prepare and publish a plan under subsection (2).

(5) Two or more local authorities may jointly prepare and publish a plan under subsection (2); but such a joint plan may be published by including it within a local well-being plan only if each local authority is a member of the public services board (see sections 47 and 49 of the 2015 Act (merging of public services boards)).

(6) A relevant body must submit to the Welsh Ministers–

(a) any part of a plan it has prepared under subsection (2) which relates to the health and well-being of carers;

(b) any other part of such a plan as may be specified by regulations.

(7) Regulations may make provision about plans prepared and published under subsection (2), including provision–

(a) specifying when a plan is to be published;

(b) about reviewing a plan;

(c) about consulting persons when preparing or reviewing a plan;

(d) about the monitoring and evaluation of services and other action set out in a plan.

Health care strategy and policy materials

England

2.13 Section 242 of the National Health Service Act 2006 imposes duties of consultation and involvement on NHS Trusts and Foundation Trusts in England:

Public involvement and consultation

242(1B) Each relevant English body must make arrangements, as respects health services for which it is responsible, which secure that users of those services, whether directly or through representatives, are involved (whether by being consulted or provided with information, or in other ways) in–

(a) the planning of the provision of those services,

(b) the development and consideration of proposals for changes in the way those services are provided, and

(c) decisions to be made by that body affecting the operation of those services.

(1C) Subsection (1B)(b) applies to a proposal only if implementation of the proposal would have an impact on–

(a) the manner in which the services are delivered to users of those services, or

(b) the range of health services available to those users.

(1D) Subsection (1B)(c) applies to a decision only if implementation of the decision (if made) would have an impact on–

(a) the manner in which the services are delivered to users of those services, or

(b) the range of health services available to those users.

2.14 As noted above, sections 116–116B of the Local Government and Public Involvement in Health Act 2007 require local authorities and clinical commissioning groups to consult, assess local needs and publish the assessment and their strategy for meeting local needs, which they must then take into account when discharging their functions.

2.15 Local authorities and clinical commissioning groups in England are required to have regard to the statutory guidance, which is *Statutory Guidance on Joint Strategic Needs Assessments and Joint Health and Wellbeing Strategies* (2013).[4]

Wales

2.16 Section 242 of the National Health Service Act 2006 imposes duties of consultation and involvement on NHS Trusts in Wales, as well as in England.

2.17 As noted above, by virtue of sections 14 and 14A of the Social Services and Well-Being (Wales) Act 2006, Local Health Boards in Wales are required to complete and publish their assessment, and a strategy, addressing (a) local needs for care and support; (b) help for carers and (c) preventative services – in relation to both children and adults. This is to

4 At www.gov.uk/government/uploads/system/uploads/attachment_data/file/223842/Statutory-Guidance-on-Joint-Strategic-Needs-Assessments-and-Joint-Health-and-Wellbeing-Strategies-March–2013.pdf.

be undertaken jointly with Local Health Boards and provision is made for co-ordination with Children and Young People's Plans:

Assessment of needs for care and support, support for carers and preventative services

14(1) A local authority and each Local Health Board any part of whose area lies within the area of the local authority must, in accordance with regulations, jointly assess–

(a) the extent to which there are people in the local authority's area who need care and support;

(b) the extent to which there are carers in the local authority's area who need support;

(c) the extent to which there are people in the local authority's area whose needs for care and support (or, in the case of carers, support) are not being met (by the authority, the Board or otherwise);

(d) the range and level of services required to meet the care and support needs of people in the local authority's area (including the support needs of carers);

(e) the range and level of services required to achieve the purposes in section 15(2) (preventative services) in the local authority's area;

(f) the actions required to provide the range and level of services identified in accordance with paragraphs (d) and (e) through the medium of Welsh.

(2) Regulations under subsection (1) may, for example, provide for the timing and review of assessments.

(3) In section 40 of the National Health Service (Wales) Act 2006 (health and well-being strategies)–

(a) after subsection (2) insert–

'(2A) The responsible bodies must take into account the most recent assessment under section 14 of the Social Services and Well-being (Wales) Act 2014 (assessment of needs for care and support, support for carers and preventative services) in the formulation or review of the strategy.

(2B) The responsible bodies must jointly publish the strategy.

(2C) The Local Health Board (or Boards) responsible for the strategy must submit to the Welsh Ministers any part of the strategy which relates to the health and well-being of carers (and if more than one Board is responsible for the strategy, they must do so jointly).';

(b) in subsection (6), after paragraph (g) insert–

'(h) the submission of the strategy or a part of the strategy, to the Welsh Ministers (including, for example, the form in which and the time by which the strategy or part is to be submitted).';

(c) in subsection (9), insert in the appropriate place–

'"carer" has the same meaning as in the Social Services and Well-being (Wales) Act 2014,'

(4) In section 26 of the Children Act 2004 (children and young people's plans), after subsection (1A) insert–

'(1AA) A local authority in Wales must take into account the most recent assessment under section 14 of the Social Services and Well-being (Wales) Act 2014 (assessment of needs for care and support, support for carers and preventative services) in the preparation and review of the plan.'

Plans following assessments of needs under section 14

14A(1) In this section, 'relevant body' means a local authority or Local Health Board which has carried out a joint assessment under section 14(1).

(2) Each relevant body must prepare and publish a plan setting out–
(a) the range and level of services the body proposes to provide, or arrange to be provided, in response to the assessment of needs under paragraphs (a) to (c) of section 14(1);
(b) in the case of a local authority, the range and level of services the authority proposes to provide, or arrange to be provided, in seeking to achieve the purposes in section 15(2) (preventative services);
(c) in the case of a Local Health Board, anything the Board proposes to do in connection with its duty under section 15(5) (Local Health Boards to have regard to the importance of preventative action when exercising functions);
(d) how the services set out in the plan are to be provided, including the actions the body proposes to take to provide, or arrange to provide, the services through the medium of Welsh;
(e) any other action the body proposes to take in response to the assessment under section 14(1);
(f) the details of anything the body proposes to do in response to the assessment jointly with another relevant body;
(g) the resources to be deployed in doing the things set out in the plan.

(3) A relevant body's plan may be published by including it within a local well-being plan published under section 39 or 44(5) of the Well-being of Future Generations (Wales) Act 2015 (the '2015 Act') by a public services board of which the body is a member.

(4) A local authority and a Local Health Board who have carried out a joint assessment together under section 14(1) may jointly prepare and publish a plan under subsection (2).

(5) Two or more local authorities may jointly prepare and publish a plan under subsection (2); but such a joint plan may be published by including it within a local well-being plan only if each local authority is a member of the public services board (see sections 47 and 49 of the 2015 Act (merging of public services boards)).

(6) A relevant body must submit to the Welsh Ministers–
(a) any part of a plan it has prepared under subsection (2) which relates to the health and well-being of carers;
(b) any other part of such a plan as may be specified by regulations.

(7) Regulations may make provision about plans prepared and published under subsection (2), including provision–
(a) specifying when a plan is to be published;
(b) about reviewing a plan;
(c) about consulting persons when preparing or reviewing a plan;
(d) about the monitoring and evaluation of services and other action set out in a plan.

CHAPTER 3

Consultation

3.1 **Introduction**

Cases

3.11 *R v Devon CC and another ex p Baker and others* [1995] 1 All ER 73, CA
The fairness principle required local authorities to consult residents before deciding to close a care home. The court set out what type of consultation fairness required, in this context

3.12 *R v North and East Devon Health Authority ex p Pow* [1997] EWHC 765 (Admin), (1997–98) 1 CCLR 280
The health authority had remained under a duty to consult despite a need for urgent action arising as a result of its own failures and its hospital closure decision would be quashed notwithstanding the practical difficulties that might ensue

3.13 *R v North and East Devon Health Authority ex p Coughlan* [2001] QB 213, (1999) 2 CCLR 285, CA
A consultation process, undertaken voluntarily, will be unlawful unless it complies with the 'Gunning criteria'

3.14 *R v Powys CC ex p Hambidge (No 2)* (1999) 2 CCLR 460, QBD
The local authority was not under a duty to consult the user of home care services before increasing charges

3.15 *R (Haringey Consortium of Disabled People and Carers Association and others) v Haringey LBC* (2002) 5 CCLR 422, QBD
The relevant guidance created a legitimate expectation of consultation before a local authority reduced grants to local charities

3.16 *R (Smith) v East Kent NHS Hospital Trust and Medway Health Authority* [2002] EWHC 2640 (Admin), (2003) 6 CCLR 251
A duty to re-consult only arises where there is a fundamental difference between the consultation proposals and the final decision

3.17 *R (Madden) v Bury MBC* [2002] EWHC 1882 (Admin), (2002) 5 CCLR 622
A decision to close to care homes was quashed when the preceding consultation process had been unlawful, owing to Bury's failure to disclose the true reasons for closure

3.18 *R (Royal Brompton and Harefield NHS Foundation Trust) v Joint Committee of Primary Care Trusts* [2012] EWCA Civ 472
Consultation was unlawful where the local authority provided consultees with inaccurate and incomplete information about the reasons for its proposed decision

continued

3.19 *R (Haggerty) v St Helens Council* [2003] EWHC 803 (Admin), (2003) 6 CCLR 352

Extraneous difficulties that limit a local authority's freedom of manoeuvre can make it lawful to undertake a process of consultation that falls well short of the usual minimum

3.20 *R (Capenhurst) v Leicester CC* [2004] EWHC 2124 (Admin), (2004) 7 CCLR 557

A voluntary consultation process, and the ensuing decision, were unlawful where the local authority had failed adequately to inform consultees of the factors that it would treat as important in reaching its decision

3.21 *R (Morris) v Trafford Healthcare NHS Trust* [2006] EWHC 2334 (Admin), (2006) 9 CCLR 648

Although a consultation process resulting in the closure of in-patient wards had been unlawful, the court refused to grant relief in a case where the public authority proposed to re-consult

3.22 *R (Smith) v North Eastern Derbyshire PCT* [2006] EWCA Civ 1291, (2006) 9 CCLR 663

Where consultation has been unlawful, relief may be withheld if it is proven that the result would inevitably have been the same

3.23 *R (Fudge) v South West Strategic Health Authority* [2007] EWCA Civ 803, (2007) 10 CCLR 599

A statutory duty to consult remained in place even where the Secretary of State had taken over the function to which the duty to consult attached; but for pragmatic reasons, relief would be refused

3.24 *R (Eisai Ltd) v NICE* [2008] EWCA Civ 438, (2008) 11 CCLR 385

Fairness required full disclosure of a computer model on which decision-making was based so as to permit the consultee to seek to undermine the validity of the model; considerations of administrative difficulty should not usually outweigh what fairness requires

3.25 *R (Boyejo) v Barnet LBC* [2009] EWHC 3261 (Admin), (2010) 13 CCLR 72

Consultation was unlawful when the decision had already been made, it did not canvass alternatives, did not sufficiently involve consultees and gave insufficient time

3.26 *R (W) v Croydon LBC* [2011] EWHC 696 (Admin), (2011) 14 CCLR 247

A statutory consultation process, with the parents of an incapacitated adult, was unlawful where the consultees had been afforded insufficient time

3.27 *R (G) v North Somerset Council* [2011] EWHC 2232 (Admin)

North Somerset had not acted unlawfully in deciding to cut the amount of direct payments and replacing direct payments with a managed care service

3.28 *R (Buckinghamshire CC) v Kingston upon Thames RLBC* [2011] EWCA Civ 457, (2011) 14 CCLR 426

A local authority was not under a statutory or common law duty to consult with another local authority before placing an individual in its area, even though that would result in a financial and administrative burden on that other local authority

3.29 *R (W) v Birmingham CC* [2011] EWHC 1147 (Admin), (2011) 14 CCLR 516

Unclear and inadequate information resulted in the consultation process being unlawful

3.30 *R (South West Care Homes Ltd) v Devon CC* [2012] EWHC 1867 (Admin)
Although failures in the consultation process were not academic, and the process had been unlawful, relief would be refused in the exercise of the court's discretion, for pragmatic reasons

3.31 *R (Royal Brompton and Harefield NHS Foundation Trust) v Joint Committee of PCT* [2012] EWCA Civ 472
The Court of Appeal re-stated the consultation principles, including that the courts will usually only grant relief where 'something has gone clearly and radically wrong'

3.32 *R (Bracking) v Secretary of State for Work and Pensions* [2013] EWCA Civ 1345, (2013) 16 CCLR 479
Consultees had had an adequate opportunity of explaining the likely effect of what was proposed on them and that was sufficient, in this case

3.33 *R (T) v Sheffield CC* [2013] EWHC 2953 QB, (2013) 16 CCLR 580
In assessing whether a consultation process was lawful, it is necessary to have careful regard to the context and all the circumstances

3.34 *R (D) v Worcestershire CC* [2013] EWHC 2490 (Admin), (2013) 16 CCLR 323
On analysis, the information provided to consultees had been accurate

3.35 *R (LH) v Shropshire Council* [2014] EWCA Civ 404, (2014) 17 CCLR 216
It was legitimate to consult on macro policy changes first but it was then necessary to consult beneficiaries of specific services that might be closed; in this case, although consultation had been unlawful, relief would be refused for pragmatic reasons

3.36 *R (Michael Robson) v Salford CC* [2013] EWHC 3481 (Admin), (2014) 17 CCLR 474
The court summarised consultation principles and concluded that, in substance, consultees had been adequately informed about what was proposed

3.37 *R (Moseley) v Haringey LBC* [2014] UKSC 56
In the circumstances of this case, it had been unlawful to consult on the basis that there was no alternative, when there were alternatives

3.38 *R (McCann) v Bridgend CBC* [2014] EWHC 4335 (Admin)
In this context, a duty to consult on alternatives to the decision proposed was imposed by the statutory code, rather than the common law

3.39 *R (Michael Robson) v Salford CC* [2015] EWCA Civ 6
The consultation materials lacked clarity but overall consultees must have known what the proposal was and what the alternative were, so that the process had been fair

3.40 *R (Forge Care Homes Ltd) v Cardiff and Vale University Health Board* [2015] EWHC 610 (Admin), (2015) 18 CCLR 39
Local Health Boards had not been under a statutory or common law duty to consult before amending their payments to care homes in respect of the tasks undertaken by registered nurses

3.41 *R (JM and NT) v Isle of Wight Council* [2011] EWHC 2911 (Admin), (2012) 15 CCLR 167
A flawed consultation resulted in decision-makers having inadequate information about risk and consequently not have 'due regard' to the needs in the PSED

3.42 *R (T) v Trafford MBC* [2015] EWHC 369 (Admin)

It is not always necessary to consult about alternative options

3.43 *R (L and P) v Warwickshire CC* [2015] EWHC 203 (Admin), (2015) 18 CCLR 458

Consultation was not required prior to making the annual budget and, in any event, the application for judicial review was out of time. A consultation process will only be unlawful because of unfairness where 'something has gone clearly and radically wrong'

3.44 *R (Morris) v Rhondda Cynon Taf CBC* [2015] EWHC 1403 (Admin), (2015) 18 CCLR 550

Fairness did not always require consultation on alternatives and, where it did, the duty applied to realistic alternatives only

3.45 *R (Sumpter) v Secretary of State for Work and Pensions* [2015] EWCA Civ 1033

A consultation process is fair if, ultimately, consultees can be expected to have understood the issues and the relevant factors

3.46 *R (Tilley) v Vale of Glamorgan Council* [2015] EWHC 3194 (Admin)

It was not unfair to fail to consult on an alternative that was not realistic and signposting consultees to additional information had been, on the facts, fair

3.47 *R (Keep Wythenshawe Special Limited) v NHS Central Manchester Clinical Commissioning Group* [2016] EWHC 17 (Admin), (2016) 19 CCLR 19

In assessing whether consultation was lawful, it is relevant to take into account the particular role that consultation is playing in the decision-making process

Introduction

3.1 A duty to consult may arise as a result of legislation, guidance or the common law duty to act fairly. In addition, public authorities often consult on a voluntary basis in order to garner useful information, forewarn the public of possible change and enhance local democracy.

3.2 The circumstances in which a duty arises as a result of legislation, or guidance, depends on the terms in which the legislation or guidance is expressed. It is a little more difficult to ascertain when a duty to consult arises by virtue of the common law duty to act fairly but:[1]

- the common law does not impose a general duty always to consult persons who may be affected by a measure;
- the common law may require a public authority to consult with a person who could be affected by the actions it proposes to undertake when that person –
  - has a legitimate expectation of being consulted as a result of possessing an interest of a kind that the courts have held to be sufficient to found such an expectation (eg the resident of a care home proposed to be closed);
  - has a legitimate expectation of being consulted as a result of a promise or established practice of consultation; or,
  - exceptionally, where a failure to consult would be conspicuously unfair;
- whether a duty arises depends on all the circumstances, in particular the statutory context, and there may be cases where a legitimate expectation of being consulted can be overridden in the public interest.

3.3 Whatever the basis of consultation, and even when consultation is undertaken voluntarily, there is a legal minimum (sometimes referred to as 'the *Gunning* criteria') which, if not met, usually (although not always) renders the consultation process unlawful and any consequential decision liable to be quashed. The public authority in question must:[2]

- undertake consultation when the proposals are still at a formative stage;
- give consultees sufficient reasons for the proposal, so as to permit intelligent consideration and response;
- give consultees adequate time for consideration and response;
- take the products of consultation conscientiously into account.

3.4 The underlying principle is that of procedural fairness. Accordingly, precisely what is required is always context sensitive.[3] For example,

- when a proposal may deprive someone of an existing benefit or advantage, or affect their enjoyment of legal rights, the standard of fairness required may be higher;[4] and

1 *R (Moseley) v Haringey LBC* [2014] UKSC 56, [2014] 1 WLR 3947 at paras 23–24, 35.
2 *R (Moseley) v Haringey LBC* [2014] UKSC 56, [2014] 1 WLR 3947 at para 25.
3 *R (Moseley) v Haringey LBC* [2014] UKSC 56, [2014] 1 WLR 3947 at para 24.
4 *R (Moseley) v Haringey LBC* [2014] UKSC 56, [2014] 1 WLR 3947 at para 26.

- a clearer explanation of the proposals may be required from the public authority, when the consultees lack relevant expertise but the proposal is likely to impinge significantly upon them;[5]
- taking the products of consultation conscientiously into account does not in general require the decision-maker carefully to analyse them.[6]

3.5 Sometimes, fairness and/or the statutory context can require public authorities to consult, not only on their preferred option but, also, on any realistic alternatives.[7]

3.6 It can also be legitimate to consult on macro policy changes and then, later, to consult beneficiaries of particular services that might be closed.[8]

3.7 Because the underlying principle is that of procedural fairness, it is ultimately for the courts to decide whether a process of consultation has been lawful and the *Wednesbury* test is not determinative.[9] However, the courts are only likely to decide that breaches of the above principles have resulted in unfairness in cases where 'something has gone clearly and radically wrong', in a way that affects at least one group of consultees.[10]

3.8 At common law, a public authority cannot avoid a quashing order, where there has been unlawful consultation, simply on the basis that its decision would probably have been the same: it has to show that 'the decision would inevitably have been the same'.[11] The Senior Courts Act 1981 now provides, however, at section 31(2A), that the High Court must refuse to grant relief 'if it appears to the court to be highly likely that the outcome for the applicant would not have been substantially different if the conduct complained of had not occurred', unless there is an 'exceptional public interest' in granting relief. Section 31(2C) imposes a similar restriction on the grant of permission to apply for judicial review. It remains to be seen how the court will approach this restriction on its traditional function.[12]

5 *R (Moseley) v Haringey LBC* [2014] UKSC 56, [2014] 1 WLR 3947 at para 26.

6 *Secretary of State for Communities and Local Government v West Berkshire DC and Reading BC* [2016] EWCA Civ 441 at para 64.

7 *R (Moseley) v Haringey LBC* [2014] UKSC 56, [2014] 1 WLR 3947 at paras 27–28, 39–41.

8 *R (LH) v Shropshire Council* [2014] EWCA Civ 404, (2014) 17 CCLR 216 at paras 21–26.

9 *R (LH) v Shropshire Council* [2014] EWCA Civ 404, (2014) 17 CCLR 216 at para 29.

10 *R (Royal Brompton and Harefield NHS Foundation Trust) v Joint Committee of PCT* [2012] EWCA Civ 472 at para 13–14; *R (L and P) v Warwickshire CC* [2015] EWHC 203 (Admin), (2015) 18 CCLR 458 at paras 18–22.

11 *R (South West Care Homes Ltd) v Devon CC* [2012] EWHC 1867 (Admin) at para 51.

12 The Bingham Centre for the Rule of Law, the Public Law Project and Justice have suggested that this duty will only arise exceptionally: *Judicial Review and the Rule of Law: An Introduction to the Criminal Justice and Courts Act 2015, Part 4* at www.biicl.org/documents/767_judicial_review_and_the_rule_of_law_-_final_for_web_19_oct_2015.pdf. However, in *R (Hawke) v Secretary of State for Justice* [2015] EWHC 3599 (Admin), as a result of section 31(2A) of the Senior Courts Act 1981 Holman J declined to grant a declaration that the Secretary of State for Justice was in breach of the PSED (under section 149 of the Equality Act 2010); instead, he indicated that his judgment was a 'declaratory judgment', following the example of Blake J in *Logan v Havering LBC* [2015] EWHC 3193 (Admin). See also *R (Enfield LBC) v Secretary of State for Transport* [2015] EWHC 3758 (Admin) at para 106 (sometimes a witness statement is required from the local authority, to establish that the test is met) and *R (HA) v The Governing Body of Hampstead School* [2016] EWHC 278 (Admin) at para 33 (these provisions may relate simply to 'technical flaws'). In *R (DAT) v West*

3.9 Despite the above, in consultation cases, a great deal of water may have flowed under the bridge by the time of the final hearing so that, unless interim relief has been secured, the courts do sometimes exercise their discretion to withhold relief (beyond declaratory relief) for pragmatic reasons.[13]

3.10 There is only a duty to re-consult when the public authority is minded to adopt a solution that is fundamentally different from the proposal consulted upon.[14]

Cases

3.11 *R v Devon CC and another ex p Baker and others* [1995] 1 All ER 73, CA

The fairness principle required local authorities to consult residents before deciding to close a care home. The court set out what type of consultation fairness required, in this context

Facts: Devon and Durham proposed to close care homes. Residents sought a judicial review on the basis that Devon and Durham had been under a duty to consult with them first, which they had not discharged.

Judgment: the Court of Appeal (Dillon, Farquharson and Simon Brown LJJ) held that Devon and Durham had been under a duty to consult but that, whilst the Devon residents had been made aware of the proposals and had been afforded adequate time to make representations, that had not been the case in Durham. As to the legal principles the court held that (1) Where a local authority proposed to close a residential home for the elderly as part of a general reorganisation of the provision of residential care for elderly people in its area, the authority owed the permanent residents of the home a duty to act fairly in making the decision to close the home, which duty included a duty to consult over the proposed closure, the reason being that the residents enjoyed an existing benefit or advantage such that it would be unfair to deprive them of it, without first consulting them. The essentials of any consultation in that context required that (i) that the residents be informed of the proposed closure of their home well in advance of the final decision on the matter; (ii) that the residents have reasonable time in which to put their objections to the proposed closure to the local authority; and (iii) that those objections be considered by the local authority. The prima facie obligation to accord procedural fairness did not mean that each individual resident had an individual right to be consulted face to face by local authority officers or groups of councillors and could be achieved by meetings held by local authority officers with the residents generally at a particular home or by views expressed through the support group.

Berkshire Council [2016] EWHC 1876 (Admin), (2016) 19 CCLR 362, Laing J found it hard to be satisfied that there was no chance of the council reaching a different decision on a reconsideration in case involving highly vulnerable children and, in any event, considered that in such a case there was an exceptional public interest in granting relief.

13 *R (Fudge) v South West Strategic Health Authority* [2007] EWCA Civ 803, (2007) 10 CCLR 599 at paras 66–67; *R (South West Care Homes Ltd) v Devon CC* [2012] EWHC 1867 (Admin) at paras 53–62.

14 *R (Smith) v East Kent NHS Hospital Trust* [2002] EWHC 2640, (2003) 6 CCLR 251 at para 45.

3.12 *R v North and East Devon Health Authority ex p Pow* [1997] EWHC 765 (Admin), (1997–98) 1 CCLR 280

The health authority had remained under a duty to consult despite a need for urgent action arising as a result of its own failures and its hospital closure decision would be quashed notwithstanding the practical difficulties that might ensue

Facts: North and East Devon needed to reduce its expenditure in the coming financial year. It first decided in February that it might be necessary to close two hospitals temporarily. In April, that was identified as the best option. In June, it determined on those closures, without prior consultation, on the ground of urgency. North and East Devon had been under a statutory duty to consult except where it was satisfied that 'a decision has to be taken without allowing time for consultation' (regulation 18 of the Community Health Councils Regulations 1996).[15]

Judgment: Moses J held that the respondent was in breach of the duty to consult because, in April, when the closure option had been identified as the optimal course, the need for closure had not been imminent and that, although quashing the closure decision would make it harder to find the necessary savings, that would not be impossible and relief should not be refused. Indeed, consultation might result in alternative strategies in that, although objectors had made their views known, they had not been included in a formal process of consultation:

> 64. There can be little doubt that by June 1997 the need to make savings required to attempt to comply with the obligations to balance the books, under section 97A of the 1977 Act, was urgent. Earlier estimates of deficit had been too optimistic. By 7th May the deficit was expected to be £2.2 million. Whatever the reason for the passage of time between February and June, the respondent says matters had become so urgent by June that it cannot be said that the decision to dispense with consultation under regulation 18(3) was irrational. For it is that ground alone, which, it is said, could justify a review of a decision under regulation 18(3), absent any suggestion of bad faith. The respondent relies upon *R v Tunbridge Wells Health Authority ex p Goodridge, Times,* 21 May 1988. In that case there was no evidence to suggest that there had been a decision to close without consultation or that the closure was urgent.
>
> 65. Mr Engelman, on behalf of the respondent, suggests that once it is clear that the need to make savings by temporary closure was urgent, it follows that the decision to dispense with consultation cannot be impugned as irrational and cannot, therefore, be reviewed. He relied upon *R v Richmond, Twickenham and Roehampton Health Authority ex p London Borough of Richmond*, unreported, 20 February 1994, a decision by Mann J. In that case no formal decision had been made under regulation 18(3), but the need for closure was described as urgent. No argument appears to have been advanced suggesting that it was the Health Authority's own fault for allowing matters to become urgent. Nevertheless, Mr Engelman suggests that it could have been advanced, and contends that absent bad faith, if the need is urgent, the decision cannot be challenged even if the Health Authority might have acted earlier at a time when consultation would have been possible.

15 SI No 640.

66. Mr Richard Gordon QC, on the other hand, relies on *R v North West Regional Health Authority ex p Daniels* [1994] COD 44, of which I also have an unreported transcript. In that case, Kennedy LJ said of the failure to consult:

> 'The District Health Authority cannot be in a better position because instead of making a proposal they allowed the situation to drift in the way I have described. In my judgment that submission is unanswerable, and neither Miss Davies nor Mr Shaw really sought to answer it.'

67. In that case, however, no relief was given because the hospital had already closed. In this case, the Respondent did not merely allow the matter to drift in the sense of doing nothing. The negotiations, in order to reach a final solution, as I have found, continued.

68. I do not think that the authorities assist. Greater help is to be found in the scheme of the regulation. Regulation 18, read as a whole, is designed to ensure that consultation does take place with a Community Health Council once a proposal of the nature it describes is under consideration. It then derogates from that provision, where a decision has to be taken without allowing time for consultation. Regulation 18, in certain cases, permits the Secretary of State to require further time for consultation; it is clearly aimed at achieving sufficient time for proper consultation. It would seriously undermine the purpose of the regulation if a Health Authority could allow time to pass to the point where matters were so urgent that there was no time left for consultation. It would permit a Health Authority, taking the view that there was only one practicable solution, to pre-empt the result of proper consultation.

...

72. In my judgment, the Health Authority erred in law in failing to appreciate the proposal temporarily to close Lynton and Winsford Hospitals was a proposal within the meaning of regulation 18(1) such as to trigger the duty to consult in April 1997. That error taints its decision of 4 June 1997 to dispense with consultation and, subject to the issue of discretion, cannot stand.

...

74. It is clear that the earlier the savings can be made the greater those savings. Nearly half the financial year has passed. Unless the hospitals are closed, it was said, the necessary savings cannot be achieved. I was told, although I could find no evidence of this, that if I grant relief it will not be possible to use the temporary closure of the hospitals as a means of making savings at all. I accept that to grant relief now will make the task of the finding the necessary savings far more difficult. But I do not accept that the evidence shows that it would be impossible. I appreciate that such savings may have to be made out of other valuable services. It has been suggested that waiting lists will be increased. Even though the task is harder, in my view the importance of the duty to consult is such that I do not think the greater burden of the task facing the Health Authority, caused by its own error in law, justifies the refusal of relief. After all, a conscientious process of consultation with an informed Community Health Council, and, not with the public at large, and which should not be confined to mere protestations of opposition, may produce alternative means of saving the £215,000 which it was hoped to achieve by the end of the financial year.

Comment: this case is not often cited, but its continued relevance probably lies in the example afforded by Moses J's strict approach to the question of relief: his approach seems to have been that where the public authority is the author of its own misfortune, only very clear evidence of insuperable difficulties would have persuaded him to decline to grant relief, notwithstanding that third parties not before the court might be adversely affected.

3.13 ***R v North and East Devon Health Authority ex p Coughlan* [2001] QB 213, (1999) 2 CCLR 285, CA**

A consultation process, undertaken voluntarily, will be unlawful unless it complies with the 'Gunning criteria'

Facts: Ms Coughlan was rendered very severely disabled by a road traffic accident. After a period of treatment at Newcourt Hospital, which North and East Devon then wished to close, she and seven other patients were moved to Mardon House hospital, with an assurance that it would be their 'home for life'. However, North and East Devon then resolved to close Mardon House. In addition, it determined that Ms Coughlan no longer met the criteria for NHS continuing healthcare, so that she had to resort to local authority residential accommodation (for which she could be charged). Ms Coughlan submitted that it was beyond the powers of a local authority to provide her with the nursing care she needed, that it was unlawful for North and East Devon to resile from its 'home for life' promise, and a breach of Article 8 ECHR, and that there had been inadequate consultation.

Judgment: the Court of Appeal (Lord Woolf MR, Mummery and Sedley LJJ) held that 'although there are criticisms to be levelled at the consultation process, and although it ran certain risks, it was not flawed by any significant non-compliance with the *Gunning criteria*' (paragraph 117). The court also said:

> 108. It is common ground that, whether or not consultation of interested parties and the public is a legal requirement, if it is embarked upon it must be carried out properly. To be proper, consultation must be undertaken at a time when proposals are still at a formative stage; it must include sufficient reasons for particular proposals to allow those consulted to give intelligent consideration and an intelligent response; adequate time must be given for this purpose; and the product of consultation must be conscientiously taken into account when the ultimate decision is taken: *R v Brent LBC ex p Gunning* (1985) 84 LGR 168.

Comment: 'Significant non-compliance' may not have been intended as a legal test, but it may be important that it is a lower threshold than that adopted in subsequent cases: see below, *R (Royal Brompton and Harefield NHS Foundation Trust) v Joint Committee of PCT* [2012] EWCA Civ 472.

3.14 ***R v Powys CC ex p Hambidge (No 2)* (1999) 2 CCLR 460, QBD**

The local authority was not under a duty to consult the user of home care services before increasing charges

Facts: Powys changed its charging policy and increased the charges it made for the 16 hours' home care that Mrs Hambidge received each week, from £10.50 to £32.70. It did not undertake general consultation in relation to its policy change, nor had it consulted any individual service user, including Mrs Hambidge.

Judgment: Jowitt J held that guidance advised that it would be good practice to consult, but that did not give rise to a duty to do so, or create any legitimate expectation. Neither did the procedural fairness principle require consultation because Mrs Hambidge did not have any legitimate expectation that her charges would never increase and she was entitled to seek a review of the level of charge she personally was asked to pay, under section 17 of the Health and Social Services and Social Security Adjudications Act 1983, under which she could not be required to pay more than a reasonable amount, having regard to her means.

Comment: the appeal was dismissed at (2000) 3 CCLR 231 by Henry, Aldous and Laws LJ, in judgments focussing on the issue of discrimination.

3.15 *R (Haringey Consortium of Disabled People and Carers Association and others) v Haringey LBC* (2002) 5 CCLR 422, QBD

The relevant guidance created a legitimate expectation of consultation before a local authority reduced grants to local charities

Facts: Haringey reduced the grants it made to charities in its area. The charities brought a judicial review submitting that Haringey had been under a duty to consult with them, but had failed to do so.

Judgment: Scott Baker J held that Haringey purported to operate under the *General Conditions of Grant Aid to Voluntary Organisations Agreement*. Because that required consultation before grants were reduced, Haringey had acted unlawfully, in breach of the charities' legitimate expectations. That unfairness was not cured by the fact that there was an internal appeals process:

> 49. Accordingly, in this case, unless there is some other way in which the relevant assistance can be provided, the rights of the claimant and her daughter will be infringed unless it is possible, using section 3 of the HRA, to construe the section compatibly with the claimant's Article 8 rights. Before considering that issue, I shall consider whether the authority has the power to provide this assistance pursuant to section 2 of the LGA as the Secretary of State contends.
>
> *Section 2 of the LGA 2000*
>
> 50. Mr Sales submits that the local authority had power to provide either accommodation or finance to secure such accommodation pursuant to section 2 of the Local Government Act 2000. The relevant provisions of section 2 are as follows.
>
> '(1) Every local authority are to have power to do anything which they consideris likely to achieve any one or more of the following –
> (a) the promotion or improvement of the economic well-being of their area;
> (b) the promotion or improvement of the social well-being of their area; and
> (c) the promotion or improvement of the environmental well-being of their area.
>
> (2) The power under subsection (1) may be exercised in relation to or for the benefit of –
> (a) the whole or any part of a local authority's are;, or
> (b) all or any persons resident or present in a local authority's area.

(3) In determining whether or how to exercise the power under subsection (1), a local authority must have regard to their strategy under section 4.

(4) The power under subsection (1) includes power for a local authority to –

(a) incur expenditure,
(b) give financial assistance to any person,
(c) enter into arrangements or agreements with any person,
(d) co-operate with, or facilitate or co-ordinate the activities of, any person,
(e) exercise on behalf of any person any functions of that person, and
(f) provide staff, goods, services or accommodation to any person.

(5) The power under subsection (1) includes power for a local authority to do anything in relation to, or for the benefit of, any person or area situated outside their area if they consider that it is likely to achieve any one or more of the objects in that subsection.

(6) Nothing in subsection (4) or (5) affects the generality of the power under subsection (1).'

Section 3 then sets certain limits to the power conferred upon the authority under section 2. The relevant provisions are as follows:

'(1) The power under section 2(1) does not enable a local authority to do anything which they are unable to do by virtue of any prohibition, restriction or limitation on their powers which is contained in any enactment (whenever passed or made).

(2) The power under section 2(1) does not enable a local authority to raise money (whether by precepts, borrowing or otherwise).'

Subsection (3) provides for the Secretary of State to made an order preventing local authorities from doing certain specified things; and subsection (5) empowers him to issue guidance about the exercise of that power which, when issued, the local authority must have regard to in the exercise of its section 2 power.

51. Mr Sales submits that this is an extremely wide power which is perfectly capable of embracing, at the very least, the provision of financial assistance for accommodation such as the claimant is seeking in this case. He points out that the power under subsection (4)(b) specifically covers the provision of financial assistance, and that section 2(2) in terms provides that the power can be exercised to the benefit of any persons resident or present in the local authority's area.

52. He submits that it would be open to the local authority to conclude, in the circumstances of this case, that the provision of financial assistance for the purpose of acquiring accommodation would be capable of promoting the social well-being of their area by benefiting two persons resident there. Mr Sales referred me to the Explanatory Notes to the Local Government Act 2000. As Lord Hope indicated in *R v A* at para 82, it is legitimate to have regard to these when construing legislation. Paragraph 15 is as follows:

> 'Together, these sections allow local authorities to undertake a wide range of activities for the benefit of their local area and to improve the quality of life of local residents, businesses and those who commute to or visit the area. This is intended to clear up much of the uncertainty which currently exists about what authorities can do. Sections 2 and 3 allow authorities to take any action, unless it is subject to statutory prohibitions, restrictions or limitations specifically set out in legislation. The intention is to broaden the scope for local authority action while

> reducing the scope for challenge on the grounds that local authorities lack specific powers.'

Mr Sales submits that this confirms that the power of this legislation is to confer very broad and general powers upon local authorities to be able to respond to the needs of local residents and businesses. He also relied upon certain paragraphs in the Guidance issued by the Secretary of State. This is entitled 'Power to Improve or Promote Economic, Social, or Environmental Well-Being.' Paragraph 7 states that 'the new power is wide-ranging and enables the local authorities to improve the quality of life, opportunity and health of their local communities'. Paragraph 10 states:

> '... the breadth of the power is such that councils can regard it as a 'power of first resort'. Rather than searching for a specific power elsewhere in statute in order to take a particular action, councils can instead look to the well-being power in the first instance ...'

53. The power conferred by section 2 is in my judgment capable of extending to the grant of financial assistance for acquiring accommodation. The question is whether there is any 'prohibition, restriction or limitation' on that power which is contained in any other enactment. Initially, Mr Sales submitted that there was no such restriction even in relation to the provision of accommodation itself. However, he has resiled from that position and has recognised that there are certain statutory provisions which are to be found both in the Housing Act 1996 and in the Immigration and Asylum Act (IAA) 1999 which would constitute limitations on the power of the authority to grant accommodation to the claimant because she is an overstayer: see Housing Act 1996 ss159 to 161 and IAA 1999 s118. The former provide that a local authority shall allocate housing accommodation only to those who are qualified to be allocated it; and the latter prevents accommodation being provided to those subject to immigration control save in special circumstances not applicable here. In addition, in my view, section 185 of the Housing Act falls into the same category (which I have considered in paragraph 9 above). However, Mr Sales contends that there is no 'prohibition, restriction or limitation' on the power of an authority to give financial assistance for the purpose of acquiring accommodation, either in these provisions or any other. He draws a distinction between, on the one hand, a case where a statute merely confers a power in a specific field so that any limitation arises simply because the power cannot be exercised outside the specified field; and, on the other, a case where the legislation in terms imposes an express restriction or limitation on the exercise of the power. Even in the latter situation, he says that it will be necessary in each case to scrutinise the legislation carefully to see whether, properly analysed, it is intended to provide a bar to its exercise at all, or whether it is merely intended to prevent the power being exercised under the particular legislation in which the restriction is to be found.

54. Mr Sales draws an analogy from the relationship between common law and statute. He referred me to the speech of Lord Wilberforce in *Shiloh Spinners v Harding* [1973] AC 691 at 725, where Lord Wilberforce said this:

> 'In my opinion where the courts have established a general principle of law or equity, and the legislature steps in with particular legislation in a particular area, it must, unless showing a contrary intention, be taken to have left cases outside that area where they were under the influence of the general law.'

A case where, as a matter of construction, the statute was held wholly to displace the common law is *Harrison v Tew* [1990] 2 AC 523. In the course of his judgment, Lord Lowry, with whose judgment the rest of their Lordships agreed, said this:

> 'One must distinguish between affirmative and negative provisions: the common law can co-exist with the statutory provision with which it is not inconsistent'.

Comment: note that in *Hambidge (No 2)* relevant guidance had not created a legitimate expectation of consultation, whereas here, it did.

3.16 *R (Smith) v East Kent NHS Hospital Trust and Medway Health Authority* [2002] EWHC 2640 (Admin), (2003) 6 CCLR 251

A duty to re-consult only arises where there is a fundamental difference between the consultation proposals and the final decision

Facts: the Trust consulted on four options for re-organising health care provision. The response to the consultation was poor and there was little support for any of the proposals. The Trust then took a decision that incorporated some elements of those four options but was not identical to any of them. The claimant, a local campaigner, sought to quash this decision, on the ground that it had been reached in breach of a statutory duty to consult on 'significant changes' to health organisation.

Judgment: Silber J held that a duty to re-consult only arises when there is a fundamental difference between the proposals on which consultation has taken place and the proposed decision:

> 45. So I approach the issue of whether there should have been re-consultation by the defendants in this case, on the proposals now under challenge on the basis that the defendants had a strong obligation to consult with all parts of the local community. The concept of fairness should determine whether there is a need to re-consult if the decision-maker wishes to accept a fresh proposal but the courts should not be too liberal in the use of its power of judicial review to compel further consultation on any change. In determining whether there should be further re-consultation, a proper balance has to be struck between the strong obligation to consult on the part of the health authority and the need for decisions to be taken that affect the running of the Health Service. This means that there should only be re-consultation if there is a fundamental difference between the proposals consulted on and those which the consulting party subsequently wishes to adopt.

3.17 *R (Madden) v Bury MBC* [2002] EWHC 1882 (Admin), (2002) 5 CCLR 622

A decision to close to care homes was quashed when the preceding consultation process had been unlawful, owing to Bury's failure to disclose the true reasons for closure

Facts: Bury decided to close two care homes for policy reasons (to reduce the amount of residential care provision in favour of alternatives such as sheltered housing) and because of its relative cost. However, when it undertook consultation about closure, Bury emphasised that one home required costly structural repairs whereas the other required costly upgrading to meet required standards for registration: concerns that were grossly exaggerated.

Judgment: Richards J held that the information that Bury provided to residents had been misleading, it had not given any indication of possible alternatives and the tenor of the exercise indicated that the principle of closure was not up for discussion: accordingly, Bury had failed to undertake lawful consultation. Relief would not be withheld because, whilst Bury would probably still have decided to close the care homes, even had it undertaken lawful consultation, 'I cannot be certain that the result would have been the same'.

3.18 *R (Royal Brompton and Harefield NHS Foundation Trust) v Joint Committee of Primary Care Trusts* [2012] EWCA Civ 472

Consultation was unlawful where the local authority provided consultees with inaccurate and incomplete information about the reasons for its proposed decision

Facts: Bury provisionally decided to close two residential care homes. It gave notice of its proposal to residents and held a series of meetings, where residents and their families were able to make their views known, before it reached its final decision. The reasons advanced publicly by Bury, for closure, were that one home had a structural fault in its foundations whilst the other did not meet registration standards, and remedying these problems would be uneconomic.

Judgment: Richards J held that the consultation had been unlawful because of Bury's failure to convey accurate information: the structural fault was very minor and Bury had failed (despite requests) to disclose the relevant survey report or even to show that report to members that made the closure decision; in relation to the other home there had been no examination of possible alternatives. The process had also been incompatible with Article 8 ECHR:

> 58. The consultation document explained in some depth the process whereby the four options had been arrived at. It set out how the centres received their individual scores, and how a short list of options had been drawn up. It noted that one of the principles adopted was that London required at least two centres due to the size of the population. It stated that the population served by London included the East of London and South East England.
>
> 59. The consultation document also explained how of the fourteen options considered only six were viable. Two of these involved three sites for London. Next, the consultation document explained how the weighted evaluation criteria had been arrived at and showed the result of applying those criteria to the six viable options:

	OPTION 2 [7 sites – 2 for London]	OPTION 6 [6 sites – 2 for London]	OPTION 8 [6 sites – 2 for London]	OPTION 10 [7 sites – 3 for London]	OPTION 12 [7 sites – 3 for London]	OPTION 14 [Top 7 sites scoring 2 for London]
Access and travel	56	14	42	14	42	14
Quality	117	117	117	117	117	156
Deliverability	66	44	22	44	22	66
Sustainability	75	75	50	75	50	50
TOTAL	314	250	213 [error: should have been 231]	250	213 [error: should have been 231]	286

60. The two lowest scoring options were options 8 and 12. The options which provided for three London centres, ie options 10 and 12, were then eliminated so that there were then four recommended options for consultation, which were described as follows:

> 'The final recommended options for consultation are:
> – Option 2 is viable as it is consistently the highest scoring potential option
> – Option 14 is retained ...
> – Option 6 is viable
> – Option 8 is viable'

61. The consultation document then set out in a box ('the London box') on the same page the reasons for preferring the two-centre option for London:

> 'LONDON
> It was recommended to the Joint Committee of Primary Care Trusts that Options 10 and 12 (which included 3 centres in London) should not form part of the public consultation for the following reasons:
> – The Joint Committee of Primary Care Trusts recommends that two designated centres is the ideal configuration for the population of London, East of England and South East England. The question of whether two centres in London is the right number will be asked during consultation.
> – The forecast activity levels for London and its catchment area (currently around 1,250 paediatric procedures per year) mean that two centres would be well placed to meet the proposed ideal number of 500 procedures a year. could only happen with three London centres if patients were diverted from neighbouring catchment areas into London. Our analysis shows this would significantly, and unjustifiably, increase travel times and impact on access for patients outside of London, South East and East of England.
> – The advice of the *Safe and Sustainable* Steering Group is that two centres, rather than three, are better placed to develop and lead a congenital heart network for London, South East and East of England according to the *Safe and Sustainable* model of care.'

62. The consultation document then turned to the question 'Which 2 centres in London?'. It set out (on pages 95–96) a table stretching across two pages, giving the scores of the three London centres, weighted as explained above, which had been the basis of its decision as to which two London centres to recommend. That table is set out below but the columns containing (1) an analysis of the evaluation criteria, (2) the individual scores given to the centres by the Kennedy Panel and (3) the weightings, have been omitted because that information has been set out above.

	GOSH weighted score	Evelina Children's Hospital weighted score	Royal Brompton weighted score
Access and travel times	42	42	42
Quality	117	156	78
Deliverability	88	66	44
Sustainability	100	100	100
Total	347	364	264

3.19 *R (Haggerty) v St Helens Council* [2003] EWHC 803 (Admin), (2003) 6 CCLR 352

Extraneous difficulties that limit a local authority's freedom of manoeuvre can make it lawful to undertake a process of consultation that falls well short of the usual minimum

Facts: St Helens declined to renew its contract with a private care home, when it concluded that the price increase required by the care home was unjustifiable and the residents could be moved safely and in a planned manner. Some residents sought a judicial review of St Helens' decision not to enter into a new contract with the home.

Judgment: Silber J held that St Helens' decision did not interfere with the residents' rights under the ECHR and was not reached in breach of its duty to consult, on the particular facts:

> 64. In any event, as I have already explained Mr Stoker's evidence shows that there has been consultation on the transfer of the claimants and how it should be achieved. Thus, there has been consultation but it is said that some relevant matters were not considered in the claimant's case. I am unable to accept Mr Skilbeck's complaint that there should have been adequate consultation but this did not take place. Five reasons individually or cumulatively lead me to that conclusion.
>
> 65. First, the Council were given seven days by Southern Cross in which to respond to its demands and consultations of the kind referred to in *Coughlan's case* would not have been possible as within this period the Council also had to consider its financial position. Secondly, the decision to close the home was that of Southern Cross and not that of the Council with the result that consultation was not required. The claimants' case is based on the erroneous assumption that it was the Council who chose to terminate the agreement. Thirdly, consultation would not have led to a different decision in respect of Southern Cross' demands because of the Council's statutory duties to take account of costs which would have led to the decision it took. Fourthly, the Council was aware that the residents were keen to stay but it was obliged to take into account their statutory duties, which as I have explained in para [16] above required them not to pay more than the Council 'would usually expect to pay' for people having the assessment needs of the claimants. Finally, as Mr Wakefield explains that even if the Council had all the information now before it when it responded to Southern Cross' demands in December 2002, it would have come to the same decision. I accept that statement as being accurate. This shows that even if proper consultation did not take place before the Council sent the letter under challenge, the Council would inevitably have reached the same decision even if proper consultation had been possible and had actually taken place.

3.20 *R (Capenhurst) v Leicester CC* [2004] EWHC 2124 (Admin), (2004) 7 CCLR 557

A voluntary consultation process, and the ensuing decision, were unlawful where the local authority had failed adequately to inform consultees of the factors that it would treat as important in reaching its decision

Facts: the claimants were service users from voluntary organisations who faced a funding cut, after a change of political control at Leicester. The new criteria were that Leicester would only fund bodies that delivered certain core services. Leicester undertook consultation, but the claimants contended that they had not been properly consulted.

Judgment: Silber J allowed the application for judicial review. Whether or not Leicester had been under a legal duty to consult, once consultation was undertaken, it had to be conducted lawfully. In this case, Leicester had not achieved that, because it had failed to make consultees aware of the criteria to be adopted and what factors would be considered decisive or of substantial importance:

> 46. It is important that any consultee should be aware of the basis on which a proposal put forward for the basis of consultation has been considered and will thereafter be considered by the decision-maker as otherwise the consultee would be unable to give, in Lord Woolf's words in *Coughlan*, either 'intelligent consideration' to the proposals or to make an 'intelligent response' to it. This requirement means that the person consulted was entitled to be informed or had to be made aware of what criterion would be adopted by the decision-maker and what factors would be considered decisive or of substantial importance by the decision-maker in making his decision at the end of the consultation process.
>
> 47. I do not think that a consultee would not have been properly consulted if he ought reasonably to have known the criterion, which the decision-maker would adopt or the factors, which would be considered decisive by the decision-maker but that the only reason why the consultee did not know these matters was because, for example, he had turned a blind eye to something of which he ought reasonably to have been aware. Thus, consultation will only be regarded as unfair if the consultee either did not know the criterion to be adopted by the decision-maker or ought not reasonably to have known of this criterion. Of course, what a consultee ought reasonably to have known about the factors, which will be considered decisive by the decision-maker depends on all the relevant circumstances, which may well be different in each case.

3.21 *R (Morris) v Trafford Healthcare NHS Trust* [2006] EWHC 2334 (Admin), (2006) 9 CCLR 648

Although a consultation process resulting in the closure of in-patient wards had been unlawful, the court refused to grant relief in a case where the public authority proposed to re-consult

Facts: Trafford decided to close inpatient wards at a local hospital.

Judgment: Hodge J quashed the decision because Trafford had not undertaken prior consultation, as required by section 11 of the Health and Social Care Act 2001. However, the court did not grant a mandatory order requiring Trafford to re-open the wards, in the light of an assurance from Trafford that it would very shortly undertake public consultation, which might lead to their re-opening.

Comment: section 11 of the Health and Social Care Act 2001 has been repealed; now, see section 242 of the National Health Service Act 2006 (and see above, 'Health care strategy and policy materials' at para 2.13).

3.22 *R (Smith) v North Eastern Derbyshire PCT* [2006] EWCA Civ 1291, (2006) 9 CCLR 663

Where consultation has been unlawful, relief may be withheld if it is proven that the result would inevitably have been the same

Facts: the Primary Care Trust (PCT) undertook a tender process which resulted in it deciding to negotiate with an American-based healthcare provider, as a preferred bidder for the provision of GP services. However, the PCT had failed to undertake public consultation, in breach of section 11 of the Health and Social Care Act 2001. At first instance, Collins J had refused to grant relief, on the basis that the claimants had an alternative remedy through the Patients' Forum and that any representations made during consultation would probably not have made any difference.

Judgment: the Court of Appeal (May and Keene LJJ) allowed the appeal, holding that the Patients' Forum was not an alternative remedy because it had no power to require the PCT to reconsider its decision and that the correct test was not whether representations were likely to have made a difference, but whether the result would *inevitably* have been the same:

> 10. I have already noted that neither Mr Pittaway nor Mr Post contended that the judge's second reason, that is that the decision would probably have been the same anyway, was alone sufficient to sustain his conclusion. That is a proper concession. Probability is not enough. The defendants would have to show that the decision would inevitably have been the same and the court must not unconsciously stray from its proper province of reviewing the propriety of the decision making process into the forbidden territory of evaluating the substantial merits of the decision. Authority for this synthesis may be found in *R v Chief Constable of Thames Valley Police ex p Cotton* [1990] IRLR 344 at 352; *Simplex GE (Holdings) Ltd and another v Secretary of State for the Environment* (1989) 57 P&CR 306 at 327; *R v Secretary of State for Environment ex p Brent London Borough Council* [1982] 1 QB 593 at 646, and see also Fordham, *Judicial Review Handbook* (4th ed) at paragraph 4.5 and Clive Lewis, *Judicial Remedies in Public Law* (3rd ed) at para 11-027. In the light of this, I think that Collins J applied a wrong principle in paragraph 27 of his judgment.

Comment: section 11 of the Health and Social Care Act 2001 has been repealed; now, see section 242 of the National Health Service Act 2006 (and see above, 'Health care strategy and policy materials' at para 2.13).

The Senior Courts Act 1981 now provides, at section 31(2A), that the High Court must refuse to grant relief 'if it appears to the court to be highly likely that the outcome for the applicant would not have been substantially different if the conduct complained of had not occurred', unless there is an 'exceptional public interest' in granting relief. It remains to be seen how the court will approach this restriction on its traditional function.

3.23 *R (Fudge) v South West Strategic Health Authority* [2007] EWCA Civ 803, (2007) 10 CCLR 599

A statutory duty to consult remained in place even where the Secretary of State had taken over the function to which the duty to consult attached; but for pragmatic reasons, relief would be refused

Facts: the Secretary of State took over from the PCT and Strategic Health Authority the planning of a scheme to provide independent sector treatment centres, selected a preferred bidder and awarded it the preferred contract.

Judgment: the Court of Appeal (Sedley, Rix and Moses LJJ) held that, notwithstanding the actions of the Secretary of State, the PCT had remained under the duty to consult, up the stage of selecting the preferred bidder, imposed by section 11 of the Health and Social Care Act 2001 and it had been in breach of that duty. However, relief would be limited to declaratory relief – it would be wholly disproportionate to undo what had been done:

> 66. In light of the Claimant's abandonment of the attempt to quash the decision, it is unnecessary for us to consider whether the failure to provide information to the Primary Care Trust in the instant appeal could possibly be said to have had anything to do with the decision of the Secretary of State. But we do believe it important to emphasise that in those cases where the obligation under section 11 may be limited, very little will be achieved by bringing proceedings for Judicial Review. In *R v Brent LBC ex p Walters* [1998] 30 HLR 328, in the context of disposal of housing by a local authority, this court rejected the suggestion that a breach of the obligation to consult should inevitably lead to the consequence that the consultation process should be re-started and the scheme of disposal be re-considered.
>
> > '... the exercise of the discretion to grant or refuse judicial review usually, and in this case certainly does, involve close attention to both the nature of the illegality of the decision and its consequences. In a case where the consultation process is impugned it is not irrelevant for the court to consider the consultation process required in the particular case and its purpose, what those entitled to be consulted actually understood, and whether compliance with the consultation process would in fact have had any significant impact on them and the decision ... where, as here, there is overwhelming evidence that the effect of Judicial Review will not be limited to requiring the authority to repeat the process in the prescribed form, but will certainly damage the interests of a large number of other individuals who have welcomed the proposals, and acted on the basis that they will be implemented, it would be absurd for the court to ignore what Schiemann LJ rightly described as the relevant 'disbenefits'. (per Judge LJ at page 381)
>
> 67. This approach, well-settled in the sphere of public law, is particularly important in this case. We acknowledge that the courts are concerned to ensure that public administration, particularly in a field as important as the National Health Service, should comply with obligations imposed by statute. Since we have had the opportunity to correct the erroneous legal view of the Department, something has been achieved. But we must recognise, also, that that opportunity has arisen in a case where the impact on the claimant and others receiving health services in Avon, Gloucestershire and Wiltshire can only be described, at this stage, as minimal. Indeed, it appears that this issue has only arisen in the wake of the more turbulent controversy as to the closure of Frenchay Hospital which has nothing whatever to do with these proceedings. Our conclusion as to the law has been reached at the cost of a disproportionate amount of time and energy, exacerbated by the burden of files containing at least one thousand documents; the costs might have been better deployed in securing and maintaining health services within the region concerned. Public law falls into disrepute if it causes an unnecessary diversion of work and resources. It is dispiriting

that we can discern little if any benefit to those in Avon, Gloucestershire and Wiltshire at having established that the Department erred in law in its views as to section 11. Others may benefit, in the future, from that conclusion, but not the claimant nor, so far as we can see, anyone within Avon, Gloucestershire and Wiltshire.

Comment: section 11 of the Health and Social Care Act 2001 has been repealed; now, see section 242 of the National Health Service Act 2006 (and see above, 'Health care strategy and policy materials' at para 2.13).

3.24 *R (Eisai Ltd) v NICE* [2008] EWCA Civ 438, (2008) 11 CCLR 385

Fairness required full disclosure of a computer model on which decision-making was based so as to permit the consultee to seek to undermine the validity of the model; considerations of administrative difficulty should not usually outweigh what fairness requires

Facts: NICE granted only limited approval for the use of a drug manufactured by Eisai. Eisai succeeded at first instance in establishing that NICE had failed to comply with anti-discrimination legislation, but not that its consultation process had been unfair. Eisai appealed on that issue, contending that it had been unfair that NICE had provided no more than a read-only computer model of the cost-effectiveness of Eisai's drug, rather than a fully executable model, that could be run with different inputs and assumptions, so as to test its reliability.

Judgment: the Court of Appeal (Tuckey, Jacob and Richards LJJ) allowed Eisai's appeal, holding that (i) the economic model was central to NICE's appraisal of the cost-effectiveness of Eisai's drug; (ii) Eisai might be able to criticise the economic model; (iii) it could only do that, if it had a fully-executable version of the model; (iv) the extra time and cost involved, and other administrative considerations, did not undermine the conclusion; that (v) balancing all the factors, including the very strong public interest involved, fairness demanded that NICE supply Eisai with a fully executable model

> 65. If fairness otherwise requires release of the fully executable version, the court should in my view be very slow to allow administrative considerations of this kind to stand in the way of its release.

3.25 *R (Boyejo) v Barnet LBC* [2009] EWHC 3261 (Admin), (2010) 13 CCLR 72

Consultation was unlawful when the decision had already been made, it did not canvass alternatives, did not sufficiently involve consultees and gave insufficient time

Facts: Barnet and Portsmouth both separately decided to terminate certain on-site, live-in services for sheltered tenants, substituting a mobile night-service, with an alarm call system.

Judgment: Deputy High Court Judge Milwyn Jarman held that Portsmouth's consultation had been inadequate in that it's 'consultation document' spoke in terms of a decision already having been made, did not canvass alternatives and failed sufficiently to involved disabled persons; also, the time afforded for representations was too short and Portsmouth had failed to take proper account of the representations made. Additionally, neither Barnet nor Portsmouth had done sufficient to draw decision-makers' attention to the duty at section 49A of the Disability Discrimination Act 1995, nor to have specific regard to the impact on those residents with a disability (cf. the residents in general) nor to take account that it might be necessary to treat such persons more favourably. Further, both authorities' conclusions, in their equalities impact assessments, that there would not be any adverse impact on residents, were *Wednesbury* unreasonable.

3.26 *R (W) v Croydon LBC* [2011] EWHC 696 (Admin), (2011) 14 CCLR 247

A statutory consultation process, with the parents of an incapacitated adult, was unlawful where the consultees had been afforded insufficient time

Facts: Croydon formed the strong provisional view that W's placement was no longer suitable and completed assessments of need to that effect. Since W lacked capacity, Croydon arranged a meeting with W's parents to discuss the assessments. However, they only disclosed the assessments to the parents a short time before the meeting. The parents objected to this late disclosure and stated that they disagreed with much of the content of the assessments. A few days later, Croydon decided to move W and he/the parents brought a judicial review.

Judgment: Ouseley J held that Croydon had not made its mind up before the meeting (although it had had a firm view), but that its consultation with the parents (required by section 4(7) of the Mental Capacity Act 2005) had been inadequate, in that it had not given the parents sufficient time before the meeting to consider the assessments and formulate their response; and by the time the parents did respond, about two weeks after the meeting, the decision had already been taken.

3.27 *R (G) v North Somerset Council* [2011] EWHC 2232 (Admin)

North Somerset had not acted unlawfully in deciding to cut the amount of direct payments and replacing direct payments with a managed care service

Facts: The claimants were two severely mentally disabled young persons, whose care had been managed by their parents, by way of direct payments. North Somerset cut the claimants' funding by 33 per cent and replaced their direct payments with a managed care service. They claimants sought a judicial review.

Judgment: Laws J dismissed the application on the basis that, factually, whilst North Somerset had reduced the budget, it was providing the same level of service and that very serious concerns had arisen about the conduct of the claimants' parents in relation to the direct payments. North Somerset had not been under a duty of consultation and any breach of the public sector equality duty (PSED) had been purely theoretical:

> 21. The burden of the evidence here is that in what plainly were difficult circumstances given the context and the background of the audit, the council have taken care to maintain the existing provision in being subject to any change yet to happen when the full further review has been completed. There is nothing in the material before me to show that a different picture emerges when one looks at the decision of May 2011. In these circum-

stances it does not seem to me there was a breach by the local authority of the procedural obligations relating to assessment or consultation either in February 2011 or in May 2011.

25. The same goes, it seems to me, for Mr Buttler's third submission which was that section 4 of the Mental Capacity Act 2005 required the council to consult the claimants' parents or carers as to whether the steps proposed to be taken in February or May 2011 were in their best interests. Such a duty however arises only if consultation is 'practicable and appropriate'. It seems to me plain that it would not have been appropriate to consult the parents given the history. Mr Buttler however submits that the carers should have been consulted. The carers in fact have continued their task as before now under the new arrangements. Their input moreover will be part of a review in due course. Though they have not been expressly consulted or their advice distinctly sought as to the changes in February or May 2011, I cannot read this in the particular circumstances as a violation of the statute.

26. The last submission made by Mr Buttler goes only to the May 2011 decision. It is that a legitimate expectation that the carers would be consulted before direct payment ceased was generated by the letter of 7 February 2011. Mr Buttler points to the terms of the letter. He says that its import is that the new temporary direct payment arrangements would continue for six months until the comprehensive review was completed. It may be that that is what was hoped would happen or indeed what the council anticipated would happen. But it seems to me that there is nothing in that letter that generates an expectation that even in the face of evidence confirming the appropriateness of a change in the arrangements such as was made in May 2011 there would be an expectation of consultation before that occurrence, and not in truth a legitimate expectation case.

3.28 *R (Buckinghamshire CC) v Kingston upon Thames RLBC* [2011] EWCA Civ 457, (2011) 14 CCLR 426

A local authority was not under a statutory or common law duty to consult with another local authority before placing an individual in its area, even though that would result in a financial and administrative burden on that other local authority

Facts: Kingston had provided SL with residential accommodation in Buckinghamshire area, so that SL was deemed to remain ordinarily resident in Kingston, for the purposes of sections 21 and 26 of the National Assistance Act (NAA) 1948, by virtue of section 24(5) of the NAA 1948 (ie for the purposes of residential accommodation). Kingston then placed SL in a supported living arrangement in Buckinghamshire, as a result of which SL became ordinarily resident in Buckinghamshire for the purposes of NAA 1948 s28 (home care) and its responsibility. Buckinghamshire sought a judicial review of the placement, on the ground that Kingston had been under a legal requirement, which it breached, to consult with Buckinghamshire before making the placement.

Judgment: the Court of Appeal (Pill, Patten and Munby LJJ) rejected Buckinghamshire's case, holding that Kingston was discharging statutory duties towards SL, to whom it also owed a duty to act fairly. The common law duty did not require Kingston to consult with Buckinghamshire, as a result of the procedural fairness principle, and it would be inconsistent with the statutory scheme for it to do so:

1) There was no legal basis for a duty of fairness towards Buckinghamshire in the form of a duty to consult it. Kingston was performing, in accordance with section 47 of the National Health Services and Community Care Act 1990 and section 29 of the 1948 Act, a duty to SL, and it was fairness to the service user that had to be at the centre of decision-making. Fairness to Buckinghamshire could arise only if performance of the duty to SL required that there should be a duty to consult it but there was no basis upon which the court could create such a duty. Such a requirement would complicate the decision-making process in relation to SL, and there would be a danger of delay and satellite litigation.

2) Co-operation in the obtaining of information was to be encouraged but an enforceable duty should not be read into the procedure. If it were to be imposed, it should be created by statute or in directions from the Secretary of State. Had Parliament intended to make provision for the protection of the financial or other interests of different authorities in the decision-making process, express provision would have been made.[16]

Comment: under the Care Act 2014, a local authority will remain responsible for service users whom it has placed in another local authority area, in residential accommodation, should those purposes move into supported housing: see paras 12.16–12.19 below.

3.29 *R (W) v Birmingham CC* [2011] EWHC 1147 (Admin), (2011) 14 CCLR 516

Unclear and inadequate information resulted in the consultation process being unlawful

Facts: in order to make necessary budgetary savings, Birmingham decided only to meet '*critical*' needs, whereas it had previously met '*critical*' and '*substantial*' needs.

Judgment: Walker J held that Birmingham's consultation and its discharge of the disability equality duty had been unlawful:

1) The material prepared for consideration on 1 and 14 March 2011 failed to address the questions which arose when considering whether the impact on the disabled of the move to 'critical only' was so serious that a less draconian alternative should be identified and funded to the extent necessary by savings elsewhere; the authority had not in any real sense moved beyond a generalised description of the likely impact and it was difficult in the circumstances to see how there could be due regard to the matters in section 49A(1) of the Disability Discrimination Act 1995 without some attempt at assessment of the practical impact on those whose needs in a particular respect fell into the substantial but not critical band; even if councillors were able to form some opinion as to the broad impact, there was not in the material any assessment of the extent to which the potential severity would or would not be reduced by such mitigating factors as were mentioned.

16 (2011) 14 CCLR 426–427.

2) The failure to address the right questions for the purposes of section 49A inevitably carried with it a conclusion that the consultation was inadequate; the consultation was also flawed because of the scope for confusion about whether the new offer related to personal or social care and because the true amount of the proposed saving for the move to critical only was not made clear until a late stage, so that consultees did not have the opportunity to assert that the sum involved in leaving the eligibility threshold unchanged could properly be found by making savings elsewhere.[17]

3.30 *R (South West Care Homes Ltd) v Devon CC* [2012] EWHC 1867 (Admin)

Although failures in the consultation process were not academic, and the process had been unlawful, relief would be refused in the exercise of the court's discretion, for pragmatic reasons

Facts: South West, a care home provider, sought a judicial review of Devon's decision to freeze the standard fees it would pay, inter alia, on the basis that Devon had failed to have due regard to the actual cost of providing care and had failed to consult.

Judgment: Singh J held that Devon had, unlawfully, failed to consult but that relief would not be granted on that account, owing to the passage of time:

> **Whether relief should be granted**
> 51. I do not accept the suggestion, in so far as it was made at the hearing before me, that the breach of the duty of consultation in this case was academic, in the sense that consultation would have made no difference to the outcome. In that regard I note what was said by the Court of Appeal in *R (Smith) v North Eastern Derbyshire Primary Care Trust* [2006] 1 WLR 3315. That was a consultation case where the learned judge at first instance had proceeded at the remedial stage on the basis that if representations had been made by the claimant, they 'probably would have made no difference'. However, the Court of Appeal held that probability is not sufficient. As May LJ said in the main judgment at paragraph 10:
>
> > 'Probability is not enough. The defendant would have to show that the decision would inevitably have been the same and the court must not unconsciously stray from its proper province of reviewing the propriety of the decision-making process into the forbidden territory of evaluating the substantial merits of the decision ...'
>
> Amongst the authorities cited for that proposition May LJ cited the important case *of R v Chief Constable of Thames Valley Police ex p Cotton* [1990] IRLR 344 at page 352, giving the judgment of Bingham LJ (as he then was). I would also note what Keene LJ had to say at paragraph 16 of the judgment in Smith.
>
> 52. Nevertheless, as the defendant submits, the court has a discretion whether to grant any remedy and, if so, what remedy. In particular, as the defendant submitted and appears to have been common ground before me, the court cannot ignore the question of possible detriment to good administration. This can arise potentially in one or both of two ways. The first is that it is expressly referred to by statute in section 31(6) of the Senior Courts Act 1981 which reads:

17 (2011) 14 CCLR 517–518.

> '(6) Where the High Court considers that there has been undue delay in making an application for judicial review, the court may refuse to grant–
> (a) leave for the making of the application; or.
> (b) any relief sought on the application.
> if it considers that the granting of the relief sought would be likely to cause substantial hardship to, or substantially prejudice the rights of, any person or would be detrimental to good administration.'

53. The second way, as the defendant submits, is that in any event, judicial review, quite apart from the questions of delay is always discretionary. One of the factors that the court will have to regard to in its discretion is the interests of good public administration (see *R v Monopolies & Mergers Commission ex p Argyll Group Plc* [1986] 2 All ER 257 at 266) in the judgment of Sir John Donaldson MR (as he then was) where he said:

> 'Good public administration requires decisiveness and finality unless there are compelling reasons to the contrary.'

54. On the facts of the present case I accept the defendant's submissions and, in the exercise of the court's discretion, would not quash the decision which is under challenge. My reasons, in brief, are as follows: first, the relevant financial year has ended on 31 March 2012. It is obvious that many transactions including, as the claimants accepted, things such as Tax Returns will have been concluded and submitted in the meantime on the understanding that the defendant authority's budget was as had been finalised in March and April of 2011 and would not be reopened now.

55. Secondly, there is a more specific type of detriment to others to which the defendants can point. This can be seen from paragraph 37 of the defendant's detailed grounds in these proceedings where they said this:

> 'A grant of relief in the present case, if it resulted in increase in care home fees for 2011/12 would cause a further and more specific detriment to good administration and hardship to third parties. At the suit of a small number of providers the defendant would have to find a very large sum overall, a windfall to those providers who appear to have been content with a decision. This in turn could necessitate recovery of the unpaid part of the increased fee from those who pay the full cost of their care through the local authority or from the relatives of those who have died in the interim. The alternative would be to place the burden on council tax payers ... the potential for hardship and distress as well as administrative inconvenience and expense is obvious.'

This part of the defendant's detailed grounds is supported by the witness statement of Jennifer Stephens, in particular paragraphs 37 to 38.

56. Thirdly, I accept the defendant's submission that this case is now extremely stale. Even if one takes the view that the grounds for making the claim first arose on 4th April 2011, the claim was commenced just inside the three-month time limit, on 1st July, and sought to overturn a decision which was in effect taken on 2nd March 2011.

57. Even if there was no undue delay, something I will put to one side for the purpose of this consideration, the original grounds were in a form which in the opinion of Mitting J did not disclose a clear and arguable challenge. On the evidence before the court it would appear that the claimants did not have the matter expedited until November 2011, after refusal of permission on the papers by Mitting J. It was not until 2nd February 2012 that the claim was amended in a skeleton argument of that date, in a form which eventually obtained permission at the oral hearing before the learned

deputy judge. By that time, as the defendants have submitted, the decision under challenge was already almost one-year-old.

58. As I have said, even if one puts to one side questions of delay, I have had regard to the principle in the Argyle case and accept the defendant's submissions that it would be detrimental to the interests of good administration to grant a quashing order in this case.

59. The final matter which I have had regard to in the exercise of the court's discretion is that, in any event, the views of the claimants on the question of fees and actual costs were well-known to the defendant. Although I have not accepted the defendant's submission that that is sufficient to mean that the duty of consultation was complied with, it is nevertheless, in my view, one factor to be taken into account in the court's exercise of discretion when it comes to the question of remedies.

60. For the claimants it was submitted that they do not seek a mandatory order requiring the court to order the defendant authority to increase the fees in question. The claimant submits that such an order would usurp the role of a public authority in making the relevant decision: so they submit the court should not hesitate to grant a quashing order. In my view, this argument is a little disingenuous, since the claimants wish there to be consultation with a view to achieving a real change in practice and not for academic reasons. If there is a real prospect of a change in practice then, in my view, for the reasons I have already given, there would be detriment to good public administration and, in the exercise of the court's discretion, I would not grant a quashing order.

61. Nevertheless, I do not accept the defendant's submission that I should refuse even declaratory relief. In my judgment it would be appropriate to grant a declaration in appropriate terms to reflect the terms of my judgment that I have accepted that the claimants succeed on their ground 3: there was an unlawful failure of consultation in the present case.

62. This would vindicate the rule of law. I note in that context the decision of Webster J in the *AMA* case, to which I have already made reference, at page 15. Granting a declaration can serve a valuable function in guiding future conduct. A declaration is a flexible and proportionate remedy: it can be tailored to fit the facts of the particular case before the court and to reflect the particular breach of public law which the court has identified. In that regard, I bear in mind the recent judgment of the Divisional Court in *R (Hurley) and Another v Secretary of State for Business Innovation and Skills* [2012] EWHC 201 (Admin), in particular at paragraph 99 (Elias LJ).

3.31 *R (Royal Brompton and Harefield NHS Foundation Trust) v Joint Committee of PCT* [2012] EWCA Civ 472

The Court of Appeal re-stated the consultation principles, including that the courts will usually only grant relief where 'something has gone clearly and radically wrong'

Facts: the Foundation Trust sought a judicial review of the major consultation undertaken by the Joint Committee of PCT into the reconfiguration of national paediatric cardiac surgical services.

Judgment: the Court of Appeal (Arden and Richards LJJ, Sir Stephen Sedley) held that the consultation had been lawful. Its judgment set out the requirements of lawful consultation, explaining that they were grounded in the fundamental principle of fairness and, also emphasising that relief would usually only be granted where '*something has gone clearly and radically wrong*' in relation to at least one group of consultees:

> 8. Apart from the statutory framework, the general law must be considered. We shall deal later in this judgment with the correct approach to an application to prevent a consultation process from taking place. At this stage, it is sufficient to describe the obligation of fairness which the law imposes on any public consultation exercise. The leading authority on this is the judgment of this court in *R v North and East Devon Health Authority ex p Coughlan* (Lord Woolf MR, Mummery and Sedley LJJ) [2001] QB 213:
>
> > '108. It is common ground that, whether or not consultation of interested parties and the public is a legal requirement, if it is embarked upon it must be carried out properly. To be proper, consultation must be undertaken at a time when proposals are still at a formative stage; it must include sufficient reasons for particular proposals to allow those consulted to give intelligent consideration and an intelligent response; adequate time must be given for this purpose; and the product of consultation must be conscientiously taken into account when the ultimate decision is taken (*R v Brent London BC ex p Gunning* (1985) 84 LGR 168).'
>
> 9. The *Coughlan* formula is a prescription for fairness. It is an aspect of fairness that a consultation document presents the issues in a way that facilitates an effective response: see, for example, *R (Capenhurst) v Leicester City Council* [2004] EWHC 2124 (Admin), (2004) 7 CCLR 557. No doubt for that reason, as will appear below, the consultation document in this case explains at length the successive criteria for change that the JCPCT applied in this case. The consultation document must be clear to the general body of applicants: see *R v Secretary of State for Transport ex p Richmond upon Thames RLBC (No 2)* [1995] Env LR 390.
>
> 10. Another aspect of fairness is that it must present the available information fairly. In this case, because the JCPCT had to collect information from the centres to present the available information it would have to make clear to the centres what information it needed. A further aspect of fairness lies in the presentation of the information on which the views of consultees should be sought. The options for change must be fairly presented. Nonetheless, a decision-maker may properly decide to present his preferred options in the consultation document, provided it is clear what the other options are: *Nichol v Gateshead Metropolitan Borough Council* (1988) 87 LGR 435.
>
> 11. The object of requiring fairness is to ensure high standards in decision-making by public bodies, and to enable responses to be made which will best facilitate a sound decision as a result. In addition, it must achieve the statutory objective of section 242(2)(b) of the National Health Service Act 2006 of engaging users.
>
> 12. If the presentation of information inaccurately would have no material adverse effect on the process of consultation, perhaps because the error is patent, the error is unlikely to amount to unfairness when taken on its own (see generally *R v Secretary of State for Transport ex p Richmond-upon-Thames RLBC (No 3)* [1995] Env LR 409). However, aspects of alleged unfairness should be reviewed both individually and in aggregate. An individual aspect of unfairness may seem trivial on its own but when seen with other aspects of unfairness it may acquire greater significance.
>
> 13. If it is alleged that a consultation process is unfair, clear unfairness must be shown. As Sullivan J pointed out in *R (Greenpeace Ltd) v Secretary of State for Industry* [2007] EWHC 311(Admin), it must be shown that the

error is such that there can be no proper consultation and that 'something [has] gone clearly and radically wrong'.

> On the other hand, it is sufficient to show that the unfairness affects only a group of the persons affected by the consultation: see *R (Medway Council and others) v Secretary of State for the Environment* [2002] EWCA 2516 (Admin). Unfairness to the general body of consultees is not required.

3.32 *R (Bracking) v Secretary of State for Work and Pensions* [2013] EWCA Civ 1345, (2013) 16 CCLR 479

Consultees had an adequate opportunity of explaining the likely effect of what was proposed on them and that was sufficient, in this case

Facts: the Secretary of State decided to close the Independent Living Fund (ILF), devolving funding for the purpose of sustaining independent living to local social services authorities. The claimant contended that consultation had been unlawful and that the Secretary of State had failed to discharge the PSED.

Judgment: The Court of Appeal (Elias, Kitchin and McCombe LJJ) held that the consultation had been adequate in that consultees had had an adequate opportunity of explaining the likely effect on them of the closure of the fund and it had not been necessary to provide them with financial information about the costs associated with closure of the ILF or to explain more than that the reason for the proposal was to achieve an integrated care system and economies of scale.

3.33 *R (T) v Sheffield CC* [2013] EWHC 2953 QB, (2013) 16 CCLR 580

In assessing whether a consultation process was lawful, it is necessary to have careful regard to the context and all the circumstances

Facts: Sheffield decided to stop paying subsidies to nurseries in relatively deprived areas where there was little prospect of making up the shortfall from fees charged to parents, so that some of the nurseries might well have to close. A judicial review was brought on the basis that Sheffield had failed to consult lawfully, had not discharged the PSED and had acted unlawfully in other, ancillary ways.

Judgment: Turner J held that Sheffield had acted lawfully. In relation to the consultation issue, he said this:

> 29. There is no dispute about the legal principles to be applied. In *R v North and East Devon HA ex p Coughlan* [2001] QB 213 the Court of Appeal held at para 108 that any consultation with respect to the decision of a public body must:
>
> i) be undertaken at a formative stage;
> ii) include sufficient reasons for the particular proposals to allow those consulted to give intelligent consideration and response;
> iii) give sufficient time for an adequate response;
> iv) must be conscientiously taken into account when the decision is taken.
>
> 30. I am satisfied that the consultation process relevant to the decision under review in this case was undertaken at a formative stage. This is an issue which is bound to be fact sensitive but the important point is that

when the process starts the ultimate decision should still be fully capable of being moulded and influenced by the response. A consultation which starts with the presentation of a fait accompli is no sort of consultation at all.

31. However, as Davies LJ pointed out in *R (Bailey and others) v London Borough of Brent* [2011] EWHC 2572 (Admin) at para 104:

> 'There cannot necessarily be easy identification of particular formative 'stages' in every decision making process...'

The Court of Appeal in that case was specifically considering the application of section 149 of the Equality Act 2010 but this observation applies equally to the common law duty to consult.

32. It is also important to put the issue of consultation into context. There will be many cases in which it will not be possible precisely to time the beginning (or even the end) of the consultation process. For example, it is by no means unusual for particular proposals to have been preceded by earlier different but related proposals upon which there has already been some level of pertinent consultation. The existence of the prior period of consultation does not, of course, obviate the need to consult further but it may have an important influence on the timing, content and duration of the process of consultation which follows.

33. This case provides an illustration of the importance of context. The issue of the future of subsidies to nurseries was the subject of dialogue and debate in January 2011. This continued as part of the subsequent Early Years Review. By December 2012, interested parties had been involved in the exchange of views and information for about two years. Even if a mechanistic approach were taken which focussed entirely on the phase of the process beginning December 2012 I consider that the matter was then still at a formative stage. The final form of the policy towards these subsidies was yet to be determined.

34. The documentation shows that over the relevant period, the defendant gave detailed reasons for the proposed curtailments of the grants. The Nurseries and other interested parties did not agree with these reasons but they were, at least, fully equipped to engage with them.

35. The time reasonably to be allowed for a response to a consultation process is, again, a highly fact sensitive issue. Once more, context is important. Where, as here, the issue upon which consultation is to take place is one in which interested parties have already been recently engaged the time reasonably required for any formal consultation period may well be shorter than in circumstances where the proposal is without precursors.

36. I am entirely satisfied that the defendant conscientiously took into account the views of those who contributed to the consultation process. The fact that the discount of 25% was reduced to 10% and the phasing out of the subsidies was postponed in 2011 is evidence that the defendant was not historically deaf to the representations it received. No doubt there will be many who are convinced that the result was a foregone conclusion but as Davies LJ observed in *Bailey* at para 194:

> 'In the field of important decisions by local authorities of a kind such as the present, nevertheless, experience teaches one that there may be many local residents who will, rightly or wrongly, assume that an announced proposal has in truth already been decided on; and that subsequent consultation or impact assessments or reports will be moulded so as to endorse a predetermined result.'

37. I do not accept that the defendant is open to legitimate criticism for failing to broaden the scope of the consultation. It was reasonable to engage primarily with the nurseries on the issue of grants. The nurseries were most directly affected by the proposals and, in any event, were in a good position to advocate the benefits of the services which they provided to those who used them. In any event, the summary of the consultation procedures set out in the consultation paper presented to Cabinet demonstrates a thorough and conscientious process the involvement of parents in which was both proportionate and timely.

38. Complaint is made that a questionnaire promulgated by the defendant on the proposals was inaptly phrased. The first question was:

> 'Do you agree that we should focus available resources on the most vulnerable children and stop the subsidy allocated to a small number of childcare providers in the city?'

I agree that this question could have been improved upon. It gave the impression that focusing on the needs of the most vulnerable children and subsidising the nurseries was inevitably a mutually exclusive choice. Also, the tone of the question was somewhat tendentious. Nevertheless, the questionnaire should not be scrutinized in a vacuum. The contents of the briefing notes and the Consultation document make it clear that the consultees were entirely familiar with the issues and options.

39. Neither am I satisfied that the fact that the nurseries are referred to as 'businesses' in some of the defendant's documentation is an indication that consultees may have been misled into thinking that these were profit making organisations. The use of the word 'business' in this context did not carry this implication and, in any event, the consultees were fully aware of the nature of the undertakings of the various providers of nursery facilities who were in receipt of the grants.

40. Taken as a whole, the consultation process in this case was fully compliant with the common law standards referred to in *Coughlan* and the challenge on this ground must fail.

3.34 *R (D) v Worcestershire CC* [2013] EWHC 2490 (Admin), (2013) 16 CCLR 323

On analysis, the information provided to consultees had been accurate

Facts: in order to achieve necessary budgetary reductions, Worcestershire concluded that, in the absence of exceptional circumstances, it would not pay a sum for home care for an adult under 65 that exceeded the net weekly cost of a care home placement. The claimant, who was significantly disabled, contended that Worcestershire had not consulted properly, or discharged its PSED under section 149 of the Equality Act 2010.

Judgment: Hickinbottom J held that whilst the claim asserted that consultees had not had adequate information on which to comment, and that decision-makers had not been informed of the likely consequences, that was on the false premise that Worcestershire's policy would result in about half of those within its scope having to choose between receiving less than was needed at home or going into residential care, whereas the reality was that, for those affected, the most likely result was that hard consideration would have to be given as to how their needs would be met more cost effectively at home and the materials for the decision-makers made it clear that hard choices would have to be made and that some service users' care package would not completely comprise their first choice of services. Accordingly, the consultation had been lawful.

3.35 *R (LH) v Shropshire Council* [2014] EWCA Civ 404, (2014) 17 CCLR 216

It was legitimate to consult on macro policy changes first but it was then necessary to consult beneficiaries of specific services that might be closed; in this case, although consultation had been unlawful, relief would be refused for pragmatic reasons

Facts: Shropshire consulted widely on a policy change, that would lead away from the provision of day centres and focus on individualised budgets, in order to make necessary budgetary savings and, also, to promote central government policy. Afterwards, Shropshire identified a number of day centres that would actually have to close.

Judgment: the Court of Appeal (Longmore, McFarlane and Lewison LJJ) held that Shropshire had been under a common law duty to consult, by reason of its duty to act fairly. The consultation it had undertaken was amply sufficient to justify its policy change, but fairness also required there to be consultation before making a decision to close an individual day centre and that had not occurred. However, given the closure of the day centre and the dispersal of its staff, the only relief granted would be declaratory:

> 28. ... From this it emerges that the duty to consult will arise when a person has an interest which the law decides is one which is to be protected by procedural fairness. Dillon LJ's reference (85F) to the observations of Deane J in *Haoucher v Minister of State for Immigration and Ethnic Affairs* (1990) 93 ALR 51, 52–3 together with his own remarks about fairness (86E-G) show that he essentially agreed with this analysis.
>
> 29. Once one appreciates that this is the source of the common law duty to consult, it must be apparent that not only is the question whether LH had an interest entitled to be protected by procedural fairness a question for the court but so also is the question whether the procedure adopted by the Council was a fair procedure. Fairness is a matter for the court not the Council to decide. If fairness requires the Council to consult about individual closures, then the Council cannot say that it can choose a method of consultation which by-passes the question whether an individual day centre should be closed.
>
> 30. Having said that I would, for my part, accept that provided the Council consults with the staff, users and relatives of a particular day centre which is to be closed, the extent to which the Council may choose to consult more widely, eg with the staff, users and relatives of other day centres in the country is essentially a matter for the Council. No doubt, if consultation with users of one day centre led to the conclusion that that day centre would not close but that another would, there would a duty to consult the users of that other day centre. But save to that extent, the principle enunciated by Clarke LJ may well be applicable, as I think Simon Brown LJ would accept in the light of what he said at page 91E-F in the *Devon* and *Durham* case.

3.36 *R (Michael Robson) v Salford CC* [2013] EWHC 3481 (Admin), (2014) 17 CCLR 474

The court summarised consultation principles and concluded that, in substance, consultees had been adequately informed about what was proposed

Facts: Salford decided to cease direct provision of transport services in order to achieve budgetary savings. In future, it would make individual transport arrangements for each eligible adult through a variety of different means, such as a 'ring and ride' service, taxis and motability vehicles. The claimants, who were both severely disabled, challenged this decision by way of judicial review.

Judgment: Deputy High Court Judge Stephen Davies dismissed the application for judicial review, holding that there was no evidence that the result of Salford's decision would be that Salford would fail to meet eligible needs for transport and the consultation duty and PSED had been discharged. Deputy High Court Judge Davies said this about consultation:

> 53. The claimants contend that the defendant was obliged at common law to undertake a proper consultation with those affected before taking the decision to withdraw the PTU service and replace it with individualised transport arrangements. The claimants contend that this duty is an aspect of the overarching common law duty to act in a procedurally fair manner. They rely on the decision of the Court of Appeal in *R v Devon CC ex p Baker* [1995] 1 All ER 73 in support of that proposition. They also draw my attention to the observations of Lord Reed JSC in *Osborn v Parole Board* [2013] 3 WLR 1020 at paras 64–72 to emphasise first that fairness is for the court and not for the decision-maker to decide, and second his explanation of the benefits to be gained from procedurally fair decision making. As to what is required in terms of consultation, they refer me to the well-known statement of Lord Woolf MR, in *R v North & East Devon HA ex p Coughlan* [2001] QB 213 at paragraph 108, where he said that:
>
>> 'It is common ground that whether or not consultation of interested parties and the public is a legal requirement, if it is embarked upon it must be carried out properly. To be proper, consultation must be undertaken at a time when proposals are still at a formative stage; it must include sufficient reasons for particular proposals to allow those consulted to give intelligent consideration and an intelligent response; adequate time must be given for this purpose; and the product of consultation must be conscientiously taken into account when the ultimate decision is taken: *R v Brent LBC ex p Gunning* (1985) 84 LGR 168.'
>
> 54. They also refer me to the analysis of the Court of Appeal, given by Arden LJ, in *R (Royal Brompton & Harefield NHS Foundation Trust) v Joint Committee of Primary Care Trusts* [2012] EWCA Civ 472 at paras 8–14. In particular they emphasise the requirement that the consultation document must present the issues in a way that facilitates an effective response, and in a way which is clear to the general body of consultees, the requirement that the available information must be presented fairly and not inaccurately, and that the unfairness need only be shown to affect a group of those affected by the consultation, as opposed to all of them.
>
> 55. Mr Greatorex in his submissions did not quarrel with the above as statements of principle. He also however emphasised para 13 of the judgment in *Royal Brompton*, where Arden LJ referred to the observations of Sullivan J (as he then was) in the *Greenpeace* case, to the effect that clear unfairness

must be shown, and that the error must show that there has been no proper consultation, and that something has gone clearly and radically wrong with the consultation process. He also referred me to the very recent decision of the Court of Appeal in *Rusal v London Metal Exchange* [2014] EWCA Civ 1271, where Arden LJ again summarised the law relating to consultation, and also stated (at paras 51–53) that the court should not ignore information which on the evidence was well known to the consultees anyway, even if not expressly referred to in the consultation document

Comment: the Court of Appeal dismissed the appeal (see below at para 3.39).

3.37 *R (Moseley) v Haringey LBC* [2014] UKSC 56

In the circumstances of this case, it had been unlawful to consult on the basis that there was no alternative, when there were alternatives

Facts: Haringey consulted on a proposal to reduce levels of council tax support, on the basis that the reductions proposed were the inevitable consequences of central government funding cuts whereas, in fact, there were realistic alternatives, including raising council tax, reducing the funding of Haringey services and using its reserves.

Judgment: the Supreme Court (Justices Hale, Kerr, Clarke, Wilson and Reed) held that, in the circumstances, Haringey's failure to alert consultees to the alternatives rendered the consultation process unfair.

Lord Wilson (with whom Lord Kerr agreed) said this:

> 23. A public authority's duty to consult those interested before taking a decision can arise in a variety of ways. Most commonly, as here, the duty is generated by statute. Not infrequently, however, it is generated by the duty cast by the common law upon a public authority to act fairly. The search for the demands of fairness in this context is often illumined by the doctrine of legitimate expectation; such was the source, for example, of its duty to consult the residents of a care home for the elderly before deciding whether to close it in *R v Devon County Council ex p Baker* [1995] 1 All ER 73. But irrespective of how the duty to consult has been generated, that same common law duty of procedural fairness will inform the manner in which the consultation should be conducted.
>
> 24. Fairness is a protean concept, not susceptible of much generalised enlargement. But its requirements in this context must be linked to the purposes of consultation. *In R (Osborn) v Parole Board* [2013] UKSC 61, [2013] 3 WLR 1020, this court addressed the common law duty of procedural fairness in the determination of a person's legal rights. Nevertheless the first two of the purposes of procedural fairness in that somewhat different context, identified by Lord Reed in paras 67 and 68 of his judgment, equally underlie the requirement that a consultation should be fair. First, the requirement 'is liable to result in better decisions, by ensuring that the decision-maker receives all relevant information and that it is properly tested' (para 67). Second, it avoids 'the sense of injustice which the person who is the subject of the decision will otherwise feel' (para 68). Such are two valuable practical consequences of fair consultation. But underlying it is also a third purpose, reflective of the democratic principle at the heart of our society. This third purpose is particularly relevant in a case like the present, in which the question was not 'Yes or no, should we close this particular care home, this particular school etc?' It was 'Required, as we are, to

make a taxation-related scheme for application to all the inhabitants of our Borough, should we make one in the terms which we here propose?'

25. In *R v Brent London Borough Council ex p Gunning* (1985) 84 LGR 168 Hodgson J quashed Brent's decision to close two schools on the ground that the manner of its prior consultation, particularly with the parents, had been unlawful. He said at p 189:

> 'Mr Sedley submits that these basic requirements are essential if the consultation process is to have a sensible content. First, that consultation must be at a time when proposals are still at a formative stage. Second, that the proposer must give sufficient reasons for any proposal to permit of intelligent consideration and response. Third,... that adequate time must be given for consideration and response and, finally, fourth, that the product of consultation must be conscientiously taken into account in finalising any statutory proposals.'

Clearly Hodgson J accepted Mr Sedley's submission. It is hard to see how any of his four suggested requirements could be rejected or indeed improved. The Court of Appeal expressly endorsed them, first in the Baker case, cited above (see pp 91 and 87), and then in *R v North and East Devon Health Authority ex p Coughlan* [2001] QB 213 at para 108. In the *Coughlan* case, which concerned the closure of a home for the disabled, the Court of Appeal, in a judgment delivered by Lord Woolf MR, elaborated at para 112:

> 'It has to be remembered that consultation is not litigation: the consulting authority is not required to publicise every submission it receives or (absent some statutory obligation) to disclose all its advice. Its obligation is to let those who have a potential interest in the subject matter know in clear terms what the proposal is and exactly why it is under positive consideration, telling them enough (which may be a good deal) to enable them to make an intelligent response. The obligation, although it may be quite onerous, goes no further than this.'

The time has come for this court also to endorse the Sedley criteria. They are, as the Court of Appeal said in *R (Royal Brompton and Harefield NHS Foundation Trust) v Joint Committee of Primary Care Trusts* [2012] EWCA Civ 472, 126 BMLR 134, at para 9, 'a prescription for fairness'.

26. Two further general points emerge from the authorities. First, the degree of specificity with which, in fairness, the public authority should conduct its consultation exercise may be influenced by the identity of those whom it is consulting. Thus, for example, local authorities who were consulted about the government's proposed designation of Stevenage as a 'new town' (*Fletcher v Minister of Town and Country Planning* [1947] 2 All ER 496 at p501) would be likely to be able to respond satisfactorily to a presentation of less specificity than would members of the public, particularly perhaps the economically disadvantaged. Second, in the words of Simon Brown LJ in the *Baker* case, at p91, 'the demands of fairness are likely to be somewhat higherwhen an authority contemplates depriving someone of an existing benefit or advantage than when the claimant is a bare applicant for a future benefit'.

27. Sometimes, particularly when statute does not limit the subject of the requisite consultation to the preferred option, fairness will require that interested persons be consulted not only upon the preferred option but also upon arguable yet discarded alternative options. For example, in *R (Medway Council and others) v Secretary of State for Transport* [2002] EWHC 2516 (Admin), [2003] JPL 583, the court held that, in consulting

about an increase in airport capacity in South East England, the government had acted unlawfully in consulting upon possible development only at Heathrow, Stansted and the Thames estuary and not also at Gatwick; and see also *R (Montpeliers and Trevors Association) v Westminster City Council* [2005] EWHC 16 (Admin), [2006] LGR 304, at para 29.

28. But, even when the subject of the requisite consultation is limited to the preferred option, fairness may nevertheless require passing reference to be made to arguable yet discarded alternative options. In *Nichol v Gateshead Metropolitan Borough Council* (1988) 87 LGR 435 Gateshead, confronted by a falling birth rate and therefore an inability to sustain a viable sixth form in all its secondary schools, decided to set up sixth form colleges instead. Local parents failed to establish that Gateshead's prior consultation had been unlawful. The Court of Appeal held that Gateshead had made clear what the other options were: see pp 455, 456 and 462. In the *Royal Brompton* case, cited above, the defendant, an advisory body, was minded to advise that only two London hospitals should provide paediatric cardiac surgical services, namely Guys and Great Ormond Street. In the Court of Appeal the Royal Brompton Hospital failed to establish that the defendant's exercise in consultation upon its prospective advice was unlawful. In its judgment delivered by Arden LJ, the court, at para 10, cited the *Gateshead* case as authority for the proposition that 'a decision-maker may properly decide to present his preferred options in the consultation document, provided it is clear what the other options are'. It held, at para 95, that the defendant had made clear to those consulted that they were at liberty to press the case for the Royal Brompton.

Lord Reed put the matter in this way:

34. I am generally in agreement with Lord Wilson, but would prefer to express my analysis of the relevant law in a way which lays less emphasis upon the common law duty to act fairly, and more upon the statutory context and purpose of the particular duty of consultation with which we are concerned.

35. The common law imposes a general duty of procedural fairness upon public authorities exercising a wide range of functions which affect the interests of individuals, but the content of that duty varies almost infinitely depending upon the circumstances. There is however no general common law duty to consult persons who may be affected by a measure before it is adopted. The reasons for the absence of such a duty were explained by Sedley LJ in *R (BAPIO Action Ltd) v Secretary of State for the Home Department* [2007] EWCA Civ 1139, [2008] ACD 20, paras 43–47. A duty of consultation will however exist in circumstances where there is a legitimate expectation of such consultation, usually arising from an interest which is held to be sufficient to found such an expectation, or from some promise or practice of consultation. The general approach of the common law is illustrated by the cases of *R v Devon County Council ex p Baker* [1995] 1 All ER 73 and *R v North and East Devon Health Authority ex p Coughlan* [2001] QB 213, cited by Lord Wilson, with which the *BAPIO* case might be contrasted.

36. This case is not concerned with a situation of that kind. It is concerned with a statutory duty of consultation. Such duties vary greatly depending on the particular provision in question, the particular context, and the purpose for which the consultation is to be carried out. The duty may, for example, arise before or after a proposal has been decided upon; it may be obligatory or may be at the discretion of the public authority; it may be restricted to particular consultees or may involve the general public; the identity of the consultees may be prescribed or may be left to the discretion of the

public authority; the consultation may take the form of seeking views in writing, or holding public meetings; and so on and so forth. The content of a duty to consult can therefore vary greatly from one statutory context to another: 'the nature and the object of consultation must be related to the circumstances which call for it' (*Port Louis Corporation v Attorney-General of Mauritius* [1965] AC 1111, 1124). A mechanistic approach to the requirements of consultation should therefore be avoided.

37. Depending on the circumstances, issues of fairness may be relevant to the explication of a duty to consult. But the present case is not in my opinion concerned with circumstances in which a duty of fairness is owed, and the problem with the consultation is not that it was 'unfair' as that term is normally used in administrative law. In the present context, the local authority is discharging an important function in relation to local government finance, which affects its residents generally. The statutory obligation is, 'before making a scheme', to consult any major precepting authority, to publish a draft scheme, and, critically, to 'consult such other persons as it considers are likely to have an interest in the operation of the scheme'. All residents of the local authority's area could reasonably be regarded as 'likely to have an interest in the operation of the scheme', and it is on that basis that Haringey proceeded.

38. Such wide-ranging consultation, in respect of the exercise of a local authority's exercise of a general power in relation to finance, is far removed in context and scope from the situations in which the common law has recognised a duty of procedural fairness. The purpose of public consultation in that context is in my opinion not to ensure procedural fairness in the treatment of persons whose legally protected interests may be adversely affected, as the common law seeks to do. The purpose of this particular statutory duty to consult must, in my opinion, be to ensure public participation in the local authority's decision-making process.

39. In order for the consultation to achieve that objective, it must fulfil certain minimum requirements. Meaningful public participation in this particular decision-making process, in a context with which the general public cannot be expected to be familiar, requires that the consultees should be provided not only with information about the draft scheme, but also with an outline of the realistic alternatives, and an indication of the main reasons for the authority's adoption of the draft scheme. That follows, in this context, from the general obligation to let consultees know 'what the proposal is and exactly why it is under positive consideration, telling them enough (which may be a good deal) to enable them to make an intelligent response': *R v North and East Devon Health Authority ex p Coughlan* [2001] QB 213, para 112, per Lord Woolf MR.

40. That is not to say that a duty to consult invariably requires the provision of information about options which have been rejected. The matter may be made clear, one way or the other, by the terms of the relevant statutory provisions, as it was in *R (Royal Brompton and Harefield NHS Foundation Trust) v Joint Committee of Primary Care Trusts* [2012] EWCA Civ 472, [2012] 126 BMLR 134. To the extent that the issue is left open by the relevant statutory provisions, the question will generally be whether, in the particular context, the provision of such information is necessary in order for the consultees to express meaningful views on the proposal. The case of *Vale of Glamorgan Council v Lord Chancellor and Secretary of State for Justice* [2011] EWHC 1532 (Admin) is an example of a case where such information was not considered necessary, having regard to the nature and purpose of that particular consultation exercise, which concerned the proposed closure of

> a specific court. In the present case, on the other hand, it is difficult to see how ordinary members of the public could express an intelligent view on the proposed scheme, so as to participate in a meaningful way in the decision-making process, unless they had an idea of how the loss of income by the local authority might otherwise be replaced or absorbed.
>
> 41. Nor does a requirement to provide information about other options mean that there must be a detailed discussion of the alternatives or of the reasons for their rejection. The consultation required in the present context is in respect of the draft scheme, not the rejected alternatives; and it is important, not least in the context of a public consultation exercise, that the consultation documents should be clear and understandable, and therefore should not be unduly complex or lengthy. Nevertheless, enough must be said about realistic alternatives, and the reasons for the local authority's preferred choice, to enable the consultees to make an intelligent response in respect of the scheme on which their views are sought.
>
> 42. As Lord Wilson has explained, those requirements were not met in this case. The consultation document presented the proposed reduction in council tax support as if it were the inevitable consequence of the Government's funding cuts, and thereby disguised the choice made by Haringey itself. It misleadingly implied that there were no possible alternatives to that choice. In reality, therefore, there was no consultation on the fundamental basis of the scheme.

Lady Hale and Lord Clark agreed with both judgments.

Comment: a slightly different approach to the existence of a consultation duty, at common law, can be found in *R (Plantagenet Alliance Ltd) v Secretary of State for Justice* [2014] EWHC 1662 (Admin) at para 98 (pre-dating *Moseley*).

3.38 *R (McCann) v Bridgend CBC* [2014] EWHC 4335 (Admin)

In this context, a duty to consult on alternatives to the decision proposed was imposed by the statutory code, rather than the common law

Facts: Ms McCann sought judicial review of Bridgend's decision to close a school without consulting adequately, including on all the alternatives to closure.

Judgment: Deputy High Court Judge Keyser allowed the application on the basis that there was a duty to consult over alternatives, but that this arose from the statutory code, rather than as a result of the fairness principle:

> 80. In my judgment, it is now clear that the defendant failed to set out in the consultation document the alternatives that had been considered and the reasons why they had been discounted. The defendant's argument at the hearing of this claim boiled down to saying that the alternatives had not been realistic or viable and therefore did not have to be identified in the consultation. In my judgment, whether or not that would be a sufficient answer in respect of consultations carried out pursuant to a common law duty or some other statutory procedure, it is not a sufficient answer under the 2013 Act and the Code. The simple requirement is to give details of 'any alternatives' that have been considered. The defendant's approach to this question seems to me to be fundamentally flawed. As I have said, apart from the '*do nothing*' option, the most obvious alternative to closing schools and opening new ones is to spend money in improving the existing schools. The documentation disclosed in the course of these proceedings

shows that the defendant clearly did give consideration, albeit at a high level of generality, to this possibility; indeed, it would have been irrational not to consider it. The defendant has formed the view that refurbishment is not a sensible option. That view may be correct, but it is not axiomatic that it is correct. The reasons why the alternative was rejected should have been stated in the consultation document. Another possible option would be to make provision on alternative sites. The defendant did not provide particulars of the alternatives it had considered; it did not even state in terms that it had considered alternative sites, and even now it is a matter of inference only that all sites considered have been identified in the course of these proceedings. Nor did the defendant even claim in the course of the statutory process that there were no other feasible or realistic options; it simply claimed that its proposal was the best option–apparently because its officers had reached that conclusion. That is not what the statutory process requires, and it undermines the clear purposes inherent in that process, because it removes from the wider public sphere the opportunity for constructive engagement with alternatives that have not been included in the proposal, and because the failure of the defendant to comply with the required discipline of clear explanation and reasoned justification of its process of reasoning is liable to compromise the intended benefits of the Code in respect of improved quality of decision-making.

3.39 *R (Michael Robson) v Salford CC* [2015] EWCA Civ 6

The consultation materials lacked clarity but overall consultees must have known what the proposal was and what the alternative were, so that the process had been fair

Facts: Salford decided to cease direct provision of transport services in order to achieve budgetary savings. In future, it would make individual transport arrangements for each eligible adult through a variety of different means, such as a 'ring and ride' service, taxis and motability vehicles. The claimants, who were both severely disabled, challenged this decision by way of judicial review.

Judgment: the Court of Appeal (Richards and Treacey LJJ, Newey J) dismissed the claimants' appeal from the decision of Deputy High Court Judge Stephen Davies. They held that the consultation had been fair in that any sensible reader of the consultation booklet would have understood that the proposal involved the withdrawal of local authority transport services from those who were assessed as able to use alternative transport arrangements so that that issue had been fairly before the consultees:

32. I have not found it easy to reach a decision on this issue. The lack of clarity in the Council's internal documentation (see eg the description of the proposal in the report to Cabinet on 11 March 2014, quoted at paragraph 9 above) seems to have been carried over into the documentation prepared for the consultation. The consultation material presented an incomplete picture by concentrating on the proposed assessment of users of the PTU services to see if alternative transport options could be used, without a clear statement that it was proposed to close the PTU itself. In consequence, Mr Wise's submission that the Council failed to consult on the closure proposal and/or that the consultation material was misleading has considerable attraction to it. In the end, however, I have reached the conclusion that that is too formalistic an analysis and that the judge was right to concentrate on

the proposed change of approach to transport arrangements for existing users and to find that the consultation process as a whole was not unfair.

33. What was important for users and their carers was not the continued existence of the PTU as such – as I have said in the context of the assessment issue, it was possible to provide the same service by other means – but the type of transport arrangements made in their case. They can have been left in no doubt that the purpose of the proposed assessments was to see if the existing service through the PTU could be replaced in each individual case by alternative arrangements. It was implicit that the PTU service would be withdrawn from those who were assessed as able to use alternative modes of transport. The reality of all this was brought home by the information that almost one half of users of the existing service were already being helped to get alternative transport to meet their needs.

34. In order to determine whether consultees were misled or were not consulted about the actual proposal, it is also necessary to have regard to the wider picture. In my view the judge was entitled to find that Mr Clemmett's witness statement was 'not sufficient to establish that those who conducted the personal visits to make the assessments were specifically tasked with making it clear to the users and their carers that the proposal *would* involve the closure of the PTU ...'. That finding did not involve the rejection of Mr Clemmett's evidence, which was unchallenged. It was simply a finding that his evidence was insufficiently detailed and specific to make good such a conclusion. Mr Clemmett's evidence taken as a whole (including the exhibited slides and media articles) does, however, provide some support for the view that consultees were aware that the proposal included closure of the PTU. The absence of any substantial evidence on behalf of the appellants that consultees were in fact misled is also highly material.

35. In *Moseley* the consultation material conveyed a positively misleading impression that other options were irrelevant. There is nothing equivalent to that in this case. In *Moseley* it was wrong to place reliance on consultees' assumed knowledge of other options for the same reason, that the message conveyed by the local authority was that other options were irrelevant. Again there is no equivalent in this case, and in my view it was open to the judge to make the finding he did that any sensible reader of the consultation booklet would have understood that the proposal involved the withdrawal of the PTU service from those who were assessed as able to use alternative transport arrangements. More generally, there is nothing in *Moseley* to cast doubt on the correctness of the legal principles by reference to which the judge directed himself in this case. The judge's conclusion on the fundamental question, that the consultation was fair, was in my view a proper one for him to reach.

3.40 *R (Forge Care Homes Ltd) v Cardiff and Vale University Health Board* [2015] EWHC 601 (Admin), (2015) 18 CCLR 39

Local Health Boards had not been under a statutory or common law duty to consult before amending their payments to care homes in respect of the tasks undertaken by registered nurses

Facts: In Wales, local health boards assessed the level of their payment for registered nursing care, in care homes, by reference to the tasks undertaken by registered nurses which only a registered nurse could perform, rather than by reference to all the tasks in fact undertaken by registered nurses, including the provision of personal care.

Judgment: Hickinbottom J held that this approach was flawed, in that the local health boards were required by section 49 of the Health and Social Care Act 2001 to pay for all the care provided by registered nurses. It was also asserted that the local health boards should have consulted and engaged in discussions. Hickinbottom J rejected that:

> 140. The nature of a public authority's duty to consult (and, in particular, the relationship between that duty and public law fairness) has recently been considered in two cases, namely by the Supreme Court in *R (Stirling) v Haringey London Borough Council* [2014] PTSR 1317, para 23 and following, per Lord Wilson JSC, and, especially, at paras 34–41 of the judgment of Lord Reed JSC with which Baroness Hale of Richmond DPSC and Lord Clarke of Stone-cum-Ebony JSC expressly agreed (at para 44), and by the Divisional Court in the proceedings concerning the remains of Richard III (*R (Plantagenet Alliance Ltd) v Secretary of State for Justice* [2015] LGR 172 (the ' Richard III case'), paras 83–98). These cases emphasise that there is no general duty on a public body to consult, that duty arising only (i) by reason of statutory provision (including, of course, that imposed in statutory guidance), and (ii) if common law fairness requires it, ie if there has been a promise or established practice to consult, or where a failure to consult would result in conspicuous unfairness. However, if and howsoever the obligation to consult arises, the full panoply of the well known *Gunning* requirements apply, ie the requirements set out by Stephen Sedley QC in *R v Brent London Borough Council ex p Gunning* (1985) 84 LGR 168, approved in that case by Hodgson J, and specifically endorsed in innumerable cases thereafter including the Court of Appeal in *R v North and East Devon Health Authority ex p Coughlan* [2001] QB 213, para 112 and the Supreme Court in the *Stirling* case [2014] PTSR 1317, para 25.
>
> 141. In this case, Mr Purchase submitted that the LHBs owed a duty to the claimants as care home providers to consult on the proposed IUM, because (i) the 2004 Circular required such consultation, and (ii) the absence of consultation resulted in conspicuous unfairness to the claimants as care home providers.
>
> 142. With regard to the 2004 Circular, he relied on the direction in para 6 requiring LHBs to 'work closely with key stakeholders', including care home providers: quoted at para 40 above. However, this does not refer to 'consultation'. A duty to consult may arise from statutory provisions that do not include the word 'consultation' (see, eg *R (Breckland District Council) v Electoral Commission Boundary Committee for England* [2009] PTSR 1611 in which the statutory scheme obliged the commission to inform persons interested of any draft proposals and take into account any representations they made). However: (i) Generally, the Welsh Ministers favour continuous engagement rather than formal consultation: see, eg, Guidance for Engagement and Consultation on Changes to Health Services issued by the Welsh Ministers, reflected to a considerable extent in the 2004 Circular. (ii) Where formal consultation is required, the statutory regime makes specific provision for it (eg section 183 of the 2006 Act requires a LHB to consult persons to whom services are provided in respect of planning and changes to those service; and regulation 27 of the Community Health Councils (Constitution, Membership and Procedures) (Wales) Regulations 2010 (SI 2010/299) (made under section 182(4) of, and Schedule 10 to, the 2006 Act) requires an LHB to consult its community health council in respect of relevant matters). In para 6 of the 2004 Circular, the Welsh Government steered clear of the concept of 'consultation'. It has to be assumed that that was deliberate.

143. The courts will be slow to add to the burden of consultation which the relevant democratically elected or otherwise accountable body has decided to impose: see, eg, the *Richard III* case [2015] LGR 172, para 98. In my judgment, although para 6 of the 2004 Circular is in the form of a direction, rather than mere guidance, it does not impose an obligation to consult. It imposes an obligation to 'work closely' together, which is a far more nebulous and ill-defined concept.

144. With regard to a common law obligation, Mr Purchase accepted that, in relation to the IUM, there was no representation or established practice that would have obliged the LHBs to consult. However, he submitted that, in all the circumstances, it was conspicuously unfair to the claimants as care home providers not to have consulted them. Those circumstances included: (i) para 45 of the 2004 Circular requires annual reviews of the FNC rate (see para 42 above). Annual reviews were avoided by tying the rate to inflation. The IUM thus departed from this guidance. However, an 'annual review' is, in my view, capable of including a review each year on the basis of pre-determined criteria. It does not necessarily require the sort of full survey performed by Laing & Buisson. However, I return to this point below. (ii) The fact that the decision has direct impact on the existing private contractual interests of the providers, affecting the price they are paid for caring for residents already in their care for a substantial period, namely five years. However, the *Stirling* case [2014] PTSR 1317 makes clear that a public authority does not have a duty to consult simply because its decision will affect private interests; and, here, the only issue is how much to pay for identified services (in respect of which the LHBs have considerable discretion). The IUM was designed merely to fix the rate at which identified services were to be provided for a fixed period. At its highest, it was to confer a commercial benefit on care home providers, not remove or derogate from a right or interest. (iii) The evidence is that the LHBs did not have adequate information to make a decision. The equality impact assessment dated 16 July 2013 suggested that there was further work to be done to understand the market and the business impact of models being considered. In para 18 of her statement dated 23 December 2014, Ms Warner accepted that the LHBs generally do not have information from the providers in respect of the differentials of nurse pay between the NHS and private market. In fact, there is evidence that the inflationary pressure on the pay of care home nurses is greater than that on NHS nurse pay: see below. However, it was for the LHBs to determine whether they did have sufficient information about such matters to enable them to make an informed decision, and their discretion as to that matter was broad. In this case, in my judgment, there is no proper basis for the contention that the LHBs were under a duty to consult properly to acquaint themselves with information concerning the private market for nurses as submitted by Mr Purchase (relying on *Secretary of State for Education and Science v Tameside Metropolitan Borough Council* [1977] AC 1014 and *R v Secretary of State for Education ex p Southwark London Borough Council* [1995] ELR 308). Furthermore, prior to these proceedings, when CFW made representations about inflation, they were not on the basis that inflationary pressures were greater in the private market than in the NHS: see, eg, the 19 June 2012 submission. In my view, the LHBs were entitled to conclude that they had sufficient information before them as to the likely inflationary pressures and that these were closely aligned to such pressures in the NHS. (iv) The decision did not take into account the fact that NHS Wales had substantially increased the number of nurses it employed, which would inevitably have had an adverse impact on care homes' ability to recruit and keep nurses at the same level of pay.

> But, again, it was for the LHBs to assess the nature of the market, and for it to determine whether it had sufficient information to make an informed decision. I am not convinced that they erred in law in deciding they had sufficient information to make such a decision. (v) Although the LHBs did not consult on the issue, they took a handful of random soundings, without full information, which compounded the sense of unfairness. Taking a random sample is of course not consultation; but I do not understand how it could compound any unfairness.
>
> 145. I am not greatly impressed by the submission on the basis of those factors. I deal with the substantive issue of whether the IUM was legally rational below; but I would have found it difficult to conclude that the claimants had suffered conspicuous unfairness by a failure to consult, on the basis of these elements alone.

Comment: the substantive issue in the case was considered in the Court of Appeal which allowed the appeal; but the Court of Appeal did not consider the consultation issue.

3.41 *R (JM and NT) v Isle of Wight Council* [2011] EWHC 2911 (Admin), (2012) 15 CCLR 167

A flawed consultation resulted in decision-makers having inadequate information about risk and consequently not have 'due regard' to the needs in the PSED

Facts: the Isle of Wight decided to change its eligibility threshold from 'Critical and Substantial' to comprise the high risk needs of persons assessed as 'Critical' and those areas of 'Substantial' needs that placed people at greatest risk of not being able to remain at home and be safe. The Isle of Wight then published a revised risk assessment tool, called 'Eligibility Review'. Two severely disabled adults sought a judicial review.

Judgment: Lang J held that the Isle of Wight's consultation had been flawed in that it failed to inform consultees about such matters as the numbers of service users whose support would be reduced, costs and savings, and what types of services would or would not be included in the new criteria. Consequently, decision-makers were deprived of important information, namely, the responses of consultees on such matters. Accordingly, the Isle of Wight had not ascertained sufficient information so as to discharge the duty of conscientious consideration, entailed by the duty to have due regard to the matters set out in the PSED.

3.42 *R (T) v Trafford MBC* [2015] EWHC 369 (Admin)

It is not always necessary to consult about alternative options

Facts: Trafford consulted on cuts to its adult social care budget, having earlier concluded, with reasons, in the context of its overall budget-setting, that it would not increase council tax or use reserves. The claimant sought a judicial review, on the basis that Trafford had failed to discharge its duty to consult about realistic alternative options.

Judgment: Stewart J dismissed the application for judicial review, holding that the main budget report made it clear that Trafford had concluded it was not realistic to increase council tax or use reserves and that, in any event, inviting the public to make alternative suggestions fairly discharged any duty to canvass alternative options:

> 36. The following can, I believe, be distilled for the present purposes from *Moseley*:
>
> (i) The inter relationship between paragraphs 27 and 28 is that *sometimes* fairness will require consultation upon discarded alternative options. Even if a consultation is statutorily required and the subject is limited to the preferred option, fairness may nevertheless require passing reference to discarded alternative options. On the facts of *Moseley* such passing reference was required. Lord Wilson approved as correct Pitchford LJ's statement that 'Consulting about a proposal does inevitably involve inviting and considering views about possible alternatives.'
>
> (ii) However, none of this undermines the opening sentence in paragraph 27 ie that it is only 'sometimes' that consultation so requires.
>
> (iii) [*Moseley* paras 37–39].
>
> > (a) In *Moseley* the statutory duty was to consult on the draft scheme. It was therefore limited to the preferred option.
> >
> > (b) A statutory duty to consult was to ensure public participation in the decision making process.
> >
> > (c) The statutory duty required, in a context with which the general public cannot be expected to be familiar, that consultees should be provided with an outline of the realistic alternatives, and an indication of the main reasons for the authority's adoption of the draft scheme.
>
> (iv) Before me there has been further debate as to whether Mostyn J in *R (L and P) v Warwickshire CC* [2015] EWHC 203 (Admin), (2015) 18 CCLR 458, paras 18–22 was correct in saying that Sullivan LJ's statement [in *R (Baird) v Environment Agency etc* [2011] EWHC 939 (Admin)] that a consultation would only be unfair as to be unlawful when something has gone 'clearly and radically wrong' survives the decision in *Moseley*. The context of that wording has to be seen in the light of what Sullivan LJ said in *Baird* which is that the test is 'whether the process is so unfair as to be unlawful.' [See also *Royal Brompton* at para 13]. It is important that the words 'clearly and radically wrong' do not indicate a 'different test, but merely (indicate) that in reality a conclusion that a consultation process has been so unfair as to be unlawful is likely to be based on a factual finding that something has gone clearly and radically wrong.' [*Baird* para 51].
>
> 37. I have come to the conclusion that in this case fairness did not require consultation upon arguable yet discarded alternative options. I say this for the following reasons:
>
> (i) I take into account the two factors in *Moseley* para 26 and I accept that there are some similarities in the statutory requirement to consult in *Moseley* and the voluntary consultation in the present case. The purpose of the voluntary consultation was to have public participation in the local authority's decision making process. Though not as clear-cut as in *Moseley*, it might be said that the context was one with which the general public may not be expected to be familiar. Nevertheless:
>
> (ii) Although the intention of the consultation was to involve the public, there was no statutory requirement to do this. Common law fairness may sometimes require consultation upon discarded alternative options. In this regard the authorities cited by Lord Wilson in *Moseley* (para 27) were *R (Medway Council and others) v Secretary of State for Transport (Medway)* [2002] EWHC 2516 (Admin) and *R (Montpeliers and Trevors Association) v Westminster City Council (Montpeliers)* [2005] EWHC 16 (Admin). It is to

be noted that both these decisions were on a single issue. In *Medway* the procedural and fairness was predicated upon a very specific basis, namely 'Knowing that the Claimant will probably and legitimately wish to advocate Gatwick as an alternative solution at a later stage in the decision making process, is it procedurally unfair of the Secretary of State to operate the consultation process in such a way that the Claimant lose their only real opportunity to present their case on Gatwick...' (para 32). In *Montpeliers* there were two consultations, one statutory and one non statutory, in relation to barriers in two London residential squares. The judge said 'Fairness required that all the various options be put to the consultees. That was never done. The same point can be put another way. The process was not fair, either in its constituent parts or overall, because some supporters of the retention of the barriers may have thought that it was not the moment to voice their views during a statutory process of making objections and likewise may have thought that there was no point in expressing views supportive of the retention of the barriers in the course of a consultation exercise which had apparently already ruled that option out of further consideration.' (para 29).

Thus the factual context in both cases was a world away from the present case, though of course these were only examples. [footnote to judgment: In *Rusal* (see below) para 40, the Court of Appeal said 'there have been exceptional cases where the courts have held that a consultation process was unfair for failure to set out alternative options'. It is not clear whether the epithet 'exceptional' survives the decision in *Moseley*.]

(iii) Further, the context of *Moseley*, though it had similarities, was different. In *Moseley*, the statutory consultation was about making people pay council tax when they were previously exempt from it. The present case involves five different consultations on differing areas of the total budget, in circumstances where there has been no (pre) determination of how and where the detailed impact of budget reductions in any particular part will fall. In this regard I also have regard to the caution endorsed by the Court of Appeal in paras 87–90 of the *Royal Brompton* case.

(iv) *Moseley* was heard on 19 June 2014 and the judgment published on 29 October 2014. The Court of Appeal heard the case of *R (United Company Rusal plc) v The London Metal Exchange* [2014] EWCA Civ 1271 on 29–30 July 2014 and published the judgment on 8 October 2014. There is nothing in *Moseley*, and in particular in paragraphs 27–28 of Lord Wilson's judgment, which detracts from para 29 of *Rusal* which provides:

> 'It is also clear from the authorities that the courts have to allow the consultant body a wide degree of discretion as to the options on which to consult: as the Divisional Court held in the *Vale of Glamorgan Council v Lord Chancellor and Secretary of State for Justice* ... at [24]:
>
> ... there is no general principle that a Minister entering into consultation must consult on all possible alternative ways in which a specific objective might arguably be capable of being achieved. It would make the process of consultation inordinately complex and time consuming if that were so....' [footnote to judgment: Permission was refused by the Supreme Court to appeal the decision in *Rusal*; see also the general statement of the Court of Appeal in *R (Robson and another) v Salford City Council* [2015] EWCA Civ 6 where Richard LJ said [22] '...the decision is largely an endorsement at Supreme Court level of principles already established at the level of the Court of Appeal...']

(v) Before presenting the proposals to the public in the way it did, the Defendant had clearly considered very carefully the alternatives of increasing council tax/using reserves. Also, information as to why these had been rejected was available to the public to some extent.

(vi) The Claimant suggests that all that was needed was something like (a) an indication that there were alternatives, (b) a rough illustration of what the alternatives might be eg increasing council tax by x%, (or less if only to mitigate the effects) and/or spending y% of unallocated reserves, (c) an account of the reasons why these had been discarded. In the circumstances of the present case, particularly given the reasoning of the Council, and the fact that this information was available and discussed during the consultation to some extent, there is a real doubt as to whether such extra steps would have made any real difference.

(vii) Overall, the Council having chosen to consult, in my judgment they were entitled lawfully to present their preferred option and to consult on the best way to achieve that.

38. All members of the Supreme Court in *Moseley* made it clear that the consultation document produced by Haringey was misleading. Lord Reed said:

> '42. As Lord Wilson has explained, those requirements were not met in this case. The consultation document presented the proposed reduction in council tax support as if it were the inevitable consequence of the Government's funding cuts, and thereby disguised the choice made by Haringey itself. It misleadingly implied that there were no possible alternatives to that choice. In reality, therefore, there was no consultation on the fundamental basis of the scheme.'

The parties are agreed that if the Defendant positively misled the public in the consultation, that would be unfair and unlawful.

> 'The Claimant alleges that the Defendant misled consultees in the present case in suggesting that there was no alternative to the cuts, relying in particular on the statement in the Social Care Information Questionnaire 'In 2015/16 Children's Services, Adult Social Care and Public Health will need to save £17.8m'. The Claimant says there was no positive suggestion anywhere in the evidence that alternatives existed to the Defendant's proposals. Rather the Defendant consulted on the erroneous basis that cuts to Adult Social Care provision must be made.
>
> I do not accept the Claimant's point. It cannot be the case that if an authority does not consult on rejected options, and only presents a preferred option for consultation, then that must be misleading. It is one thing positively to mislead as in Moseley. It is quite another for the Council, in all the circumstances of the case, to have and to put forward, after careful and detailed consideration, a point of view that circumstances dictated that it was not realistic to increase council tax or to use reserves and therefore to focus the consultation on savings in services.'

3.43 *R (L and P) v Warwickshire CC* [2015] EWHC 203 (Admin), (2015) 18 CCLR 458

Consultation was not required prior to making the annual budget and, in any event, the application for judicial review was out of time. A consultation process will only be unlawful because of unfairness where 'something has gone clearly and radically wrong'

Facts: judicial review was sought on the basis that Warwickshire had failed lawfully to consult on budgetary reductions affecting services for disabled children.

Judgment: Mostyn J dismissed the application, holding that Warwickshire had not been under a common law duty to undertake consultation before fixing its annual budget because (i) it had not promised to consult, (ii) it had not created an established practice of consultation and (iii) the failure to consult did not lead to conspicuous unfairness. In any event, the date of the relevant decision was the date of the full council meeting that approved the budget and the application for judicial review was out of time. In addition, Mostyn J held that the *'clearly and radically wrong'* test survives the *Moseley* decision:

> 18. So these are the principles to be applied in working out whether a duty to consult arises or not. Let us assume that it does. The next question is how it should be carried out. Plainly the answer is that the consultation must be carried out fairly. In *R (Baird) v Environment Agency and Arun District Council* [2011] EWHC 939 (Admin), at paras [50]–[51] Sullivan LJ stated that a consultation will only be so unfair as to be unlawful when something has gone 'clearly and radically wrong'. This strong test was affirmed in *R (Royal Brompton and Harefield NHS Foundation Trust) v Joint Committee of Primary Care Trusts* [2012] EWCA Civ 472, 126 BMLR 134 by Arden LJ at para [13].
>
> 19. There has been a debate before me whether this remains the test following the recent decision of the Supreme Court in *R (Moseley) v Haringey London Borough Council* [2014] UKSC 56, [2014] 1 WLR 3947, which was a case concerning a statutory consultation on the implementation in Haringey of a council tax reduction scheme in the light of the withdrawal by the government of the council tax benefit scheme and the passing on of its operation (with less money) to local authorities. It was said that the consultation was unfair because it in effect applied Henry Ford's prescription about the Model T: 'any customer can have a car painted any color that he wants so long as it is black'. Haringey only consulted on its sole proposal, which was to pass on the cut, and did not set out any alternatives (such as keeping it at the old level and paying for it by cutting other services or by increasing council tax).
>
> 20. At para [27] Lord Wilson stated that 'fairness will require that interested persons be consulted not only upon the preferred option but also upon arguable yet discarded alternative options'. As I read his judgment he did not seek to alter the high test propounded by Sullivan LJ for a case where the duty was imposed at common law. Rather, to my mind, he applied it as the consultation there had gone clearly and radically wrong by presenting the people with Henry Ford's single choice alone. Nor do I read Lord Reed's judgment as altering that high test. He expressed his analysis of the relevant law in a way which 'lays less emphasis upon the common law duty to act fairly, and more upon the statutory context and purpose of the particular duty of consultation with which we are concerned' (para [34]). At paras [37] and [38] he stated:
>
>> '[37] Depending on the circumstances, issues of fairness may be relevant to the explication of a duty to consult. But the present case is not in my opinion concerned with circumstances in which a duty of fairness is owed, and the problem with the consultation is not that it was 'unfair' as that term is normally used in administrative law. In the present context, the local authority is discharging an important function in relation to local government finance, which affects its residents generally. The statutory obligation is, 'before making a scheme', to consult any major precepting authority, to publish a draft scheme, and, critically, to

'consult such other persons as it considers are likely to have an interest in the operation of the scheme'. All residents of the local authority's area could reasonably be regarded as 'likely to have an interest in the operation of the scheme', and it is on that basis that Haringey proceeded.

[38] Such wide-ranging consultation, in respect of the exercise of a local authority's exercise of a general power in relation to finance, is far removed in context and scope from the situations in which the common law has recognised a duty of procedural fairness. The purpose of public consultation in that context is in my opinion not to ensure procedural fairness in the treatment of persons whose legally protected interests may be adversely affected, as the common law seeks to do. The purpose of this particular statutory duty to consult must, in my opinion, be to ensure public participation in the local authority's decision-making process.'

21. Therefore, Lord Reed was saying that for this particular statutory consultation the legislative intention was that the people should in a meaningful way 'participate' in the decision-making process. That is a distance away from what the common law is doing when it imposes a duty to consult. Rather, it is imposing a requirement that the decision-making process is fair not that the consultees should (at least up to a point) actually be decision-makers as well.

22. My view is supported by the decision of Richards LJ in *R (Robson) v Salford City Council* [2015] EWCA Civ 6 (20 January 2015) where he stated at para [22] that 'in fact the decision in Moseley is largely an endorsement at Supreme Court level of principles already established at the level of the Court of Appeal ...'. Plainly he thought that the high test of Sullivan LJ was still applicable where the common law had imposed the duty.

3.44 *R (Morris) v Rhondda Cynon Taf CBC* [2015] EWHC 1403 (Admin), (2015) 18 CCLR 550

Fairness did not always require consultation on alternatives and, where it did, the duty applied to realistic alternatives only

Facts: Rhondda decided to cease funding full-time nursery education for three-year-olds, for budgetary reasons. The claimants sought a judicial review, submitting that Rhondda's consultation had been inadequate, in that Rhondda had failed to provide consultees with fair and accurate information about the proposal and had failed to invite views on possible alternatives. They also submitted that the decision would result in Rhondda failing to discharge its duty under section 22 of the Children Act 2006, to secure sufficient childcare for working parents.

Judgment: Patterson J dismissed the application for judicial review holding that the consultation did invite comment on the only two realistic alternatives, which was sufficiently fair; and that the duty at section 22 of the Children Act 2006 was a strategic duty which permitted local authorities to take into account their resources. Patterson J reviewed the authorities on consultation:

Discussion and conclusions

62. In my judgment the case of *Moseley*, as has been said, generally states the previous principles on consultation. That means that once a consultation has been embarked upon for it to be fair it has to:

i) let those with a potential interest in the subject matter know clearly what the proposal of the public authority is;
ii) explain why the proposal is under positive consideration;
iii) give the consultees sufficient information so that they can make an informed response to the proposal under consideration;
iv) allow sufficient time for those consultees to be able to submit their informed response;
v) conscientiously consider the product of the consultation and take that into account when reaching and taking the final decision.

63. As *R (Royal Brompton and Harefield NHS Foundation Trust) v Joint Committee of Primary Care Trust* [2012] EWCA Civ 472 makes clear at [10]:

> 'Another aspect of fairness is that it must present the available information fairly. In this case, because the JCPCT had to collect information from the centres to present the available information it would have to make clear to the centres what information it needed. A further aspect of fairness lies in the presentation of the information on which the views of consultees should be sought. The options for change must be fairly presented. Nonetheless, a decision-maker may properly decide to present his preferred options in the consultation document, provided it is clear what the other options are: *Nichol v Gateshead Metropolitan Borough Council* (1988) 87 LGR 435.'

As part of presenting information in a clear way, the decision maker may present his preferred option. Part of the available information to be presented to the public may be alternative options for change. What is an alternative option will depend on the factual and context specific circumstances of the consultation in question.

64. The case of *Robson* [2015] EWCA Civ 6 concerned a consultation exercise by Salford City Council to close its passenger transport unit which provided a transport service for disabled adults between their homes and adult day centres and to make alternative transport arrangements. The closure formed part of a package of cost cutting measures and was budgeted to save £600,000 a year. The consultation exercise was criticised on the basis that the information contained in the consultation booklet was materially misleading, that it presented an incomplete picture by concentrating on the users of the passenger transport unit service to see if alternative transport options could be used. The Court of Appeal found that what was important was the type of transport arrangements made in the case of service users. To do that regard had to be had for the wider picture. When that was done there had been no significant misleading of the consultees which was the case in *Moseley*.

65. The case of *R (L and P) v Warwickshire CC* [2015] EWHC 203 (Admin), (2015) 18 CCLR 458 confirms the political nature of budgetary considerations and how a court has to be cautious about trespassing over the line which is the boundary of a democratically made decision. The case before Mostyn J involved cuts to be made to the integrated disability service which would be implemented when its 'local offer' to set out social care services was approved. Mostyn J found that the case did not come remotely close to conspicuous unfairness amounting to an abuse of power. It was a case where the budget was regularly and constitutionally set by a local authority in the present climate of austerity. All democratic procedures and safeguards were followed. That ground of challenge failed on the basis of delay but, had he considered the merits, Mostyn J said that he would have found firmly against the consultation exercise being unfair.

66. The case of *T* (supra) was a challenge to budget cuts made to Trafford's adult social care budget which, it was contended, directly affected the claimant who had a diagnosis of autism and learning disabilities, was extremely vulnerable and would be at risk should any of his support be reduced. The issue was whether the defendant was under a common law duty to include information about realistic alternative options in its consultation on the proposed cuts to adult social care. Stewart J emphasised at [32(iv)] and [32(v)] in commenting on the decision in *Moseley*:

> '(iv) (paragraph 27) 'Sometimes, particularly when statute does not limit the subject of the requisite consultation to the preferred option, fairness will require that interested persons be consulted not only upon the preferred option but also upon arguable yet discarded alternative options.'
>
> (v) (paragraph 28) 'But, even when the subject of the requisite consultation is limited to the preferred option, fairness may nevertheless require passing reference to be made to arguable yet discarded alternative options.' He then refers in support of this to two authorities, one of which is the *Royal Brompton* case.'

67. In the circumstances of the case before him Stewart J concluded that fairness did not require consultation on arguable but discounted alternative options. Where there was an intention to have public participation in the decision making process and its context was one with which the public may not be familiar fairness can sometimes require that a consulting body consult upon possible alternative ways in which a specific objective might be capable of being met but that was not a general principle. The defendant had considered carefully increasing council tax and using Council reserves and there was information available to some extent as to why that was rejected. There was a real doubt in the case before Stewart J that an indication of alternatives, what they might be and why they had been discarded would have made any real difference. The Local Authority was entitled to consult on its preferred option and the best way to achieve that but was not under any duty to do more.

68. After the decision in M*oseley* it is clear that the issue of fairness in a consultation exercise is very context specific. The three cases that the claimant refers to illustrate that point. The case of T is the most similar to that before me but given that all judgments have turned on their factual context I cannot derive any universal principle or principles of application that assist here. That being the case I turn to the application of the law to the facts in the specific consultation exercise carried out.

3.45 *R (Sumpter) v Secretary of State for Work and Pensions* [2015] EWCA Civ 1033

A consultation process is fair if, ultimately, consultees can be expected to have understood the issues and the relevant factors

Facts: Mr S sought a judicial review of the Secretary of State for Work and Pensions's decision to replace disability living allowance with the personal independence payment (PIP), on the basis that the consultation process had been unfair and unlawful, in that (1) the Secretary of State for Work and Pensions had not made it clear that he intended to reduce the threshold condition for enhanced mobility PIP to an inability to walk more than 20 metres and had prejudged that issue, and (2) it had not been made clear that re-allocation of resources from physically impaired claimants, to non-physically impaired claimants, meant that the PIP criteria were significantly more restrictive than the higher rate disability living allowance (DLA) mobility criteria, which would cause substantial numbers of claimants to lose their entitlement.

Judgment: the Court of Appeal (Patten, McCombe and Gloster LJJ) held that overall the consultation process had been fair and, in that the Secretary of State for Work and Pensions had ultimately made his proposals clear and he had not prejudged any issues, and in that it should have been obvious from the Secretary of State for Work and Pensions's impact tables that 280,000 fewer people were predicted to receive enhanced rate mobility under the PIP, compared with those on DLA higher rate mobility. McCombe LJ said this on behalf of the Court of Appeal:

> 49. The applicable law was not seriously in issue, either before the judge or before us. Before Hickinbottom J the principles were uncontroversial and he set them out in the passage of the judgment to which I have referred. Equally, before us, while both parties said that the starting point on the law relating to challenges to public authority consultations is now to be found in the Supreme Court decision in *R (Moseley) v Haringey LBC* [2014] 1 WLR 3497 (decided after the judge gave his judgment) both acknowledged that in *R (Robson) v Salford City Council* [2015] EWCA Civ 6 at [22], Richards LJ said that the decision in Moseley was largely an endorsement by the Supreme Court of principles already established in this court and was an illustration of the application of those principles.
>
> 50. The overriding principle is that consultations must be 'fair', an easy concept to state, but sometimes rather less easy to apply in practice. The application of the duty is 'intensely case-sensitive' (per Arden LJ in *R (United Company Rusal PLC) v The London Metal Exchange* [2014] EWCA Civ 1271 at [28], a case in which (as we were told) the Supreme Court, since Moseley, has refused permission to appeal to that court.

3.46 *R (Tilley) v Vale of Glamorgan Council* [2015] EWHC 3194 (Admin)

It was not unfair to fail to consult on an alternative that was not realistic and signposting consultees to additional information had been, on the facts, fair

Facts: Vale of Glamorgan decided, in principle, to close libraries, unless it was possible to develop community-led libraries.

Judgment: Elisabeth Laing J held that it had not been unfair of the Vale of Glamorgan not to consult on the possible alternative option, of making financial savings by reducing library opening hours, or to draw attention to the disadvantages of community-led libraries because (i) reduced library opening hours was not, on the facts, a realistic alternative that could produce the necessary savings; (ii) sufficient information had been given about the proposals to permit an informed response, including a signpost to a review which referred to the disadvantages of community-led libraries; and (iii) in any event, in relation to both complaints, the consultation document included a box for additional comments, which could have been utilised to make either complaint.

3.47 *R (Keep Wythenshawe Special Limited) v NHS Central Manchester Clinical Commissioning Group* [2016] EWHC 17 (Admin), (2016) 19 CCLR 19

In assessing whether consultation was lawful, it is relevant to take into account the particular role that consultation is playing in the decision-making process

Facts: campaigners challenged changes to acute hospital care, claiming that the consultation process had been flawed, that it had been unlawful not to re-consult (given that the decision ultimately adopted diverged from the consultation proposals and that the ultimate decisions had been irrational).

Judgment: Dove J held that the consultation process had been lawful, the failure to re-consult had been lawful and the resulting decision rational. He drew attention to a particular factor, relevant to assessing the standard of fairness to be expected from a consultation process, and in particular relevant to whether a failure to re-consult was lawful, as follows:

> 71. Firstly, the role that the consultation is playing in the decision-making process must be considered. At one end of the spectrum a consultation could perform the function of a referendum, or an exercise in direct democracy, determining the decision for the public body through a popular vote. At the other end of the spectrum the purpose of the consultation may be simply to elicit views about a proposal to which regard will be had as an influence on the decision but which (even if it produced an overwhelming majority of opinion opposed to the authority's proposal) could not be binding upon the authority. Another dimension is that in some circumstances the consultation may be taking place in the context of a staged decision-making process and may be part of a sequence of consultations to be undertaken during that process. The requirements of fairness will be shaped by the needs of the stage that the decision-taking has reached and the recognition that there will be further consultation and further decisions to be made later in the process. The role that the consultation will play in the decision-making process will be an influence upon the requirements of fairness in terms, for instance, of the nature and extent of the information necessary for the consultation to be considered fair, and also the manner in which the outcome of the consultation is considered when the decision is reached.

CHAPTER 4

Guidance

continued

4.27 *R (Forest Care Home Limited) v Pembrokeshire CC* [2010] EWHC 3514 Admin, (2011) 14 CCLR 103

The greater the deviation from statutory guidance, the more compelling the justification must be

4.28 *R (Mohammed Mohsan Ali) v Newham LBC* [2012] EWHC 2970 (Admin), (2012) 15 CCLR 715

Cogent reasons were required for departing from non-statutory but national, expert guidance

4.29 *R (Torbay Quality Care Forum Ltd) v Torbay Council* [2014] EWHC 4321 (Admin)

A simple disagreement with non-statutory guidance did not amount to a good enough reason for diverging from it

4.30 *R (KM) v Northamptonshire CC* [2015] EWHC 482 (Admin)

It could be appropriate to construe a local authority's policy as 'fleshed out' by statutory guidance, but not where there was inconsistency between the two

Introduction and principles

4.1 Directions and guidance are a means by which central government exercises control over the implementation of legislation in order to promote consistency (but also flexibility, where local considerations justify divergence from guidance), accountability and the maintenance of high standards. Local authorities may publish guidance to their own officers, and the public, for similar reasons.

4.2 Public authorities may be required to follow directions, or to 'act under' guidance or take guidance into account, by legislation[1] or the common law.[2] At common law, guidance may be a relevant consideration it would be irrational to disregard.[3]

4.3 When local authorities publish their own guidance or policy, as to how they will exercise a broad statutory discretion, it is usually implicit in the legislation that they will not entirely fetter their discretion, so as to preclude them considering an exceptional case on its merits; however, legislation that entitles an authority to promulgate rules may be construed as entitling it to promulgate bright line rules.[4]

4.4 Lawful guidance can be an essential element in securing the coherent, transparent and consistent performance of administrative discretions[5] but its precise effect depends on all the circumstances, including in particular the statutory context.

4.5 If guidance or policy is sufficiently clear (and, generally, its meaning is a question for the court, in which the *Wednesbury* principle plays no part[6]), it usually gives rise to a legal obligation, recently expressed as 'a requirement of good administration', that it will be followed by the authority that has published the guidance, at least until the guidance or policy changes.[7]

4.6 It is in general unnecessary for the guidance to include an express proviso that the public authority will, ultimately, consider each case on its merits, it being generally implicit that a public authority will apply a policy expressed in absolute or unqualified terms in a manner that does not fetter its discretion.[8] It will not usually be unlawful to deviate from unlawful guidance and, in addition, guidance may be quashed insofar as it

1 See, for example, section 7 of the Local Authority Social Services Act 1970 and section 78 of the Care Act 2014.

2 *Mandalia v Secretary of State for the Home Department* [2015] UKSC 59, [2015] 1 WLR 4546 at para 31.

3 *R (Coglan) v Chief Constable of Greater Manchester Police* [2004] EWHC 2801 (Admin) at paras 46–48.

4 *R (Hillsden) v Epping DC* [2015] EWHC 98 (Admin) at paras 27–39.

5 *R (Alconbury Developments Ltd) v Secretary of State for the Environment, Transport, and the Regions* [2001] UKHL 23, [2003] 2 AC 295 at para 143; *R(Lumba) Secretary of State for the Home Department* [2011] UKSC 12, [2012] 1 AC 245 at para 34.

6 *Mandalia v Secretary of State for the Home Department* [2015] UKSC 59, [2015] 1 WLR 4546 at para 31.

7 *Mandalia v Secretary of State for the Home Department* [2015] UKSC 59, [2015] 1 WLR 4546 at paras 29–31.

8 *R (West Berkshire DC) v Secretary of State for Communities and Local Government* [2016] EWCA Civ 441, [2016] PTSR 982 at para 21.

is unlawful (for example, if it is ultra vires relevant legislation or incompatible with the European Convention on Human Rights (ECHR)).[9]

4.7 A person affected by an administrative policy is not for that reason alone entitled to be consulted before the public authority changes its policy but he or she may be entitled to be consulted, as a result of legislation, guidance or the common law: see chapter 3 above on Consultation.

4.8 Directions are mandatory, unless they are *ultra vires*, whereas public authorities may diverge from guidance, if they have a sufficiently cogent reason.[10]

4.9 Whether a reason for a public authority diverging from guidance is sufficiently cogent is a context sensitive and evaluative question, that depends on:

- the terms of the legislation (eg whether it imposes a duty to 'act under', or simply to have regard to, the guidance);[11] and
- all the circumstances of the case, in particular the extent to which the guidance is expert, well-reasoned and intended to be normative.[12]

4.10 A cogent reason is usually exceptional circumstances or local factors not contemplated by the guidance.

4.11 The decision of a public authority will usually be unlawful if, in breach of legislation or the common law, it disregards intra vires guidance, including by:[13]

- misunderstanding it (the proper construction of policy generally being a hard-edged question for the court[14]); or by
- acting differently than advised by the guidance simply because the public authority disagrees with it (rather than because of genuine exceptional circumstances or special local factors not contemplated by the guidance).

4.12 However, a public authority may sometimes be able to justify its divergence from guidance by reference to reasons advanced by it in litigation, rather than considered contemporaneously.[15]

4.13 The Senior Courts Act 1981 now provides, at section 31(2A), that the High Court must refuse to grant relief 'if it appears to the court to be highly likely that the outcome for the applicant would not have been substantially different if the conduct complained of had not occurred', unless there is an 'exceptional public interest' in granting relief. Section 31(3C) imposes

9 *R (A) v Secretary of State for Health* [2009] EWCA Civ 225, [2010] 1 WLR 279 at para 78; *Gillick v West Norfolk and Wisbech Area Health Authority* [1985] UKHL 7, [1986] AC 112; *R (West Berkshire DC) v Secretary of State for Communities and Local Government* [2016] EWCA Civ 441, [2016] PTSR 982 at para 22.

10 *R v North Derbyshire Health Authority ex p Fisher* (1997–8) 1 CCLR 150, QBD at 155G–K.

11 *R v Islington LBC ex p Rixon* (1997–8) 1 CCLR 119, QBD at 123F–K.

12 *R (Mohammed Mohsan Ali) v Newham LBC* [2012] EWHC 2970 (Admin), (2012) 15 CCLR 715 at paras 39–41.

13 *R v North Derbyshire Health Authority ex p Fisher* (1997–8) 1 CCLR 150, QBD at 155G–K and at 165J–166B.

14 *Mandalia v Secretary of State for the Home Department* [2015] UKSC 59, [2015] 1 WLR 4546 at para 31.

15 *R (X) v Tower Hamlets LBC* [2013] EWCA Civ 904 at para 38.

a similar restriction on the grant of permission to apply for judicial review. It remains to be seen[16] how the court will approach this restriction on its traditional function but the provision is potentially relevant in cases where the claimant submits that a decision is unlawful owing to the local authority's failure to take into account guidance, or act under statutory guidance.

Statutory basis of adult social care guidance

4.14 The basis for statutory guidance relating to adult social care is primarily section 78 of the Care Act 2014, which provides, inter alia, that 'A local authority must act under the general guidance of the Secretary of State in the exercise of functions given to it by this Part or by regulations under this Part' (section 78(1)).

4.15 The current statutory guidance under the Care Act 2014 is the *Care and Support Statutory Guidance.*[17]

4.16 In addition, the Department of Health has published non-statutory guidance, also known as departmental guidance, including *Care Act Factsheets.*[18]

4.17 More widely, section 7 of the Local Authority Social Services Act (LASSA) 1970 remains in force, making provision in relation to directions and guidance as follows:

> **Local authorities to exercise social services functions under guidance of Secretary of State.**
>
> 7(1) Local authorities shall, in the exercise of their social services functions, including the exercise of any discretion conferred by any relevant enactment, act under the general guidance of the Secretary of State.
>
> (1A) Section 78 of the Care Act 2014 applies instead of this section in relation to functions given by Part 1 of that Act or by regulations under that Part.

16 The Bingham Centre for the Rule of Law, the Public Law Project and Justice have suggested that this duty will only arise exceptionally: *Judicial Review and the Rule of Law: An Introduction to the Criminal Justice and Courts Act 2015, Part 4* at www.biicl.org/documents/767_judicial_review_and_the_rule_of_law_-_final_for_web_19_oct_2015.pdf. However, in *R (Hawke) v Secretary of State for Justice* [2015] EWHC 3599 (Admin), as a result of section 31(2A) of the Senior Courts Act 1981 Holman J declined to grant a declaration that the SSJ was in breach of the PSED (under section 149 of the Equality Act 2010); instead, he indicated that his judgment was a 'declaratory judgment', following the example of Blake J in *Logan v Havering LBC* [2015] EWHC 3193 (Admin). See also *R (Enfield LBC) v Secretary of State for Transport* [2015] EWHC 3758 (Admin) at para 106 (sometimes a witness statement is required from the public authority to establish that the test is met) and *R (HA) v The Governing Body of Hampstead School* [2016] EWHC 278 (Admin) at para 33 (these provisions may relate simply to 'technical flaws'). In *R (DAT) v West Berkshire Council* [2016] EWHC 1876 (Admin), (2016) 19 CCLR 362, Laing J found it hard to be satisfied that there was no chance of the council reaching a different decision on a reconsideration in case involving highly vulnerable children and, in any event, considered that in such a case there was an exceptional public interest in granting relief.

17 Department of Health, Updated 24 March 2016.

18 www.gov.uk/government/publications/care-act–2014-part–1-factsheets/care-act-factsheets-–2).

Directions by the Secretary of State as to exercise of social services functions

7A(1) Without prejudice to section 7 of this Act, every local authority shall exercise their social services functions in accordance with such directions as may be given to them under this section by the Secretary of State.

(2) Directions under this section
(a) shall be given in writing; and
(b) may be given to a particular authority, or to authorities of a particular class, or to authorities generally.

4.18 The expression 'social services functions' is defined for the purposes of LASSA 1970 s7 as all those functions set out in Schedule 1 to LASSA 1970, which include functions relating to adults and, also, to children under, inter alia, the Children Act 1989 and the Children Act 2004.

In Wales, codes of practice and statutory guidance have been issued under sections 145 and 169 of the Social Services and Well-being (Wales) Act 2014.[19]

Cases

4.19 *R v North Yorkshire CC ex p William Hargreaves* (1997–8) 1 CCLR 104, QBD

An assessment that failed to take into account the service user's preferences, incompatibly with the statutory guidance, was unlawful

Facts: a dispute arose between Mr Hargreaves and North Yorkshire as to what form suitable respite care ought to take for Mr Hargreaves' intellectually impaired sister, Beryl Hargreaves. North Yorkshire had experienced great difficulty in communicating with Ms Hargreaves, exacerbated by Mr Hargreaves' overly protective actions. However, Ms Hargeaves had demonstrated an ability to express preferences and there was some evidence that her preferences were not identical to her brother's.

Judgment: paragraphs 3.15 and 3.25 of the statutory guidance at the time, 'The Policy Guidance', required local authorities to involve the individual service user in the assessment process and take account of their preferences. At 112H, Dyson J held that:

> ... the Respondent made its decision without taking into account the preferences of Miss Hargreaves on the issue in question. It must follow that the decision was unlawful in the sense that it was made in breach of paragraphs 3.16 and 3.25 of the Policy Guidance.

Comment: no doubt, had it been impossible or impracticable to ascertain Ms Hargreaves' preferences, North Yorkshire's failure to do so would have been lawful because it would have had a cogent reason for departure from the statutory guidance.

19 These are collated at http://gov.wales/topics/health/socialcare/act/code-of-practice/?lang=en.

4.20 **R v Islington LBC ex p Rixon (1997–8) 1 CCLR 119, QBD**

A local authority acts unlawfully if it fails to comply in substance with statutory guidance issued under section 7 of the Local Authority Social Services Act 1970, or fails to take into account non-statutory/departmental guidance

Facts: the applicant was a severely mentally and physically disabled 24-year-old man, whose mother considered that inadequate provision had resulted in him losing skills acquired at his special needs school and failing to develop his full potential. It was common ground that Islington's assessment and care plan failed to address comprehensively the applicant's needs and failed to comply with relevant central government guidance.

Judgment: Sedley J held that Islington had acted unlawfully in failing to 'act under' statutory guidance and in failing properly to take into account non-statutory guidance:

> This section, therefore, creates a positive duty to arrange for recreational and 'gateway' educational facilities for disabled persons. It is, counsel agree, a duty owed to the individual and not simply a target duty. I will come later to the question of its legal ambit and content. It introduces in turn section 7(1) of the Local Authority Social Services Act 1970:
>
> > *Local authorities shall, in the exercise of their social services functions, including the exercise of any discretion conferred by any relevant enactment, act under the general guidance of the Secretary of State.*
>
> (By an amendment introduced into the statute, section 7A *requires* local authorities to exercise their social services functions in accordance with any such *directions* as may be given to them by the Secretary of State.)
>
> What is the meaning and effect of the obligation to 'act under the general guidance of the Secretary of State'? Clearly guidance is less than direction, and the word 'general' emphasises the non-prescriptive nature of what is envisaged. Mr McCarthy, for the local authority, submits that such guidance is no more than one of the many factors to which the local authority is to have regard. Miss Richards submits that, in order to give effect to the words 'shall ... act', a local authority must follow such guidance unless it has and can articulate a good reason for departing from it. In my judgment Parliament in enacting section 7(1) did not intend local authorities to whom ministerial guidance was given to be free, having considered it, to take it or leave it. Such a construction would put this kind of statutory guidance on a par with the many forms of non-statutory guidance issued by departments of state. While guidance and direction are semantically and legally different things, and while 'guidance does not compel any particular decision' (*Laker Airways Ltd v Department of Trade* [1967] QB 643, 714 per Roskill LJ), especially when prefaced by the word 'general', in my view Parliament by section 7(1) has required local authorities to follow the path charted by the Secretary of State's guidance, with liberty to deviate from it where the local authority judges on admissible grounds that there is good reason to do so, but without freedom to take a substantially different course.
>
> ...
>
> A failure to comply with the statutory policy guidance is unlawful and can be corrected by means of judicial review: *R v North Yorkshire County Council ex p Hargreaves* (1997) 1 CCLR 104 (Dyson J, 30 September 1994). Beyond this, there will always be a variety of factors which the local authority is required on basic public law principles to take into account. Prominent among these will be any recommendations made in the particular case by a

review panel: *R v Avon County Council ex p M* [1994] 2 FLR 1006 (Henry J). In contradistinction to statutory policy guidance, a failure to comply with a review panel's recommendations is not by itself a breach of the law; but the greater the departure, the greater the need for cogent articulated reasons if the court is not to infer that the panel's recommendations have been overlooked.

A second source of considerations which manifestly must be taken into account in coming to a decision is the practice guidance issued by the Department of Health. This currently takes the form of a Practitioners' Guide entitled 'Care Management and Assessment', which sets out 'a set of principles' derived from 'current views of practice'. The guidance breaks care management down into a series of stages, moving through communication and assessment to assembly of a care plan, and then on to the implementation, monitoring and periodic review of the plan. An element critical to the present case, step 4, is described thus:

> 'The next step is to consider the resources available from statutory, voluntary, private or community sources that best meet the individual's requirements. The role of the practitioner is to assist the user in making choices from these resources, and to put together an individual care plan.'

...

The care plan, as Mr McCarthy readily admits, does not comply either with the policy guidance or the practice guidance issued by central government. There has been a failure to comply with the guidance contained in paragraph 3.24 of the policy document to the effect that following assessment of need, the objectives of social services intervention as well as the services to be provided or arranged should be agreed in the form of a care plan. For the reasons which I have given, if this statutory guidance is to be departed from it must be with good reason, articulated in the course of some identifiable decision-making process even if not in the care plan itself. In the absence of any such considered decision, the deviation from the statutory guidance is in my judgment a breach of the law; and so *a fortiori* is the reduction of the Flexiteam service from 3 hours as originally agreed, whatever the activity, to 3 hours swimming or 1 hours at home. I cannot accept Mr McCarthy's submission that the universal knowledge that no day centre care was available for Jonathan was so plainly the backdrop of the section 2 decision that there was no need to say so. It is one thing for it to have been a backdrop in the sense of a relevant factor, but another for it to have been treated as an immoveable object. The want of any visible consideration of it disables the respondent from showing that it was taken into account in the way spelt out in the *Gloucestershire* case. I do, however, accept Mr McCarthy's submission that Miss Richards' further contention that the respondent has failed to consider alternatives to day centre care for Jonathan comes so late that there has been no opportunity to file evidence about it. Further, the whole situation in relation to day centre provision is about to change, making this element marginal save perhaps by way of fallback.

The care plan also fails at a number of points to comply with the practice guidance on, for example, the contents of a care plan, the specification of its objectives, the achievement of agreement on implementation on all those involved, leeway for contingencies and the identification and feeding back of assessed but still unmet need. While such guidance lacks the status accorded by section 7 of [Local Authority Social Services Act 1970], it is, as I have said, something to which regard must be had in carrying out the statutory functions. While the occasional lacuna would not furnish evidence of

> such a disregard, the series of lacunae which I have mentioned does, in my view, suggest that the statutory guidance has been overlooked.
>
> In such a situation I am unable to accede to Mr McCarthy's submission that the failures to follow the policy guidance and practice guidance are beyond the purview of the court. What he can, I think, legitimately complain of is the fact that both of these submissions, in their present formulation, have emerged for the first time in the presentation of the applicant's case in court and were not adumbrated earlier. While he has not suggested that the lateness of the points has prevented material evidence from being placed before the court, Mr McCarthy may be entitled to rely on it in resisting any consequential relief, and I will hear him in due course on this.

Comment: this is a generally, although not universally, accepted statement of the legal consequences of failing to 'act under' statutory guidance, or properly take into account non-statutory guidance. Sedley J's decision turned on the language of section 7(1) of the Local Authority Social Services Act 1970; but section 78 of the Care Act 2014 contains the same duty, to 'act under the general guidance of the Secretary of State'; and there continues to be relevant non-statutory guidance. So this decision should have continued relevance.

Perhaps more questionable is whether there is such a great difference in the approach to statutory and non-statutory guidance as Sedley J indicates, or whether there is a continuum which recognises that a statutory duty to 'act under' guidance tends to require an especially good reason for any departure, but that each set of guidance is to some extent different in what it requires by way of response. It may be that even a substantial departure from statutory guidance can, in principle, be justified by a sufficiently cogent reason; whereas it may be very difficult to justify a local departure from some non-statutory guidance, expertly formulated and intended to have a normative effect across England and Wales.

4.21 *R v North Derbyshire Health Authority ex p Fisher* (1997–8) 1 CCLR 150, QBD

Acting contrary to guidance because of a simple disagreement with the guidance is tantamount to failing to take it into account

Facts: North Derbyshire adopted practices which, on analysis, were designed to defer making additional funding available for the prescription of Beta-Interferon (for the treatment of Multiple Sclerosis), despite the fact that the NHS executive had issued guidance advising all NHS purchasing bodies to do so.

Judgment: Dyson J held:

> In my judgment Mr Elvin and Mr Seys Llewellyn are right. If the Circular provided no more than guidance, albeit in strong terms, then the only duty placed upon health authorities would be to take it into account in the discharge of their functions. They would be susceptible to challenge only on *Wednesbury* principles if they failed to consider the Circular, or they misconstrued or misapplied it whether deliberately or negligently: see *Grandsden & Co Ltd and Another v Secretary of State for the Environment and Another* (1985) 54 P&CR 86, 93–94.
>
> ...

> Mr Seys Llewellyn emphasised two points. First the respondents were under a statutory duty not to overspend: see section 97(1)(a) of the 1977 Act and the Department of Health Circular HC(91)25. Secondly, clinical decisions must always be taken with due regard to the resources available: see, for example, *R v Cambridge Health Authority* [1995] 1 WLR 898. I unreservedly accept both propositions as correct. But on the facts of this case, they do not assist the respondents. The respondents had funds available, but chose not to allocate them. As for clinical decisions, they were not for the respondents to take, and it is no part of the applicant's case to suggest that they were.
>
> I conclude therefore that the policy was unlawful because it was not a proper application of the guidance contained in the Circular, and the respondents did not properly take into account the essential requirements of the Circular in adopting and maintaining their policy. In my judgment, the respondents were aware from an early stage that they were not properly applying or taking account of the Circular. They knew that their own policy amounted to a blanket ban on Beta-Interferon treatment. A blanket ban was the very antithesis of national policy, the aim of which was to target the drug appropriately at patients who were most likely to benefit from treatment. They knew from as early as 12 January 1996 that, if there was no imminent prospect of a trial, it might be difficult to 'hold the line'. Most revealingly of all, the note of the meeting of that date spoke about the possibility of 'creative constraints'. This is surprising language to find in the context of health care.
>
> What they had in mind at this early stage was using the possibility of a trial as a creative means of avoiding the implementation of national policy. The reason was plainly that the respondents disagreed with that policy. I fear that 'creative' is a euphemism for 'disingenuous'. The prospect of a trial served its purpose as a creative constraint until that prospect disappeared. Thereafter the respondents resorted to other unacceptable and inconsistent excuses in seeking to hold the line, and hang on to their unsustainable position. My conclusion on this issue, based on the reasons that I have given, is sufficient to dispose of this application, subject to questions of relief.

4.22 *R v Sutton LBC ex p Tucker* (1997–8) 1 CCLR 251, QBD

In failing to undertake long-term planning the local authority had acted inconsistently with the statutory guidance and therefore unlawfully

Facts: the applicant's daughter, who was severely disabled and experienced substantial communication difficulties, had remained in hospital for two years after she was ready to be discharged, because of Sutton's failure to complete an assessment and care plan that addressed its long-term obligations so as to enable her discharge.

Judgment: Hidden J accepted the applicant's submission that Sutton had acted unlawfully by failing to 'act under' statutory guidance:

> Mr Gordon submitted that Sutton had acted unlawfully in having no lawful care plan which would show exactly the points of disagreement between Mrs Tucker and Sutton which would identify unmet need and would set out clearly the objectives for Therese and the criteria for meeting such objectives. Had there been such a care plan the efforts or lack of efforts of the Local Authority would have been transparent. Again I find Mr Gordon is right in his criticisms of the document which is put forward as a care

> plan in that, as he correctly submits, there are no stated overall objectives in terms of long term obligations, carers' obligations or service providers, there is no criteria for the measurement of objectives because the objectives themselves are not recorded in any care plan.

Hidden J declined to exercise his discretion to refuse relief on the basis that the family had had an alternative remedy through the statutory complaints procedure:

> As to whether I should in my discretion refuse relief on the basis of any alternate remedy, I find there is here a discrete point of law to be decided as to whether or not the respondent has acted unlawfully in failing to make a service provision decision under section 47(1)(b) of the National Health Service and Community Care Act 1990. That decision involves consideration of the statutory guidance issued under section 7 of the Local Authority Social Services Act 1970 and the non-statutory guidance as well. In particular it requires consideration of paragraphs 3.24 and 3.41 of the statutory policy guidance. In that situation I hold that the applicant is not precluded from making this application for judicial review by the availability of any other remedy such as the complaints procedure under section 7B of LASSA or the default powers under section 7D. I have to consider in relation to available remedies or avenues of redress, as they were referred to by Simon Brown LJ in *R v Devon County Council ex p Baker*, the question of which avenue is the more convenient, expeditious and effective. I am quite satisfied that judicial review is here the avenue to be preferred on those bases. I do not consider the default powers to be an alternative remedy where there is a discrete point of law (see *ex parte S*). If the matter were to go by the complaints procedure under section 7A Mrs Tucker as a non-legally aided person would be forced to argue points of law before a non-qualified body. That could not be convenient, expeditious or effective. There is, in fact, no true alternative remedy. The position might be otherwise if the case were founded simply on *Wednesbury* irrationality or if it were a Children Act case (see *ex parte T* at pages 814F and 815C). I am further satisfied that there is here a clear failure to follow the guidance given in paragraphs 3.24 and 3.41 of the policy guidance which is clearly binding on local authorities and the respondent in particular. The respondent had discharged its duty under section 47(1)(a) of the 1990 Act to carry out an assessment of the applicant's needs by 13th April 1994. I find that the respondent is in clear breach of its duty under section 47(1)(b) in that it has still not made the decision which is called for by that section. There is still no service provision decision. Equally there is no care plan, as Mr Eccles accepts, in that there is still no provision for Therese's long term placement and therefore for her discharge from National Health Service care.

Comment: section 72 of the Care Act 2014 will introduce a system of appeals. Consultation on that system closed on the 30 March 2015.[20] It can be expected that judicial review will be permitted only very exceptionally, in cases that fall within the appeal system. Otherwise, Hidden J's approach will continue to be relevant, although there are a number of other decisions that offer a different slant on the 'alternative remedy' issue.[21]

20 *Care Act 2014: Consultation on draft regulations and guidance to implement the cap on care costs and policy proposals for a new appeals system for care and support*: www.gov.uk/government/uploads/system/uploads/attachment_data/file/400757/2903104_Care_Act_Consultation_Accessible_All.pdf.

21 *R (Cowl) v Plymouth CC* [2001] EWCA Civ 1935, (2002) 2 CCLR 42 and *R (F, J, S, R) v Wirral BC* [2009] EWHC 1626 (Admin), (2009) 12 CCLR 452. See also para 7.97 below.

4.23 *R v Secretary of State for Health ex p Pfizer Limited* (1999) 2 CCLR 270, QBD

Central government guidance was ultra vires

Facts: Concerned about a potential drain on NHS resources, the Secretary of State promulgated Circular No 1998/158, which advised doctors not to prescribe Viagra 'other than in exceptional circumstances', cleared in advance with the Standing Medical Advisory Committee.

Judgment: Collins J held that the purpose of the Circular was to cause GPs to act contrary to their professional obligation to give their patients such treatment as they considered to be necessary and appropriate, and contrary to their duty of care under paragraph 12 of Schedule 2 to the National Health Service (General Medical Services) Regulations 1992;[22] therefore, it was unlawful. Viagra was manufactured in France and the Circular was also in breach of Article 7 of Directive 89/105/EC, insofar as it amounted to a restriction on the use of a medicinal product which was not accompanied by 'reasons based on objective and verifiable criteria'.

Comment: while local authorities must 'act under' statutory guidance and take into account non-statutory guidance, their primary obligation of course is to act as required by legislation. If guidance is ultra vires legislation, local authorities must act consistently with the legislation, not the guidance, which can, itself, be challenged by way of judicial review and quashed.

4.24 *R v Birmingham CC ex p Killigrew* (2000) 3 CCLR 109, QBD

An assessment that failed to consider up-to-date medical evidence and the views of the GP and carers, incompatibly with the statutory guidance, was unlawful

Facts: Birmingham had provided the claimant with 12 hours' care each day, in the light of her severe disability. It then moved the claimant to better adapted accommodation and reduced her hours of care to three and a half hours during weekdays, with some additional care over the weekend. The decision was unreasoned. After the issue of a judicial review, Birmingham undertook an assessment, which concluded that the hours should be increased to six hours each day, and which gave as its reason that, under the existing arrangements, little direct care was provided for most of the day.

Judgment: Hooper J held that it was notable that the reduction in the hours of care coincided with a decision that two carers rather than one needed to be provided, to comply with manual handling requirements, and that it was important that the reduction in hours was not driven by the economic consequences of that decision. In any event, Birmingham's assessment was unlawful for two reasons: (1) it contained no proper analysis of why 12 hours care had been provided, why that was no longer necessary and what would be done if an emergency arose, (2) in breach of the statutory guidance, Birmingham had failed to take into account up-to-date medical evidence and the views of the GP and the claimant's carers.

22 SI No 635.

4.25 *R v Merton, Sutton and Wandsworth Health Authority ex p Perry, Andrew and Harman* (2000) 3 CCLR 378, QBD

The decision to close a long-stay hospital for learning disabled adults was unlawful because of a failure first of all to assess the needs of residents, as advised by non-statutory guidance

Facts: the health authority decided to close Orchard Hill, a long-stay hospital for people with profound learning disabilities, on economic grounds, despite having promised residents a 'home for life'.

Judgment: Jackson J held that the health authority's decision-making process was unlawful for two reasons: (1) it failed to take into account its promises of a 'home for life' (notwithstanding the failure of consultees to raise this matter), (2) inconsistently with the non-statutory guidance, on page 2 of *HSG (92)42*, it had failed to undertake individual assessments of the residents' future care needs.

4.26 *R (Munjaz) v Mersey Care NHS Trust* [2005] UKHL 58

The status of the Mental Health Act 1983 Code of Practice was such that any divergence from it would be unlawful, unless it was undertaken with great care and for cogent reasons

Facts: Mr Munjaz complained that his seclusion, whilst a psychiatric patient at a high security mental hospital, was unlawful in that the hospital's policy departed from the Mental Health Act 1983 Code of Practice and in that it was incompatible with the ECHR.

Judgment: the House of Lords (Lords Bingham, Steyn, Hope, Scott and Brown) held that a hospital should only depart from the Code with great care and for cogent reasons, but that was the case here:

> 21. It is in my view plain that the Code does not have the binding effect which a statutory provision or a statutory instrument would have. It is what it purports to be, guidance and not instruction. But the matters relied on by Mr Munjaz show that the guidance should be given great weight. It is not instruction, but it is much more than mere advice which an addressee is free to follow or not as it chooses. It is guidance which any hospital should consider with great care, and from which it should depart only if it has cogent reasons for doing so. Where, which is not this case, the guidance addresses a matter covered by section 118(2), any departure would call for even stronger reasons. In reviewing any challenge to a departure from the Code, the court should scrutinise the reasons given by the hospital for departure with the intensity which the importance and sensitivity of the subject matter requires. [Lord Bingham of Cornhill]

Further, properly operated, the hospital's policy would prevent any possible breach of rights under Articles 3, 5 or 8 ECHR.

4.27 *R (Forest Care Home Limited) v Pembrokeshire CC* [2010] EWHC 3514 (Admin), (2011) 14 CCLR 103

The greater the deviation from statutory guidance, the more compelling the justification must be

Facts: Forest Care Home Limited challenged Pembrokeshire's methodology for assessing the cost of providing care accommodation locally, the fact that it took into account its own limited resources and the steps it took to prevent Forest Care Home Limited seeking a contribution from residents.

Judgment: Hickinbottom J allowed the application for judicial review, making these observations in relation to the relevant guidance:

> 28. By section 7 of the Local Authority Social Services Act 1970, in performing its functions, the Council must 'act under' the general guidance of the relevant Minister or, in respect of a devolved function, the Welsh Ministers. Following guidance is not mandatory: but an authority can only depart from it for good reason. If it deviates from guidance without a considered and cogently-reasoned decision, it acts unlawfully and in a manner which is amenable to judicial review *(R v London Borough of Islington ex p Rixon* (1997–98) 1 CCLR 119, especially at page 71; and *R (Munjaz) v Mersey Care National Health Service Trust* [2005] UKHL 58, especially per Lord Bingham at paragraph 21 and per Lord Hope at paras 68 to 69). Sedley J (as he then was) encapsulated the proper approach to guidance in *Rixon* as follows:
>
> > '... [W]hile 'guidance' does not compel any particular decision..., especially when prefaced by the word 'general', in my view Parliament by section 7(1) has required authorities to follow the path charted by the Secretary of State's guidance, with liberty to deviate from it where the local authority judges on admissible grounds that there is good reason to do so ...'
>
> With that I respectfully agree.
>
> 29. The learned judge went on to insert a restriction on the authority's ability to deviate from the guidance, namely: '... but without the freedom to take a substantially different course'. I hesitate to do anything but agree with that too, because of the eminence of (now) Sedley LJ as an administrative lawyer and the fact that the point is not going to be determinative in this claim: but it seems to me, as a matter of principle, Parliament has given the relevant decision-making power to the local authority and, despite the terms of section 7 of the 1970 Act, it would be open to an authority to depart even substantially from guidance if it had sufficiently compelling grounds for so doing. However, certainly, the more the proposed deviation from guidance, the more compelling must be the grounds for departure from it.

4.28 *R (Mohammed Mohsan Ali) v Newham LBC* [2012] EWHC 2970 (Admin), (2012) 15 CCLR 715

Cogent reasons were required for departing from non-statutory but national, expert guidance

Facts: Newham decided to provide tactile paving in its area (to assist visually impaired persons), but in accordance with standards and specifications that fell short of those recommended in non-statutory guidance issued by the Department of Transport.

Judgment: Kenneth Parker J held that the national guidance was the product of a highly expert analysis, was issued against the background of the equality duty and was set out in imperative terms, owing to the long-term need to achieve an acceptable level of uniformity and consistency throughout localities: in all the circumstances, Newham had not had sufficiently good reasons to depart from this guidance.

Comment: a good example illustrating that court decisions in this area are context sensitive. Although the guidance in this case was not statutory, it was intrinsically so persuasive and so clearly intended to be normative that only cogent reasons justified a departure from it.

4.29 *R (Torbay Quality Care Forum Ltd) v Torbay Council* [2014] EWHC 4321 (Admin)

A simple disagreement with non-statutory guidance did not amount to a good enough reason for diverging from it

Facts: the Forum brought a challenge to the level of care home fees that Torbay determined it would pay.

Judgment: Deputy High Court Judge Lambert allowed the application for judicial review on the basis that the mathematical adopted by Torbay had been irrational and because Torbay had no justification for departing from the advice in the non-statutory guidance to disregard third party contributions when assessing the usual cost of care – it had simply disagreed with that advice:

> 60. *R (Bevan and Clarke) v Neath* [2012] LGR 728 contains the sage lesson that although amenable to judicial review decisions in relation to the particular statutory duty here involved are generally to be left to the decision maker and the decision maker alone is to decide on the manner and intensity of the inquiry to be undertaken into any relevant factor. The second lesson is that the weight to be given to a relevant factor is for the decision maker and not for the court in the absence of irrationality. This approach is endorsed by the Court of Appeal in *R (Members of the Committee of Care North East Northumberland) v Northumberland County Council* (2014) 17 CCLR 117 where it is stressed that the Circular contains guidance and is not to be equated with a statutory duty and as would be expected in a case of guidance it does not prescribe any particular methodology which local authorities must adopt in order to have due regard to the actual costs of providing care. When considering the force of a submission that a local authority has taken either insufficient steps to equip itself with relevant information or has generated incorrect information for itself it is plainly important to remember as was stressed by the Court of Appeal that provided some inquiry into the relevant factor to which due regard has to be paid is made by the decision maker then 'it is generally for the decision maker to decide on the manner and intensity of the inquiry to be undertaken into the relevant factor': see per Beatson J in *R (Bevan and Clarke LLP) v Neath Port Talbot CBC* (2012) 15 CCLR 294 at paragraph 56. Previous decisions in different statutory contexts will not support the need for any particular form of analysis in the current situation. Some authorities will produce an arithmetical calculation; others may look at a number of comparables. I accept, of course, from *Northumberland* that carrying out an arithmetical calculation is but one way of having 'due regard for the actual cost of providing care' but is not the only legally permissible way. The extent to which judges in other cases have been prepared to delve in great detail into the facts is something which I approach with great caution in this case. The paradigm notion I have adopted is that of Beatson J in *Bevan and Clarke* as endorsed by Sullivan LJ and Aikens LJ in their specific comments in

Northumberland. Borrowing further from *Bevan and Clarke* I remind myself that in judicial review the court will be particularly circumspect in engaging with the conclusions of the primary decision maker in relation to complex economic and technical questions. The normal setting of fee rates is a matter involving economic and financial assessment and a degree of expertise in how this sector operates. There is also a judgment to be made about the proper allocation of scarce resources: see Supperstone J in *R (Care North East) v Northumberland* (2013) 16 CCLR 276 at paragraph 58. It seems to me that this is the type of case where traditional judicial review principles in relation to administrative decisions must be honoured scrupulously. It is not the type of case where the boundaries of judicial review should be rolled back at all, particularly not by a judge at first instance. In the course of assessing the facts in this case I have tried very hard to reach a conclusion which would allow me to say that the intensity of the inquiry here being dealt with by the decision maker was a matter for them and that I should leave well alone. With regret for the consequences, but with no real hesitation as to the principle I must honour I consider that the Claimant's first ground is well made out. If the decision maker treads the path of economic modelling then it seems to me it cannot proceed with a model that is significantly flawed. I was careful to take into account the fact that one person's flawed mathematical model might be another person's best estimate. I took heavily into account the fact that the intensity and nature of the inquiry which is required of the local authority is primarily a matter for the decision maker. But if the local authority chooses to adopt a mathematical model some scrutiny of this is available on general public law principles. Those principles require, it seems to me, that wherever possible the merits of the decision remain with the decision maker. But here the merits of the decision are so fundamentally flawed by adopting the unnecessary weighting which no-one can explain as being necessary that the decision to employ this falls fairly and squarely within the scope of judicial review as being a decision which no reasonable decision taker properly directing themselves on the facts could take. In the end no matter what epithet is used to describe the decision, whether it not adding up or being beyond the bounds of logic or all reasonableness the decision does, it seems to me, fall within that narrow band of decisions which can properly be the subject of judicial review. The deployment of the weighted average makes no sense in the first place and has no reasonable application in the model. There may, perhaps, have been some explanation for this but there is none which I can now scrutinise. The presence of an inexplicable weighting within the mathematical model shows it to be a matter of fact which no reasonable decision taker could properly take into account.

4.30 *R (KM) v Northamptonshire CC* [2015] EWHC 482 (Admin)

It could be appropriate to construe a local authority's policy as 'fleshed out' by statutory guidance, but not where there was inconsistency between the two

Facts: Mr KM sought a judicial review of aspects of Northamptonshire's charging policy relating to home care services.

Judgment: Gilbart J held that he was prepared to read Northamptonshire's charging policy as fleshed out by the statutory guidance but that could not be done, in this case, because Northamptonshire's policy was inconsistent with the statutory guidance.

CHAPTER 5

The public sector equality duty

continued

5.47 *R (Domb) v Hammersmith & Fulham LBC* [2009] EWCA Civ 941

The local authority had acted lawfully by providing decision-makers with an impact assessment and information about their duties under the disability equality duty and related legislation, and giving careful consideration to the objections of disabled persons and the potential adverse impacts upon them, notwithstanding a failure to include reference to gender and race issues in the formal report, since the impact assessment rationally concluded that there was no significant risk of adverse consequences in those regards

5.48 *R (JL) v Islington LBC* [2009] EWHC 458 (Admin), (2009) 12 CCLR 322

The local authority had not discharged the disability equality duty because there was no audit trail or other documentation demonstrating a proper approach

5.49 *Pieretti v Enfield LBC* [2010] EWCA Civ 1104, (2010) 13 CCLR 650

The disability equality duty applied to all local authority functions, including under sections 184 and 202 of the Housing Act 1996

5.50 *R (W) v Birmingham CC* [2011] EWHC 1147 (Admin), (2011) 14 CCLR 516

A generalised consideration of the likely impact, without any real assessment of the practical effect of what appeared to be a significant restriction of eligibility for care services, resulted in a local authority failing to have 'due regard' to the needs identified in the PSED

5.51 *R (McDonald) v Kensington & Chelsea RLBC* [2011] UKSC 33, (2011) 14 CCLR 341

It had been unnecessary explicitly to refer to the disability equality duty when undertaking a community care assessment and it could not be inferred that the disability equality duty had been disregarded

5.52 *Barnsley MBC v Norton* [2011] EWCA Civ 834, (2011) 14 CCLR 617

It was a breach of the disability equality duty to fail to consider the needs of a disabled occupier before evicting her

5.53 *JG and MB v Lancashire CC* [2011] EWHC 2295 (Admin), (2011) 14 CCLR 629

It was legitimate to make a macro budgetary decision, likely to adversely affect disabled persons, on the basis that the council was not committed to any specific initiative until consultation and compliance with the PSED had been undertaken

5.54 *R (Rajput) v Waltham Forest LBC, R (Tiller) v East Sussex CC* [2011] EWCA Civ 1577, (2012) 15 CCLR 147

Where the potential impact of changes to service provision on elderly and disabled individuals was obvious, as was the justification (a budgetary saving) and decision-makers had been advised of their duty under the disability equality duty and the factual background, and plainly understood them, their balancing of risks and benefits discharged their duty under the disability equality duty, notwithstanding any express reference to the legislation

5.55 *R (JM and NT) v Isle of Wight Council* [2011] EWHC 2911 (Admin), (2012) 15 CCLR 167

A flawed consultation resulted in decision-makers having inadequate information about risk and consequently not have 'due regard' to the needs in the PSED

5.56 *R (D, S) v Manchester CC* [2012] EWHC 17 (Admin), (2012) 15 CCLR 603

While the local authority had not undertaken a formal impact assessment, in substance it had discharged the PSED

5.57 *R (South West Care Homes Ltd) v Devon CC* [2012] EWHC 2967 (Admin)

The PSED was breached by a failure to consider measures of mitigation and of the proper management of risk

5.58 *R (D) v Worcestershire CC* [2013] EWHC 2490 (Admin), (2013) 16 CCLR 323

Notwithstanding shortcomings in the equality impact assessment and an absence of qualitative and quantative data, decision-makers were informed of the risks and mitigating measures and had in substance discharged the PSED

5.59 *R (Bracking) v Secretary of State for Work and Pensions* [2013] EWCA Civ 1345, (2013) 16 CCLR 479

Owing to a failure to draw the Minister's attention to the possible adverse consequences for disabled persons, and her legal duties under the PSED, the PSED had been breached

5.60 *R (T) v Sheffield CC* [2013] EWHC 2953 QB, (2013) 16 CCLR 580

Too fine a level of analysis risks descending into an impermissible appeal of the merits

5.61 *R (Michael Robson) v Salford CC* [2014] EWHC 3481 (Admin), (2014) 17 CCLR 474

Some parts of the assessment were not as detailed and rigorous as they could have been but in the round the PSED was discharged

5.62 *R (Aspinall and others) v Secretary of State for Work and Pensions* [2014] EWHC 4134 (Admin)

The Secretary of State had clearly demonstrated an awareness of the potential adverse effect on disabled people, of closing the Independent Living Fund and the application for judicial review was a misconceived attempt to persuade the court to engage in micro-management

5.63 *R (MA) v Secretary of State for Work and Pensions* [2014] EWCA Civ 13, [2014] PTSR 584

The Secretary of State had had regard to the risks to disabled persons and budgetary considerations, he was aware of his legal duties and had, in substance, discharged the PSED

5.64 *R (Michael Robson) v Salford CC* [2015] EWCA Civ 6

Notwithstanding imperfections in its approach, viewed more widely, the evidence may show that a local authority had had proper regard to the PSED

5.65 *R (Tilley) v Vale of Glamorgan Council* [2015] EWHC 3194 (Admin)

A failure to discharge the PSED was immaterial in the context of a decision that would not require any particular service being terminated

5.66 *R (Mark Logan) v Havering LBC* [2015] EWHC 3193 (Admin)

The only relief granted would be declaratory, in a case where a lawful EIA had been drawn to the attention of some, but not all, councillors, when the Council reached a decision in full council

5.67 *R (Hawke) v Secretary of State for Justice* [2015] EWHC 3599 (Admin)

Where section 31(2A) of the Senior Courts Act 1981 applies the court may not grant a declaration but it may furnish the parties with a 'declaratory judgment'

5.68 *R (DAT) v West Berkshire Council* [2016] EWHC 1876 (Admin), (2016) 19 CCLR 362

A budgetary decision was unlawful because the report to members failed to set out or accurately summarise the PSED but, otherwise, the material before members was lawful

Introduction

5.1 The statutory machinery is considered in detail below. The core provision is section 149 of the Equality Act 2010 which creates the public sector equality duty (PSED). The key provision is section 149(1):

> **Public sector equality duty**
>
> **149**(1) A public authority must, in the exercise of its functions, have due regard to the need to–
>
> (a) eliminate discrimination, harassment, victimisation and any other conduct that is prohibited by or under this Act;
>
> (b) advance equality of opportunity between persons who share a relevant protected characteristic and persons who do not share it;
>
> (c) foster good relations between persons who share a relevant protected characteristic and persons who do not share it.

5.2 The aim of the PSED is to promote equality, by eliminating conduct such as discrimination and by promoting equality of opportunity and good relations between persons who share a 'relevant protected characteristic' and persons who do not.

5.3 In the context of health and social care, the effect of the PSED is that, whenever they formulate policy, or make decisions in individual cases, public authority decision-makers must have due regard to the need to advance the equality of opportunity of disabled, elderly, young and otherwise vulnerable service users and to promote good relations between them and others. This imposes a positive duty to have due regard to the need to provide services that will place service users on a level footing with those who do not share their 'relevant protected characteristic'.

5.4 In an age of seemingly constant change, at the policy and individual level, largely driven by budgetary considerations, a particular effect of the PSED is to require decision-makers carefully to assess the risks that may arise from a proposed change, how they can be mitigated, what monitoring should take place and whether those risks can be justified, having due regard to the need to advance equality of opportunity between vulnerable service users and others. It is this aspect of the PSED that the case-law has focussed on, thus far.

5.5 Accordingly (although the court will uphold decision-making which '*in substance*' integrates the core considerations underlying the PSED into its decision-making), local authorities and health bodies should:[1]

- advise decision-makers in writing of all the facets of the statutory duty in section 149 of the Equality Act 2010 (see para 5.14 below);
- ensure that the reports provided to decision-makers include a robust, critical assessment of the potential risks, as well as information about the mitigating steps proposed, alternative options, plans for monitoring and further decision-making if risks do materialise and the justification for the course proposed;
- advise decision-makers in writing that they are under a personal duty to discharge the PSED. Usually, this involves considering any equality impact assessment (EIA) in full, the responses to any consultation

1 *R (Bracking) v Secretary of State for Work and Pensions* [2013] EWCA Civ 1345, (2013) 16 CCLR 479 at para 25.

exercise and the information referred to in the preceding bullet points, in the light of the PSED;
- advise decision-makers in writing that they have to decide whether, treating the objectives in the PSED as important considerations, what is proposed is justifiable, or whether the plan should be modified or even abandoned.

5.6 None of this means that local authorities and health bodies cannot make budget cuts, or take other decisions that are adverse to, or do not fully promote, the interests of vulnerable persons who possess a 'relevant protected characteristic', but the PSED operates as a restraining influence, or ever-present conscience. And, whilst the PSED is an obligation of process rather than end result, the process, diligently undertaken, should result in modified or even reversed outcomes in some cases.

5.7 In principle, the PSED applies to decision-making in individual cases. That can make a real difference in other contexts beyond adult social care, where the needs of persons susceptible to inequality are not so well catered for within the relevant statutory machinery itself. In the social care context, however, case-law indicates that a social worker, and even a policy maker, may comply with the PSED simply by undertaking assessment and care planning that complies with the legislation and relevant guidance, on the basis that this already, in substance, incorporates the PSED.[2] That logic may apply now with greater force, given the over-arching duty in section 1 of the Care Act 2014 to promote every individual's well-being, and the detailed provision for assessing and meeting needs in the Care Act 2014, the statutory instruments made under it and the *Care and Support Statutory Guidance*, which have, themselves, been through a detailed impact assessment process.[3]

5.8 Much of the case-law relating to the PSED process has been summarised recently by McCombe LJ on behalf of the Court of Appeal in *R (Bracking) v Secretary of State for Work and Pensions*[4] as follows:

> 25. Two lever arch files of authorities were placed before the court which included some thirteen cases in which relevant duties and the requirements placed on public authorities have been considered. Fortunately the principles were not significantly in dispute between the parties. I summarise the points identified, which are not, I think, different in substance from those summarised by the Judge in paragraph 32 of his judgment.
>
> 26.(1) As stated by Arden LJ in *R (Elias) v Secretary of State for Defence* [2006] 1 WLR 3213; [2006] EWCA Civ 1293 at [274], equality duties are an integral and important part of the mechanisms for ensuring the fulfilment of the aims of anti-discrimination legislation.
>
> (2) An important evidential element in the demonstration of the discharge of the duty is the recording of the steps taken by the decision maker in seeking to meet the statutory requirements: *R (BAPIO Action Ltd) v Secretary of State for the Home Department* [2007] EWHC 199 (QB) (Stanley Burnton J (as he then was)).

2 *R (McDonald) v Kensington & Chelsea RLBC* [2011] UKSC 33, (2011) 14 CCLR 341; *R (AM) v Birmingham CC* [2009] EWHC 688 (Admin), (2009) 12 CCLR 407; *R (Rajput) v Waltham Forest LBC* [2011] EWCA Civ 1577, (2012) 15 CCLR 147.

3 www.legislation.gov.uk/ukia/2014/407/pdfs/ukia_20140407_en.pdf.

4 [2013] EWCA Civ 1345, (2013) 16 CCLR 479.

(3) The relevant duty is upon the Minister or other decision maker personally. What matters is what he or she took into account and what he or she knew. Thus, the Minister or decision maker cannot be taken to know what his or her officials know or what may have been in the minds of officials in proffering their advice: *R (National Association of Health Stores) v Department of Health* [2005] EWCA Civ 154 at [26–27] per Sedley LJ.

(4) A Minister must assess the risk and extent of any adverse impact and the ways in which such risk may be eliminated before the adoption of a proposed policy and not merely as a 'rearguard action', following a concluded decision: per Moses LJ, sitting as a Judge of the Administrative Court, in *Kaur & Shah v LB Ealing* [2008] EWHC 2062 (Admin) at [23–24].

(5) These and other points were reviewed by Aikens LJ, giving the judgment of the Divisional Court, in *R (Brown) v Secretary of State for Work and Pensions* [2008] EWHC 3158 (Admin), as follows:

i) The public authority decision maker must be aware of the duty to have 'due regard' to the relevant matters;
ii) The duty must be fulfilled before and at the time when a particular policy is being considered;
iii) The duty must be 'exercised in substance, with rigour, and with an open mind'. It is not a question of 'ticking boxes'; while there is no duty to make express reference to the regard paid to the relevant duty, reference to it and to the relevant criteria reduces the scope for argument;
iv) The duty is non-delegable; and
v) Is a continuing one.
vi) It is good practice for a decision maker to keep records demonstrating consideration of the duty.

(6) '[G]eneral regard to issues of equality is not the same as having specific regard, by way of conscious approach to the statutory criteria.' (per Davis J (as he then was) in *R (Meany) v Harlow DC* [2009] EWHC 559 (Admin) at [84], approved in this court in *R (Bailey) v Brent LBC* [2011] EWCA Civ 1586 at [74–75].)

(7) Officials reporting to or advising Ministers/other public authority decision makers, on matters material to the discharge of the duty, must not merely tell the Minister/decision maker what he/she wants to hear but they have to be 'rigorous in both enquiring and reporting to them': *R (Domb) v Hammersmith & Fulham LBC* [2009] EWCA Civ 941 at [79] per Sedley LJ.

(8) Finally, and with respect, it is I think, helpful to recall passages from the judgment of my Lord, Elias LJ, in *R (Hurley & Moore) v Secretary of State for Business, Innovation and Skills* [2012] EWHC 201 (Admin) (Divisional Court) as follows:

(i) At paragraphs [77–78]

'[77] Contrary to a submission advanced by Ms Mountfield, I do not accept that this means that it is for the court to determine whether appropriate weight has been given to the duty. Provided the court is satisfied that there has been a rigorous consideration of the duty, so that there is a proper appreciation of the potential impact of the decision on equality objectives and the desirability of promoting them, then as Dyson LJ in *Baker* (para [34]) made clear, it is for the decision maker to decide how much weight should be given to the various factors informing the decision.

[78] The concept of 'due regard' requires the court to ensure that there has been a proper and conscientious focus on the statutory criteria, but if that is done, the court cannot interfere with the decision simply because it would have given greater weight to the equality implications

of the decision than did the decision maker. In short, the decision maker must be clear precisely what the equality implications are when he puts them in the balance, and he must recognise the desirability of achieving them, but ultimately it is for him to decide what weight they should be given in the light of all relevant factors. If Ms Mountfield's submissions on this point were correct, it would allow unelected judges to review on substantive merits grounds almost all aspects of public decision making.'

(ii) At paragraphs [89–90]

'[89] It is also alleged that the PSED in this case involves a duty of inquiry. The submission is that the combination of the principles in *Secretary of State for Education and Science v Tameside Metropolitan Borough Council* [1977] AC 1014 and the duty of due regard under the statute requires public authorities to be properly informed before taking a decision. If the relevant material is not available, there will be a duty to acquire it and this will frequently mean than some further consultation with appropriate groups is required. Ms Mountfield referred to the following passage from the judgment of Aikens LJ in Brown (para [85]):

> '... the public authority concerned will, in our view, have to have due regard to the need to take steps to gather relevant information in order that it can properly take steps to take into account disabled persons' disabilities in the context of the particular function under consideration.'

[90] I respectfully agree ...'

...

60. In the end, drawing together the principles and the rival arguments, it seems to me that the 2010 Act imposes a heavy burden upon public authorities in discharging the PSED and in ensuring that there is evidence available, if necessary, to demonstrate that discharge. It seems to have been the intention of Parliament that these considerations of equality of opportunity (where they arise) are now to be placed at the centre of formulation of policy by all public authorities, side by side with all other pressing circumstances of whatever magnitude.

5.9 Laing J has added a gloss to paragraph 60 of *Bracking* as follows:[5]

39. In paragraph 60 of *Bracking* McCombe LJ said, 'In the end, drawing together the principles and the rival arguments, it seems to me that section 149 imposes a heavy burden on public authorities, in discharging the PSED and in ensuring that there is the evidence available, if necessary, to demonstrate their discharge. It seems to me to have been the intention of Parliament that these considerations of equality of opportunity (where they arise) are now to be placed at the centre of formulation of policy by all public authorities, side by side with all other pressing circumstances of whatever magnitude'.

40. Paragraph 60 of *Bracking* recognises that there may be circumstances in which the evidence it refers to is not necessary, and that there may be circumstances in which considerations of equality do not arise. These are important provisos. Nonetheless, it seems to me, also, that if and in so far as paragraph 60 suggests that public authorities must give equal weight to equality considerations and to other 'pressing circumstances of whatever magnitude' it is not supported by the language of section 149, and is

5 In *R (DAT) v West Berkshire Council* [2016] EWHC 1876 (Admin), (2016) 19 CCLR 362.

inconsistent both with the passage from *Hurley* which is cited with apparent approval in paragraph 26(8) of *Bracking*, and with *Baker*. I consider, therefore, that paragraph 60 of *Bracking* cannot have been intended to have that effect.

5.10 It is also notable that at para 89 of *R (Staff Side of the Police Negotiating Board) v Secretary of State for Work and Pensions*,[6] Elias LJ, McCombe J and Sales J concluded that, where the Secretary of State had not personally considered the PSED, it was sufficient that her department had done so, when making the recommendation that she had accepted.

5.11 As the cases show:

- whether or not there has been a breach of the PSED is a highly fact-specific, evaluative question. The principles are important; excessive citation of authority is deprecated;[7]
- an unduly forensic analysis may distract from asking whether in substance the PSED has been discharged and may in some cases amount to an inappropriate attack on the merits of the underlying decision;[8]
- in some contexts it may be important to focus on the different strands of the PSED but in other contexts there may be no practical difference between them;[9]
- as is the case with consultation, a local authority is entitled to reach a macro budgetary decision on the basis that implementation will be subject to discharge of the PSED;[10]
- whilst there is a 'duty of inquiry' implicit in the duty to have 'due regard' the courts do not appear to have defined that duty in terms that extend it beyond the usual *Tameside* duty of undertaking a level and manner of enquiry that satisfies the *Wednesbury* test;[11]
- provided rigorous consideration has been given to the duty, so that there is a proper appreciation of the potential impact of the decision on equality objectives and the desirability of promoting them, it is for the decision-maker to decide how much weight should be given to the various factors informing the decision (subject to *Wednesbury*);[12]

6 [2011] EWHC 3175 (Admin).

7 *R (Bracking) v Secretary of State for Work and Pensions* [2013] EWCA Civ 1345, (2013) 16 CCLR 479 at para 25; *R (DAT) v West Berkshire Council* [2016] EWHC 1876 (Admin), (2016) 19 CCLR 362 at para 41.

8 *R (Bailey) v Brent LBC* [2011] EWCA Civ 1586 at para 102; *R (Greenwich Community Law Centre) v Greenwich LBC* [2012] EWCA Civ 496 at para 20; *R (Copson) v Dorset Healthcare University NHS Foundation Trust* [2013] EWHC 732 (Admin) at para 57(4); *R (MA) v Secretary of State for Work and Pensions* [2013] EWHC 2213 (QB) at paras 72–74, 86; *R (MA) v Secretary of State for Work and Pensions* [2014] EWCA Civ 13, [2014] PTSR 594 at paras 85–92; *R (Aspinall and others) v Secretary of State for Work and Pensions* [2014] EWHC 4134 (Admin) at paras 16–24.

9 *R (MA) v Secretary of State for Work and Pensions* [2014] EWCA Civ 13, [2014] PTSR 584 at para 91.

10 *JG and MB v Lancashire CC* [2011] EWHC 2295 (Admin), (2011) 14 CCLR 629 at paras 43–45.

11 *R (Hurley and Moore) v Secretary of State for Business, Innovation and Skills* [2012] EWHC 201 (Admin) at para 89.

12 *R (Brown) v Secretary of State for Work and Pensions* [2008] EWHC 3158 (Admin), [2009] PTSR 1506 at para 82; *R (Hurley and Moore) v Secretary of State for Business, Innovation and Skills* [2012] EWHC 201 (Admin) at paras 77–78; *R (DAT) v West Berkshire Council* [2016] EWHC 1876 (Admin), (2016) 19 CCLR 362 at paras 39–41.

- where the future is uncertain it can be sufficient to make a rational judgment about the future and then monitor the outcome with a view to making necessary adjustments.[13]

5.12 The Equality and Human Rights Commission has published useful guidance for anyone involved in budget cuts and service reductions: *Making fair financial decisions: Guidance for decision-makers*.[14] It would make sense for reports to decision-makers expressly to draw attention to this guidance.

5.13 The Senior Courts Act 1981 now provides, at section 31(2A), that the High Court must refuse to grant relief 'if it appears to the court to be highly likely that the outcome for the applicant would not have been substantially different if the conduct complained of had not occurred', unless there is an 'exceptional public interest' in granting relief. Section 31(3C) imposes a similar restriction on the grant of permission to apply for judicial review. It remains to be seen[15] how the court will approach this restriction on its traditional function but the provision is potentially relevant, in particular, in cases where the claimant submits that a decision is unlawful owing to the local authority's failure to discharge the PSED.

Statutory machinery

5.14 Many cases refer to the disability equality duty (DED), at section 49A of the Disability Discrimination Act (DDA) 1995. The critical provisions are now to be found in Chapter 1 of Part 11 of the Equality Act 2010, where section 149 is central (although one needs to go back to Chapter 1 of Part 2 for extended definitions of the various 'protected characteristics' and to Chapter 2 of Part 2 for definitions of different types of discrimination and other forms of prohibited conduct).

13 *R (Unison) v Lord Chancellor* [2015] EWCA Civ 935, [2016] ICR 1 at para 121.

14 January 2015: www.equalityhumanrights.com/sites/default/files/publication_pdf/Making%20Fair%20Financial%20Decisions%20Guidance%20for%20Decision%20Makers%20January%202015.pdf.

15 The Bingham Centre for the Rule of Law, the Public Law Project and Justice have suggested that this duty will only arise exceptionally: *Judicial Review and the Rule of Law: An Introduction to the Criminal Justice and Courts Act 2015, Part 4* at http://www.biicl.org/documents/767_judicial_review_and_the_rule_of_law_-_final_for_web_19_oct_2015.pdf. However, in *R (Hawke) v Secretary of State for Justice* [2015] EWHC 3599 (Admin), as a result of section 31(2A) of the Senior Courts Act 1981 Holman J declined to grant a declaration that the Secretary of State for Justice was in breach of the PSED (under section 149 of the Equality Act 2010); instead, he indicated that his judgment was a 'declaratory judgment' , following the example of Blake J in *R (Logan) v Havering LBC* [2015] EWHC 3193 (Admin). See also *R (Enfield LBC) v Secretary of State for Transport* [2015] EWHC 3758 (Admin) at para 106 (sometimes a witness statement is required from the public authority to establish that the test is met) and *R (HA) v The Governing Body of Hampstead School* [2016] EWHC 278 (Admin) at para 33 (these provisions may relate simply to 'technical flaws'). In *R (DAT) v West Berkshire Council* [2016] EWHC 1876 (Admin), (2016) 19 CCLR 362, Laing J found it hard to be satisfied that there was no chance of the council reaching a different decision on a reconsideration in case involving highly vulnerable children and, in any event, considered that in such a case there was an exceptional public interest in granting relief.

5.15 Section 149 provides, in full, as follows:

Public sector equality duty

149(1) A public authority must, in the exercise of its functions, have due regard to the need to–
(a) eliminate discrimination, harassment, victimisation and any other conduct that is prohibited by or under this Act;
(b) advance equality of opportunity between persons who share a relevant protected characteristic and persons who do not share it;
(c) foster good relations between persons who share a relevant protected characteristic and persons who do not share it.

(2) A person who is not a public authority but who exercises public functions must, in the exercise of those functions, have due regard to the matters mentioned in subsection (1).

(3) Having due regard to the need to advance equality of opportunity between persons who share a relevant protected characteristic and persons who do not share it involves having due regard, in particular, to the need to–
(a) remove or minimise disadvantages suffered by persons who share a relevant protected characteristic that are connected to that characteristic;
(b) take steps to meet the needs of persons who share a relevant protected characteristic that are different from the needs of persons who do not share it;
(c) encourage persons who share a relevant protected characteristic to participate in public life or in any other activity in which participation by such persons is disproportionately low.

(4) The steps involved in meeting the needs of disabled persons that are different from the needs of persons who are not disabled include, in particular, steps to take account of disabled persons' disabilities.

(5) Having due regard to the need to foster good relations between persons who share a relevant protected characteristic and persons who do not share it involves having due regard, in particular, to the need to–
(a) tackle prejudice, and
(b) promote understanding.

(6) Compliance with the duties in this section may involve treating some persons more favourably than others; but that is not to be taken as permitting conduct that would otherwise be prohibited by or under this Act.

(7) The relevant protected characteristics are–
age;
disability;
gender reassignment;
pregnancy and maternity;
race;
religion or belief;
sex;
sexual orientation.

(8) A reference to conduct that is prohibited by or under this Act includes a reference to–
(a) a breach of an equality clause or rule;
(b) a breach of a non-discrimination rule.

(9) Schedule 18 (exceptions) has effect.

Who is under the PSED and when?

5.16 The duty arises whenever a 'public authority' exercises its 'functions' (section 149(1)) and whenever a body that is not a 'public authority' exercises a 'public function' (section 149(2)).

As far as concerns public authorities:

- a 'public authority' includes a local authority[16] (see section 150 and Schedule 19);
- a local authority's 'functions' are 'all the duties and powers of a local authority; the sum total of the activities Parliament has entrusted to it. Those activities are its functions': *Hazell v Hammersmith & Fulham LBC*;[17]
- in the social care context, the most obvious functions to which the PSED applies are the formulation of policy and internal guidance and decisions affecting numbers of people (for example, to close a care home or day centre); when discharging functions of that kind, local authorities must discharge the PSED;
- when making macro budgetary or policy decisions local authorities may undertake a relatively broad, high-level discharge of the PSED, subject to more focussed consideration later on before specific implementing measures are taken;[18]
- whereas, in principle, the PSED also applies to decision-making in the case of individuals, social workers who assess needs and undertake care planning in accordance with the Care Act 2014, the statutory instruments and the *Care and Support Statutory Guidance* would not usually have to do anything more than that, lawfully to assess needs and undertake care planning.[19]

5.17 As far as concerns bodies that 'exercise public functions':

- section 150(5) provides that 'A public function is a function that is a function of a public nature for the purposes of the Human Rights Act 1998';
- section 73 of the Care Act 2014 legislates that a private or social sector provider is exercising a function of a public nature if, on the basis of payments or arrangements made by a local authority, it provides care and support to an adult, or support to a carer, (i) in the course of providing personal care where the adult is living; or (ii) residential accommodation together with nursing or personal care.

It is important that the PSED is discharged as part of the decision-making process but the court will probably not quash a decision when a later

16 The complete list, in Schedule 19, includes Ministers of the Crown, most government departments, most NHS bodies and many regulatory bodies.

17 [1992] 2 AC 1 at 29F.

18 *JG and MB v Lancashire CC* [2011] EWHC 2295 (Admin), (2011) 14 CCLR 629 paras 43–45.

19 *R (McDonald) v Kensington & Chelsea RLBC* [2011] UKSC 33, (2011) 14 CCLR 341; *R (AM) v Birmingham CC* [2009] EWHC 688 (Admin), (2009) 12 CCLR 407; *R (Rajput) v Waltham Forest LBC* [2011] EWCA Civ 1577, (2012) 15 CCLR 147

assessment, undertaken in good faith, demonstrates that it would be pointless to grant relief.[20]

Who are the beneficiaries of the PSED?

5.18 There are two, slightly different, groups:

- the first part of the Equality Act 2010, and section 149(1)(a) (both concerned with 'prohibited conduct'), apply to all persons who have a 'protected characteristic', as defined at sections 4–12 of the Equality Act 2010 (age, disability, gender re-assignment, marriage and civil partnership, pregnancy and maternity, race, religion or belief, sex and sexual orientation; however, they only apply to persons who have the protected characteristic of marriage or civil partnership in relation to work issues because the parts of the Equality Act 2010 covering services and public functions, premises and education do not apply to those characteristics[21]);
- section 149(1)(b) and (c), and following, apply to all persons who have a 'relevant protected characteristic', as defined at section 149(7) – that is, any of the 'protected characteristics' at sections 4–12 of the Equality Act 2010, aside from marriage and civil partnership status.

What is 'due regard'?

5.19 The duty to 'have due regard' to the needs identified in section 149(1) can be understood as meaning that the public authority must give such consideration to those needs as is appropriate.

5.20 Thus, the greater the risk that a policy or decision will affect one or more persons with a 'relevant protected characteristic', the more careful and searching the public body must be in its scrutiny of what that impact may entail, how it may be mitigated and monitored and on what basis it may be justified: greater scrutiny is required when deciding to close care homes or day centres, than when deciding what stationery to buy.

5.21 The judgment of McCombe LJ in the *Bracking* case, set out above at para 5.8, explains the PSED with particular reference to the duty to have 'due regard'. As McCombe LJ explains, whilst the question of what weight should be attributed to relevant matters is ultimately a matter for the local authority, 'the concept of 'due regard' requires the court to ensure that there has been a proper and conscientious focus on the statutory criteria'.

5.22 Having said that, the statutory criteria, as supplemented by the statutory instruments, guidance, codes of practice and technical guidance, comprise an abundance of relevant factors so plentiful that, superimposed on a complex factual matrix, generally results in any half-decent lawyer being able to point to one or more considerations that a local authority has failed explicitly, or even implicitly, to deal with. The courts have discouraged an unduly forensic analysis and, without using these words, intimated sometimes that relief might only be granted when something has gone seriously

20 *R (West Berkshire DC) v Secretary of State for Communities and Local Government* [2016] EWCA Civ 441, [2016] PTSR 982 at paras 86–87.

21 See Equality Act 2010 ss28(1)(a), 32(1)(b), 84(1)(b), 90.

wrong, so that the local authority has not in substance given proper and conscientious consideration to the more important issues in the case.[22] In addition, the courts have articulated a series of limiting principles (see para 5.11 above) and the Senior Courts Act 1981 has been restrictively revised (see para 5.13 above). The context and scale of any potential impact seem to be powerful considerations, in this regard.

The first 'need'

5.23 The first need is to have due regard to the need to eliminate discrimination, harassment, victimisation and any other conduct prohibited by or under the Equality Act 2010 (section 149(1)(a)).

5.24 In practice, this means that a local authority must satisfy itself that what it proposes to do:

- does not amount to discrimination that is made unlawful by Chapter 2 of Part 1, in particular 'direct discrimination' (section 13), 'disability discrimination' (section 15) or 'indirect discrimination' (section 19);
- does not involve a failure to make 'reasonable adjustments' (section 20);
- does not involve positive action in circumstances where that is not permitted (section 159); and
- does not tolerate a continuing course of offensive conduct (see paragraph 3.9 of *Equality Act 2010 Technical Guidance on the Public Sector Equality Duty: England* (8/14)).[23]

The second 'need'

5.25 This is the need to advance equality of opportunity between persons who share a 'relevant protected characteristic' and those who do not (section 149(1)(b)).

5.26 This need is particularly relevant in the social care context, in that many adults and children who share a 'relevant protected characteristic' are under-represented in certain activities and do not have the same opportunities to enjoy a fulfilling life, as others do, so that positive action is needed if that level of inequality is to be redressed or mitigated.

5.27 The second 'need', at section 149(1)(b), is expanded upon in section 149(3) and (4) as follows:

> (3) Having due regard to the need to advance equality of opportunity between persons who share a relevant protected characteristic and persons who do not share it involves having due regard, in particular, to the need to–

22 *R (Bailey) v Brent LBC* [2011] EWCA Civ 1586, [2012] BLGR 530 at para 102; *R (Hurley) v Secretary of State for Business, Innovation and Skills* [2012] EWHC 201 (Admin), [2012] HRLR 13 at para 87; *R (Zaccheus 2000 Trust) v Secretary of State for Work and Pensions* [2013] EWCA Civ 1202, [2013] PTSR 1427 at paras 60 and 64; *R (Unison) v Lord Chancellor* [2015] EWCA Civ 935, [2016] ICR 1 at para 116; *R (CPAG) v Secretary of State for Work and Pensions* [2011] EWHC 2616 (Admin) at paras 57, 76 and 79.

23 At www.equalityhumanrights.com/publication/technical-guidance-public-sector-equality-duty-england.

(a) remove or minimise disadvantages suffered by persons who share a relevant protected characteristic that are connected to that characteristic;
(b) take steps to meet the needs of persons who share a relevant protected characteristic that are different from the needs of persons who do not share it;
(c) encourage persons who share a relevant protected characteristic to participate in public life or in any other activity in which participation by such persons is disproportionately low.

(4) The steps involved in meeting the needs of disabled persons that are different from the needs of persons who are not disabled include, in particular, steps to take account of disabled persons' disabilities.

5.28 The 'disadvantages' referred to in section 149(3)(a) include exclusion, rejection, lack of opportunity, lack of choice or barriers to accessing services (see paragraph 3.19 of the *Equality Act 2010 Technical Guidance on the Public Sector Equality Duty: England* (8/14)).[24]

5.29 The different needs referred to in section 149(3)(b) include:

- needs that are intrinsic to the 'relevant protected characteristic', in the sense that a young disabled person may need different services, in order to participate in education, training or work, than an able-bodied person (this is also covered by section 149(4)); and
- 'social needs' that have arisen in consequence of treatment by society, in the sense that members of a particular group may have been discouraged from taking up certain opportunities.

5.30 The reference to 'public life' and other activities, in section 149(3)(c) is a reference to employment, professions, sporting and cultural activities, voting, membership of bodies such as school councils and residents' associations and being appointed to public office. 'Participation' requires consideration to be given to the overall numbers and, also, to whether persons with a 'relevant protected characteristic' are involved in the running and decision-making.

The third 'need'

5.31 The third need is to foster good relations between persons who share a 'relevant protected characteristic' and those who do not (section 149(1)(c)).

5.32 That is expanded upon in section 149(5):

(5) Having due regard to the need to foster good relations between persons who share a relevant protected characteristic and persons who do not share it involves having due regard, in particular, to the need to–
(a) tackle prejudice, and
(b) promote understanding.

5.33 So, if a local authority plans to provide supported accommodation for mental patients in a street where the neighbours object, that would be a good opportunity to have regard to this need (and see paragraph 3.39 of

24 www.equalityhumanrights.com/publication/technical-guidance-public-sector-equality-duty-england.

the *Equality Act 2010 Technical Guidance on the Public Sector Equality Duty: England* (8/14)).[25]

Positive action

5.34 It follows, as explained at Chapter 4 of the *Equality Act 2010 Technical Guidance on the Public Sector Equality Duty: England* (8/14)[26] that positive action may be lawful when triggered by the thought process required by section 149:

> **When is positive action lawful?**
> It will be lawful for a relevant body to take positive action where it reasonably thinks that people who share a protected characteristic (section 158):
> a) experience a disadvantage connected to that characteristic; or
> b) have needs that are different from the needs of persons who do not share that characteristic; or
> c) have disproportionately low participation in an activity compared to those who do not share that protected characteristic.
>
> Action may be taken when any one or all of these conditions exist. Sometimes the conditions will overlap – for example, people sharing a protected characteristic may be at a disadvantage which may also give rise to a different need or may be reflected in their low level of participation in particular activities.
>
> **What action is lawful?**
> Where the conditions above apply, the relevant body may take any action which is proportionate to meet the aims stated in the Act. Those aims are:
> - enabling or encouraging persons who share the protected characteristic to overcome or minimise that disadvantage
> - meeting those needs, or
> - enabling or encouraging persons who share the protected characteristic to participate in that activity.
>
> Positive action is not the same as positive discrimination, which is unlawful. The difference between the two is explained in the Code of Practice on Services, Public Functions and Associations.

Complying with the PSED in practice

5.35 This is dealt with fully at Chapter 5 of the *Equality Act 2010 Technical Guidance on the Public Sector Equality Duty: England* (8/14):[27]

> 5.1 Chapter 2 explains that to 'have due regard' to the three aims in the general equality duty a relevant body must consciously consider the need to do the things set out in the general equality duty in exercising any of its functions which are subject to the duty.
>
> 5.2 A body subject to the duty will find the principles in section 2.21 of Chapter 2 useful in deciding what action it needs to take to ensure it is

25 www.equalityhumanrights.com/publication/technical-guidance-public-sector-equality-duty-england.

26 www.equalityhumanrights.com/publication/technical-guidance-public-sector-equality-duty-england.

27 www.equalityhumanrights.com/publication/technical-guidance-public-sector-equality-duty-england.

complying with the general equality duty on a continuing basis. In summary those principles are:

- knowledge of the duty
- timeliness
- real consideration
- sufficient information
- non-delegable
- review, and
- evidence of consideration.

5.3 Listed authorities will need to ensure that they also comply with the mandatory steps set out in the specific duty regulations, covered in Chapter 6 of this guidance. The specific duties are intended to enable better performance of the general equality duty.

5.4 In order to decide what action to take a body subject to the duty could ask itself a series of questions. The sections in this chapter suggest how these questions could be answered:

1. How will it assess the relevance of the duty to the functions it exercises?
See: Identifying the relevance of the general equality duty to the functions of a body subject to the duty (paras 5.5–5.14)

2. How will it gather the information it needs to enable it to comply with the duty?
See: Ensuring a sound evidence base (paras 5.15–5.34)

3. How will it ensure that those exercising those functions understand their obligations under the duty?

4. How will it ensure that the duty is complied with both before and during any decision-making process?

5. How will it integrate rigorous and substantive consideration of the duty into the operation of its functions and its decision-making processes?
See: Ensuring due regard in decision making (paras 5.35–5.50)

6. How will it show it has complied with the duty?
See: Providing evidence of compliance (paras 5.51–52).

Listed authorities should also refer to Chapter 6.

7. How will it build compliance with the duty into its commissioning or procurement/dealing with third parties?
See: Meeting the duty in relation to other bodies (paras 5.53–5.64)

8. What review mechanisms will it put in place to ensure that compliance with the duty is continuing?
See: Ensuring a sound evidence base (at paras 5.15–5.18).

Specific duties

5.36 In England, a Minister of the Crown may impose specific duties on the public authorities listed in Part 1 of Schedule 19 to the Equality Act 2010. The list includes Ministers of the Crown, most government departments, most NHS bodies, the Care Quality Commission (CQC), Monitor and local authorities. (There is a similar list for Welsh public authorities, in Part 2 of Schedule 19).

5.37 Specific duties are imposed by the Equality Act 2010 (Disability) Regulations 2010,[28] which require the listed public authorities to:

- publish information to demonstrate their compliance with the PSED (regulation 3);
- publish one or more equality objectives which it thinks it should achieve to do any of the things mentioned in the PSED (regulation 4).

5.38 Further information and advice is provided at Chapter 6 of the *Equality Act 2010 Technical Guidance on the Public Sector Equality Duty: England* (8/14).[29]

Enforcement

5.39 The Equality and Human Rights Commission (EHRC) has a range of enforcement powers, under sections 8, 10 and 32 of the Equality Act 2006, that it may exercise in relation to (i) the PSED, (ii) the specific duties.

5.40 Any individual with an interest in the matter may make an application for judicial review, on the basis that local authority decision-making is undermined by a failure to discharge the PSED. However, a judicial review claim cannot be made in respect of the specific duties, as these can only be enforced by the EHRC.

Statutory instruments

5.41 Of the statutory instruments made under Equality Act 2010, the most important are:

- the Equality Act 2010 (Disability) Regulations 2010[30] (these contain provisions expanding on when a person is and is not disabled (etc), provisions about auxiliary aids or services and reasonable adjustments and other matters);
- the Equality Act 2010 (Specific Duties) Regulations 2011 (see above).[31]

Guidance, codes and technical guidance

5.42 There is guidance, statutory codes of practice and technical guidance:

- the full range is to be found on the website of the Equality and Human Rights Commission;[32]
- the most important statutory code of practice, for present purposes is the *Services, Public Functions and Associations Statutory Code Of Practice*;[33]

28 SI No 2128.

29 www.equalityhumanrights.com/publication/technical-guidance-public-sector-equality-duty-england.

30 SI No 2128.

31 SI No 2260.

32 www.equalityhumanrights.com/legal-and-policy/legislation/equality-act–2010/equality-act-guidance-codes-practice-and-technical-guidance#cop.

33 www.equalityhumanrights.com/publication/services-public-functions-and-associations-statutory-code-practice.

- there is also useful technical guidance on the PSED for England,[34] Scotland,[35] and Wales;[36]
- and *The Essential Guide to the Public Sector Equality Duty*.[37]

Cases

5.43 *R (Chavda) v Harrow LBC* [2007] EWHC 3064 (Admin), (2008) 11 CCLR 187

A local authority failed to discharge the disability equality duty when it failed to draw the decision-makers' attention to the duties imposed thereby

Facts: Three local residents in receipt of community care services sought a judicial review of Harrow's decision, taken for budgetary reasons, to change its eligibility criteria from substantial and critical, to critical only.

Judgment: Deputy High Court Judge Mackie QC held that Harrow's decision-making was unlawful because the decision-makers had not been referred to the disability equality duty (a forerunner of the PSED) at section 49A of the DDA 1995: it was not sufficient to mention a 'potential conflict with the DDA'; decision-makers had to be informed what their duties under the disability equality duty were. If that had been done, there would have been a written record of it.

5.44 *R (Eisai Ltd) v NICE* [2007] EWHC 1941 (Admin), (2007) 10 CCLR 368

Since decision-makers had not been advised about their statutory duties, and their consideration of the issues did not disclose an awareness of or consideration of such duties, their formulation of policy and decision-making were unlawful

Facts: NICE granted only limited approval for the use of a drug manufactured by Eisai. Eisai succeeded at first instance in establishing that NICE had failed to comply with anti-discrimination legislation, but not that its consultation process had been unfair (although the Court of Appeal later allowed Eisai's appeal on that issue).

Judgment: Dobbs J held, on the discrimination issue, that NICE had failed to have due regard to the likely effect of its decision on minority groups, in breach of its duties under the Race Relations Act 1976 and the Disability Discrimination Act 1995:

> 94. Junior Counsel for NICE was listed as a member of the panel, presumably in the role of independent legal advisor. [7b/33a/178]. It is the more surprising therefore, that there was no discussion or advice given during the hearing about relevant anti-discrimination legislation or even human

34 www.equalityhumanrights.com/publication/technical-guidance-public-sector-equality-duty-england.

35 www.equalityhumanrights.com/publication/technical-guidance-public-sector-equality-duty-scotland.

36 www.equalityhumanrights.com/publication/technical-guidance-public-sector-equality-duty-wales.

37 www.equalityhumanrights.com/publication/essential-guide-public-sector-equality-duty-0.

rights legislation, given that the issue of discrimination had been raised. There is no reference whatever within the body of the decision to any of the duties and obligations of the authority with regard to discrimination. It appears that no consideration was given as to how these duties might impact on the Guidance. Instead of looking at how NICE as a public body could itself promote equal opportunity, having accepted that the Guidance could have a discriminatory effect if applied slavishly, the approach taken was to leave it to others to sort out in the hope and expectation that they would. (Para 4.7). That, in my judgement, is not good enough, particularly given the lack of substance in the justification advanced by Professor Stevens and taking into account the ramifications of the Guidance.

95. The issue of the atypical groups is dealt with in an unsatisfactory way in the Guidance. This creates confusion and the potential for discrimination. In Paragraph 4.3.13 (Para 80) there is reference to the interpretation of the MMSE scores being difficult for the atypical groups. However, this is said not to disadvantage them at entry level. There is then specific reference as to what should happen to those with learning disabilities. The position of those with marked language problems, who the Guidance had previously identified as being 'different', is left up in the air. The reference to the discontinuation level does not clarify for the clinician the position with respect to those with marked language difficulties who fall outside the 'normal' parameters. [CB/6/167]. There is potential for further confusion with regard to those with learning disabilities. While it is said that learning disability specialists should be responsible for the initiation of treatment, it does not indicate clearly whether such specialists are to use MMSE tests as a guide, or are free to make assessments with no reference to MMSE tests at all or whether only a diagnosis by the specialist of 'moderate' AD will attract mandatory funding. Contrast with this the assistance given in the quoted passage from the Guidelines cited in paragraph 81. Given that the 2006 Guidance, in contrast with the 2001 Guidance, excluded those with mild AD from its recommendation, it is particularly important that the Guidance is clear and free from ambiguity.

96. Following the reasoning above, I take the view that the approach of the Appeal Panel was flawed, in that no proper consideration was given to NICE's duties as a public authority to promote equal opportunities and to have due regard to the need to eliminate discrimination. It was unreasonable and unlawful to overlook that responsibility. A similar view is taken of the Guidance, particularly as there is no evidence that before issuing the Guidance the 'due diligence' duties were considered or complied with or that any thought was given to present or imminent obligations under anti-discrimination law. (See 2007 Action Plan [9/44/154]) Despite the publication of the Action Plan in January 2007 and the invitation of the Alzheimer's Society to NICE in a letter dated 4 January 2007 to consider amendment of the Guidance in the light of its discriminatory impact, nothing was done [15/1/7]. In my judgment the Guidance has failed to avoid discrimination against the relevant groups.

5.45 *R (AM) v Birmingham CC* [2009] EWHC 688 (Admin), (2009) 12 CCLR 407

Discharge of the community care assessment and planning process also discharged the disability equality duty

Facts: AM, who was severely disabled, obtained a place at university. He sought a fully adapted toilet facility including a hoist. That provision would have been expensive and Birmingham decided that, because AM was continent, it was unlikely that he would need to use it during the day. Accordingly, Birmingham resolved to provide only a certain amount of additional personal care. AM sought a judicial review but was granted permission only to argue that Birmingham had failed to discharge its duty under section 49A of the Disability Discrimination Act 1995.

Judgment: Cranston J dismissed the application, holding that in substance the community care assessment process had resulted in Birmingham having due regard to the need to promote equality of opportunity in education and due regard to the other obligations owed to disabled persons.

5.46 *R (Boyejo) v Barnet LBC* [2009] EWHC 3261 (Admin), (2010) 13 CCLR 72

Not only had the local authorities done insufficient to draw the decision-makers' attention to their duty under the disability equality duty, the impact assessments, concluding that there would not be any adverse consequences, were Wednesbury *irrational*

Facts: Barnet and Portsmouth both separately decided to terminate certain on-site, live-in warden services for sheltered tenants, substituting a mobile night-service and an alarm call system.

Judgment: Deputy High Court Judge Milwyn Jarman held that Portsmouth's consultation had been inadequate in that it's '*consultation document*' spoke in terms of a decision already having been made, did not canvass alternatives and failed sufficiently to involve disabled persons; also, the time afforded for representations was too short and Portsmouth had failed to take proper account of the representations made. Additionally, neither Barnet nor Portsmouth had done sufficient to draw decision-makers' attention to the duty at section 49A of the Disability Discrimination Act 1985, nor to have specific regard to the impact on those residents with a disability (cf. the residents in general) of the proposed change, nor to take account that it might be necessary to treat such persons more favourably. Further, both authorities' conclusions, in their equalities impact assessments, that there would not be *any* adverse impact on residents, were *Wednesbury* unreasonable.

5.47 *R (Domb) v Hammersmith & Fulham LBC* [2009] EWCA Civ 941

The local authority had acted lawfully by providing decision-makers with an impact assessment and information about their duties under the disability equality duty and related legislation, and giving careful consideration to the objections of disabled persons and the potential adverse impacts upon them, notwithstanding a failure to include reference to gender and race issues in the formal report, since the impact assessment rationally concluded that there was no significant risk of adverse consequences in those regards

Facts: Hammersmith decided to reduce local council tax by three per cent. It then decided to introduce a charging regime for home care services. Ms Domb sought a judicial review, inter alia, on the basis that Hammersmith had failed to discharge its duties under equalities legislation.

Judgment: the Court of Appeal (Lord Clarke MR, Sedley and Rix LJJ) held that, in the circumstances of that case, the three per cent Council Tax cut had to be treated as a given, so that the only realistic options for consideration were charging or raising the eligibility threshold. It was obvious that the introduction of charging would adversely impact on the users of home care services but there was no evidence that the local authority did not have due regard to the relevant equality duties as a matter of substance as well as form: not only had a careful consultation been carried out, in which the principled opposition to a charging scheme had been stressed and reported on in the report to cabinet, but the report advised decision-makers of the thrust of their duty under the disability equality duty and underlined in the strongest terms that the issue required decision makers to take care before they acted. Smaller points on the detail of the impact assessment and/or report did not lead to the conclusion that there had been any material failure of due regard. The failure to make specific mention of the racial and gender equality duties in the report was not a serious flaw, given the evidence that there would be no disproportionate adverse impact on racial groups and women. The Court left open the question whether the equality duties fell to be discharged when macro budgetary decisions were made, that impinged on later decision-making of the kind in the present case.

Rix LJ said this on the jurisprudence:

> 52. Our attention has been drawn to a number of authorities on the need to have due regard to equality duties, in particular *R (Elias) v Secretary of State for Defence* [2005] EWHC 1435 (Admin) (Elias J), [2006] EWCA Civ 1293, [2006] 1 WLR 3213, *R (Chavda) v London Borough of Harrow* [2007] EWHC 3064 (Admin), (2008) 11 CCLR 187 (HHJ Mackie QC), *R (Baker) v Secretary of State for Communities and Local Government* [2008] EWCA Civ 141, [2008] LGR 239, *R (Brown) v Secretary of State for Work and Pensions* [2008] EWHC 3158 (Admin), and *R (Meany, Glynn and Sanders) v Harlow District Council* [2009] EWHC 559 (Admin) (Davis J). I find the greatest help in the judgments of Dyson LJ in Baker (dealing with the RRA 1976) at paras 30ff and of Scott Baker LJ in Brown (dealing with the DDA 1995) at paras 89/96, where each of them summarises what is involved in the duty to have 'due regard'. For present purposes I take from those summaries in particular the observations that there is no statutory duty to carry out a formal impact assessment; that the duty is to have due regard, not to achieve results or to refer in terms to the duty; that due regard does not exclude paying regard to countervailing factors, but is 'the regard that is appropriate in all the circumstances'; that the test of whether a decision maker has had due regard is a test of the substance of the matter, not of mere form or box-ticking, and that the duty must be performed with vigour and with an open mind; and that it is a non-delegable duty.
>
> 53. No authority has been cited as being of particular relevance to the facts of our case. I note, however, that *Chavda* concerned the activities of councils with respect to their provision of social services. In *Chavda*, where Harrow restricted home care services to people with critical needs only, there was a total failure to mention the DDA 1995 duty in any of the documents produced for Harrow's decision makers. There was no effort proactively to seek the views of the disabled or to refer to the duty in the planning stages of the consultation. There was no equality impact assessment. Harrow nevertheless submitted that it had observed its duty in substance, and had

engaged in consultation and other ways with the disabled. However, what Judge Mackie considered as critical was that '*There is no evidence that this legal duty and its implications were drawn to the attention of the decision-takers who should have been informed not just of the disabled as an issue but of the particular obligations which the law imposes*' (at para 40). However, I cannot say that I derive any assistance from that, very different, case.

Sedley LJ added this important observation:

79. Members are heavily reliant on officers for advice in taking these decisions. That makes it doubly important for officers not simply to tell members what they want to hear but to be rigorous in both inquiring and reporting to them. There are aspects of the evaluation, quoted by Rix LJ, which strike me as Panglossian – for example the ignoring of actual outcome in favour of 'planned outcome' and the limiting of consequential risk to the possibility that charges would not be introduced – and parts of the report to members which present conclusions without the data needed to evaluate them.

5.48 *R (JL) v Islington LBC* [2009] EWHC 458 (Admin), (2009) 12 CCLR 322

The local authority had not discharged the disability equality duty because there was no audit trail or other documentation demonstrating a proper approach

Facts: JL suffered from autism and received 1,248 hours of support each year. Islington then changed its eligibility criteria, as a result of which disabled children with 'high needs' (such as JL) received only 624 hours each year. Islington later added a small number of additional hours to enable some respite provision to be made. JL sought a judicial review.

Judgment: Black J held that Islington had not undertaken a genuine assessment of JL's needs but simply applied their new eligibility policy, that an eligibility policy could not be used to determine whether or not a local authority was under a duty to act under section 20 of the Children Act 1989 (which imposed an absolute duty) and that Islington's policy was flawed in a number of respects, in particular in that it had the effect of excluding needs that Islington would have decided it was necessary to meet (under section 2 of the Chronically Sick and Disabled Persons Act 1970). In addition, Islington had failed to discharge its duty under section 49A of the Disability Discrimination Act 1995 when drawing up its criteria:

115. The claimants submit that by imposing a maximum of 12 hours for provision, in order to assist in one of the local authority's stated aims, ie to make provision to more disabled people, the local authority may have extended opportunity for some disabled people (those who are less disabled) but may also have curtailed it for others (the more disabled). They argue that this is not consistent with the objectives in section 49A(c), (d) and (f), to which the local authority should have had due regard.

116. The local authority protests that the criteria were designed to promote those objectives. Its intention was, it says, to ensure that the most support went to those families with the highest needs; the greater the disability, the more substantial would be the service provision. This is the scheme that it built into the criteria. If there is any discrimination, it says, then it is against people who are not disabled, not against people who are.

117. The local authority response misses the point, in my view. This case itself is a clear example of the problem. The imposition of a cap on support at 12 hours a week led to a huge reduction in the assistance provided to JL. That had the capacity to render him and his family less able to cope with his disability and, therefore, to diminish his equality of opportunity vis a vis able bodied people and to discourage rather than encourage his participation in public life. Whether it did or not is not a matter upon which I wish to express an opinion; further assessment will be necessary to determine that. However, it is possible to see that, depending on a family's particular circumstances, the result of the ceiling on support might be to deprive a child of features of his support which were critical to his functioning, especially if he was particularly needy. The saving in hours may have enabled the local authority to improve the lot of another, perhaps less, disabled child and secured greater equality of opportunity for him but that does not remove the disadvantage to the more disabled child ...

121. The local authority submits that it has had regard to section 49A. However, there is no audit trail confirming that the local authority has complied with its DDA duty or even had reference to it at all. The local authority has produced no documentation to demonstrate a proper approach to the question. There is no evidence that a proper impact assessment was carried out to see how the proposals were likely to affect particular groups of disabled children ...

5.49 *Pieretti v Enfield LBC* [2010] EWCA Civ 1104, (2010) 13 CCLR 650

The disability equality duty applied to all local authority functions, including under sections 184 and 202 of the Housing Act 1996

Facts: Enfield found that Mr and Mrs Pieretti had become intentionally homeless on account of their failure to pay rent. However, Enfield had been presented with evidence that Mr and Mrs Pierretti had been significantly depressed. Mr and Mrs Pieretti contended that Enfield had breached section 49A of the Disability Discrimination Act 1995, by failing to enquire into whether their ability to pay rent had been undermined by their illness.

Judgment: the Court of Appeal (Mummery, Longmore and Wilson LJJ) held that Enfield had been in breach of the disability equality duty by failing to make further enquiry into a feature of the evidence that raised a real possibility that Mr and Mrs Pieretti were disabled in a sense relevant to whether they could fairly be adjudged to have become homeless intentionally:

33. But the law does not require that in every case decision-makers under s184 and s202 must take (active) steps to inquire into whether the person to be subject to the decision is disabled and, if so, is disabled in a way relevant to the decision. That would be absurd. What, then, is the extent of their duty under s49A(1)(d)? No doubt the aspect of the duty under s49A(1) specified at (d) would have been easier to understand if it had been formulated as 'to take *due* steps to take account of disabled persons' disabilities ...'. 'Due' means 'appropriate in all the circumstances' (see *R (Baker) v Secretary of State for Communities and Local Government* [2008] EWCA Civ 141, per Dyson LJ at [31]) so the simple task would have been to survey all the circumstances and then to ask what steps it would be appropriate to take in the light of them. Instead, however, the aspect of the duty specified at (d) is to 'have due regard to ... the need to take' such steps. In

R (Brown) v Secretary of State for Work and Pensions [2008] EWHC 3158 (Admin) the Divisional Court of the Queen's Bench Division (Scott Baker and Aikens LJJ), at [84], described the phraseology of s49A(1)(d) as 'convoluted'. The court helpfully proceeded, at [90] to [96], to identify six general principles referable to the duty to have 'due regard' in all six of the aspects specified in the subsection, including, second, that it demanded 'a conscious approach' and, third, that it should be performed 'in substance, with rigour and with an open mind'.

34. For practical purposes, however, I see little difference between a duty to 'take due steps to take account' and the duty under s49A(1)(d) to 'have due regard to ... the need to take steps to take account'. If steps are not taken in circumstances in which it would have been appropriate for them to be taken, ie in which they would have been due, I cannot see how the decision-maker can successfully claim to have had due regard to the need to take them.

35. In my view, therefore, the reviewing officer was in breach of her duty under s49A(1)(d) if she failed to take due steps to take account of a disability on the part of the appellant. In the context of her duty of review under s202 of the Act of 1996 I would refine the question as follows: did she fail to make further inquiry in relation to some such feature of the evidence presented to her as raised a real possibility that the appellant was disabled in a sense relevant to whether he acted 'deliberately' within the meaning of subsection (1) of s191 of the Act of 1996 and, in particular, to whether he acted 'in good faith' within the meaning of subsection (2) thereof?

Comment: in other specific homelessness contexts, it has been held that the similar duty (to treat the best interests of children as a primary consideration, under section 11(2) of the Children Act 2004) did not apply: *Huzrat v Hounslow LBC*;[38] *Mohamoud v Kensington & Chelsea RLBC*.[39]

5.50 *R (W) v Birmingham CC* [2011] EWHC 1147 (Admin), (2011) 14 CCLR 516

A generalised consideration of the likely impact, without any real assessment of the practical effect of what appeared to be a significant restriction of eligibility for care services, resulted in a local authority failing to have 'due regard' to the needs identified in the PSED

Facts: in order to make necessary budgetary savings, Birmingham decided only to meet 'critical' needs, whereas it had previously met 'critical' and 'substantial' needs.

Judgment: Walker J held that Birmingham's consultation and its discharge of the disability equality duty had been unlawful: the material prepared for decision-makers failed to identify the risk of adverse consequences in practical terms or give any idea of how the potential severity of the proposal could be mitigated. Accordingly, the decision-makers had not had 'due regard' to the needs identified in the PSED.

38 [2013] EWCA Civ 1865.
39 [2015] EWCA Civ 789.

5.51 *R (McDonald) v Kensington & Chelsea RLBC* [2011] UKSC 33, (2011) 14 CCLR 341

It had been unnecessary explicitly to refer to the disability equality duty when undertaking a community care assessment and it could not be inferred that the disability equality duty had been disregarded

Facts: Ms McDonald had limited mobility and a small, neurogenic bladder, which caused her to have to urinate several times a night. Kensington initially provided Ms McDonald with a commode and a night-time carer. It then assessed her need using different language, as being for incontinence pads and absorbent sheets. Ms McDonald sought a judicial review.

Judgment: the Supreme Court (Walker, Hale, Brown, Kerr and Dyson JJSC, Hale JSC dissenting) held that (i) Kensington's decision was not a practice, policy or procedure for the purposes of section 21 of the Disability Discrimination Act 1995 and even if it was, it was justified; and (ii) given that Kensington was discharging a function under a statute concerned with the welfare of disabled persons it was superfluous for it to refer to the disability equality duty and 'absurd' to suggest that its failure to have done so was evidence that it had disregarded the disability equality duty.

5.52 *Barnsley MBC v Norton* [2011] EWCA Civ 834, (2011) 14 CCLR 617

It was a breach of the disability equality duty to fail to consider the needs of a disabled occupier before evicting her

Facts: Barnsley was entitled to possession of the Norton family's dwelling and brought possession proceedings. The Norton family defended possession proceedings on the public law ground that the daughter of the family was disabled, but Barnsley had breached its disability equality duty under section 49A of the Disability Discrimination Act 1995.

Judgment: the Court of Appeal (Maurice Kay, Carnwath and Lloyd LJJ) held that Barnsley had been in breach of the disability equality duty, by failing to have due regard to the needs of the disabled daughter before and during the possession proceedings: because the disability equality duty applied to all the local authority's functions. In all the circumstances, it was right to make a possession order, but Barnsley should have considered the need to secure suitable accommodation for the disabled daughter and her own small baby and were required to do so now.

Comment: as this case shows, whilst the disability equality duty/PSED is often relevant to policy decisions, it can also be relevant to decisions in individual cases although, it seems, the court has expressed satisfaction that ordinary community care procedures do, in themselves, result in substantial compliance with those duties.

5.53 *JG and MB v Lancashire CC* [2011] EWHC 2295 (Admin), (2011) 14 CCLR 629

It was legitimate to make a macro budgetary decision, likely to adversely affect disabled persons, on the basis that the council was not committed to any specific initiative until consultation and compliance with the PSED had been undertaken

Facts: in order to make necessary budgetary savings, Lancashire determined to reduce its adult social services expenditure and to undertake consultation on specific money-saving initiatives, including changing the eligibility threshold from moderate to substantial. That decision was made later, after consultation and an equalities impact assessment.

Judgment: Kenneth Parker J held that it had been lawful for Lancashire to take a preliminary budgetary decision, knowing that implementation of the budget was likely to adversely affect disabled persons, but not committing itself to any specific initiative until consultation and compliance with the PSED had been achieved which, later, had been achieved:

> 43. In relation to the statutory duties under section 49A DDA, the leading guidance as to the relevant principles has been given by the Court of Appeal in *R (Baker) v Secretary of State for Communities and Local Government* [2008] EWCA Civ 141 at paras 31–40 and by the Divisional Court in *R (Brown) v Secretary of State for Work and Pensions* [2008] EWHC 3158 (Admin) at paras 79–96. A number of principles emerge as follows:
>
> i) The statutory duty under Section 49A DDA is not one to achieve a particular substantive result (whether to promote equality or otherwise) but to have 'due regard' to the need to achieve these goals. Due regard is regard that 'is appropriate in all the circumstances' (*Baker* at para 31 by Dyson LJ (as he then was)).
>
> ii) The public authority must also pay regard to any countervailing factors which, in the context of the function being exercised, it is proper and reasonable for the public authority to consider. The weight to be given to the countervailing factors is a matter for the public authority, not the court, unless the assessment by the public authority is unreasonable or irrational (*Baker* at para 34, *Brown* at para 82).
>
> iii) A failure to make explicit reference to the statute does not show that the duty has not been performed (*Brown* at para 93). It is immaterial whether or not the decision-maker was even aware of the duty provided that in substance he had due regard to the matters specified in it (*Baker* at paras 36, 37, 40 and 46).
>
> iv) There is no obligation in the DDA to carry out a formal EIA (*Brown* at para 89) although such an EIA is a helpful way of demonstrating that the statutory duty has been complied with.
>
> 44. Mr Ian Wise QC, who appeared on behalf of the Claimants, laid emphasis on a number of other propositions that can be derived from the case-law as follows:
>
> i) Due regard must be given 'before and at the time that a particular policy that will or might affect disabled people is being considered by the public authority in question' (*Brown* at para 91).
>
> ii) Due regard to the duty must be 'an essential preliminary' to any important policy decision not a 'rearguard action following a concluded decision' (*R (BAPIO Action Limited) v Secretary of State for the Home Department* [2007] EWCA Civ 1139 at para 3 by Sedley LJ).
>
> iii) Put another way, consideration of the duty must be 'an integral part of the formulation of a proposed policy, not justification for its adoption' (*R (Kaur) and others v Ealing LBC* [2008] EWHC 2062 (Admin) at para 24 by Moses J (as he then was)).
>
> iv) 'Due regard' means specific regard by way of conscious approach to the specified needs (*R (Meany) v Harlow District Council* [2009] EWHC

559 (Admin) at para 74; *R (Boyejo) v Barnet LBC* [2009] EWHC 3261 (Admin) at para 58).

v) If a risk of adverse impact is identified consideration should be given to measures to avoid that impact before fixing on a particular solution (*Kaur* at para 44).

45. Mr Wise also relied heavily on the recent decision in *R (WM and others) v Birmingham City Council* [2011] EWHC 1147 (Admin). In that case Birmingham decided to restrict eligibility for adult social care only to those individuals with critical needs. Taking its decision, Birmingham produced several equality impact assessments which purported to show due regard to the disability equality duty. However, Walker J held that due regard had not in fact been shown and quashed the decision. The thrust of that decision was that although Birmingham City Council had been aware of the need to pay due regard it had not, in fact, sought to carry out an assessment of the practical impact on those whose needs in a particular respect fell into the substantial band but not into the critical band. Thus the Judge said:

> 'I readily accept that throughout the process the Council was giving consideration to how to address the needs of the disabled. In that sense its decisions taken in relation to adult social care were decisions which were relevant to its performance of the Section 49A duty. That is not the same thing, however, as doing what Section 49A seeks to ensure, namely to consider the impact of a proposed decision and ask whether a decision with that potential impact would be consistent with the need to pay due regard to the principles of disability equality.' (para 179)

5.54 *R (Rajput) v Waltham Forest LBC, R (Tiller) v East Sussex CC* [2011] EWCA Civ 1577, (2012) 15 CCLR 147

Where the potential impact of changes to service provision on elderly and disabled individuals was obvious, as was the justification (a budgetary saving) and decision-makers had been advised of their duty under the disability equality duty and the factual background, and plainly understood them, their balancing of risks and benefits discharged their duty under the disability equality duty, notwithstanding any express reference to the legislation

Facts: the local authorities decided to change the level of provision they made in connection with sheltered housing (East Sussex) and day centres (Waltham Forest). Those decisions were challenged on the basis that the local authorities had failed to discharge their duty under section 49 of the Disability Discrimination Act 1995.

Judgment: the Court of Appeal (Carnwath, Rimer and Jackson LJJ) held that the East Sussex decision-maker had been asked to make a decision whether to reduce service provision for elderly and disabled individuals in order to achieve budgetary savings. All the relevant facts were before him and the risks were obvious. His decision that the budgetary savings were justified did, in the circumstances, discharge his duty under the PSED in substance, despite his failure expressly to refer to the duty and to explain how he had discharged it.

5.55 *R (JM and NT) v Isle of Wight Council* [2011] EWHC 2911 (Admin), (2012) 15 CCLR 167

A flawed consultation resulted in decision-makers having inadequate information about risk and consequently not have 'due regard' to the needs in the PSED

Facts: the Isle of Wight decided to change its eligibility threshold from 'Critical and Substantial' to comprise the high risk needs of persons assessed as 'Critical' and those areas of 'Substantial' needs that placed people at greatest risk of not being able to remain at home and be safe. The Isle of Wight then published a revised risk assessment tool, called 'Eligibility Review'. Two severely disabled adults sought a judicial review.

Judgment: Lang J held that the Isle of Wight's consultation had been flawed in that it failed to inform consultees about such matters as the numbers of service users whose support would be reduced, costs and savings, and what types of services would or would not be included in the new criteria. Consequently, decision-makers were deprived of important information, namely, the responses of consultees on such matters. Accordingly, the Isle of Wight had not ascertained sufficient information so as to discharge the duty of conscientious consideration, entailed by the duty to have due regard to the matters set out in the PSED.

5.56 *R (D, S) v Manchester CC* [2012] EWHC 17 (Admin), (2012) 15 CCLR 603

While the local authority had not undertaken a formal impact assessment, in substance it had discharged the PSED

Facts: Manchester decided to reduce its adult social care budget by £17M over two years and the claimants sought a judicial review, on the basis that Manchester had failed to discharge its duty under section 49A of the Disability Discrimination Act 1995.

Judgment: Ryder J held that Manchester had acted lawfully: it had consulted extensively and taken into account the responses, in particular, of disabled and elderly persons; it had considered the impact of its proposals on such persons and the countervailing factors that justified the course proposed; decision-makers were advised about the PSED; the macro budget was subject to implementation in the light of more specific consultation and further consideration of the PSED in the light of specific initiatives; accordingly, Manchester clearly discharged the PSED, notwithstanding their failure to undertake a formal impact assessment:

> 59. *General*: I have already commented that the budget strategy was as a matter of principle lawful and in accordance with good practice. Save as respects whether due regard was had to the public sector equality duty or rather the DDA 1995 duty, the claimants do not suggest otherwise. Good governance demands that a budget is not only an estimate of planned spending, it is also a projection based upon foreseeable risks which includes a contingency for uncertainties. Where risk assessments are incomplete or inchoate and/or financial circumstances are such that predictions are necessarily less certain, the contingency becomes all the more important. Here it was crucial. Were this not to be the case, budgets of many public bodies

would be impugned by the erroneous elision of uncertainty with unfairness and/or illegality. That is not in any way to suggest that the public sector equality duty or its predecessor do not apply to budgetary decisions: they categorically do, but where flexibility is built into the budget so that subsequent corporate decisions and decisions relating to individuals can still lawfully be made by reference to the potential impact of the proposals on the persons affected then it is possible for the duty to be complied with i.e. there is nothing wrong in principle with such an approach and nothing inconsistent with the duties under the DDA 1995 or the EA [Equality Act] 2010.

60. In this regard I find myself in agreement with Kenneth Parker J in *JG and MB v Lancashire CC* [2011] EWHC 2295 (Admin) at [48] to [51] in particular at [50] albeit in the different factual circumstances of that case:

> 'The economic reality was that to meet imperative needs of reducing expenditure it would be extraordinarily difficult to avoid an adverse effect on adult social care. But there remained flexibility as to how any such effect on disabled persons could be minimised and mitigated ...'

61. I respectfully agree that this view of principle is reinforced by the application of the perspective provided by Ouseley J in *R (Fawcett Society) v Chancellor of the Exchequer* [2010] EWHC 3522 (Admin) at [15] to local government budgets. This was helpfully summarised by Kenneth Parker J in the *Lancashire* case at [52]:

> 'in my view it was sensible, and lawful, for the defendant first to formulate budget proposals and then, at the time of developing the policies that are now under challenge, to consider the specific impact of proposed policies that might be implemented within the budgetary framework.'

5.57 *R (South West Care Homes Ltd) v Devon CC* [2012] EWHC 2967 (Admin)

The PSED was breached by a failure to consider measures of mitigation and of the proper management of risk

Facts: South West, a care home provider, sought a judicial review of Devon's decision as to the standard fees it would pay.

Judgment: Deputy High Court Judge Milwyn Jarman held that Devon was in breach of the PSED:

52. Accordingly the council submits there was sufficient regard to impact on elderly and disabled residents. The Fee Structure Proposal report merely put a figure on the homes which were at risk of closure, a risk which in general terms had already been considered in the EIA [Equality Impact Assessment]. The exercise in which it was engaged did not involve the assessment of needs or the cutting of services or curtailment of choice but merely the calculation of cost.

53. In my judgment that approach fails to have due regard, in substance or with rigour or with an open mind, to the need to eliminate discrimination and to promote equality of opportunity amongst elderly or disabled residents. The council in carrying out this exercise failed to ask itself what it could do in respect of those needs. It is not good enough to say that the needs of individual residents had been or would be assessed under section 47 of the 1990 Act. In particular, even if most if not all homes identified in the Fee Structure Proposal report as at risk of closure would close in any

event, there was no proper consideration of mitigation measures or proper management of such closures in setting the fees. The EIA should have been reconsidered having regard to this information. Having regard to the procedure adopted in the case of the structured closure of one home is not a sufficient regard to deal with this identified risk. Furthermore, there was no proper consideration in my judgment of the staff costs of engaging and interacting with those residents suffering from dementia.

5.58 *R (D) v Worcestershire CC* [2013] EWHC 2490 (Admin), (2013) 16 CCLR 323

Notwithstanding shortcomings in the equality impact assessment and an absence of qualitative and quantative data, decision-makers were informed of the risks and mitigating measures and had in substance discharged the PSED

Facts: in order to achieve necessary budgetary reductions, Worcestershire concluded that, in the absence of exceptional circumstances, it would not pay a sum for home care for an adult under 65 that exceeded the net weekly cost of a care home placement. The claimant, who was significantly disabled, contended that Worcestershire had not consulted properly, or discharged the PSED.

Judgment: in relation to the PSED issue, Hickinbottom J held that since the subject matter was the provision of services to persons with protected characteristics it was likely that Worcestershire had had due regard to the needs of such persons and that, in any event, whilst criticisms could be made of the equality impact assessment, and whilst there was an absence of qualitative or quantative data, the decision-makers had adequate information before them to appreciate how service users might be adversely affected, how the policy sought to address that and the alternative options that had been considered. Hickinbottom J summarised the legal principles in this way:

93. The relevant propositions of law for the purposes of this claim are as follows.

i) Section 149(1) sets out a number of statutory goals, eg the elimination of discrimination and the advancement of equality of opportunity. Section 149(3) sets out sub-goals in respect of the goal of advancement of equality of opportunity, eg the removal or minimisation of disadvantages suffered and the taking of steps to meet the needs of a relevant person. However, the provisions do not impose a duty on an authority to take any particular steps or to achieve any particular result or goal; nor, reciprocally, do they give direct rights to an individual with a protected characteristic. An authority merely has a duty to have due regard to the need to achieve the statutory goals.

ii) 'Due regard' is merely proper or appropriate regard in all the circumstances (*R (Baker) v Secretary of State for Communities and Local Government* [2008] EWCA Civ 141 at [31]).

iii) Determining whether the decision-maker has had due regard to the relevant statutory need or goal is an exercise (a) which is fact-sensitive, being dependent upon all the circumstances of the particular case (*R (Harris) v London Borough of Haringey* [2010] EWCA Civ 703 at [40], and *R (Bailey) v London Borough of Brent* [2011] EWCA Civ 1586 at [75] and [83]); (b) which looks at substance, not form (*R (Domb) v London*

Borough of Hammersmith & Fulham [2009] EWCA Civ 941); (c) for which a mere general awareness of the duty is insufficient: it requires 'a conscious directing of the mind to the obligations' (*R (Meany) v Harlow District Council* [2009] EWHC 559 (Admin) at [74] per Davis J (as he then was), approved in *Bailey*); (d) which requires consideration of specific goals in play and an analysis of the relevant material with those goals in mind (*Harris* at [40]); (e) which requires 'rigour and an open mind' (*R (Brown) v Secretary of State for Work and Pensions* [2008] EWHC 3158 (Admin)) at [92]); and (e) which must be performed before or at the time the particular policy is considered, it being 'an essential preliminary' to any important policy decision not a 'rearguard action following a concluded decision' (*R (BAPIO Action Ltd) v Secretary of State for the Home Department* [2007] EWCA Civ 1139).

iv) If the risk of adverse impact is identified, consideration should be given to measures to avoid that impact before fixing on a particular solution (*R (Kaur) v London Borough of Ealing* [2008] EWHC 2062 (Admin)).

v) The court's role in considering whether the decision-maker has erred in paying due regard to the relevant goals has been the subject of consideration in a number of recent cases, which have tended to consider two options: (a) the court considers whether any regard was taken by the decision-maker, and if so, whether the decision was *Wednesbury* unreasonable; or (b) the court takes it own view of what is due regard in all the circumstances. I am afraid I have found that debate somewhat arid. The law, as I understand it, was set out by Elias LJ in *R (Hurley and Moore) v Secretary of State for Business Innovation and Skills* [2012] EWHC 201 (Admin) at [77]–[78]:

> '77. ... I do not accept that this means that it is for the court to determine whether appropriate weight has been given to the duty. Provided the court is satisfied that there has been a rigorous consideration of the duty, so that there is a proper appreciation of the potential impact of the decision on equality objectives and the desirability of promoting them, then as Dyson LJ in *Baker* (at [34]) made clear, it is for the decision-maker to decide how much weight should be given to the various factors informing the decision.
>
> 78. The concept of 'due regard' requires the court to ensure that there has been a proper and conscientious focus on the statutory criteria, but if that is done, the court cannot interfere with the decision simply because it would have given greater weight to the equality implications of the decision than did the decision-maker. In short, the decision-maker must be clear precisely what the equality implications are when he puts them in the balance, and he must recognise the desirability of achieving them, but ultimately it is for him to decide what weight they should be given in the light of all relevant factors. If [the claimant's] submissions on this point were correct, it would allow unelected judges to review on substantive merits grounds almost all aspects of public decision-making.'

That being a judgment of a Divisional Court, it is binding on me. However, with respect to judges who might have taken a different view from it, in my judgment (a) it is in accordance with principle; (b) it is in accordance with authorities of the higher courts such *Domb* (especially at [72]), *Baker* (at [34]) and *Brown* (at [82]), as well as recent judgments of this court (*R (D and S) v Manchester City Council* [2012] EWHC 17 (Admin) at [52]), and *R (S and KF) v Secretary of State for Justice* [2012]

EWHC 1810 (Admin); and (c) I do not consider that *Meany* (at [72]), which seems to have been used to support an alternative approach (see *JM* at [104] and *Williams* at [18] and [24]–[25]), does, on a proper reading, support any different approach. In my judgment, the exposition of Elias LJ in *Hurley and Moore,* upon which I could not improve and which I gratefully adopt, is clearly correct. It requires the court to consider whether the decision-maker approached the question correctly, in line with the law set out above; but, if he does so, the weight given to the consideration is entirely a matter for him.

…

95. I will deal with those in turn. However, before I do, it is worthwhile marking that this ground is particularly challenging for the claimant for the following reasons (which, in part, reflect the analysis and comments of Davis LJ in *R (Bailey) v London Borough of Brent* [2011] EWCA Civ 1586 at [102] and of His Honour Judge Keyser QC in *R (Copson) v Dorset Healthcare University NHS Foundation Trust* [2103] EWHC 732 (Admin) at [57], for which I am grateful):

i) The claimant has the burden of showing that the relevant public authority has failed to comply with its PSED.

ii) The Policy, which the Cabinet determined should be adopted, was specifically in respect of the provision of services to persons with a relevant protected characteristic (ie disability), and the relevant protected characteristic was the reason for the provision of services to them. Indeed, the very decision for the Cabinet was in relation to the proper balance between a diminution in choice and control of those with the relevant protected characteristic (ie adult community care service users) in favour of a reduction of public expenditure. As Judge Keyser astutely comments, it does not necessarily follow that the Cabinet had due regard to the need to advance equality of opportunity; but the subject matter of the Cabinet's decision makes the claimant's contention that the Cabinet failed to have due regard rather less plausible.

iii) Whether an authority has complied with its PSED is fact-specific. This is not a case where the PSED was simply ignored. As I have indicated (see paragraph 43 above), not only was an EIA commissioned, the Council set up an EIA Working Group to oversee and contribute to the EIA, in the context of the consultation responses, and it met a number times. At each meeting, it considered the requirements of the PSED, and in particular the need to advance equality of opportunity for disabled people. The Council's Equality and Diversity Manager (Ms Sandra Bannister), who was a member of that group, states:

> 'Throughout the decision-making exercise Due Regard was given to the need to advance equality of opportunity…' (26 June 2013 Statement, paragraph 22))

iv) As again referred to in paragraph 43 above, Ms Bannister accepts that the EIA could have been fuller; but (a) an EIA is not a statutory requirement – it is merely a tool whereby decision-makers might inform their efforts to comply with their PSED – and it is thus wrong to subject it to minute forensic or exegetical analysis (see *Domb* at [52] per Rix LJ, *Bailey* at [102] per Davis LJ, and *Copson* at [57(6)] per Judge Keyser); and (b) Ms Bannister considered that, reading all the material the Cabinet had before it, the potential adverse impact for disabled people affected by the policy was clear:

'... a small number of individuals are likely to be adversely impacted by the Policy because it will result in them not receiving their first choice as to provision to meet their eligible needs...'.

v) Although perhaps not a factor of great weight, the Cabinet was concerned that adult community service users aged over 65 were the subject of the additional restriction on community care packages of a usual maximum expenditure not exceeding the equivalent residential care costs; and were concerned that this was unfair as between disabled adults of different ages on the basis of age. That was factor is favour of the Policy.

5.59 *R (Bracking) v Secretary of State for Work and Pensions* [2013] EWCA Civ 1345, (2013) 16 CCLR 479

Owing to a failure to draw the Minister's attention to the possible adverse consequences for disabled persons, and her legal duties under the PSED, the PSED had been breached

Facts: the Secretary of State decided to close the Independent Living Fund (ILF), devolving funding for the purpose of sustaining independent living to local social services authorities. The claimant contended that consultation had been unlawful and that the Secretary of State had failed to discharge the PSED.

Judgment: The Court of Appeal (Elias, Kitchin and McCombe LJJ) held that consultation had been adequate in that consultees had had an adequate opportunity of explaining the likely effect on them of the closure of the fund and it had not been necessary to provide them with financial information about the costs associated with closure of the ILF or to explain more than that the reason for the proposal was to achieve an integrated care system and economies of scale. As far as concerned the PSED, the material presented to the Minister signally failed to draw her attention to the possible adverse consequences for disabled individuals and her legal duties; the majority (Elias LJ dissenting) held that it could not be inferred from the evidence that, nonetheless, the Minister had herself personally appreciated such matters. McCombe LJ summarised the legal principles on behalf of the Court of Appeal at paragraph 25 (set out above at para 5.8).

5.60 *R (T) v Sheffield CC* [2013] EWHC 2953 QB, (2013) 16 CCLR 580

Too fine a level of analysis risks descending into an impermissible appeal of the merits

Facts: Sheffield decided to stop paying subsidies to nurseries in relatively deprived areas where there was little prospect of making up the shortfall from fees charged to parents, so that some of the nurseries might well have to close. A judicial review was brought on the basis that Sheffield had failed to consult lawfully, had not discharged the PSED and had acted unlawfully in other, ancillary ways.

Judgment: Turner J held that Sheffield had acted lawfully. In relation to the PSED, he said this:

55. I am of the view that the defendant in this case fulfilled its duties under section 149. In doing so I bear in mind the observations of the Court of Appeal in *Bailey* in which Davis LJ held at para 102:

'Councils cannot be expected to speculate on or to investigate or to explore such matters ad infinitum; nor can they be expected to apply, indeed they are to be discouraged from applying, the degree of forensic analysis for the purpose of an EIA and of consideration of their duties under s149 which a QC might deploy in court. The outcome of cases such as this is ultimately, of course, fact specific ... All the same, in situations where hard choices have to be made it does seem to me that to accede to the approach urged by Miss Rose in this case would, with respect, be to make effective decision-making on the part of local authorities and other public bodies unduly and unreasonably onerous.'

56. In *R (Greenwich Community Law Centre) v Greenwich London Borough Council* [2012] EWCA Civ 496 Elias LJ held at para 30:

'I would emphasise the need for the court to ask whether as a matter of substance there has been compliance; it is not a tick box exercise. At the same time the courts must ensure that they do not micro-manage the exercise.'

57. In *R (Branwood) v Rochdale MBC* [2013] EWHC 1024 (Admin), Haddon-Cave J remarked at para 60:

'In my judgment, the claimant's argument runs counter to the direction of travel of authorities in this area: which is to discourage challenges based on minute criticisms of EIAs, or elaborate inquisitions of possible permutations of equality ... It is not the law that public authorities must set out s149 verbatim, collect, analyse and record each scrap of data with regard to every single protected group and then analyse each such group *seriatim* against every limb of s149, looking at endless permutations and combinations. A sense of proportionality and reality is required. The basic test is simple: whether 'in substance ... due regard' has been had to the relevant statutory need. This straightforward test should be the touchstone, both for those seeking to fulfil the PSED duties and those seeking to challenge.'

5.61 *R (Michael Robson) v Salford CC* [2014] EWHC 3481 (Admin), (2014) 17 CCLR 474

Some parts of the assessment were not as detailed and rigorous as they could have been but in the round the PSED was discharged

Facts: Salford decided to cease direct provision of transport services in order to achieve budgetary savings. In future, it would make individual transport arrangements for each eligible adult through a variety of different means, such as a 'ring and ride' service, taxis and motability vehicles. The claimants, who were both severely disabled, challenged this decision by way of judicial review.

Judgment: Deputy High Court Judge Stephen Davies dismissed the application for judicial review, holding that there was no evidence that the result of Salford's decision would be that Salford would fail to meet eligible needs for transport and the consultation duty and PSED had been discharged. Deputy High Court Judge Davies said this about the PSED:

62. I was taken by Mr Wise QC and Mr Suterwalla to s149, who emphasised: (1) the mandatory nature of the obligation imposed by the section; (2) the

specific obligation to have due regard to the need to take steps to meet the different needs of (in this case) disabled adults from non-disabled adults and, in particular, to take steps which take account of disabled adults' disabilities. As to point (2), they submitted that this was far from being a vague or a general exhortation, but a hard edged requirement to have regard to the need to identify how the needs of disabled adults differed from those of non-disabled adults and to ascertain what steps could and should be undertaken to meet those needs.

63. I was also referred by them to the decision of the Divisional Court in *Brown v Secretary of State for Work & Pensions* [2008] EWHC 3158 (Admin), where Aikens LJ: (a) held that the obligation to have 'due regard' meant to have proper and appropriate regard for the goals set out in the (predecessor) section [para 82]; (b) held that in order to comply with that obligation it was necessary to have due regard to the need to gather relevant information [para 85]; (c) identified a number of relevant principles as to how that duty should be fulfilled in practice, including a duty to exercise the duty in substance, as opposed to box ticking, with rigour and with an open mind [paras 90–96].

64. I was also referred by Mr Wise QC and Mr Suterwalla to the decision of the Court of Appeal in *R (Bracking) v Secretary of State for Work & Pensions* [2013] EWCA Civ 1345 and, in particular, the eight relevant principles identified by McCombe LJ at para 26 of his judgment. The claimants particularly emphasised: (a) principle 4, the need to assess the risk and extent of any adverse impact and means of elimination before adopting the policy and not as a rearguard action; (b) principle 6, the need to have specific conscious, as opposed to merely general, regard; (c) principle 8, the need for a proper and conscientious focus on the statutory criteria, and the need to make inquiry.

65. Mr Greatorex did not contest these principles. He did however remind me, by reference to these authorities, that it is a duty to have regard, not a duty to achieve a particular result, and that weight was a matter for the decision maker and not the court. He also referred me to the decision of the Court of Appeal in *Bailey v Brent LBC* [2011] EWCA Civ 1586, to the effect that: (a) the decision is a fact-sensitive one [para 83]; (b) s149 does not require the decision maker to speculate, investigate or explore *ad infinitum*, or to apply the degree of forensic analysis which a QC would deploy in court [para 102]. He also submitted that, although recommended as advisable, there was no positive obligation to undertake or to record the result of a formal equality impact assessment, so that I should have regard to the totality of the process, and not limit myself to conducting a forensic analysis of the words used in the impact assessment.

66. Mr Greatorex also submitted that in a case such as the present, which was concerned exclusively with disabled persons, it could not possibly be said that the defendant had overlooked its duty to have due regard to the impact of its decision on disabled persons. Mr Wise QC and Mr Suterwalla countered by submitting that this illustrated the danger of adopting a general approach, as opposed to the focussed rigorous approach which was required, particularly by reference to the need to have due regard to the need to take mitigating steps.

Comment: the Court of Appeal dismissed the ensuing appeal (see below at para 5.64).

5.62 *R (Aspinall and others) v Secretary of State for Work and Pensions* [2014] EWHC 4134 (Admin)

The Secretary of State had clearly demonstrated an awareness of the potential adverse effect on disabled people, of closing the Independent Living Fund and the application for judicial review was a misconceived attempt to persuade the court to engage in micro-management

Facts: following the decision in *Bracking* (para 5.59 above) the Secretary of State for Work and Pensions reconsidered whether to close the Independent Living Fund (ILF) and to transfer funding to local authorities in England and to devolved administrations in Scotland and Wales. Having considered further evidence, the Secretary of State for Work and Pensions decided again to close the ILF. The claimants sought a judicial review on the basis that the Secretary of State for Work and Pensions had failed to comply with the PSED, in particular in that, in making his decision, the Secretary of State for Work and Pensions had not known enough about the likely impact on the 18,000 people who would be affected and/or had not done enough to find out.

Judgment: Andrews J dismissed the application for judicial review, holding that the Secretary of State for Work and Pensions had a clear awareness of the adverse effect on disabled people, that would follow from closing the ILF, and that the application for judicial review was a misconceived attempt to persuade the court to micro-manage the information-gathering aspect of the PSED:

> 16. Mr Chamberlain QC, who appeared with Ms Apps on behalf of the Defendant, submitted that as the duty relating to information is a duty to *'have due regard to the need to take steps to gather relevant information'* and not an independent information-gathering duty, it suffices if the decision maker, having considered the matter, reasonably believes he has sufficient material on which to discharge the PSED. I do not accept that submission, which would lead to the iniquitous result that a decision taken on the basis of inadequate information could be upheld on the basis that a Minister reasonably (but mistakenly) believed he had sufficient information to discharge the PSED.
>
> 17. In *Hurley and Moore*, Elias LJ accepted the submission that the combination of the Tameside principle and the duty of 'due regard' under s149 of the 2010 Act required public authorities to be properly informed before taking a decision. His observation that further information-gathering was unnecessary if the public body *properly* considers that it can exercise its duty with the material it has, must be read in that context. 'Properly' connotes that the public body has sufficient relevant material and therefore does not need to gather more, even if a further consultation or evidence-gathering exercise would result in it being even better informed.
>
> 18. A decision cannot be impugned if it was taken on sufficient information, even if additional relevant information might have been obtained, but the decision maker has taken the reasonable view that such additional information would not materially add to his store of relevant knowledge. That is so even if that view, in hindsight, turns out to have been mistaken. However, if the decision maker is not in fact properly informed, it is no answer to the challenge to say that he reasonably believed that he was. The question whether the information gathered and considered by the defendant was

adequate for the purpose of performing his statutory duty is a matter for the court to decide.

19. In *Hurley and Moore* Elias LJ also made it clear (at [87]) that:

> 'it is quite hopeless to say that the duty has not been complied with because it is possible to point to one or other piece of evidence which might be considered relevant which was not specifically identified in the EIA. I suspect that virtually every decision could be challenged on that basis...'

He specifically endorsed the observations of Davis LJ in *R (Bailey) v London Borough of Brent* [2011] EWCA Civ 1586 at [102] that decision-makers:

> 'cannot be expected to speculate on or to investigate or to explore such matters ad infinitum; nor can they be expected to apply, indeed they are to be discouraged from applying, the degree of forensic analysis for the purpose of an EIA and of consideration of their duties under s.149 which a QC might deploy in court'.

20. In *R (Zaccheus 2000 Trust) v Secretary of State for Work and Pensions* [2013] EWCA Civ 1202, Sullivan LJ endorsed those observations, and those of Underhill J at first instance to the effect that the court is not concerned with a drafting competition. EIAs (Equality Impact Analyses, now known as Equality Analyses or EAs) are not legal documents. Their purpose is to evidence that due regard has been had to the specified factors. Sullivan LJ stated that in almost every case, it would be possible to say that one or more of the specified factors could, with advantage, have been considered in greater detail, but the fact that criticisms can properly be made of an EIA does not mean that the public authority exercising the function will have failed to have due regard to the specified factors [66].

21. In that case, the criticism of the EIA was remarkably similar to that in the present case, in that it was said that no attempt had been made to quantify the impact of the decision (restricting the increases in housing benefit to the consumer price index). The EIA had stated, with reasons, why it was not possible to provide estimates on the distribution of losses because the precise impact depended on various (imponderable) factors including whether landlords decided to restrict rent increases. The Court of Appeal held that the lack of quantification in the EIA did not lead to the conclusion that there was a failure to have due regard to the specified factors. Moreover, although the analysis in the EIA was limited, and more could have been said, the Court of Appeal did not accept that the information which was provided was irrelevant or uninformative.

22. In *R (Greenwich Community Law Centre) v London Borough of Greenwich* [2012] EWCA Civ 496, Elias LJ at [30] held that the court should ask:

> 'whether as a matter of substance there has been compliance; it is not a tick box exercise. At the same time the courts must ensure that they do not micro-manage the exercise.' (emphasis added)

23. The duty to have 'due regard' is not a duty to achieve a result, but a duty to have regard to the need to achieve the relevant goals. As McCombe LJ made clear in Bracking No 1 at [26], citing with approval an earlier passage in the judgment of Elias LJ in *Hurley and Moore* at [77]–[78], the concept of 'due regard' requires the court to ensure that there has been a proper and conscientious focus on the statutory criteria, but if that is done, the court cannot interfere with the decision simply because it would have given a different weight to the equality implications than the decision maker did. The decision maker must be clear precisely what the equality implications are when he puts them in the balance, and he must recognise the desirability

of achieving them, but ultimately it is for him to decide what weight they should be given in the light of all relevant factors.

24. It is of importance to highlight this in the present case, because the decision to close the ILF has understandably engendered very strong feelings among those who may be adversely affected by it. However, no challenge has been made to the Minister's decision on the basis that it was *Wednesbury* unreasonable. It was common ground before me that if the court was satisfied that there was due compliance with the PSED, this claim for judicial review must fail. It is no part of the court's function to express a view as to the quality or correctness of the decision. It can only decide whether the decision was taken lawfully.

5.63 *R (MA) v Secretary of State for Work and Pensions* [2014] EWCA Civ 13, [2014] PTSR 584

The Secretary of State had had regard to the risks to disabled persons and budgetary considerations, he was aware of his legal duties and had, in substance, discharged the PSED

Facts: the Secretary of State for Work and Pensions introduced the 'bedroom tax'. This reduced the amount of housing benefit payable where the number of bedrooms in the property exceeded a permitted number, although discretionary housing benefit might then be received. The scheme posed an obvious risk to disabled adults and children who needed a bedroom of their own, thus taking the household over the bedroom limit (although some provision had been made to mitigate that risk).

Judgment: the Court of Appeal (Lord Dyson MR, Longmore and Ryder LJJ) held that the evidence showed that the Secretary of State was well aware of the serious impact that the bedroom tax might have, that there had been wide consultation, that the Secretary of State had carefully considered the responses, considered mitigating steps and whether more funds could be made available so that, in substance, he had discharged the PSED. Having cited at length from the decision of McCombe J in the *Bracking* case (set out above at para 5.8) Lord Dyson MR said this:

Breach of the PSED

The claimants' case

85 The argument advanced by Mr Westgate (ably supported by Ms Mountfield) is in substance the same as that which was rejected by the Divisional Court. The principal complaint is that the history of the evolution of the policy discloses no focused analysis such as section 149 requires. There was no analysis of disability-related matters. The equality impact assessment of June 2012 did not indicate the numbers of disabled persons with housing needs which would not be met under the new regime.

86. At para 83 of his judgment, Laws LJ set out a number of detailed matters which the claimants submitted the Secretary of State should have investigated. I give as an example: '(e) the ability of disabled people, and of children and their families, to cope with the effects of the Regulation, including difficulties they may face in taking compensatory steps (eg working, taking in a lodger, moving, requesting DHPs)'. At para 86, Laws LJ said that these criticisms were 'an attempt to persuade the court to 'micro-manage' the policy-making process'. They looked very like a list of objections to the policy 'under the guise of a litany of matters left unconsidered. That is all

but an assault on the outcome – the terms of regulation B13 – rather than the process'.

87. Mr Westgate rejects this criticism of his case. He also says that there was no specific consideration by the Secretary of State (or the Divisional Court) of whether the requirements of section 149(1)(b), (3)(a) or (b), (4) or (6) were satisfied. There is no evidence that during the legislative process the Secretary of State even had his attention drawn to his obligation to have due regard to the need to advance equality of opportunity between disabled and non-disabled persons. This is an obligation that is distinct from the obligation to have due regard to the need to eliminate discrimination. The decision-maker cannot give due regard to the need to advance equality of opportunity without having first given informed consideration to what the barriers to equality of opportunity are, and what if anything could be done to address or diminish them. In relation specifically to section 149(6), there was no evidence that the Secretary of State had considered what particular steps he could have taken to meet the needs of disabled persons which were different from those of non-disabled persons.

88. Mr Westgate submits that, even if the minister had a vague awareness that he owed legal duties to the disabled, that would not suffice: see per Elias LJ quoted in the *Bracking* case [2014] Eq LR 60, para 77. The Secretary of State was bound to have due regard to the impact of the proposed scheme on disabled persons who, by reason of their disability, had a need for an additional room.

89, Ms Mountfield also submits that, in relation to the needs of those who were not under-occupying and the extent to which DHPs could prevent or mitigate inequality of opportunity, the Secretary of State failed to conduct a sufficiently focused and evidenced consideration of an obviously relevant statutory equality need. There was no evidence of any contemporaneous regard to the circumstances of those disabled persons who were deemed by the bedroom criteria to be under-occupying, but were not in fact under-occupying for disability reasons. The equality impact assessment stated in terms that the impact of DHPs had not been assessed.

90. Finally, Ms Mountfield submits that the Secretary of State could not lawfully rely on DHPs to solve the problem without conducting a proper analysis of whether local authorities were to be given the means to do so.

Conclusion on PSED

91. I would reject these submissions. I agree that it is insufficient for the decision-maker to have a vague awareness of his legal duties. He must have a focused awareness of each of the section 149 duties and (in a disability case) their potential impact on the relevant group of disabled persons. In some cases, there will be no practical difference between what is required to discharge the various duties even though the duties are expressed in conceptually distinct terms. It will depend on the circumstances. I am not persuaded that on the facts of this case there was any practical difference between what was required by the various duties. I did not understand any such difference to be suggested by Mr Westgate or Ms Mountfield.

92. The history of the evolution of the policy which I have set out at paras 15–36 above shows that the Secretary of State well understood that there are some disabled persons who, by reason of their disabilities, have a need for more space than is deemed to be required by their non-disabled peers. The question of how this special need should be accommodated in the proposed new scheme was the subject of wide consultation of interested parties and considered in great detail by the Secretary of State and Parliament.

The particular issue of whether (i) there should be sub-categories who were to be excluded from the application of the bedroom criteria, (ii) their claims should be dealt with by DHPs or (iii) there should be a combination of these two solutions was considered at great length. So too was the question of whether there would be sufficient money available for DHPs and whether the adequacy of the DHP fund should be kept under review. This was all part of the decision-making process. In my view, it is clear that, in conducting this process, the Secretary of State did have due regard to his statutory duties. It was obvious that he was aware of the serious impact that the bedroom criteria would have on disabled persons who, by reason of their disability, had an actual need for more accommodation than they would be deemed to need by those criteria. That is why so much effort was devoted to seeking a solution to the problem. The PSED challenge is not concerned with the lawfulness or even the adequacy of the solution that was adopted. It is only concerned with the lawfulness of the process. In my view, the process did not breach the Secretary of State's PSED.

5.64 *R (Michael Robson) v Salford CC* [2015] EWCA Civ 6

Notwithstanding imperfections in its approach, viewed more widely, the evidence may show that a local authority had had proper regard to its PSED

Facts: Salford decided to cease direct provision of transport services in order to achieve budgetary savings. In future, it would make individual transport arrangements for each eligible adult through a variety of different means, such as a 'ring and ride' service, taxis and motability vehicles. The claimants, who were both severely disabled, challenged this decision by way of judicial review.

Judgment: the Court of Appeal (Richards and Treacey LJJ, Newey J) dismissed the claimants' appeal from the decision of Deputy High Court Judge Stephen Davies, holding that Salford had not been under a duty to undertake an impact assessment but had done so and had ascertained sufficient information to discharge its duty of inquiry: application for judicial review, holding that there was no evidence that the result of Salford's decision would be that Salford would fail to meet eligible needs for transport and the consultation duty and PSED had been discharged:

38. There is no dispute as to the principles governing the application of section 149. We were referred to a convenient summary at paragraph 26 of the judgment of McCombe LJ in *R (Bracking) v Secretary of State for Work and Pensions* [2013] EWCA Civ 1345, (2013) 16 CCLR 479. Mr Wise pointed in particular to subparagraph (2), where it is said that an important evidential element in the demonstration of the discharge of the duty is the recording of the steps taken by the decision-maker in seeking to meet the statutory requirements; to subparagraph (4), where it is stated that the public authority "must assess the risk and extent of any adverse impact and the ways in which such risk may be eliminated before the adoption of a proposed policy and not merely as a 'rearguard action', following a concluded decision"; and to subparagraph (8), which quotes from the judgment of Elias LJ in *R (Hurley and Moore) v Secretary of State for Business, Innovation and Skills* [2012] EWHC 201 (Admin), [2012] HRLR 13. The quoted passages include these:

'78. The concept of 'due regard' requires the court to ensure that there has been a proper and conscientious focus on the statutory criteria,

> but if that is done, the court cannot interfere with the decision simply because it would have given greater weight to the equality implications of the decision than did the decision maker. In short, the decision maker must be clear precisely what the equality implications are when he puts them in the balance, and he must recognise the desirability of achieving them, but ultimately it is for him to decide what weight they should be given in the light of all relevant factors ...
>
> 89. It is also alleged that the PSED in this case involves a duty of inquiry. The submission is that the combination of the principles in *Secretary of State for Education and Science v Tameside MBC* [1977] AC 1014 and the duty of due regard under the statute requires public authorities to be properly informed before taking a decision. If the relevant material is not available, there will be a duty to acquire it and this will frequently mean that some further consultation with appropriate groups is required. Ms Mountfield referred to the following passage from the judgment of Aikens LJ in *Brown* (para 85) [*R (Brown) v Secretary of State for Work and Pensions* [2008] EWHC 3158 (Admin), [2009] PTSR 1506]:
>
> ... the public authority concerned will, in our view, have to have due regard to the need to take steps to gather relevant information in order that it can properly take steps to take into account disabled persons' disabilities in the context of the particular function under consideration.
>
> 90. I respectfully agree ....'

39. In *Bracking* itself it was held that there was a breach of the duty, essentially because of the absence of hard evidence that the minister had had a focused regard to the potentially very grave impact upon individuals in the relevant group of disabled persons. As McCombe LJ put it at paragraph 63, 'what was put before the minister did not give to her an adequate flavour of the responses received indicating that independent living might well be put seriously in peril for a large number of people'.

40. As to the reference to *Brown* in the passage quoted from *Hurley and Moore*, it is also relevant to note paragraph 89 of the judgment of Aikens LJ in *Brown*:

> 'Accordingly, we do not accept that either section 49A(1) in general, or section 49A(1)(d) in particular, [ie the statutory predecessor to section 149 of the Equality Act 2010] imposes a statutory duty on public authorities requiring them to carry out a formal disability equality impact assessment when carrying out their functions. At the most it imposes a duty on a public authority to consider undertaking an assessment, along with other means of gathering information, and to consider whether it is appropriate to have one in relation to the function or policy at issue, when it will or might have an impact on disabled persons and disability.'

41. The only other authority to which we were referred on the issue is *R (Bailey) v Brent London Borough Council* [2011] EWCA Civ 1586, [2012] LGR 530, especially for the statement of Pill LJ at paragraph 83 that '[w]hat observance of [the] duty requires of decision-makers is fact-sensitive; it inevitably varies considerably from situation to situation, from time to time and from stage to stage'; and the observation of Davis LJ at paragraph 102 that, where the council was fully apprised of its duty under section 149 and had the benefit of a most careful report and impact assessment, it 'cannot be expected to speculate on or to investigate or to explore such matters ad infinitum'.

42. The appellants' essential case is that the Council failed to comply with its legal obligation to gather sufficient information, to analyse the adverse impacts of the closure of the PTU on users of the existing service, and to consider ways in which any disadvantage to them could be mitigated. It is submitted in particular that the Community Impact Assessment was inadequate for the purpose. That document is summarised at paragraph 41 of the judge's judgment. As he states, it begins with a summary and continues in five sections to address what is being impact assessed (Section A), whether an assessment is required (Section B), the results of the consultation (Section C), potential impacts and how they will be addressed (Section D), and an action plan and review (Section E). The judge then sets out what he considers to be the most relevant points from Sections C3, D and E. I will not repeat that material.

…

47. I accept Mr Oldham's submissions. In my judgment the Council did have due regard to the matters identified in section 149 in relation to the disabled adults potentially affected by the decision to close the PTU. That largely follows from the conclusions I have reached on the assessment issue and the consultation issue. Through the carrying out of individual transport assessments and a lawful consultation exercise, it had obtained sufficient information to discharge the duty of inquiry for the purposes of section 149. The information obtained was analysed in the Community Impact Assessment. It may be that the imperfections of that document went even further than was acknowledged by the judge, but in my view he was entitled to find on the basis of the document taken as a whole that the Council had proper regard to the section 149 matters. I do not accept the submission that a greater degree of analysis was required. The judge was also right to look at the matter more widely, as he did in paragraph 71 of his judgment, and to find that in its decision-making process as a whole the Council was evidently aware of the potential adverse impacts on disabled adult service users and was actively considering steps to meet the needs of such persons and to eliminate, reduce or mitigate those impacts. It seems to me that everything the Council did to ensure the discharge of its duty towards those persons under section 2 of the Chronically Sick and Disabled Persons Act 1970 also helped to ensure the discharge of its public sector equality duty towards them. The case advanced by Mr Wise does appear to me to go wider than the relevant ground of appeal but even if the full width of the case is entertained it should in my judgment fail.

5.65 *R (Tilley) v Vale of Glamorgan Council* [2015] EWHC 3194 (Admin)

A failure to discharge the PSED was immaterial in the context of a decision that would not require any particular service being terminated

Facts: Vale of Glamorgan decided, in principle, to close libraries, unless it was possible to develop community-led libraries.

Judgment: Elisabeth Laing J held that, whilst the Cabinet Report had failed to draw attention to the equality impact assessments, or to analyse the potential adverse impacts of library closures, that failure to discharge the PSED did not vitiate the decision, since there had not been an operative decision to close any library and no person had delegated authority to do so. The flaws in the process could be remedied before any closure decision was made.

5.66 *R (Mark Logan) v Havering LBC* [2015] EWHC 3193 (Admin)

The only relief granted would be declaratory, in a case where a lawful EIA had been drawn to the attention of some, but not all, councillors, when the council reached a decision in full council

Facts: Havering decided to replace the previous 100 per cent reduction for those eligible for council tax support because of their lack of resources with an 85 per cent reduction. Mr Logan sought a judicial review claiming, inter alia, that Havering had breached the PSED.

Judgment: the EIA was not defective, but there was insufficient evidence to support the conclusion that due regard was had to the assessment by those who took the decision: the decision was taken by the full council, comprising 54 councillors, but the EIA had not been circulated to all of them. However, the only relief necessary to vindicate the public interest and the claimant's rights was declaratory. On the topic of section 31(2A) of the Senior Courts Act 1981, Blake J said this:

> 55. In my judgment, any consideration of whether the outcome was highly likely to have been substantially the same even if due regard had been had to the PSED should normally be based on material in existence at the time of the decision and not simply post-decision speculation by an individual decision maker. Any other course runs the risk of reducing the importance of compliance with duties of procedural fairness and statutory or other requirements that certain matters be taken into account and others disregarded. Indeed, it would undermine the efficacy of judicial review as an instrument to ensure that the rule of law applies to decision making by public authorities, by deterring claimants from bringing a case or the court from granting permission by a declaration by a decision maker who has failed to obey the law to the effect that obedience would have made no difference. Whatever else Parliament may have intended to achieve by this legislation, I cannot infer that it included so draconian a modification of constitutional principles. It may well be that the new provision was only intended to apply to somewhat trivial procedural failings that could be said to be incapable of making a material difference to the decision made. If recourse can be had to the drafting history and statements of sponsoring Ministers to assess the purpose of the legislation and the mischief to be cured there may be material support for such a conclusion. Such an approach is permissible without impugning Parliamentary privilege where the issues of justification, proportionality and compatibility with European norms are engaged (see for example *Age UK* [2009] EWHC 2336 (Admin) at [42] to [59]).
>
> 56. I recognise that there is evidence at the time of the decision pointing to the proposition that due regard to the PSED by all decision takers would not have made a difference: there was a pressing economic case to increase revenue by reducing the scheme; the cabinet properly advised by its officers after considering all options supported the scheme without any evidence of dissent; there were no dissentient voices in the debate before the full council where the cabinet recommendation was adopted without a division; no council member has stated that he was unaware of the EIA and would have opposed the new scheme if s/he had been.
>
> 57. In the end, I do not propose to refuse relief on the basis of a conclusion that these indicators when taken alongside the other evidence before me made it 'highly unlikely' that the full Council would have done other

than adopt the recommendation of the cabinet. This is because, for other reasons, I have concluded that it is not just and convenient for a formal declaration to be granted to the claimant in respect of this point.

58. At the conclusion of the hearing, I invited the parties to make submissions on whether the terms of SCA 1981 s31(2A) 'any relief' precluded the court giving a declaratory judgment. The defendant was prepared to concede not in this case, whilst reserving the position for the future. I am satisfied that 'relief' in that section must be read alongside the definition of relief set out in section 31(1) that does not include a declaratory judgment and whatever the outcome of the 'highly likely' assessment, permission having been granted there are no restraints on the court delivering its judgment on the issue.

59. Such a course might not have been open, if the debate had been at the permission stage where SCA 1981 s31(3D) precludes the grant of permission 'if it appears to the High Court to be highly likely that the outcome for the applicant would not have been substantially different.' I do not rejoice in the prospect of having to make such assessments in cases like the present at the permission stage. It seems to me to have the potential for increasing the length, cost and complexity of the proceedings and bringing an unwelcome constraint on the court's flexible assessment of the interests of justice. In the absence of clear pointers at the time that the flaw was a technical one that made no difference, the court will inevitably be drawn into some degree of speculation or second guessing the decision of the public authority that has the institutional competence to make it.

5.67 *R (Hawke) v Secretary of State for Justice* [2015] EWHC 3599 (Admin)

Where section 31(2A) of the Senior Courts Act 1981 applies the court may not grant a declaration but it may furnish the parties with a 'declaratory judgment'

Facts: Mrs Hawke, who was seriously disabled, was unable realistically and at proportionate cost, to visit her husband Mr Hawke, who was a prisoner. Mr and Mrs Hawke claimed that the Secretary of State for Justice was acting unlawfully by not detaining Mr Hawke closer to their home.

Judgment: Holman J held that there was negligible, if any, evidence to show that the Secretary of State for Justice had had any real regard to the PSED when formulating the relevant Prison Service Instruction (PSI) or when making decisions about Mr and Mrs Hawke but that, in any event, even if he had done, it was highly unlikely that he would do more than the PSI already provided for, namely, allow for 'accumulated visits'. Accordingly, he applied the new provisions in section 31(2A) and (2B) of the Senior Courts Act 1981:

55. Today Mr Straw has appeared again to present his submissions, as has Ms Slarks to present her contrary submissions. The issue arises from the impact and effect of section 31(2A) and (2B) of the Senior Courts Act 1981 as inserted by the Criminal Justice and Courts Act 2015. These particular inserted provisions took effect from 13 April 2015, which was before the date of commencement of the present proceedings. They provide as follows:

(2A) The High Court–

(a) must refuse to grant relief on an application for judicial review, and

(b) may not make an award under subsection (4) [which relates to damages] on such an application,

if it appears to the court to be highly likely that the outcome for the applicant would not have been substantially different if the conduct complained of had not occurred.

(2B) The court may disregard the requirements in subsection (2A)(a) and (b) if it considers that it is appropriate to do so for reasons of exceptional public interest.'

56. The essential submission of Ms Slarks is that subsection (2A) is directly in point in this case, and that there are no reasons of exceptional public interest such that it may be disregarded pursuant to subsection (2B).

57. It seems to me, first, that the word 'relief' where it appears in subsection (2A)(a) must refer back to the word 'relief' where it appears in subsection 31(1). In that subsection the relevant forms of 'relief' are identified, and they include 'a declaration'. So far as is material to the present case, therefore, it seems to me that I should read subsection (2A)(a) as if it read 'must refuse to grant a declaration ... ' The words of paragraph(a) are of course mandatory and completely binding upon me, if the gateway words at the conclusion of subsection (2A) appear to me to be made out. I have already said at paragraph 47 above:

> 'However neither claimant has suffered any loss as a result, since even if the Secretary of State for Justice or his staff or officials had fully and duly discharged their duties under that section, the outcome would have been, and will still be, the same.'

58. I do not resile in any way at all from what I said in that paragraph. Accordingly, it seems to me crystal clear that it does indeed appear to me to be highly likely that the outcome for the claimants would not have been substantially different if the conduct complained of, namely the failure to have due regard to the public sector equality duty as section 149 requires, had not occurred.

59. Mr Straw seeks to avoid that particular conclusion by arguing as follows (this is in fact the second of his four main submissions today). He says that, bearing in mind the intention of Parliament behind section 149, the duty under that section is a freestanding, explicit statutory duty. He says that it is, or would be, 'an important outcome' for the claimants to establish by declaration that there has been a breach of that duty. With respect to the ingenuity of Mr Straw, however, it seems to me that that particular submission is circular; and if I acceded to it, it would effectively negative the impact and intended effect of section 31(2A), and I do not accept that submission.

60. Mr Straw submits also (this was his first numbered submission today) that section 149 of the Equality Act is an important statutory provision, intended to create a positive duty on public authorities to have due regard to all the matters elaborated in that section. He says that it is important that effect be given to it by making it an 'enforceable duty'. He submits that it would 'emasculate that section' if I declined in the present case to grant a declaration or construed section 31(2A) as preventing me from doing so. I cannot accept that submission either. Of course, I fully accept that the public sector equality duty is a very important statutory duty indeed, bearing down on all public authorities. That, indeed, was made very clear by the Court of Appeal in *Bracking*, if indeed it was not already clear. Even a formal declaration itself is not 'enforceable' against a public authority, and does not give rise to any additional or subsequent remedies. The added provisions in section 31 are recently enacted and appear to me

to be entirely general and unqualified in their reach and impact, subject to subsection (2B). If Parliament had wanted in some way to 'ring fence' the public sector equality duty under section 149 of the Equality Act from the reach and impact of section 31(2A), it could easily have done so by some suitable words of exception. It seems to me, however, that the reach and purpose of the added subsection (2A) is quite clear and is general, and I should not seek to cut down or limit its scope.

61. My attention has been drawn to some words of Blake J in *Logan v London Borough of Havering* [2015] EWHC 3193 (Admin) in which he gave judgment on 6 November 2015. It is clear, however, from paragraph 57 of his judgment in that case that there were 'other reasons' why in any event he concluded that it was not appropriate to make a formal declaration, and accordingly his words are in fact obiter. It is to be noted that in any event he concluded his judgment at paragraph 61 by saying:

> '[The claimant] will obtain no personal benefit from a declaration. Following the grant of permission, a useful public purpose has been achieved for the future, if the defendant accepts the conclusions in this judgment on the requirements to have due regard ...'

62. He thus was making what he had described as 'a declaratory judgment' at paragraph 58 of his judgment, without making any formal declaration.

63. In my view, the facts and circumstances of the present case fall fair and square within the embargo in section 31(2A), subject only to the exception in subsection (2B) to which I now turn. In relation to this, Mr Straw submits that this is a case in which the embargo should be disregarded and that 'it is appropriate to do so for reasons of exceptional public interest'. He stresses, first, the considerable importance of the statutory public sector equality duty. I fully recognise the importance of that duty, but it is only one of hundreds if not thousands of statutory duties upon the whole spectrum of public authorities. There is nothing in fact in section 149 to elevate the public sector equality duty to some specially prestigious position above many other no less important statutory duties upon public authorities. It does not seem to me that there is about the present case some 'exceptional public interest', although there is obviously significant public interest.

64. Mr Straw submits, however, that if the claimants in this case cannot get a declaration then no one can get a declaration who cannot show that the outcome for them would have been substantially different. Essentially, that is the intended purpose and effect of subsection (2A). I agree with him that if my judgment stands, then it may be difficult for individual claimants, who cannot show that the outcome for them would have been substantially different if the conduct complained of had not occurred, to obtain a freestanding declaration that there has been a breach of section 149. That, as I say, appears to me to be the intended purpose and effect of these recently added provisions. But it is not an absolute and inevitable effect. Just to take two possible examples: If even after a 'declaratory judgment' a public authority persisted in failing to discharge its public sector equality duty under section 149, then there may come a time when, on proof of that failure, a claimant may be able successfully to persuade the court that enough is enough and that the exceptional public interest under subsection (2B) has become engaged. Alternatively (without in any way deciding the point), it may be that if a body such as the Equality Commission, which has very express responsibilities in this field, reached a considered decision that a public authority was in such continuing breach of the public sector equality duty that it was necessary to obtain a formal declaration from the court, then such a body may be able to persuade the court that the exception in subsection (2B) is

engaged, even though, by the nature of the body, it would not be able to show that the outcome for it would have been substantially different.

65. So, for these reasons, I am clear, now that it has been drawn to my attention, that section 31(2A) of the Senior Courts Act 1981 does apply in this case and that the exception under subsection (2B) is not established. I am therefore forbidden by statute from granting the declaration which in paragraph 47 above I had previously contemplated granting. The formal outcome of the case will therefore be, not as I expressed it under the heading 'Outcome' in paragraph 48 above, but that the whole of the claim for judicial review is dismissed.

66. I nevertheless conclude this judgment by repeating what I said in paragraph 45 above: that I am not satisfied on the facts and in the circumstances of this case that the Secretary of State for Justice or his officials of staff have given the positive due regard which section 149 of the Equality Act 2010 requires, and on the facts and in the circumstances of this case, there has been a failure by the Secretary of State for Justice to discharge his duties under that section. I intend those words to represent 'a declaratory judgment' of the kind contemplated by Blake J in paragraphs 58 and 61 of his judgment in *Logan*. I am confident that the Secretary of State for Justice or appropriately senior officials will consider and take heed of what I have said.

5.68 *R (DAT) v West Berkshire Council* [2016] EWHC 1876 (Admin), (2016) 19 CCLR 362

A budgetary decision was unlawful because the report to members failed to set out or accurately summarise the PSED but, otherwise, the material before members was lawful

Facts: West Berkshire passed a budget which included reduced funding for its short breaks services.

Judgment: Laing J held that the council had failed to comply with the PSED in one respect but otherwise had lawfully discharged their duty:

35. 'Due regard' is such regard as is appropriate in all the circumstances. Dyson LJ (as he then was) said in *R (Baker) v Secretary of State for Communities and Local Government* [2008] EWCA Civ 141, [2009] PTSR 809 at para 31:

> 'In my judgment, it is important to emphasise that the section 71(1) duty [Race Relations Act 1976 – one of the equality duties which was replaced by section 149] is not a duty to achieve a result, namely to eliminate unlawful racial discrimination or to promote equality of opportunity and good relations between persons of different racial groups. It is a duty to have due regard to the need to achieve these goals. The distinction is vital. Thus the inspector did not have a duty to promote equality of opportunity between the applicants and persons who were members of different racial groups; her duty was to have due regard to the need to promote such equality of opportunity. She had to take that need into account, and in deciding how much weight to accord to the need, she had to have due regard to it. What is due regard? In my view, it is the regard that is appropriate in all the circumstances. These include on the one hand the importance of the areas of life of the members of the disadvantaged racial group that are affected by the inequality of opportunity and the extent of the inequality; and on the other hand, such countervailing factors as are relevant to the function which the decision-maker is performing.'

36. At paragraph 36 of his judgment, Dyson LJ rejected a submission that the inspector's failure to refer expressly to section 71 was decisive (section 71 is one of the statutory predecessors of section 149). He said, at paragraph 37, that the question was whether the duty had been complied with in substance. Just as the repetition of a mantra referring to the provision did not of itself show that section 71 had been complied with, so a failure to refer to the provision did not show that the duty was not discharged. In my judgment this approach was approved by the House of Lords in *R v (McDonald) v Kensington and Chelsea RLBC* [2011] UKSC 33, [2011] 4 All ER 881 per Lord Brown at paragraphs 23 and 24. *Baker* was a case about a decision of a planning inspector, and *McDonald* concerned a local authority's decision to reduce the provision of care to a disabled woman. Neither case, as Mr Broach reminded me, was a challenge to a decision to cut a service which affected many people, but I do not consider that this can undermine the two principles to which Dyson LJ referred.

37. There is an apparent tension, if not a conflict, however, between those two principles and a trend in some of the other cases on the equality duties, exemplified most recently in *R (Bracking) v Secretary of State for Work and Pensions* [2013] EWCA Civ 1345, [2014] Eq LR 60 and in *Hotak v Southwark London Borough Council* [2015] UKSC 30, [2015] 2 WLR 1341. That general trend is to expound principles (often without relevant argument) which impose requirements on public bodies which are not expressly present in the language of section 149. In *Bracking*, at paragraph 25, McCombe LJ (with whom Kitchin LJ agreed) recorded that two lever arch files of authorities had been put before the court, including 13 on the equality duties. 'Fortunately', he said, 'the relevant principles are not significantly in dispute between the parties'. He gave a summary of those principles at paragraph 26 of the judgment. Principle 5(i), for example, that 'The... decision maker must be aware of the duty to have regard to relevant matters' is inconsistent with *Baker*, and to some extent inconsistent with principle 5(iii). Principle 6 '...general regard to issues of equality is not the same as having specific regard, by way of conscious approach to the statutory criteria' is also, on one reading, inconsistent with *Baker*.

38. At paragraph 26(8) the Court of Appeal cited, with apparent approval, paragraphs 77 and 78 of *Hurley*. In paragraph 77 of *Hurley* Elias LJ said, 'Provided the court is satisfied that there has been a rigorous consideration of the duty, so that there is a proper appreciation of the potential impact of the decision on equality objectives and the desirability of promoting them, then, as Dyson LJ in *Baker*... made clear, it is for the decision maker to decide how much weight should be given to the various factors informing the decision'. In paragraph 78, he said, 'The concept of 'due regard' requires the court to ensure that there has been a proper and conscientious focus on the statutory criteria... In short, the decision maker must be clear precisely what the equality implications are when he puts them in the balance....'.

39. In paragraph 60 of *Bracking* McCombe LJ said, 'In the end, drawing together the principles and the rival arguments, it seems to me that section 149 imposes a heavy burden on public authorities, in discharging the PSED and in ensuring that there is the evidence available, if necessary, to demonstrate their discharge. It seems to me to have been the intention of Parliament that these considerations of equality of opportunity (where they arise) are now to be placed at the centre of formulation of policy by all public authorities, side by side with all other pressing circumstances of whatever magnitude'.

40. Paragraph 60 of *Bracking* recognises that there may be circumstances in which the evidence it refers to is not necessary, and that there may be circumstances in which considerations of equality do not arise. These are important provisos. Nonetheless, it seems to me, also, that if and in so far as paragraph 60 suggests that public authorities must give equal weight to equality considerations and to other 'pressing circumstances of whatever magnitude' it is not supported by the language of section 149, and is inconsistent both with the passage from *Hurley* which is cited with apparent approval in paragraph 26(8) of *Bracking*, and with *Baker*. I consider, therefore, that paragraph 60 of *Bracking* cannot have been intended to have that effect.

41. The practical question, or questions, posed by section 149 in relation to a particular decision will depend on the nature of the decision and on the circumstances in which it is made. It is clear from the authorities that the fundamental requirement imposed by section 149 is that a decision maker, having taking reasonable steps to inquire into the issues, must understand the impact, or likely impact, of the decision on those of the listed equality needs which are potentially affected by the decision. On appropriate facts, this may require no more than an understanding of the practical impact on the people with protected characteristics who are affected by the decision (see, for example, paragraph 91 of *R (MA) v Secretary of State for Work and Pensions* [2014] EWCA Civ 13, [2014] PTSR 614, and paragraph 92, 'In my view it was clear that, in conducting this process, the Secretary of State did have due regard to his statutory duties. It was obvious that he was aware of the serious impact of the bedroom criteria would have on disabled people'). Further, where an impact is obvious, as a matter of common sense, but its extent is inherently difficult to predict, there may be 'nothing wrong in making a reasonable judgment and then monitoring the outcome with a view to making any adjustments that may seem necessary: the section 149 duty is ongoing' (per Underhill LJ at paragraph 121 of *R (Unison) v Lord Chancellor (No 3)* [2015] EWCA Civ 935, [2016] 1 CMLR 25.

Discussion

Decision 1

42. I am conscious of the intense pressures, financial, and of timing, to which the decisions 1 and 2 were a response. I cannot ignore the time constraints which affected the Council in making decision 1, given, in particular, the tight framework for making a decision on the budget, the 47 different areas in which cuts were proposed in Phase 1, and the unexpected and late further reduction in Government funding which forced the Council to initiate the Phase 2 consultation. I do not, I hope, understate any of those factors. They are, however, not relevant to the legality issue, in my judgment. The only question on that issue is whether, in substance, members were given the help they needed on the legal issues which they had to consider before making a cut to the funding for short breaks.

43. These factors are relevant to the section 149 issue to some extent, because they are the background against which I must decide whether or not the Council had 'due regard' to the listed equality needs. The local authority context is also relevant to the question of due regard in a further way. The full council, unlike a government minister, is a collective body. It is made up of councillors, who (apart from members of the executive) are not full-time politicians. Those who are not retired, or not in work, often have full-time jobs outside local government. They fulfil important public duties part-time, often at meetings in the evening, often after a full day's work. They are entitled to expect, and very often are given, excellent help

by full-time expert officers to understand the policy and legal issues which will equip them to make lawful decisions. I readily accept Mr Knafler's submission, based on paragraph 36 of the judgment of Baroness Hale in *R (Morge) v Hampshire County Council* [2011] UKSC 2, [2011] 1 WLR 268, that courts should not impose too demanding a standard on officers' reports. Councillors are democratically elected. They do a difficult and at times unpopular job under tight time constraints. Parliament has given them, and not the courts, the job of making difficult decisions such as setting the annual revenue budget for their area. I also accept his submission that officers are entitled, if they can, to simplify and make concrete, for the purposes of the decision at issue, what may be complex legal issues. It may not always help councillors to give them the text of a statute. A pithy summary, if it is accurate, is often much more use.

44. I also accept that Mr Knafler's submissions that the Council discharged the duty of reasonable inquiry imposed by section 149 by consulting with providers and parents/carers, and that the materials provided by officers to members (the summary of the consultation and the collection of the verbatim comments) could, in the circumstances of this case, and given the inherent future uncertainties, and the information gathered by officers from providers, have enabled members to understand the likely practical impact of the cut in funding on parents carers and children. I reject Mr Broach's various submissions, based on a variety of different suggested deficiencies in the gathering and analysis of the relevant information by officers (for example on the question of unmet need), that the material could not have given members the necessary factual understanding. I bear in mind the warning of Laws LJ in *R (MA) v Secretary of State for Work and Pensions* [2013] EWHC (QB) 2213, [2013] PTSR 1521 at paragraph 86, of the dangers of the court 'micromanaging' decision making by public bodies.

45. The difficult question in this case is whether, despite that provision by officers to members of the necessary factual information, the Council failed to have due regard to the listed needs. I am conscious that this is a question of substance, not form. The problem is that while members were given the text of section 149, they were directed, in four places in the documents (in two cases in text adjacent to the recitation of section 149(1)), to the formula to which I have referred above. That would have been fine if the formula accurately encapsulated, for the purposes of the decision about short breaks, the effect of section 149. However, first, the formula is not tailored to that decision, and seems to be a general formula devised for all the 47 decisions. Second, it does not accurately capture the effect of section 149 in the context of that decision.

46. As I have found, members had the factual material which would have enabled them to have due regard to the statutory needs. However, they were directed to look at that material in a way that did not help them to focus on the right question, but, instead, told them to focus on an irrelevant, or at best, only partly relevant, question. Had the report only included the text of section 149(1), it might not have made councillors' lives easy, but I could have been satisfied that they had considered the right question. The flaw in the presentation of the material is that the repeated use of the formula to which I have referred, twice with the text of section 149(1), and twice on its own. That way of presenting the equality issues unavoidably suggests that the formula is equivalent to, or a substitute for, the statutory considerations, and it is not. It does not satisfy me that members asked themselves the right question when they looked at the material officers had so diligently assembled.

CHAPTER 6

Discrimination

6.1 **Introduction and statutory machinery**

Cases

6.10 *Croydon LBC v Moody* (1999) 2 CCLR 92, CA
Psychiatric evidence that there was a real prospect of a tenant's behaviour improving was relevant to whether it was reasonable to make a possession order

6.11 *North Devon Homes Ltd v Brazier* [2003] EWHC 574 (Admin), (2003) 6 CCLR 245
The fact that an eviction would not be justified under the Disability Discrimination Act 1995 was highly relevant to whether it would be reasonable to order possession and, in this case, it would not be

6.12 *Manchester CC v Romano* [2004] EWCA Civ 834, [2005] 1 WLR 2775
A possession order could be granted in favour of a local authority against a disabled secure tenant if the local authority believed it was justified in seeking possession to avoid endangering the health or safety of any neighbours and if it was reasonable in all the circumstances for the local authority to hold that opinion

6.13 *Lewisham LBC v Malcolm* [2008] UKHL 43, (2008) 11 CCLR 573
In this case, the tenant's breach of contract was not caused by his disability; the landlord had not sought possession for a reason connected with his disability and, in any event, he had not been treated differently than a tenant without that disability who had committed the same breach

6.14 *R (Gill) v Secretary of State for Justice* [2010] EWHC 364 (Admin), (2010) 13 CCLR 193
The Secretary of State had unlawfully failed to make reasonable adjustments so that a prisoner with a learning disability could undertake offending behaviour work that was comprehensible and meaningful for him

6.15 *Thomas-Ashley v Drum Housing Association Ltd* [2010] EWCA Civ 265, [2010] 2 P&CR 17
A covenant against keeping pets did not discriminate against a disabled tenant

6.16 *R (McDonald) v Kensington & Chelsea RLBC* [2011] UKSC 33, (2011) 14 CCLR 341
It had been unnecessary explicitly to refer to the disability equality duty when undertaking a community care assessment and it could not be inferred that the disability equality duty had been disregarded

continued

6.17 *Commissioner of Police for the Metropolis v ZH* [2013] EWCA Civ 69, (2013) 16 CCLR 109

The police had failed to make 'reasonable adjustments' by moderating their approach to physical restraint in the case of a young adult who suffered from severe autism

6.18 *Akerman-Livingstone v Aster Communities Ltd* [2015] UKSC 15, [2015] AC 1399

The court should not ordinarily determine summarily a possession claim on disability discrimination grounds that appear to be substantial because, unlike defences under the ECHR, it was not the case that a tenant's rights under the Equality Act 2010 would almost always be outweighed by the landlord's property rights

Introduction and statutory machinery

6.1 Persons with 'protected characteristics' are protected from direct and indirect discrimination.

6.2 The persons subject to protection are those who share the 'protected characteristics' of age, disability, gender re-assignment, marriage and civil partnership[1], pregnancy and maternity, race, religion or belief, sex and sexual orientation (see sections 4–12 of the Equality Act 2010).

6.3 'Direct discrimination' is addressed at section 13:

Direct discrimination

13(1) A person (A) discriminates against another (B) if, because of a protected characteristic, A treats B less favourably than A treats or would treat others

...

(3) If the protected characteristic is disability, and B is not a disabled person, A does not discriminate against B only because A treats or would treat disabled persons more favourably than A treats B.

6.4 This wording is broad enough to cover discrimination against the carer of a person with a 'protected characteristic', where the discrimination is because of that 'protected characteristic'.[2]

6.5 'Disability discrimination' is addressed at section 15:

Discrimination arising from disability

15(1) A person (A) discriminates against a disabled person (B) if –

(a) A treats B unfavourably because of something arising in consequence of B's disability, and

(b) A cannot show that the treatment is a proportionate means of achieving a legitimate aim.

(2) Subsection (1) does not apply if A shows that A did not know, and could not reasonably have been expected to know, that B had the disability.

6.6 'Disability' is defined at section 6, for these purposes, as a physical or mental impairment that has a substantial and long-term adverse effect on a person's ability to carry out normal day-to-day activities. Further provision is made in Schedule 1.

6.7 'Indirect discrimination' is addressed at section 19:

Indirect discrimination

19(1) A person (A) discriminates against another (B) if A applies to B a provision, criterion or practice which is discriminatory in relation to a relevant protected characteristic of B's.

(2) For the purposes of subsection (1), a provision, criterion or practice is discriminatory in relation to a relevant protected characteristic of B's if –

1 However, persons who have the protected characteristic of marriage or civil partnership are only protected in relation to work issues because the parts of the Equality Act 2010 covering services and public functions, premises and education do not apply to those characteristics.

2 See *Coleman v Law* [2010] 1 CMLR 28, [2010] ICR 242 (the protection of the Equal Treatment Framework Directive 2000/78/EC protected from direct discrimination and harassment employees who were not themselves disabled but who were associated with disabled persons (eg where the parent of a disabled child is treated less favourably than other parents of non-disabled children)).

(a) A applies, or would apply, it to persons with whom B does not share the characteristic,
(b) it puts, or would put, persons with whom B shares the characteristic at a particular disadvantage when compared with persons with whom B does not share it,
(c) it puts, or would put, B at that disadvantage, and
(d) A cannot show it to be a proportionate means of achieving a legitimate aim.

6.8 There are many other anti-discrimination provisions, including, in particular, a duty at section 29 on those providing services to the public or exercising a public function to make 'reasonable adjustments', as defined in sections 20–22. The duty to make 'reasonable adjustments' includes the following core definition:

Duty to make adjustments

20(1) ...
(2) The duty comprises the following three requirements.
(3) The first requirement is a requirement, where a provision, criterion or practice of A's puts a disabled person at a substantial disadvantage in relation to a relevant matter in comparison with persons who are not disabled, to take such steps as it is reasonable to have to take to avoid the disadvantage.
(4) The second requirement is a requirement, where a physical feature puts a disabled person at a substantial disadvantage in relation to a relevant matter in comparison with persons who are not disabled, to take such steps as it is reasonable to have to take to avoid the disadvantage.
(5) The third requirement is a requirement, where a disabled person would, but for the provision of an auxiliary aid, be put at a substantial disadvantage in relation to a relevant matter in comparison with persons who are not disabled, to take such steps as it is reasonable to have to take to provide the auxiliary aid.

6.9 Case-law often considers the duty of managers of premises not to discriminate against occupiers, inter alia, by evicting them, in section 35:

Management

35(1) A person (A) who manages premises must not discriminate against a person (B) who occupies the premises –
(a) in the way in which A allows B, or by not allowing B, to make use of a benefit or facility;
(b) by evicting B (or taking steps for the purpose of securing B's eviction);
(c) by subjecting B to any other detriment.

Cases

6.10 *Croydon LBC v Moody* (1999) 2 CCLR 92, CA

Psychiatric evidence that there was a real prospect of a tenant's behaviour improving was relevant to whether it was reasonable to make a possession order

Facts: Croydon brought possession proceedings against Mr Moody as a result of his being a nuisance and annoyance to neighbours. There was evidence from a consultant psychiatrist that that had been caused by a deterioration in Mr Moody's personality disorder, but his condition was susceptible to, and he had agreed to, medical treatment. The recorder rejected the evidence of a psychiatrist and found that Mr Moody had acted deliberately,

Judgment: the Court of Appeal (Evans, Chadwick LJJ) held that the recorder should have taken into account the psychiatrist's evidence because a real prospect of Mr Moody's behaviour improving was relevant to whether it was reasonable to order possession. In addition, it seemed wrong to disregard what consequences would ensue for Mr Moody, if he were evicted.

6.11 *North Devon Homes Ltd v Brazier* [2003] EWHC 574 (Admin), (2003) 6 CCLR 245

The fact that an eviction would not be justified under the Disability Discrimination Act 1995 was highly relevant to whether it would be reasonable to order possession and, in this case, it would not be

Facts: North Devon Homes (NDH) brought possession proceedings against Ms Brazier because of her nuisance towards neighbours: keeping them awake at night by banging and shouting, using foul language and making rude gestures towards them. On the evidence, this was caused by mental illness.

Judgment: David Steel J refused to make a possession order because any eviction would be discriminatory, in breach of section 22 of the Disability Discrimination Act 1995, in that there was no evidence that NDH had ever formed the opinion that Ms Brazier's eviction was necessary in order not to endanger the health or safety of any person and there was no evidence that the nuisance towards the neighbours went beyond discomfort and endangered the health or safety of any person:

> 23. Whilst I accept that fact of unlawfulness under the 1995 Act would not necessarily be determinative of the application under the Housing Act, nonetheless it seems to me that this passage is based upon a misconception. The Act does not bar evictions: only those which are not justified by the specific circumstances set out in section 24. The respondent, having adopted a proper review of the situation in accordance with the express terms of the Act, may conclude in the future that the health and safety of her neighbours are prejudiced and thus steps should be taken to evict the appellant. But this situation has not arisen.
>
> 24. As I see it, the fact that the 'eviction' of the appellant is not justified by the terms of the Act and is thus unlawful is a highly relevant consideration in the exercise of the discretion:
>
> (i) Whilst it may be true that 'the degree of misbehaviour' is significant, without much prospect of it 'abating', the fact remains that the 1995 Act furnishes its own code for justified eviction which requires a higher threshold.
>
> (ii) Against that background, the court is accordingly being invited to exercise its discretion by way of promotion of unlawful conduct: compare section 57.
>
> (iii) Furthermore, the limitations on interference with the appellant's right to respect for her home are set out in the 1995 Act. It is appropriate for the powers accorded by the 1988 Act to be read in a compatible manner: see section 3 of the Human Rights Act 1998.

25. For these reasons, I conclude that it was not appropriate to make an order for possession in this case and the appeal is allowed.

6.12 *Manchester CC v Romano* [2004] EWCA Civ 834, [2005] 1 WLR 2775

A possession order could be granted in favour of a local authority against a disabled secure tenant if the local authority believed it was justified in seeking possession to avoid endangering the health or safety of any neighbours and if it was reasonable in all the circumstances for the local authority to hold that opinion

Facts: Manchester obtained possession orders against two tenants on the grounds of neighbour nuisance. The tenants both suffered from a recognised mental illness and appealed on the basis that their eviction was in breach of the Disability Discrimination Act 1995.

Judgment: the Court of Appeal (Brooke and Jacob LJJ, Sir Martin Nourse) dismissed the appeals, holding that whilst seeking possession was subjecting a disabled tenant to 'any other detriment' within the meaning of section 22(3)(c) of the Disability Discrimination Act 1995, so that if the reason for such action related to the disability of the tenant it would be unlawful unless it could be justified pursuant to section 24(2) of the 1995 Act. When considering whether a landlord's treatment of a disabled tenant was justified under section 24(3)(a) of the 1995 Act the court should ask, first, whether the landlord held the opinion that it was necessary to seek possession in order that the health of an individual person or persons would not be put at risk, and, secondly, whether that opinion was objectively justified by reference to the facts known to the landlord at the time he embarked on the alleged discriminatory treatment. If a tenant could prove that the landlord's conduct in seeking possession amounted to unlawful discrimination that would be a relevant factor when the court was determining, pursuant to section 84(2)(a) of the Housing Act 1985, whether it was reasonable to make an order for possession. In both these cases Manchester had been justified in seeking a possession order so as to protect the health of neighbours:

69. In the present appeals, the council must prove that if it did not take this action someone's health or safety would be endangered. It does not have to prove that that person's health or safety has actually been damaged. The World Health Organisation has since 1948 adopted the following definition of the word '*health*': '*Health is a state of complete physical, mental and social well-being and not merely the absence of disease or infirmity.*'

70. If health is endangered, that state is put at risk. The statute does not use the words '*seriously endangered*', and when interpreting the 1995 Act compatibly with the Convention for the Protection of Human Rights and Fundamental Freedoms scheduled to the Human Rights Act 1998, it is necessary to bear in mind not only the Convention rights of the disabled person but also the Convention rights of his neighbours. It may be useful in this context to compare the evidence given by Mr Schofield, the owner-occupier of the house next door to Ms Romano, with the approach of the Grand Chamber of the European Court of Human Rights in *Hatton v United Kingdom* (2003) 37 EHRR 611.

6.13 *Lewisham LBC v Malcolm* [2008] UKHL 43, (2008) 11 CCLR 573

In this case, the tenant's breach of contract was not caused by his disability; the landlord had not sought possession for a reason connected with his disability and, in any event, he had not been treated differently than a tenant without that disability who had committed the same breach

Facts: Mr Malcolm was a secure tenant of Lewisham but Lewisham brought possession proceedings against him, on the ground that he had sub-let his flat. Mr Malcolm defended proceedings on the basis that he was a disabled person, that the sub-letting flowed from his disability and that it would be incompatible with sections 22 and 24 of the Disability Discrimination Act 1995 to make a possession order.

Judgment: the House of Lords (Lords Bingham and Scott, Lady Hale, Lord Brown and Lord Neuberger: Lady Hale partially dissenting) held that it would not amount to discrimination in breach of the Disability Discrimination Act 1995 to make a possession order against Mr Malcolm, albeit that he was a disabled person: first, on the facts, Mr Malcolm had not sub-let because of his disability; second, the landlord had not sought possession for a reason that related to Mr Malcolm's disability but because he had sub-let his flat; and third, the correct comparator for deciding whether Mr Malcolm had been treated less favourably than others was a person without a mental disability who had sub-let in breach of contract: such a tenant would also have been evicted, so there was no discrimination; fourth, since the landlord had not known of Mr Malcolm's disability, that could not have played a part in the landlord's thinking and statutory discrimination could not have occurred.

Comment: section 15 of the Equality Act 2010 (not in force at the time) requires an adjusted approach, providing that the tenant's actions do, on the facts, stem from their '*disability*' and the landlord knew, or reasonably ought to have known, of the disability: where the tenant's actions arise out of their disability it will be unlawful to treat them unfavourably unless that is a proportionate means of achieving a legitimate aim. That seems to by-pass the need to identify a specific comparator in the way chosen in *Malcolm*: see *Akerman-Livingstone v Aster Communities Ltd*, below at para 6.18.[3]

6.14 *R (Gill) v Secretary of State for Justice* [2010] EWHC 364 (Admin), (2010) 13 CCLR 193

The Secretary of State had unlawfully failed to make reasonable adjustments so that a prisoner with a learning disability could undertake offending behaviour work that was comprehensible and meaningful for him

Facts: Mr Gill was a life-sentence prisoner who had served more than twice his tariff. The Parole Board was unwilling to direct his release or recommend transfer to open conditions until he had completed offending behaviour programmes. However, having a learning disability, Mr Gill had been unable to complete such programmes.

3 [2015] UKSC 15, [2015] 2 WLR 721.

Judgment: Cranston J allowed Mr Gill's application for judicial review, holding that:

1) Applying the approach identified by Blake J in *R (Lunt) v Liverpool City Council* [2009] EWHC 2356 (Admin):

> i) The Secretary of State has policies, practices and procedures regarding access to offender behaviour programmes;
> ii) Those policies, practices and procedures include a statement that IQ in the region of 80 or below may prevent meaningful engagement with the material in a programme, and this makes it difficult or impossible for inmates with a learning disability like the claimant's to make use of the offending behaviour work within the same period as other prisoners. The claimant has been prevented from making use of offending behaviour courses because of his learning disability;
> iii) Therefore the Secretary of State came under a duty to take such steps as were reasonable in all the circumstances to change those practices so that the claimant could access offending behaviour work in the same way as prisoners who are not disabled;
> iv) The Secretary of State has failed to take such steps and to consider what steps could be taken, including for instance alternative means of enabling the claimant to undertake offending behaviour work, additional aids and services, or transfer;
> v) The failure is not justified. It is no answer to raise the spectre of ruinous costs if the Secretary of State had to offer adapted courses to all prisoners with limited intellectual abilities. This case is concerned with this particular claimant.

2) The Secretary of State had failed, without good reason, to comply with his own policies regarding completion of offending behaviour work, and making reasonable adjustments for prisoners with disabilities.

3) *(Obiter)* The issue in this case concerns a purely governmental function, the continued detention of the claimant, and is not concerned with the provision of a service within section 19 of the Disability Discrimination Act 1995.

6.15 *Thomas-Ashley v Drum Housing Association Ltd* [2010] EWCA Civ 265, [2010] 2 P&CR 17

A covenant against keeping pets did not discriminate against a disabled tenant

Facts: Ms Thomas-Ashley kept a dog in breach of her tenancy agreement. The dog caused a nuisance by barking and the landlord brought possession proceedings. Ms T-A's defence was that she suffered from bi-polar mood disorder, her dog was critical to her health and the possession proceedings discriminated against her on the ground of disability, in breach of sections 24A and 24D the Disability Discrimination Act 1995.

Judgment: the Court of Appeal (The Chancellor, Thomas LJ and Sir Scott Baker) held that the covenant against keeping animals did not discriminate against Ms T-A on account of her disability or make it unreasonably difficult for her to enjoy the premises; in addition, it would be unreasonable to expect Ms T-A's landlord to remove that covenant because, if he did so, his own lease would become liable to forfeiture.

6.16 *R (McDonald) v Kensington & Chelsea RLBC* [2011] UKSC 33, (2011) 14 CCLR 341

It had been unnecessary explicitly to refer to the disability equality duty when undertaking a community care assessment and it could not be inferred that the disability equality duty had been disregarded

Facts: Ms McDonald had limited mobility and a small, neurogenic bladder, which caused her to have to urinate several times a night. Kensington initially provided Ms McDonald with a commode and a night-time carer. It then assessed her need using different language, as being for incontinence pads and absorbent sheets. Ms McDonald sought a judicial review.

Judgment: the Supreme Court (Walker, Hale, Brown, Kerr and Dyson JJSC, Hale JSC dissenting) held that (i) Kensington's decision was not a practice, policy or procedure for the purposes of section 21 of the Disability Discrimination Act 1995 and even if it was, it was justified:

> 21. Mr Cragg's argument under these provisions, if I understand it, is that, in substituting incontinence pads for a night-time carer to meet the appellant's night-time toileting need, the respondents are manifesting or applying:
>
> > 'a practice, policy or procedure which makes it: (a) impossible or unreasonably difficult for disabled persons to receive any benefit that is or may be conferred, or (b) unreasonably adverse for disabled persons to experience being subjected to any detriment to which a person is or may be subjected, by the carrying-out of a function by the authority'
>
> within the meaning of section 21E(1), so that, as provided by section 21E(2), it is their duty 'to take such steps as it is reasonable, in all the circumstances of the case, for the authority to have to take in order to change that practice, policy or procedure so that it no longer has that effect'. If that be right, then, by virtue of section 21D(2)(a) and 21B(1), a failure to comply with that duty constitutes unlawful discrimination by the respondents against the appellant unless the respondents can show pursuant to section 21D(2)(b) that this failure is justified under section 21D(5), namely that its acts are 'a proportionate means of achieving a legitimate aim'.
>
> 22. The argument to my mind is hopeless. In the first place I find it impossible to regard the respondents' decision in this case as the manifestation or application of anything that can properly be characterised as a 'practice, policy or procedure' within the meaning of this legislation. Rather, in taking the impugned decision, the respondents were doing no more and no less than their statutory duty as fully described under issue one above. Secondly, even were that not so, it follows from all that I have already said (not least with respect to Article 8.2) that the respondents' acts here must be regarded as constituting 'a proportionate means of achieving a legitimate aim' within the meaning of section 21D(5) (even assuming that there were otherwise steps which it would have been reasonable for them to take to change their practice, policy or procedure within the meaning of section 21E(2)). Here again, therefore, I agree with the views of the court below except only that, whereas Rix LJ was merely 'sceptical as to whether any relevant policy or practice for the purposes of section 21E(1) exists in this case' (para 73), I am clear that it does not.

6.17 *Commissioner of Police for the Metropolis v ZH* [2013] EWCA Civ 69, (2013) 16 CCLR 109

The police had failed to make 'reasonable adjustments' by moderating their approach to physical restraint in the case of a young adult who suffered from severe autism

Facts: ZH, who suffered from severe autism, epilepsy and learning disabilities, became fixated by the water at a local swimming pool and would not move away from the poolside. His carers knew that if he was touched he might jump into the pool. The swimming pool manager called the police who after a brief conversation with the carers, established that ZH was autistic, went up to him and touched him. ZH then jumped into the pool (he was fully clothed at the time). The police then pulled ZH out of the pool and restrained him before taking him, soaking wet and agitated, to the police station. ZH sued.

Judgment: the Court of Appeal (Lord Dyson MR, Richards and Black LJJ) held that the first instance judge had been entitled to conclude that the police had breached ZH's rights under Articles 3, 5 and 8 ECHR, and that they were guilty of assault and false imprisonment and a breach of section 21B of the Disability Discrimination Act 1995. The police defence under the Mental Capacity Act 2005 failed: while sections 4–6 of that Act permitted certain acts to be done in connection with the care and treatment of persons lacking capacity if it is in their best interests, those statutory defences were pervaded by concepts of reasonableness, practicability and appropriateness, which were lacking in this case: the police could and should have consulted with ZH's carers about how best to handle him and could not have had a reasonable belief that their actions were in his best interests:

> 61. The judge first dealt with the reasonable adjustments pleaded at para 33 (i), (ii) and (vi) which all related to consulting the carers. He concluded that it was 'practicable and appropriate, indeed essential, that the police informed themselves properly before taking any action which led to the application of force on [ZH]' (para 134). In effect, he repeated what he had said earlier in relation to the MCA issues. Importantly, he rejected the defence submission that (i) there was no evidence that the police intended to restrain ZH in advance of his coming out of the water and (ii) it was not reasonable to expect the officers to consult the carers beforehand (para 135). He said:
>
> > 'The duty to consult the carers arose from the outset, and the duty to make reasonable adjustments was a continuing obligation throughout. In any event, as I have found, the police did decide, by means of a very brief discussion, to lift ZH from the water to the poolside leading as was entirely foreseeable, to virtually immediate restraint.'
>
> 62. The judge also accepted ZH's case on each of the other pleaded reasonable adjustments and rejected in its entirety the plea of justification. As regards justification, he held that it was not necessary in order to avoid endangering the health or safety of anyone (including ZH) to have carried on without seeking information and advice from the carers.
>
> …

67. I do not find it necessary to make detailed observations as to the scope of the duty to make reasonable adjustments. What is reasonable will depend on the facts of the particular case. Section 21E(2) states in terms that it is the duty of the authority to take such steps as it is reasonable *in all the circumstances of the case* to have to make to change the practice, policy or procedure so that (relevantly for the present case) it no longer has detrimental effect. I accept that police officers are not required to make medical diagnoses. They are not doctors. But the important feature of the present case is that, even before they restrained ZH, they knew that he was autistic and epileptic. They knew (or ought to have known) that autistic persons are vulnerable and have limited understanding. Further, I see no basis for holding that the duty to make reasonable adjustments is not a continuing duty. In my view, the judge was entitled to reach the conclusion that he did on this issue. It was a decision on the particular facts of this case. I reject the submission that his decision makes practical policing unduly difficult or impossible.

6.18 *Akerman-Livingstone v Aster Communities Ltd* [2015] UKSC 15, [2015] AC 1399

The court should not ordinarily determine summarily a possession claim on disability discrimination grounds that appear to be substantial because, unlike defences under the ECHR, it was not the case that a tenant's rights under the Equality Act 2010 would almost always be outweighed by the landlord's property rights

Facts: Mr Akerman-Livingstone had a severe distress disorder and defended possession proceedings on the basis that they involved discrimination against him on the ground of his disability, contrary to section 15 of the Equality Act 2010. The county court judge made a possession order on the basis that such a defence fell to be considered in the same way as a defence under Article 8 ECHR, ie with the effect that a possession order would almost always be a proportionate means of achieving the twin aims of vindicating the local authority's property rights and enabling the authority to comply with its statutory duties in the allocation and management of its housing stock. He concluded that the defendant did not have a seriously arguable case and that there was no need for a full trial, so he made the possession order. A High Court judge and the Court of Appeal dismissed the defendant's appeals.

Judgment: the Supreme Court (Neuberger, Hale, Clarke, Wilson and Hughes JJSC) held that because of various recent factual developments in the case, a trial judge would be bound to conclude that a possession order would be proportionate. However, the substantive right to equal treatment protected by section 35(1)(b) of the Equality Act 2010 was different from and stronger than the rights protected by Article 8 ECHR; once the possibility of disability discrimination was made out, the burden was on the landlord to show that there was no unfavourable treatment because of something arising in consequence of the tenant's disability contrary to section 15(1)(a), or that an order for possession was a proportionate means of achieving a legitimate aim under section 15(1)(b); that it could not be taken for granted that the aim of vindicating the landlord's property rights would almost always prevail over a tenant's right to have due allowances made for the consequences of his disability; that where social housing was involved the aim of enabling the local authority to comply with its statutory housing duties might have to give way to the equality rights of a particular disabled person; that, therefore, although such a claim could be dealt with summarily under CPR 55.8(1), that would not normally be an appropriate course if the claim were genuinely disputed on grounds which appeared to be substantial, where disclosure or expert evidence might be required; and that, accordingly, the judge in the county court had misdirected himself in his approach to the claim for possession.

Part II

CHAPTER 7

An overview of the Care Act 2014 and the Social Services and Well-being (Wales) Act 2014

The Care Act 2014

Introduction

7.1 Adult social care in England is now largely governed by the Care Act 2014. The preamble to the Act describes it as:

> An Act to make provision to reform the law relating to care and support for adults and the law relating to support for carers; to make provision about safeguarding adults from abuse or neglect; to make provision about care standards; to establish and make provision about Health Education England; to establish and make provision about the Health Research Authority; to make provision about integrating care and support with health services; and for connected purposes.

7.2 The Care Act 2014 is accompanied by a detailed Explanatory Note,[1] which provides a useful overview of its content. In short:

- Part 1 of the Care Act 2014 sets out the general responsibilities of local authorities for care and support, and safeguarding, in relation to adults, carers and children becoming adults. Some sections came into force on the 1 October 2014 (eg for the purpose of allowing regulations to be made) but most of Part 1 came into force on the 1 April 2015. A few provisions are not yet in force, at all or fully, most notably those relating to the cap on care costs based on sections 15 and 16;
- Part 2 makes further provision in relation to care standards and the work of the Care Quality Commission. Some sections came into force on the 1 October 2014 (eg for the purpose of allowing regulations to be made) but most of Part 2 came into force on the 1 April 2015;
- Part 3 deals with health care and sets up Health Education England, Local Education and Training Boards and the Health Research Authority. It also makes provision for further integration of health and social care. Again, some sections came into force on the 1 October 2014 (eg for the purpose of allowing regulations to be made), but most of Part 3 came into force on the 1 April 2015.

Key terms

7.3 The Care Act 2014 applies to:

- an 'adult', defined at section 2(8) as 'a person aged 18 or over'; and
- a 'carer', defined in section 10(3) as 'an adult who provides or intends to provide care for another adult', which includes 'providing practical or emotional support' (section 10(11));
- a 'child ... likely to have needs for care and support after becoming 18' (section 58);
- a 'child's carer', defined as 'an adult (including one who is a parent of the child) who provides or intends to provide care for the child [otherwise than under a contract or as voluntary work]' (section 60);

1 Explanatory Notes are admissible aids to the construction of legislation: see *R v Montila* [2004] UKHL 50, [2001] 1 WLR 3141 at paras 32–36.

- a 'young carer', defined as 'a person under 18 who provides or intends to provide care for an adult [otherwise than under a contract or as voluntary work]' (section 63(6).

7.4 'A child', 'child's carer' and 'young carer' are considered below under 'children in transition' at para 8.25 onwards.

The well-being duty

Section 1(1)

7.5 Section 1(1) imposes a general duty on local authorities: 'the general duty of a local authority, in exercising a function under this Part in the case of an individual, is to promote that individual's well-being'.

7.6 As to the 'functions' exercisable under Part 1 of the Act, '"functions" embraces all the duties and powers of a local authority; the sum total of the activities Parliament has entrusted to it. Those activities are its functions': *Hazell v Hammersmith & Fulham LBC.*[2]

7.7 Clause 1(1) of the Care Bill had referred to 'adults' and the change of focus to 'individuals' makes it plain that both 'adults' and 'carers' are within the scope of section 1.

7.8 The expression 'general duty' was considered in *R (G) v Barnet LBC*,[3] for the purposes of section 17 of the Children Act 1989 which states:

> 17(1) It shall be the general duty of every local authority (in addition to the other duties imposed on them by this Part)–
> (a) to safeguard and promote the welfare of children within their area who are in need; and
> (b) so far as is consistent with that duty, to promote the upbringing of such children by their families, by providing a range and level of services appropriate to those children's needs.

On behalf of the majority, Lord Hope said:

> 91. I think that the correct analysis of section 17(1) is that it sets out duties of a general character which are intended to be for the benefit of children in need in the local social services authority's area in general. The other duties and the specific duties which then follow must be performed in each individual case by reference to the general duties which section 17(1) sets out. What the subsection does is to set out the duties owed to a section of the public in general by which the authority must be guided in the performance of those other duties ...
>
> As Mr Goudie for the defendants accepted, members of that section of the public have a sufficient interest to enforce those general duties by judicial review. But they are not particular duties owed to each member of that section of the public of the kind described by Lord Clyde in *R v Gloucestershire County Council ex p Barry* [1997] AC 584, 610 which give a correlative right to the individual which he can enforce in the event of a failure in its performance.

7.9 The purpose of section 1(1) is to define the purpose of the legislation, by making it clear that 'the well-being of the individual is paramount and that local authorities must promote the individual's well-being in decisions

2 [1992] 2 AC 1 at 29F.
3 [2003] UKHL 57, [2004] 2 AC 208.

made with and about them. These principles (found in section 1 as a whole) implement the Law Commission's recommendation for a 'single unifying purpose around which adult social care is organised' (para 3.7 of the *Draft Care and Support Bill*).[4]

7.10 The importance of giving effect to the statutory purpose was underlined by Laws J in *R v Somerset CC ex p Fewings*:[5]

> ... where a statute does not by express words define the purposes for which the powers it confers are to be exercised, the decision-maker is bound nevertheless to ascertain and apply the aims intended, since no statute can be purposeless: and therefore unless the Act's true purpose is correctly understood the decision-maker, who is Parliament's delegate, is at risk of using powers to an end for which they were never given him. If he does so, he exceeds his authority as surely as if he transgresses the plainest statutory language ...

7.11 The *Care and Support Statutory Guidance* addresses the well-being duty at Chapter 1. It explains the purpose of the well-being principle as being to place the individual at the heart of the assessment and planning process:

> 1.7 Promoting wellbeing involves actively seeking improvements in the aspects of wellbeing set out above when carrying out a care and support function in relation to an individual at any stage of the process from the provision of information and advice to reviewing a care and support plan. Wellbeing covers an intentionally broad range of the aspects of a person's life and will encompass a wide variety of specific considerations depending on the individual.
>
> 1.8 A local authority can promote a person's wellbeing in many ways. How this happens will depend on the circumstances, including the person's needs, goals and wishes, and how these impact on their wellbeing. There is no set approach – a local authority should consider each case on its own merits, consider what the person wants to achieve, and how the action which the local authority is taking may affect the wellbeing of the individual.
>
> 1.9 The Act therefore signifies a shift from existing duties on local authorities to provide particular services, to the concept of 'meeting needs' (set out in sections 8 and 18–20 of the Act). This is the core legal entitlement for adults to care and support, establishing one clear and consistent set of duties and power for all people who need care and support.

7.12 The word 'promote' in section 1(1) suggests that, while the advancement of well-being is of great importance, there can be countervailing considerations.

7.13 The possibility of countervailing considerations is recognised in case-law in similar contexts, for example, under section 17 of the Children Act 1989, where there is a general duty to 'promote' the welfare of children in need; under section 55 of the Borders, Citizenship and Immigration Act 2009, where there is a duty to exercise immigration functions having regard to the need to 'promote' the welfare of children in the United Kingdom; and under section 1 of the National Health Service Act 2006, where there is a duty to continue to 'promote' a comprehensive health service.

4 Presented to Parliament by the Secretary of State for Health by Command of Her Majesty, July 2012, The Stationery Office, Cm 8386.

5 [1995] 1 All ER 513 at 524H–525C.

7.14 One major countervailing consideration is expressly set out in the Act: the duty to promote well-being is not of limitless consequence because, by virtue of sections 13 and 18 of the Act, the duty to meet needs only extends to those needs for care and support that are assessed as meeting the eligibility criteria. In other cases, the Act empowers local authorities to provide services. Section 1 applies to the exercise of that power, and will require serious consideration of the matters set out at sections 1(1), (2) and (3), but will not convert it into a duty or require local authorities to disregard the reason why the eligibility criteria exist, which is to achieve an equitable distribution of the bulk of the resources expected to be available.

7.15 Otherwise, leaving aside resources, the general tenor of section 1 seems to indicate that local authorities should not be astute to identify countervailing considerations that justify failing to make provision that promotes the individual's well-being to the fullest possible extent.

7.16 Many parts of the statutory machinery expressly invoke the well-being principle, most notably the Care and Support (Eligibility Criteria) Regulations 2015:[6]

> **Needs which meet the eligibility criteria: adults who need care and support**
>
> **2**(1) An adult's needs meet the eligibility criteria if–
> (a) the adult's needs arise from or are related to a physical or mental impairment or illness;
> (b) as a result of the adult's needs the adult is unable to achieve two or more of the outcomes specified in paragraph (2); and
> (c) as a consequence there is, or is likely to be, a significant impact on the adult's well-being.

Section 1(2)

7.17 'Well-being' has an extended definition, at section 1(2):

> **1**(2) 'Well-being', in relation to an individual, means that individual's well-being so far as relating to any of the following–
> (a) personal dignity (including treatment of the individual with respect);
> (b) physical and mental health and emotional well-being;
> (c) protection from abuse and neglect;
> (d) control by the individual over day-to-day life (including over care and support, or support, provided to the individual and the way in which it is provided);
> (e) participation in work, education, training or recreation;
> (f) social and economic well-being;
> (g) domestic, family and personal relationships;
> (h) suitability of living accommodation;
> (i) the individual's contribution to society.

7.18 The consequence of section 1(2) would seem to be that the factors enumerated have become statutorily relevant considerations, such that a failure to have regard to any one of them will result in a decision being amenable to judicial review, at least if the consideration was material, on the facts, on the ground that there has been a failure to have regard to a relevant consideration (in accordance with the usual principle, that 'if the [public

6 SI No 313.

authority] takes into account matters irrelevant to his decision or refuses or fails to take account of matters relevant to his decision ... the court may set his decision aside': *R (Alconbury Developments Limited) v Secretary of State for the Environment, Transport and the Regions*.[7]

Conclusion on the well-being duty in section 1

7.19 The general thrust of sections 1(1) and (2), is that local authorities are to adopt a holistic approach and promote the well-being of the individual as a whole, in ways that range from protecting him from abuse or neglect to promoting his participation in work and recreation and his social and economic well-being; from promoting his well-being in domestic, family and personal relationships, to enhancing his contribution to society.

7.20 These provisions afford a guiding vision of what it is to be an individual, for these purposes, and of the required relationship between the local authority and the individual. The individual is to be seen, as far as possible, as being autonomous, unique and expansive in their interests. The local authority should, as far as possible, place the individual and their views at the heart of the social care process.

7.21 Although directed at the welfare of children, rather than the well-being of adults, the judgment of Lord Justice Munby on behalf of the Court of Appeal in *Re G (Children)*[8] is relevant in this context:

> 25. If then the welfare of the child is paramount, two obvious questions arise: first, what do we mean by welfare; and, second, by reference to what standard or yardstick is welfare to be assessed?
>
> 26. 'Welfare', which in this context is synonymous with 'well-being' and 'interests' (see Lord Hailsham LC *in In re B (A Minor) (Wardship: Sterilisation)* [1988] AC 199, 202), extends to and embraces everything that relates to the child's development as a human being and to the child's present and future life as a human being. The judge must consider the child's welfare now, throughout the remainder of the child's minority and into and through adulthood. The judge will bear in mind the observation of Sir Thomas Bingham MR in *Re O (Contact: Imposition of Conditions)* [1995] 2 FLR 124, 129, that:
>
>> 'the court should take a medium-term and long-term view of the child's development and not accord excessive weight to what appear likely to be short-term or transient problems.'
>
> That was said in the context of contact but it surely has a wider resonance. How far into the future the judge must peer – and with modern life expectancy a judge dealing with a young child today may be looking to the 22nd century – will depend upon the context and the nature of the issue. If the dispute is about whether the child should go on a school trip the judge will be concerned primarily with the present rather than the future. If the question is whether a teenager should be sterilised the judge will have to think a very long way ahead indeed.
>
> 27. In *Re McGrath (Infants)* [1893] 1 Ch 143, 148, Lindley LJ said:
>
>> 'The dominant matter for the consideration of the court is the welfare of the child. But the welfare of a child is not to be measured by money only, nor by physical comfort only. The word welfare must be taken in

7 [2001] UKHL 23, [2003] 2 AC 295 at para 10.
8 [2012] EWCA Civ 1233, [2013] ELR 25.

its widest sense. The moral and religious welfare of the child must be considered as well as its physical well-being. Nor can the ties of affection be disregarded.'

Those words are as true today as a century ago. Evaluating a child's best interests involves a welfare appraisal in the widest sense, taking into account, where appropriate, a wide range of ethical, social, moral, religious, cultural, emotional and welfare considerations. Everything that conduces to a child's welfare and happiness or relates to the child's development and present and future life as a human being, including the child's familial, educational and social environment, and the child's social, cultural, ethnic and religious community, is potentially relevant and has, where appropriate, to be taken into account. The judge must adopt a holistic approach. As Thorpe LJ once remarked (*In re S (Adult Patient: Sterilisation)* [2001] Fam 15, 30), 'it would be undesirable and probably impossible to set bounds to what is relevant to a welfare determination.'

28. To this I would add two points.

29. I have referred to the child's happiness. Very recently, Herring and Foster have argued persuasively (*'Welfare means rationality, virtue and altruism'*, (2012) 32 Legal Studies 480), that behind a judicial determinations of welfare there lies an essentially Aristotelian notion of the *'good life'*. What then constitutes a *'good life'*? There is no need to pursue here that age-old question. I merely emphasise that happiness, in the sense in which I have used the word, is not pure hedonism. It can include such things as the cultivation of virtues and the achievement of worthwhile goals, and all the other aims which parents routinely seek to inculcate in their children.

30. I have also referred to the child's familial, educational and social environment, and his or her social, cultural, ethnic and religious community. The well-being of a child cannot be assessed in isolation. Human beings live within a network of relationships. Men and women are sociable beings. As John Donne famously remarked, '*No man is an Island* ...' Blackstone observed that 'Man was formed for society'. And long ago Aristotle said that 'He who is unable to live in society, or who has no need because he is sufficient for himself, must be either a beast or a God'. As Herring and Foster comment, relationships are central to our sense and understanding of ourselves. Our characters and understandings of ourselves from the earliest days are charted by reference to our relationships with others. It is only by considering the child's network of relationships that their well-being can be properly considered. So a child's relationships, both within and without the family, are always relevant to the child's interests; often they will be determinative.

31. I should add that there has been no suggestion in the present case that the interests of any of the five children with whom we are concerned are or may be in conflict with the interests of any of the others. We are therefore not concerned with the point about the application of section 1(a) of the 1989 Act in such a situation which, although raised before them, their Lordships avoided deciding in *Birmingham City Council v H (A Minor)* [1994] 2 AC 212 but which the lower courts have had to consider on a number of occasions: see *Birmingham City Council v H (No 2)* [1993] 1 FLR 883, *Re T and E (Proceedings: Conflicting Interests)* [1995] 1 FLR 581, *In re A (Children) (Conjoined Twins: Surgical Separation)* [2001] Fam 147, and *Re S (Relocation: Interests of Siblings)* [2011] EWCA Civ 454, [2011] 2 FLR 678.

32. So much for welfare, how is it to be assessed? The answer was provided by Lord Upjohn in *J v C* [1970] AC 668, 722:

'the law and practice in relation to infants ... have developed, are developing and must, and no doubt will, continue to develop by reflecting and adopting the changing views, as the years go by, of reasonable men and women, the parents of children, on the proper treatment and methods of bringing up children; for after all that is the model which the judge must emulate for ... he must act as the judicial reasonable parent.'

33. Lord Upjohn's reference to changing views is crucial. The concept of welfare is, no doubt, the same today as it was in 1925, but conceptions of that concept, to adopt the terminology of Professor Ronald Dworkin, or the content of the concept, to adopt the corresponding terminology of Lord Hoffmann (*see Birmingham City Council v Oakley* [2001] 1 AC 617, 631), have changed and continue to change. A child's welfare is to be judged today by the standards of reasonable men and women in 2012, not by the standards of their parents in 1970, and having regard to the ever changing nature of our world: changes in our understanding of the natural world, technological changes, changes in social standards and, perhaps most important of all, changes in social attitudes.

34. If the reasonable man or woman is receptive to change he or she is also broad-minded, tolerant, easy-going and slow to condemn. We live, or strive to live, in a tolerant society increasingly alive to the need to guard against the tyranny which majority opinion may impose on those who, for whatever reason, comprise a small, weak, unpopular or voiceless minority. Equality under the law, human rights and the protection of minorities, particularly small minorities, have to be more than what Brennan J in the High Court of Australia once memorably described as '*the incantations of legal rhetoric*'.

Mandatory relevant considerations

7.22 In addition, section 1(3) requires local authorities to exercise their functions under Part 1 of the Care Act 2014 having regard to a checklist of factors:

1(3) In exercising a function under this Part in the case of an individual, a local authority must have regard to the following matters in particular–

(a) the importance of beginning with the assumption that the individual is best-placed to judge the individual's well-being;

(b) the individual's views, wishes, feelings and beliefs;

(c) the importance of preventing or delaying the development of needs for care and support or needs for support and the importance of reducing needs of either kind that already exist;

(d) the need to ensure that decisions about the individual are made having regard to all the individual's circumstances (and are not based only on the individual's age or appearance or any condition of the individual's or aspect of the individual's behaviour which might lead others to make unjustified assumptions about the individual's well-being);

(e) the importance of the individual participating as fully as possible in decisions relating to the exercise of the function concerned and being provided with the information and support necessary to enable the individual to participate;

(f) the importance of achieving a balance between the individual's well-being and that of any friends or relatives who are involved in caring for the individual;

(g) the need to protect people from abuse and neglect;

(h) the need to ensure that any restriction on the individual's rights or freedom of action that is involved in the exercise of the function is kept to the minimum necessary for achieving the purpose for which the function is being exercised.

7.23 The *Care and Support Statutory Guidance* provides advice about these relevant factors, at Chapter 1, in particular:

> 1.15 All of the matters listed above must be considered in relation to every individual, when a local authority carries out a function as described in this guidance. Considering these matters should lead to an approach that looks at a person's life holistically, considering their needs in the context of their skills, ambitions, and priorities – as well as the other people in their life and how they can support the person in meeting the outcomes they want to achieve. The focus should be on supporting people to live as independently as possible for as long as possible.
>
> 1.16 As with promoting wellbeing, the factors above will vary in their relevance and application to individuals. For some people, spiritual or religious beliefs will be of great significance, and should be taken into particular account. Local authorities should consider how to apply these further principles on a case-by-case basis. This reflects the fact that every person is different and the matters of most importance to them will accordingly vary widely.
>
> 1.17 Neither these principles, nor the requirement to promote wellbeing, require the local authority to undertake any particular action. The steps a local authority should take will depend entirely on the circumstances. The principles as a whole are not intended to specify the activities which should take place. Instead, their purpose is to set common expectations for how local authorities should approach and engage with people.

7.24 The matters set out in 'the checklist' at section 1(3) are explicitly made into statutorily relevant considerations, so that a decision will be unlawful if it disregards one of those considerations, unless, perhaps, on particular facts, that consideration was not material: but that seems far-fetched in the case of section 1(3), which sets out a series of fundamental considerations that appear plainly intended always to be, at the very least, taken into account.

7.25 The conventional approach to relevant considerations is that it is a matter of law which considerations are legally relevant;[9] but that it is then a question of judgment for the authority, what weight to attribute to the relevant consideration, when deciding what course of action to take. For example, in *Tesco Stores Limited v Secretary of State for the Environment*,[10] Lord Keith said:

> It is for the courts ... to decide what is a relevant consideration. If the decision maker wrongly takes the view that some consideration is not relevant, and therefore has no regard to it, his decision cannot stand and he must be required to think again. But it is entirely for the decision maker to attribute to the relevant considerations such weight as he thinks fit, and the court will not interfere unless he has acted unreasonably in the *Wednesbury* sense.

9 *R (Khatun) v Newham LBC* [2004] EWCA Civ 55, [2005] QB 37.

10 [1995] 1 WLR 759 at 764G–H.

7.26 That is not, however, the only approach. In *R v East London and The City Mental Health NHS Trust ex p von Brandenburg,*[11] Sedley LJ said that 'The principle that the weight to be given to such facts is a matter for the decision-maker, moreover, does not meant that the latter is free to dismiss or marginalise things to which the structure and policy of the Act attach obvious importance'. It may be that the courts will treat the considerations in section 1(3) as requiring not just to be taken into account but, also, to be accorded very significant weight.

7.27 From a different angle, Aikens LJ explained what it meant to 'have due regard' to the disability equality duty at section 49A of the Disability Discrimination Act 1995 in *R (Brown) v Secretary of State for Work and Pensions*[12] and, while the language and the statutory context is somewhat different, it may be that the courts will adopt this approach to the important considerations in section 1(3):

> 90. Subject to these qualifications, how, in practice, does the public authority fulfil its duty to have 'due regard' to the identified goals that are set out in section 49A(1) of the 1995 Act? An examination of the cases to which we were referred suggests that the following general principles can be tentatively put forward. First, those in the public authority who have to take decisions that do or might affect disabled people must be made aware of their duty to have 'due regard' to the identified goals: compare, in a race relations context, *R (Watkins-Singh) v Governing Body of Aberdare Girls' High School* [2008] 3 FCR 203, para 114, per Silber J. Thus, an incomplete or erroneous appreciation of the duties will mean that 'due regard' has not been given to them: see, in a race relations case, the remarks of Moses LJ in *R (Kaur) v Ealing London Borough Council* [2008] EWHC 2062 (Admin) at [45].
>
> 91. Secondly, the 'due regard' duty must be fulfilled before and at the time that a particular policy that will or might affect disabled people is being considered by the public authority in question. It involves a conscious approach and state of mind. On this compare, in the context of race relations: the *Elias* case [2006] 1 WLR 3213, para 274, per Arden LJ. Attempts to justify a decision as being consistent with the exercise of the duty when it was not, in fact, considered before the decision, are not enough to discharge the duty: compare, in the race relations context, the remarks of Buxton LJ in *C's* case [2009] 2 WLR 1039, para 49.
>
> 92. Thirdly, the duty must be exercised in substance, with rigour and with an open mind. The duty has to be integrated within the discharge of the public functions of the authority. It is not a question of 'ticking boxes'. Compare, in a race relations case the remarks of Moses LJ in *Kaur's* case, paras 24–25.
>
> 93. However, the fact that the public authority has not mentioned specifically section 49A(1) in carrying out the particular function where it has to have 'due regard' to the needs set out in the section is not determinative of whether the duty under the statute has been performed: see the judgment of Dyson LJ in *Baker's* case [2009] PTSR 809, para 36. But it is good practice for the policy or decision maker to make reference to the provision and any code or other non-statutory guidance in all cases where section 49A(1) is in play. 'In this way the [policy or] decision maker is more likely to ensure that the relevant factors are taken into account and the scope for argument as to whether the duty has been performed will be reduced': *Baker's* case, para 38.

11 [2001] EWCA Civ 239, [2002] QB 235 at para 4.

12 [2008] EWHC 3158 (Admin).

94. Fourthly, the duty imposed on public authorities that are subject to the section 49A(1) duty is a non-delegable duty. The duty will always remain on the public authority charged with it. In practice another body may actually carry out practical steps to fulfil a policy stated by a public authority that is charged with the section 49A(1) duty. In those circumstances the duty to have 'due regard' to the needs identified will only be fulfilled by the relevant public authority if (i) it appoints a third party that is capable of fulfilling the 'due regard' duty and is willing to do so; and (ii) the public authority maintains a proper supervision over the third party to ensure it carries out its 'due regard' duty: compare the remarks of Dobbs J in *R (Eisai Ltd) v National Institute for Health and Clinical Excellence* [2007] EWHC 1941 (Admin) at [92] and [95].

95. Fifthly, and obviously, the duty is a continuing one.

96. Sixthly, it is good practice for those exercising public functions in public authorities to keep an adequate record showing that they had actually considered their disability equality duties and pondered relevant questions. Proper record-keeping encourages transparency and will discipline those carrying out the relevant function to undertake their disability equality duties conscientiously. If records are not kept it may make it more difficult, evidentially, for a public authority to persuade a court that it has fulfilled the duty imposed by section 49A(1): see the remarks of Stanley Burnton J in *R (BAPIO Action Ltd) v Secretary of State for the Home Department* [2007] EWHC 199 (Admin) at [69]; those of Dobbs J in the *Eisai* case [2007] EWHC 1941 (Admin) at [92] and [94]; and those of Moses LJ in *Kaur's* case, para 25.

Preventative services

7.28 Section 2 of the Care Act 2014 imposes a duty on local authorities to provide or arrange for the provision of services aimed at preventing or reducing adults' needs for care and support, and carers' needs for support, in their area. That duty can be discharged jointly with other local authorities.

7.29 The *Care and Support Statutory Guidance* addresses preventative services at Chapter 2, noting at paragraph 2.1 that:

> 2.1 It is critical to the vision in the Care Act that the care and support system works to actively promote wellbeing and independence, and does not just wait to respond when people reach a crisis point. To meet the challenges of the future, it will be vital that the care and support system intervenes early to support individuals, helps people retain or regain their skills and confidence, and prevents need or delays deterioration wherever possible.

7.30 The Guidance goes on to explain that there are three levels of preventative services:

i) primary services aimed at individuals with no particular needs, to maintain their health and promote their well-being;
ii) secondary services aimed in a targeted manner at individuals with an increased risk of developing needs; and
iii) tertiary services aimed at minimising the effect of disability or deterioration on people with established or complex conditions.

In addition, there are intermediate care and re-ablement services.

7.31 Sections 9(6) and 10(8) require local authorities assessing adults and carers to consider the assistance that preventative services might afford.

Section 24(2) requires local authorities to provide advice and information about preventative services to persons for whom it has decided not to provide care and support/support.

7.32 The Care and Support (Preventing Needs for Care and Support) Regulations 2014:[13]

- allows charges to be levied for preventative services, provided the charge does not reduce the adult's income below the amount specified in regulation 7 of the Care and Support (Charging and Assessment of Resources) Regulations 2014;[14]
- does not allow charges for (i) 'community equipment' costing £1,000.00 or less; (ii) intermediate care and re-ablement services for up to six weeks; (iii) services provided to a carer intended to prevent or delay the development by the carer of needs for support or to reduce the carer's needs for support which, consist of provision made directly to the adult needing care; and (iv) services for adults suffering from variant Creuttzfeldt-Jacob disease.

Information and advice

7.33 Section 4 of the Care Act 2014 requires local authorities to establish and maintain a service for providing people in its area with information and advice relating to care and support for adults and support for carers: thus, local authorities may provide information and advice themselves, or make arrangements with an independent body to do so. They may also perform the duty jointly with other local authorities (section 4(6)). The *Care and Support Statutory Guidance* advises, in fact, that local authorities should foster a 'mixed economy' of provision, including independently provided advice (paragraph 3.14).

7.34 The duty to provide information and advice is owed (i) to every person, whether they are an adult, or a carer, or some other person; (ii) whether or not the person seeking advice resides in the local authority's area (or, for example, is contemplating moving into the local authority's area); (iii) whether or not the person seeking advice has any 'eligible needs'.

7.35 Sections 4(2) and(3) stipulate what areas the information and advice must cover:

> 4(2) The service must provide information and advice on the following matters in particular–
> (a) the system provided for by this Part and how the system operates in the authority's area,
> (b) the choice of types of care and support, and the choice of providers, available to those who are in the authority's area,
> (c) how to access the care and support that is available,
> (d) how to access independent financial advice on matters relevant to the meeting of needs for care and support, and
> (e) how to raise concerns about the safety or well-being of an adult who has needs for care and support.
> (3) In providing information and advice under this section, a local authority must in particular–

13 SI No 2673.
14 SI No 2672.

(a) have regard to the importance of identifying adults in the authority's area who would be likely to benefit from financial advice on matters relevant to the meeting of needs for care and support, and
(b) seek to ensure that what it provides is sufficient to enable adults–
  (i) to identify matters that are or might be relevant to their personal financial position that could be affected by the system provided for by this Part,
  (ii) to make plans for meeting needs for care and support that might arise, and
  (iii) to understand the different ways in which they may access independent financial advice on matters relevant to the meeting of needs for care and support.

7.36 The detail of how much and what information and advice to provide is, to an extent, and inevitably, left to local authorities. However, the terms of section 4(2) and (3) suggest that detailed advice and information is required; as does:

- the duty in section 4(4) to ensure that advice is 'accessible to, and proportionate to the needs of, those for whom it is being provided'; and
- the duty to provide, not just 'information' but also 'advice' (paragraph 3.8 of the *Care and Support Statutory Guidance* states that 'In this section of guidance, the term 'information' means the communication of knowledge and facts regarding care and support. 'Advice' means helping a person to identify choices and/or providing an opinion or recommendation regarding a course of action in relation to care and support'); and
- Chapter 3 of the *Care and Support Statutory Guidance*, in particular at paragraphs 3.17 and 3.24, which set out in some detail what should be covered.

7.37 The *Care and Support Statutory Guidance* provides detailed advice about different methods of providing advice at paragraphs 3.25–3.35; the importance of access to financial information and advice, at paragraphs 3.36–3.52; and about adult safeguarding, at paragraphs 3.53–3.54. Finally, advice is give about the need to adopt and publish an information and advice strategy (paragraphs 3.62–3.70).

Promoting integration with health etc.

7.38 Section 3 of the Care Act 2014 requires local authorities to exercise their functions under Part 1 so as to ensure the integration of care and support provision with health, health-related and housing provision where that would benefit adults and carers in their area.

7.39 This requirement meshes with section 13N of the National Health Service Act 2006, which imposes the obverse duty on clinical commissioning groups.

7.40 This topic is addressed at Chapter 15 of the *Care and Support Statutory Guidance*, which:

- gives examples of how local authorities and clinical commissioning groups should consider collaborating on planning; commissioning; the provision of assessment, information and advice; the delivery of

care/support; pooled budgets and integrated management (building on their existing duty to collaborate on the preparation of Joint Strategic Needs Assessments and Joint Health and Well-Being Strategies);
- draws attention to the breadth of the integration, co-operation and partnership duties and powers under the Care Act 2014 (see below).

7.41 Further provision is made under:
- section 12(7) of the Care Act 2014 (combined assessments);
- section 22 of the Care Act 2014 and the Care and Support (Provision of Health Services) Regulations 2014 (prohibition on local authorities providing health care subject to limited exceptions; joint working on NHS Continuing Healthcare cases)(and see also regulation 7 of The Care and Support (Assessment) Regulations 2014);
- section 74 of, and Schedule 3 to the Care Act 2014 and the Care and Support (Discharge from Hospital) Regulations 2014 (the hospital discharge machinery).

Co-operating generally

7.42 Section 6(1) of the Care Act 2014 mirrors section 10 of the Children Act 2004, in that it requires local authorities and 'relevant partners' to co-operate with each other in the exercise of their functions relevant to adults with needs for care and support and carers. As the Explanatory Note points out, this does not confer any new functions but relates to co-operation in the exercise of existing functions.

7.43 'Relevant partners' include district councils, county councils, NHS bodies, Ministers of the Crown exercising functions relating to social security, employment and training and prison, chief officers of police for the area, probation service providers and any other body specified in regulations (section 6(7)).

7.44 Local authorities are also required to co-operate with such other persons as it considers appropriate, such as care services providers, primary health care providers, social housing providers (section 6(2) and (3)), although such persons are not required to co-operate with local authorities.

7.45 Local authorities are required to make arrangements for ensuring co-operation between adult social care officers, housing officers, the director of children's services and the director of public health (section 6(4)).

7.46 All the above duties have a purpose:

> **6**(6) The duties under subsections (1) to (4) are to be performed for the following purposes in particular–
> (a) promoting the well-being of adults with needs for care and support and of carers in the authority's area,
> (b) improving the quality of care and support for adults and support for carers provided in the authority's area (including the outcomes that are achieved from such provision),
> (c) smoothing the transition to the system provided for by this Part for persons in relation to whom functions under sections 58 to 65 are exercisable,
> (d) protecting adults with needs for care and support who are experiencing, or are at risk of, abuse or neglect, and (e) identifying

lessons to be learned from cases where adults with needs for care and support have experienced serious abuse or neglect and applying those lessons to future cases.

7.47 Co-operation is addressed at Chapter 15 of the *Care and Support Statutory Guidance*, which

- reminds local authorities that where they are not required actively to promote integration with health service, for example under section 3, they always remain under a co-operation duty, for the benefit of adults and carers in need of care and support/support in their area and that this can be achieved in a number of ways: by information sharing, or providing staff or services, for example;
- makes a particular point about the importance of co-operation between social services and housing departments 'given that housing and suitability of living accommodation play a significant role in support a person to meet their needs and can help to delay that person's deterioration' (paragraph 15.24);
- draws attention to the breadth of the integration, co-operation and partnership obligations under the Act.

Co-operating in specific cases

7.48 Where a local authority requests co-operation from a 'relevant partner' or from any other local authority, in relation to an adult, carer, carer of a child or young carer, the relevant partner/other local authority must comply with the request unless it considers that so doing would be incompatible with its own duties or would otherwise have an adverse effect on the exercise of its functions (section 7(1)).

7.49 The obverse is also true: a local authority must co-operate, on the same basis, when requested by a 'relevant partner' or any other local authority (section 7(2)).

7.50 'Relevant partners' for these purposes are the same bodies specified in section 6(7) (above).

7.51 Any person who decides not to comply with one of these requests for co-operation has to provide written reasons (section 7(3)).

7.52 Co-operation in specific cases is addressed in the *Care and Support Statutory Guidance* at Chapter 15, which:

- explains that co-operation should be a part of the general, strategic thinking of local authorities and their partners but that sometimes there will be individual cases where more specific forms of co-operation will be required, for example, by requesting and providing specific services for an individual, for example, when an individual is moving from one area to another;
- reminds local authorities of the breadth of their integration, co-operation and partnership obligations.

Involvement/independent advocates/relevance of the Mental Capacity Act 2005

7.53 As indicated above, a major purpose of the 'well-being' duty in section 1(1) and (2), and the statutory relevant factors in section 1(3), is to place the individual and their views, wishes, feelings and beliefs at the heart of the social care process.

7.54 That principle is activated by a series of more concrete provisions, including but by no means limited to provisions that require local authorities to:

- provide information and advice (section 4);
- promote diverse and high quality services (section 5);
- focus an assessment on the well-being duty (sections 9(4) and 10(5)(c)) and involve the adult, any carer and any other person the adult asks to be involved or, where the adult lacks capacity, who appears to be interested in their welfare (section 9(5) and 10(7));
- arrange supported self-assessments (regulation 2 of the Care and Support (Assessment) Regulations 2014[15]) and, in any event, to take into account the individual's wishes and preferences and the outcome they seek (regulation 3);
- involve the adult, the carer and other relevant persons in the preparation of a care and support/support plan and 'take all reasonable steps to reach agreement with the adult or carer for whom the plan is being prepared about how the authority should meet the needs in question' (sections 25(3)–(5)).

7.55 As it is put in the *Care and Support Statutory Guidance*:

> *Supporting the person's involvement in the assessment*
> 6.30. Putting the person at the heart of the assessment process is crucial to understanding the person's needs, outcomes and wellbeing, and delivering better care and support. The local authority must involve the person being assessed in the process as they are best placed to judge their own wellbeing. In the case of an adult with care and support needs, the local authority must also involve any carer the person has (which may be more than one carer), and in all cases, the authority must also involve any other person requested. The local authority should have processes in place, and suitably trained staff, to ensure the involvement of these parties, so that their perspective and experience supports a better understanding of the needs, outcomes and wellbeing.
>
> 6.31. Where local authorities identify that an adult is unable to effectively engage in the assessment process independently, it should seek to involve somebody who can assist the adult in engaging with the process and helping them to articulate their preferred outcomes and needs as early as possible. This will include some people with mental impairments who will nevertheless have capacity to engage in the assessment alongside the local authority. They may require assistance whereby the local authority provides an assessment, tailored to their circumstances, their needs and their ability to engage. They should be supported in understanding the assessment process and assisted to make decisions wherever possible.

15 SI No 2827.

6.32. Where there is concern about a person's capacity to make a specific decision, for example as a result of a mental impairment such as dementia, acquired brain injury or learning disabilities, then an assessment of capacity should be carried out under the Mental Capacity Act 2005. Those who may lack capacity will need extra support to identify and communicate their needs and make subsequent decisions, and may need an Independent Mental Capacity Advocate. The more serious the needs, the more support people may need to identify their impact and the consequences. Professional qualified staff, such as social workers, can advise and support assessors when they are carrying out an assessment with a person who may lack capacity.

7.56 By virtue of section 67 of the Care Act 2014, there are to be 'independent advocates' for adults, carers, children in transition and child carers who lack the capacity to participate in care planning or would experience substantial difficulty in participating. The underlying purpose is to do everything possible, even in difficult cases, to ensure that the individual is at the heart of the social care process. A failure to appoint an 'independent advocate', in breach of section 67(2) of the Care Act 2014, will almost certainly make the resultant assessment unlawful.[16]

7.57 Section 67 of the Care Act 2014 provides that:

- where a local authority is required by a 'relevant provision' to 'involve' an individual, but it appears that the individual would experience 'substantial difficulty' in participating;
- it must arrange for an 'independent advocate' to 'represent and support the individual for the purpose of facilitating the individual's involvement';
- unless the local authority is satisfied that there is an appropriate person (not engaged in providing care or treatment for the individual in a professional or paid capacity) to undertake the 'independent advocate' function. However, this exception is itself dis-applied by regulation 4 of The Care and Support (Independent Advocacy Support) (No 2) Regulations 2014[17] when either (i) the NHS is likely to accommodate the individual in hospital for at least 28 days or in a care home for least eight weeks; or (ii) the local authority and the potentially appropriate person disagree on a material issue but agree that the individual should have an 'independent advocate'.

7.58 The 'relevant provisions' are defined in section 67(3):

67(3) The relevant provisions are–
(a) section 9(5)(a) and (b) (carrying out needs assessment);
(b) section 10(7)(a) (carrying out carer's assessment);
(c) section 25(3)(a) and (b) (preparing care and support plan);
(d) section 25(4)(a) and (b) (preparing support plan);
(e) section 27(2)(b)(i) and (ii) (revising care and support plan);
(f) section 27(3)(b)(i) and (ii) (revising support plan);
(g) section 59(2)(a) and (b) (carrying out child's needs assessment);
(h) section 61(3)(a) (carrying out child's carer's assessment);
(i) section 64(3)(a) and (b) (carrying out young carer's assessment).

16 *R (SG) v Haringey LBC* [2015] EWHC 2579 (Admin), (2015) 18 CCLR 444.
17 SI No 2824.

7.59 Section 68 of the Care Act 2014 requires independent advocates to be appointed in adult safeguarding cases: that requirement is addressed in chapter 24 below on Safeguarding.

7.60 The Care and Support (Independent Advocacy Support) (No 2) Regulations 2014[18] regulate both local authorities and advocates as follows:

- regulation 2 sets out the requirements to be met for a person to be treated by the local authority as an independent advocate. The local authority must obtain an enhanced criminal record certificate and satisfy themselves that the independent advocate is fully independent of the local authority, not engaged on a professional or paid basis with the adult or carer and appropriately trained, experienced and competent, with integrity/of good character and appropriately supervised. On this basis it is hard to imagine an independent advocate being anyone other than a member of high quality, professional organisation (of which there are a number in existence);
- regulation 3 sets out the matters that a local authority must have regard to, when determining whether an individual would have 'substantial difficulty' in participating in the exercise of relevant local authority functions;
- regulation 5 sets out in some detail:
  - how independent advocates are to discharge their functions, so as to understand all the relevant circumstances; to involve the individual as much as possible; to communicate 'the individual's views, wishes or feelings' and to assist the individual to make decisions and, if they wish, to challenge the local authority's decisions;
  - that independent advocates are entitled to examine and take copies of the individual's records with their consent (if they have capacity) or if that is in their best interests (if they lack capacity);
  - that where the individual lacks capacity, the independent advocate is to communicate their views, wishes and feelings to the extent that they are able to ascertain them;
  - that where the individual lacks capacity, the independent advocate is to challenge a decision made by a local authority if they consider that it is inconsistent with the local authority's general duty in section 1 of the Act to promote the individual's wellbeing;
- regulation 6 sets out how the local authority is to assist independent advocates, take into account and respond to their representations;
- regulation 7 provides that when combined assessments take place (eg for an adult and their carer) the local authority must arrange for both individuals subject to the assessment to share the same independent advocate, or to have separate independent advocates if there is a conflict of interest.

7.61 Chapter 7 of the *Care and Support Statutory Guidance* addresses independent advocacy, expressing the core principle in this way:

> 7.6 Local authorities must involve people in decisions made about them and their care and support or where there is to be a safeguarding enquiry or SAR. Involvement requires the local authority helping people to understand

18 SI No 2889.

> how they can be involved, how they can contribute and take part and sometimes lead or direct the process. People should be active partners in the key care and support processes of assessment, care and support and support planning, review and any enquiries in relation to abuse or neglect. No matter how complex a person's needs, local authorities are required to involve people, to help them express their wishes and feelings, to support them to weigh up options, and to make their own decisions.
>
> 7.7 The duty to involve applies in all settings, including for those people living in the community, in care homes or, apart from safeguarding enquiries and SARs, in prisons, for example.

7.62 The Guidance contains brief advice about the relationship between independent advocacy under the Care Act 2014 and under the Mental Capacity Act 2005:

> 7.9 Many of the people who qualify for advocacy under the Care Act will also qualify for advocacy under the Mental Capacity Act 2005. The same advocate can provide support as an advocate under the Care Act and under the Mental Capacity Act. This is to enable the person to receive seamless advocacy and not to have to repeat their story to different advocates. Under whichever legislation the advocate providing support is acting, they should meet the appropriate requirements for an advocate under that legislation.

7.63 Provision is made for the appointment of Independent Mental Capacity Advocates by:

- sections 35–41 of the Mental Capacity Act 2005;
- the Mental Capacity Act 2005 (Independent Mental Capacity Advocates) (General) Regulations 2006 and, in Wales, by the Mental Capacity Act 2005 (Independent Mental Capacity Advocates) (Wales) Regulations 2007;
- the Mental Capacity Act 2005 (Independent Mental Capacity Advocates) (Expansion of Role) Regulations 2006; and
- Chapter 10 of the Mental Capacity Act Code of Practice.

7.64 For present purposes, it is sufficient to replicate the 'Quick Summary' in the Code:

> **Quick summary**
>
> *Understanding the role of the IMCA service*
>
> • The aim of the IMCA service is to provide independent safeguards for people who lack capacity to make certain important decisions and, at the time such decisions need to be made, have no-one else (other than paid staff) to support or represent them or be consulted.
>
> • IMCAs must be independent.
>
> *Instructing and consulting an IMCA*
>
> • An IMCA must be instructed, and then consulted, for people lacking capacity who have no-one else to support them (other than paid staff), whenever:
>
> – an NHS body is proposing to provide serious medical treatment, or
> – an NHS body or local authority is proposing to arrange accommodation (or a change of accommodation) in hospital or a care home, and
> – the person will stay in hospital longer than 28 days, or
> – they will stay in the care home for more than eight weeks.
>
> • An IMCA may be instructed to support someone who lacks capacity to make decisions concerning:

– care reviews, where no-one else is available to be consulted
– adult protection cases, whether or not family, friends or others are involved Ensuring an IMCA's views are taken into consideration

• The IMCA's role is to support and represent the person who lacks capacity. Because of this, IMCAs have the right to see relevant healthcare and social care records.

• Any information or reports provided by an IMCA must be taken into account as part of the process of working out whether a proposed decision is in the person's best interests.

7.65 The wider relevance of the Mental Capacity Act 2005 is considered below in chapter 23.

Market oversight and provider failure

7.66 Business failure can be large-scale (think Southern Cross) or localised, but in both cases places service users at risk. The statutory machinery for supervising the financial viability of registered care providers (whether that is home care, care home or other forms of registrable provision) and catering for their business failure, so as to safeguard the welfare of service users, is at:

- sections 19 and 48–57 of the Care Act 2014;
- the Care and Support (Market Oversight Information) Regulations 2014;[19]
- the Care and Support (Market Oversight Criteria) Regulations 2015;[20]
- the Care and Support (Business Failure) Regulations 2015;[21]
- the Care and Support (Cross-border Placements) (Business Failure Duties of Scottish Local Authorities) Regulations 2014;[22]
- the Care and Support (Cross-border Placements and Business Failure: Temporary Duty) (Dispute Resolution) Regulations 2014;[23] and
- Chapter 5 of the *Care and Support Statutory Guidance*.

7.67 Sections 53–57 of the Care Act 2014, together with the Care and Support (Market Oversight Information) Regulations 2014 and the Care and Support (Market Oversight Criteria) Regulations 2015, contain a scheme for supervising the financial viability of registered care providers and alerting local authorities to likely business failures.

7.68 Essentially, they contain provision for the Care Quality Commission (CQC) to identify major providers which, because of their size, geographic location, specialism or other factors, would be difficult for one or more local authorities to replace, and where national oversight is required.

7.69 CQC must then assess the financial viability of such organisations (which are required to provide specified information to the CQC) and report to relevant local authorities, if it considers that they are likely to succumb to business failure (sections 55(1) and 56).

19 SI No 2822.
20 SI No 314.
21 SI No 301.
22 SI No 2839.
23 SI No 2843.

7.70 CQC also has power to require the provider to develop a plan for how to mitigate or eliminate a significant risk to its financial sustainability and to arrange for, or require the provider to arrange for, a person with appropriate expertise to undertake an independent review of the business (section 55(2)).

7.71 Local authorities have a duty to take action in response to business failure, or indeed any service interruption, whether or not a business falls within the CQC regime and sections 48–52 contain machinery for ensuring continuity of care in the event of business failure.

7.72 Section 48 of the Care Act 2014 provides that where any registered care provider is unable to continue to undertake a regulated activity because of business failure (defined at regulation 2 of the Care and Support (Market Oversight Criteria) Regulations 2015), the local authority is under a temporary duty to meet the needs for care and support/support being provided to adults/carers in the local authority area, so far as it is not already required to do so.

7.73 In other words, where a local authority is already under a statutory duty to meet needs, that duty continues irrespective of the business failure of a particular provider; the function of section 48 is to impose a duty where none previously existed, for example, towards self-funders or individuals funded by other local authorities.

7.74 That duty arises as soon as the local authority becomes aware of the business failure (section 52). It applies whether or not:

- the adult is ordinarily resident in the local authority's area;
- the local authority or some other local authority made the arrangements;
- the local authority has undertaken any form of assessment;
- any of the needs meet the eligibility criteria (so long as they do not require the provision of services excluded under sections 21–23 of the Care Act 2014: services for certain persons subject to immigration control, health care and housing: sections 52(7)–(8)).

7.75 The duty continues for as long as the local authority considers necessary. However:

- the local authority need not meet needs in the same way as the registered care provider did (section 52(2)); although
- it must involve the adult, the carer and other relevant persons when deciding how to meet needs (section 52); and
- the local authority may charge, but not for the provision of information and advice and only for the cost of meeting needs (section 48(5)).

7.76 Further provision is made in section 48, and in sections 49–52, for ordinary residence and cross-border disputes, and for Wales and Northern Ireland.

7.77 Of course, as paragraph 5.25 of the *Care and Support Statutory Guidance* points out, local authorities may be required or entitled to meet needs, by virtue of sections 18 and 20 of the Care Act 2014, whenever there is a service interruption and for whatever reason.

7.78 The Guidance provides useful practical advice, including a reminder to local authorities always to keep their 'ear to the ground', by dialogue with local providers, to anticipate and possibly remedy any potential business failure or service interruption.

Promoting diversity and quality

7.79 The Care Act 2014 imposes a duty on local authorities to promote a diverse and good quality market in local care and support/support services:

> 5(1) A local authority must promote the efficient and effective operation of a market in services for meeting care and support needs with a view to ensuring that any person in its area wishing to access services in the market–
> (a) has a variety of providers to choose from who (taken together) provide a variety of services;
> (b) has a variety of high quality services to choose from;
> (c) has sufficient information to make an informed decision about how to meet the needs in question.

7.80 The rest of section 5 sets out the considerations that local authorities must take into account and makes provision for joint working with other local authorities to discharge this duty.

7.81 This 'market shaping' duty is addressed at Chapter 4 of the *Care and Support Statutory Guidance*, which expresses the core duty in this way:

> 4.6 **Market shaping** means the local authority collaborating closely with other relevant partners, including people with care and support needs, carers and families, to facilitate the whole market in its area for care, support and related services. This includes services arranged and paid for by the state through the authority itself, those services paid by the state through direct payments, and those services arranged and paid for by individuals from whatever sources (sometimes called 'self-funders'), and services paid for by a combination of these sources. Market shaping activity should stimulate a diverse range of appropriate high quality services (both in terms of the types, volumes and quality of services and the types of provider organisation), and ensure the market as a whole remains vibrant and sustainable.
>
> 4.7 The core activities of market shaping are to engage with stakeholders to develop understanding of supply and demand and articulate likely trends that reflect people's evolving needs and aspirations, and based on evidence, to signal to the market the types of services needed now and in the future to meet them, encourage innovation, investment and continuous improvement. It also includes working to ensure that those who purchase their own services are empowered to be effective consumers, for example by helping people who want to take direct payments make informed decisions about employing personal assistants. A local authority's own commissioning practices are likely to have a significant influence on the market to achieve the desired outcomes, but other interventions may be needed, for example, incentivising innovation by user-led or third sector providers, possibly through grant funding.

7.82 The Guidance also emphasises the importance of adopting published strategies:

> 4.52 Commissioning and market shaping should be fundamental means for local authorities to facilitate effective services in their area and it is important that authorities develop evidence-based local strategies for how they exercise these functions, and align these with wider corporate planning. Local

authorities should have in place published strategies that include plans that show how their legislative duties, corporate plans, analysis of local needs and requirements (integrated with the Joint Strategic Needs Assessment and Joint Health and Wellbeing Strategy), thorough engagement with people, carers and families, market and supply analysis, market structuring and interventions, resource allocations and procurement and contract management activities translate (now and in future) into appropriate high quality services that deliver identified outcomes for the people in their area and address any identified gaps.

4.53 Since 2007 there has been a duty on local authorities and latterly clinical commissioning groups, through health and wellbeing boards, to undertake Joint Strategic Needs Assessments (JSNA). JSNA is a process that assesses and maps the needs and demand for health and care and support, supports the development of joint Health and Wellbeing Strategies to address needs, understands community assets and informs commissioning of local health and care and support services that together with community assets meet needs.

4.54 Market shaping and commissioning intentions should be cross-referenced to JSNA, and should be informed by an understanding of the needs and aspirations of the population and how services will adapt to meet them. Strategies should be informed and emphasise preventative services that encourage independence and wellbeing, delaying or preventing the need for acute interventions. Statutory guidance on JSNA and Joint Health and Wellbeing Strategies was published in March 2013. The ambition is for market shaping and commissioning to be an integral part of understanding and delivering the whole health and care economy, and to reflect the range and diversity of communities and people with specific needs, in particular:

- people needing care and support themselves (through for example, consumer research);
- carers;
- carer support organisations;
- health professionals;
- care and support managers and social workers (and representative organisations for these groups);
- relevant voluntary, user and other support organisations;
- independent advocates;
- the wider local population;
- provider organisations (including where appropriate housing providers); and
- other tiers of local government.

Assessing and meeting needs under the Care Act 2014 in outline

7.83 Detailed consideration of the statutory machinery and case-law is set out below. In barest outline, however, the essential machinery is as follows:

- sections 9 and 10 impose a duty on local authorities to assess the needs for care and support that an adult might have, or the needs for support that a carer might have. The assessment must be written and provided to the adult/carer (section 12(3) and (4));
- section 13 requires the local authority to determine (in writing, providing a copy to the adult/carer) whether any needs for care and support meet the eligibility criteria, what can done to meet those needs and

whether the adult/carer is ordinarily resident in the local authority's area;

- section 14 requires the local authority to undertake a financial assessment, for charging purposes;
- sections 24, 25 and 26 require care and support plans, or support plans, including provision of a personal budget for adults, to be compiled in writing and provided to the adult/carer;
- sections 18 and 19 impose a duty to meet an adult's 'eligible' needs for care and support, and a carer's needs for support, if they are ordinarily resident in the local authority's area and certain other conditions are fulfilled; they also confer a power to meet needs for care and support, or support, in certain circumstances. The new national eligibility criteria are to be found in the Care and Support (Eligibility Criteria) Regulations 2015;
- section 8 provides that needs may be met by providing accommodation in a care home or some other type of premises; by providing care and support at home or in the community; or by providing counselling/social work, goods and facilities or information, advice and advocacy. Sections 22 and 23 exclude the provision of health care or simple housing and section 21 limits provision to persons subject to immigration control.

The pre-legislative and legislative process of the Care Act 2014

7.84 The pre-legislative process of the Care Act 2014 was as follows:

- 11 May 2011, the Law Commission published its report called *Adult Social Care* (Law Com No 326), recommending a major overhaul of adult social care legislation;[24]
- July 2011, the Dilnot Commission published *Fairer Care Funding: the Report of the* Commission *on Funding of Care and Support;*[25]
- July 2012, the Secretary of State for Health published material indicating agreement with the recommendations of the Law Commission and the Dilnot Commission:
  - *Caring for our future: progress report on funding;*[26]
  - *Reforming the law for adult care and support: the Government's response to Law Commission report 326 on adult social care;*[27]
  - the White Paper, *Caring for our future: reforming care and support;*[28]
  - The *Draft Care and Support Bill;*[29]

24 http://lawcommission.justice.gov.uk/publications/1460.htm.

25 www.dilnotcommission.dh.gov.uk/our-report.

26 www.dh.gov.uk/health/2012/07/scfunding/.

27 www.dh.gov.uk/health/files/2012/07/2900021-Reforming-the-Law-for-Adult-Care_ACCESSIBLE.pdf.

28 Cm 8378: www.dh.gov.uk/health/2012/07/careandsupportwhitepaper/.

29 Presented to Parliament by the Secretary of State for Health by Command of Her Majesty (July 2012, The Stationery Office, Cm 8386), for the purposes of consultation and pre-legislative scrutiny: www.dh.gov.uk/health/2012/07/careandsupportbill/.

- 6 March 2014 there was published the Joint Committee on the Draft Care and Support Bill – Report.[30] This included a section-by-section analysis of the draft Bill. Videos of oral evidence[31] and transcripts of the written and oral evidence[32] have been retained.
- that was followed by a government publication, *The Care Bill explained including a response to consultation and pre-legislation scrutiny on the Draft Care and Support Bill.*[33]

7.85 The legislative process was as follows:

- the Care Bill was introduced into the House of Lords and had its first reading on the 9 May 2013, its third reading on the 29 October 2013;
- it had its first reading in the House of Commons on the 30 October 2013;
- after a number of debates and a Committee Stage, received Royal Assent on the 14 May 2014.[34]

Repeals and transitional provisions for the Care Act 2014

7.86 Parts of the Care Act 2014 came into force on the 1 September 2014, largely for the purpose of making regulations, and the great majority of the Care Act 2014 came into force on the 1 April 2015, the most notable exception being the cap on care costs in sections 15 and 16 of the Act and provisions flowing from that cap.

7.87 For detailed repeals and transitional provisions, see:

- Update on final Orders under the Care Act 2014;[35]
- the *Care and Support Statutory Guidance*, Chapter 23 and Annex I;
- Health Research Authority (Transfer of Staff, Property and Liabilities) and Care Act 2014 (Consequential Amendments) Order 2014;[36]
- Care and Support (Miscellaneous Amendments) Regulations 2015;[37]
- Care Act 2014 and Children and Families Act 2014 (Consequential Amendments) Order 2014;[38]
- Care Act 2014 (Transitional Provision) Order 2015;[39]

30 www.publications.parliament.uk/pa/jt201213/jtselect/jtcare/143/14302.htm.

31 www.parliament.uk/business/committees/committees-a-z/joint-select/draft-care-and-support-bill/further-information-page/.

32 www.parliament.uk/business/committees/committees-a-z/joint-select/draft-care-and-support-bill/publications/.

33 www.gov.uk/government/uploads/system/uploads/attachment_data/file/228864/8627.pdf.

34 Full copies of the debates and reports are available at http://services.parliament.uk/bills/2013–14/care/stages.html; all the Bill papers (including briefing papers, written submissions from outside bodies and impact assessments) are available at http://services.parliament.uk/bills/2013–14/care/documents.html.

35 www.gov.uk/government/uploads/system/uploads/attachment_data/file/413386/Guidance_and_Orders_Note_-_final.pdf.

36 SI No 3090.

37 SI No 644.

38 SI No 914.

39 SI No 995.

- Care Act 2014 (Health Education England and the Health Research Authority) (Consequential Amendments and Revocations) Order;[40]
- Care Act 2014 (Commencement No 4) Order 2015;[41]
- Care Act 2014 (Consequential Amendments) (Secondary Legislation) Order 2015; and
- Care Act 2014 (Commencement No 5) Order 2016.

The cap on care costs and associated means-testing

7.88 The Care Act 2014 contains provision for a lifetime cap on care costs, in sections 15 and 16, which was to be set at £72,000.00, whether those costs were incurred in care homes or by way of home care. 'Hotel costs' associated with care provision were to be excluded from the cap, but were to be made subject to a separate cap of £12,000.00 per annum. This change was due to be brought into force in April 2016, but that has now been deferred until 2020.

7.89 In addition, the Care Act 2014 contains provision for means testing, under section 17. Section 17 has been largely in force since the 1 October 2014 and the 1 April 2015, but the provisions that mesh with the care cap provisions are not in force. More widely, the government's intention had been to use regulations to raise the 'upper limit' to £118,000 and the 'lower limit' to £17,000, so that only those with assets worth more than £118,000.00 would have to pay the full price, whereas all those with assets of between £17,000 and £118,500, who met the eligibility criteria for care, would be entitled to some financial support according to a sliding scale. This change was also due to be brought into force in April 2016, but that also has now been deferred until 2020.

7.90 There is a government fact sheet about these changes.[42]

Secondary legislation under the Care Act 2014

7.91 The key secondary legislation is as follows:

- Care and Support (Assessment) Regulations 2014;[43]
- Care and Support (Business Failure) Regulations 2014;[44]
- Care and Support (Charging and Assessment of Resources) Regulations 2014;[45]
- Care and Support (Children's Carers) Regulations 2014;[46]
- Care and Support (Deferred Payment) Regulations 2014;[47]
- Care and Support (Direct Payments) Regulations 2014;[48]

40 SI No 137.
41 SI No 993.
42 www.gov.uk/government/uploads/system/uploads/attachment_data/file/268683/Factsheet_6_update__tweak_.pdf.
43 SI No 2827.
44 SI No 301.
45 SI No 2672.
46 SI No 305.
47 SI No 2671.
48 SI No 2871.

- Care and Support (Discharge of Hospital Patients) Regulations 2014;[49]
- Care and Support (Disputes Between Local Authorities) Regulations 2014;[50]
- Care and Support (Ordinary Residence) (Specified Accommodation) Regulations 2014;[51]
- Care and Support (Personal Budget: Exclusion of Costs) Regulations 2014;[52]
- Care and Support (Preventing Needs for Care and Support) Regulations 2014;[53]
- Care and Support (Provision of Health Services) Regulations 2014;[54]
- Care and Support (Sight-impaired and Severely Sight-impaired Adults) Regulations 2014;[55]
- Care and Support and After-care (Choice of Accommodation) Regulations 2014;[56]
- Care and Support (Independent Advocacy Support) (No 2) Regulations 2014.[57]

7.92 The other secondary legislation is as follows:

- Care Act 2014 (Consequential Amendments) (Secondary Legislation) Order 2014;[58]
- Care Act 2014 (Health Education England and the Health Research Authority) (Consequential Amendments and Revocations) Order 2015;[59]
- Care Act 2014 (Transitional Provision) Order 2015;[60]
- Care Act 2014 and Children and Families Act 2014 (Consequential Amendments) Order 2014;[61]
- Care and Support (Cross-border Placements and Business Failure: Temporary Duty) (Dispute Resolution) Regulations 2014;[62]
- Care and Support (Cross-border Placements) (Business Failure Duties of Scottish Local Authorities) Regulations 2014;[63]
- Care and Support (Isles of Scilly) Order 2014;[64]
- Care and Support (Market Oversight Criteria) Regulations 2014;[65]
- Care and Support (Market Oversight Information) Regulations 2014;[66]

49 SI No 2823.
50 SI No 2829.
51 SI No 2828.
52 SI No 2840.
53 SI No 2673.
54 SI No 2821.
55 SI No 2854.
56 SI No 2670.
57 SI No 2889.
58 SI No 643.
59 SI No 137.
60 SI No 995.
61 SI No 914.
62 SI No 2843.
63 SI No 2828.
64 SI No 642.
65 SI No 314.
66 SI No 2822.

- Care and Support (Miscellaneous Amendments) Regulations 2014;[67]
- False or Misleading Information (Specified Care Providers and Specified Information) Regulations 2015;[68]
- Health Education England (Transfer of Staff, Property and Liabilities) Order 2015;[69]
- Health Education England Regulations 2014;[70]
- Health Research Authority (Transfer of Staff, Property and Liabilities) and Care Act 2014 (Consequential Amendments) Order 2014.[71]

Guidance

7.93 The Care Act 2014 has a specific statutory basis for guidance, at section 78 of the Care Act 2014, which provides, inter alia, that 'A local authority must act under the general guidance of the Secretary of State in the exercise of functions given to it by this Part or by regulations under this Part' (section 78(1)).

7.94 The current statutory guidance under the Care Act 2014 is *Care and Support Statutory Guidance*.[72]

7.95 In addition, the Department of Health (DoH) has published Care Act Factsheets.[73]

7.96 For the principles and case-law on guidance, see chapter 4 above.

Forthcoming appeals provisions

7.97 The government has created a power in the Care Act 2014, at section 72, to introduce an appeals procedure by way of regulations, in relation to all or many decisions made under Part 1 of the Care Act 2014. The government completed a consultation process on this in March 2015.[74]

Publicly available resources

7.98 The Social Care Institute for Excellence has published a suite of resources commissioned by the Department of Health in partnership with the Local Government Association, Association of Directors of Adult Social Services and the Care Providers Alliance to support those commissioning and providing care and support in implementing the Care Act 2014.[75]

67 SI No 644.
68 SI No 988.
69 SI No 137.
70 SI No 3215.
71 SI No 3090.
72 DoH, March 2016.
73 www.gov.uk/government/publications/care-act–2014-part–1-factsheets/care-act-factsheets-–2.
74 www.gov.uk/government/uploads/system/uploads/attachment_data/file/400757/2903104_Care_Act_Consultation_Accessible_All.pdf.
75 www.scie.org.uk/care-act–2014/.

7.99 The College of Social Work has published *The College of Social Work Guide to the Social Work Practice Implications of the Care Act 2014.*[76]

The Social Services and Well-being (Wales) Act 2014

7.100 Wales has passed its own legislation in this area, the Social Services and Well-being (Wales) Act 2014. It received Royal Assent on 1 May 2014 and came fully into force on 6 April 2016.

7.101 The Social Services and Well-being (Wales) Act 2014 is:

- based on the White Paper, *Sustainable Social Services for Wales: A Framework for Action*;[77]
- supplemented by regulations, codes and guidance;[78]
- surrounded by further information, including an *Explanatory Memorandum* and details of the legislative process, available on the Welsh Assembly website.[79]

7.102 As noted above, there is a useful Explanatory Note.[80] Explanatory Notes are admissible aids to the construction of legislation: see *R v Montila*.[81]

76 www.tcsw.org.uk/uploadedFiles/TheCollege/Policy/2014%2005%2029%20Care%20Act%20Practice%20Implications.pdf.

77 http://gov.wales/docs/dhss/publications/110216frameworken.pdf.

78 For the current state of play, see www.ccwales.org.uk/the-act/. For the codes and guidance, see http://gov.wales/topics/health/socialcare/act/code-of-practice/?lang=en.

79 www.senedd.assembly.wales/mgIssueHistoryHome.aspx?IId=5664.

80 www.legislation.gov.uk/anaw/2014/4/contents.

81 [2004] UKHL 50, [2001] 1 WLR 3141 at paras 32–36.

CHAPTER 8

Community care assessments

continued

Urgent cases

8.51 *R (AA) v Lambeth LBC* [2001] EWHC 741 (Admin), (2002) 5 CCLR 36
The court is entitled to order a local authority to provide services pending assessment, even where the local authority does not consider that the criteria for interim provision are met

8.52 *R (Alloway) v Bromley LBC* [2004] EWHC 2108 (Admin), (2005) 8 CCLR 61
Services may be provided pending completion of a re-assessment even in cases where there have been prior assessments

Nature of an assessment

8.53 *R v Avon CC ex p M* (1999) 2 CCLR 185, [1994] 2 FCR 259, QBD
An assessment must also encompass psychological needs and an authority had to have strong reasons for diverging from the cogently reasoned conclusions of a complaints panel

8.54 *R v Bristol CC ex p Penfold* (1997–8) 1 CCLR 315, QBD
An assessment must fully explore needs

8.55 *R v Haringey LBC ex p Norton* (1997–8) 1 CCLR 168, QBD
An assessment must explore social and recreational needs, not just social care needs

Assessment process

8.56 *R v North Yorkshire CC ex p William Hargreaves* (1997–8) 1 CCLR 104, QBD
Account must be taken of the service user's views even where they are difficult to ascertain, for whatever reason

8.57 *R v Islington LBC ex p Rixon* (1997–8) 1 CCLR 119, QBD
Assessments are central; they must comply in substance with statutory guidance and demonstrably have regard to relevant departmental guidance

8.58 *R v Kensington and Chelsea RLBC ex p Kujtim* (1999) 2 CCLR 340, CA
Local authorities are required to re-assess the possible needs of persons, even after their service has been terminated as a result of persistent, unequivocal misconduct, if it appears that they intend to conduct themselves properly

8.59 *R v Birmingham CC ex p Killigrew* (2000) 3 CCLR 109, QBD
An assessment contain an explanation for its decision and take into account up-to-date medical evidence and evidence from carers

8.60 *R v Newham LBC ex p Patrick* (2001) 4 CCLR 48, QBD
Referring a homeless woman with care needs to a housing charity did not amount to a discharge of the duty to assess or meet her needs

8.61 *R (A and B) v East Sussex CC and the Disability Rights Commission* [2003] EWHC 167 (Admin), (2003) 6 CCLR 194
Local authorities were under a duty to assess the needs and take into account the preferences of persons even when those persons have substantial communication difficulties, including by consulting carers as to how it is best to communicate

8.62 *R (Heffernan) v Sheffield CC* [2004] EWHC 1377 (Admin), (2004) 7 CCLR 350
An assessment that was incompatible with the eligibility criteria was unlawful

8.63 *R (B) v Lambeth LBC* [2006] EWHC 639 (Admin), (2006) 9 CCLR 239

The function of judicial review is to pronounce upon the lawfulness or otherwise of public decision-making, not to investigate its merits

8.64 *R (Ireneschild) v Lambeth LBC* [2007] EWCA Civ 234, (2007) 10 CCLR 243

It was unnecessary in the particular circumstances to allow the applicant to comment on a medical adviser's adverse report before completing the assessment; assessments are iterative and should not be too finely scrutinised

8.65 *R (AM) v Birmingham CC* [2009] EWHC 688 (Admin), (2009) 12 CCLR 407

A properly completed assessment also discharges the disability equality duty

8.66 *R (B) v Cornwall CC* [2009] EWHC 491 (Admin), (2009) 12 CCLR 381

A local authority must fully involve the service user and other relevant persons but is ultimately required to undertake its own assessment

8.67 *R (F, J, S, R) v Wirral BC* [2009] EWHC 1626 (Admin), (2009) 12 CCLR 452

Minor criticisms of assessments, not likely to result in changed services, should be brought through a complaints procedure

8.68 *R (SG) v Haringey LBC* [2015] EWHC 2579 (Admin), (2015) 18 CCLR 444

The failure to appoint an independent advocate, under section 67(2) of the Care Act 2014, for a vulnerable adult, who spoke no English and was illiterate, and who suffered from PTSD, insomnia, depression and anxiety, rendered the assessment unlawful

Introduction

8.1 The main purpose of an assessment is identified at paragraph 6.5 of the *Care and Support Statutory Guidance*:

> 6.5 The aim of the assessment is to identify what needs the person may have and what outcomes they are looking to achieve to maintain or improve their wellbeing. The outcome of the assessment is to provide a full picture of the individual's needs so that a local authority can provide an appropriate response at the right time to meet the level of the person's needs. This might range from offering guidance and information to arranging for services to meet those needs. The assessment may be the only contact the local authority has with the individual at that point in time, so it is critical that the most is made of this opportunity.

8.2 As this indicates, the purpose of an assessment goes well beyond identifying what 'eligible needs' an adult or carer might have, that a local authority is required to meet.

8.3 Experience shows that the main causes of litigation in this particular context are where a local authority:

- fails to start an assessment, even though the low statutory threshold has arisen, requiring an assessment;[1]
- fails to make immediately necessary provision pending completion of an assessment;[2]
- fails to complete an assessment within a reasonable period: paragraph 6.29 of the Guidance states that an assessment –

  > ... should be carried out over an appropriate and reasonable timescale, taking into account the urgency of needs and a consideration of any fluctuation in those needs,

  and that local authorities:

  > ... should inform the individual of an indicative timescale over which their assessment will be conducted and keep the individual informed throughout the assessment process;
- completes an unlawful assessment, on the basis of which inadequate services are offered, for example, by failing to involve relevant persons, failing to take into account relevant material or reaching unreasoned or irrational conclusions.[3]

8.4 That said, applications for judicial review of assessment-related failures generally only succeed when the claimant establishes a clear breach of the legal parameters (see chapter 27 for more on judicial review). The courts tend to:

- focus on the substance of the issue, rather than on the detail of what remains, even now, a highly complex and detailed scheme that cannot always be perfectly adhered to;

1 See, under the previous regime, *R v Bristol CC ex p Penfold* (1997–8) 1 CCLR 315.

2 See, under the previous regime, *R (AA) v Lambeth LBC* [2001] EWHC 741 (Admin), (2002) 5 CCLR 36.

3 See, again under the previous regime, *R v North Yorkshire CC ex p William Hargreaves* (1997–8) 1 CCLR 104 and *R v Islington LBC ex p Rixon* (1997–8) 1 CCLR 119.

- defer to professional evaluation and judgment, by adopting a relatively generous reading of the assessment material;
- manifest a strong appreciation that the function of judicial review is to correct legal errors and not to engage with factual disputes or ongoing monitoring of local authority activity, particularly bearing in mind the availability of alternative remedies (currently, alternative dispute resolution (ADR) and the statutory complaints procedure (see para 7.97 below)),[4] especially where the challenge is perceived to be fact-specific or focussed on relatively minor aspects of the assessment process or as being little more than a challenge to the merits of the local authority assessment (see paras 27.8–27.9 and 27.15–27.28 below). That tendency is likely to increase as a result of:
  - the enactment of section 31(2A) of the Senior Courts Act 1981, which provides that the High Court must refuse to grant relief 'if it appears to the court to be highly likely that the outcome for the applicant would not have been substantially different if the conduct complained of had not occurred', unless there is an 'exceptional public interest' in granting relief (see para 3.8 above and para 27.10 below); and
  - the forthcoming statutory appeals procedure (see para 7.97 above).

8.5 The courts tend to involve themselves more readily on issues of interim relief, in order to hold the ring or create a situation of stability; where significant errors of law may be involved; where something appears to have gone seriously awry in the assessment process and where significant numbers of people may be involved; but again the court is likely to hold back when it perceives there to be a suitable alternative remedy and that tendency is likely to increase for the reasons set out above in para 8.4.

Legislative and administrative framework

8.6 The statutory duty to assess the needs of adults and carers, and in some cases, children, is set out in the Care Act 2014 at sections 9–13 (adults and carers), 58–59 (children's needs after they turn 18), 60–62 (children's carers) and 63–64 (young carers). Aspects of the Care Act 2014 that concern children/young persons are addressed later at 'children in transition' (see para 8.25 below).

8.7 In relation to adults and carers, the two crucial assessment steps, before the care planning process starts, are to:

- assess in writing the adult's needs for care and support (the 'needs assessment') and the carer's needs for support (the 'carer's assessment' (under sections 9–12); then
- (i) 'determine' in writing which of those needs are 'eligible needs'; (ii) 'consider' what could be done to meet those needs; (iii) 'ascertain' whether the adult wishes the local authority to meet those needs; and

4 See, in particular, *R (Ireneschild) v Lambeth LBC* [2007] EWCA Civ 234, (2007) 10 CCLR 243 and *R (F, J, S, R) v Wirral BC* [2009] EWHC 1626, (2009) 12 CCLR 452.

(iv) 'establish' whether the adult/carer is ordinarily resident in the local authority's area (section 13).

Assessment key features

8.8 Key features of the statutory duty to assess adults and carers, found in the Care Act 2014 itself, are:

A low threshold

- the threshold is low: the duty to assess arises 'where it appears to a local authority' that an adult, or carer, 'may have needs' for 'care and support' (adult) or 'support' (carer) (sections 9(1) and 10(1)). The possibility that a need may exist must no doubt be a realistic one, but the threshold is on any view low;
- the duty requires an assessment to be completed 'regardless of the authority's view' of 'the level of the adult's needs for care and support'/ 'the level of the carer's needs for support' or 'the level of the adult's financial resources'/'the level of the carer's financial resources or of those of the adult needing care' (sections 9(2) and 10(4)). In other words, the duty to assess will arise even though –
  - it seems plain that none of the adult's or carer's needs will amount to 'eligible needs' or, indeed, needs that the local authority is at all likely to exercise a power to address;
  - it seems plain that the adult's or carer's means will exceed the 'financial limit' (see paras 11.10–11.15 below).

A free service

- A local authority may not charge for undertaking any form of assessment under the Care Act 2014 (see para 11 8 below).

Matters to be covered

- the assessment of an adult must include an assessment of the impact of the adult's needs for care and support on their 'well-being' (as defined in section 1(2)), the 'outcomes' the adult wishes to achieve in day-to-day life and whether, and if so to what extent, the provision of care and support could contribute to the achievement of those outcomes (section 9(4)). This emphasises the importance of assessing what it is that the adult wants to do with his or her life;
- the assessment of a carer must include an assessment of whether the carer is able, and is likely to continue to be able, to provide care; whether they are willing, and are likely to continue to be willing to do so; the impact of the carer's needs for support on their 'well-being' (as defined in section 1(2)); the 'outcomes' the carer wishes to achieve in day-to-day life and whether, and if so to what extent, the provision of care and support could contribute to the achievement of those outcomes (section 10(5)); and the local authority must take into account whether the carer works, or wishes to do so and is participating in education, training or recreation, or wishes to do so (section 10(6)). This emphasises the

importance of ensuring that carers do not become trapped in a caring role.

Process

Legislation

- the local authority must *involve* the adult and any carer and any person whom the adult asks to be involved or, where the adult lacks capacity, who appears to the authority to be interested in the adult's welfare (sections 9(5) and 10(7)). The importance of ensuring effective participation and involvement is further emphasised and provided for in regulation 3 of the Care and Support (Assessment) Regulations 2014 and at paragraphs 6.30–6.53 of the *Care and Support Statutory Guidance*;
- it is implicit in the Act that, in assessing an adult's needs, the local authority must disregard any support being provided by a carer, although such support (willingly provided) may be taken into account later, during the care and support planning stage and that is spelled out at paragraph 6.15 of the Guidance;
- when carrying out an assessment, a local authority must also consider whether matters other than the provision of care and support might contribute to the achievement of the outcomes the adult/carer wishes to achieve and whether the adult/carer might benefit from 'anything which might be available in the community', under section 2 (preventative measures) or under section 4 (information and advice) (section 9(6) and section 10(8));
- the local authority is required to provide and retain 'a written record' of adult's and carer's assessments (section 12(3) and (4));
- a local authority may undertake 'combined assessments' (adult's and carer's) and/or 'joint assessments' (with other agencies) (section 12(5), (6) and (7));
- in the case of an adult the local authority must make, and provide, a written and reasoned determination 'whether any of the needs meet the eligibility criteria' (section 13(1) and (2)) and, if so, it must (i) 'consider' 'what could be done to meet those needs'; (ii) 'ascertain' 'whether the adult wants to have those needs met by the local authority' and (iii) 'establish' 'whether the adult is ordinarily resident in the local authority's area' (section 13(2));
- in the case of a carer the local authority must make a written and reasoned determination 'whether any of the needs meet the eligibility criteria' (section 13(1)) and, if so, it must (i) 'consider' 'what could be done to meet those needs'; and (ii) 'establish' 'whether the adult needing care is ordinarily resident in the local authority's area' (section 13(3));
- where none of the adult's needs meet the eligibility criteria, the local authority must give him or her written advice and information about 'what can be done to meet or reduce the needs' and 'to prevent or delay the development of needs for care and support, or the development of needs for support, in the future' (section 13(4) and (5));
- section 67 provides that where an individual would experience substantial difficulty in participating in the assessment process, the local authority must appoint an independent advocate. Paragraph 6.23 of

the Guidance states that from the time of first contact 'local authorities should consider whether the individual would have substantial difficulty in being involved in the assessment process and if so consider the need for independent advocacy' and paragraphs 6.33–6.34 and Chapter 7 contain further advice. The Care and Support (Independent Advocacy Support) (No 2) Regulations 2014, regulate both local authorities and advocates;[5]

- a local authority need not carry out an assessment when it is refused (section 11(1)) although it remains under a duty to do so when the adult lacks capacity to refuse the assessment and the local authority is satisfied that it would be in their best interests to carry out the assessment, or that they are experiencing or at risk of abuse or neglect (section 11(2)). Otherwise, the obligation to carry out an assessment revives when, after a refusal, an assessment is requested, or the circumstances change (sections 11(3), (4), (5) and (7));
- assessments may be delegated (section 79(1); paragraph 6.99 and Chapter 18 of the Guidance).

Regulations

8.9 The assessment duties in the Care Act 2014 are supplemented by duties found in the Care and Support (Assessment) Regulations 2014, which provide that:

- local authorities are required to facilitate a 'supported self-assessment' where the adult or child concerned wishes and has the capacity/competence (regulation 2);
- assessments are to be conducted in a manner which is 'appropriate and proportionate to the needs and circumstances of the individual to whom it relates' and 'ensures that the individual is able to participate in the process as effectively as possible' (regulation 3);
- where the level of an individual's needs fluctuates, the local authority must take into account their circumstances over an appropriate period of time (regulation 3(3) of the Care and Support (Assessment) Regulations 2014 and paragraphs 6.58–6.59 of the Guidance);
- the local authority must provide information about the assessment process, wherever practicable before it commences (regulation 3(4) and (5));
- assessments must consider the impact of the needs of the individual on 'any person who is involved in caring for the individual' and 'any person the local authority considers to be relevant'; they must also consider the impact of providing care on child carers (regulation 4);
- local authorities must ensure that every person undertaking assessments 'has the skills, knowledge and competence to carry out the assessment in question' and 'is appropriately trained' and, where appropriate, seeks an expert view (regulation 5). Further 'An assessment which relates to an individual who is deafblind must be carried out by a person who has specific training and expertise relating to individuals

5 This has teeth: an assessment completed without having engaged an independent advocate, in breach of section 67, was held to be unlawful in *R (SG) v Haringey LBC* [2015] EWHC 2579 (Admin), (2015) 18 CCLR 444.

who are deafblind' (regulation 6). These provisions, together with the Guidance, also in effect require persons who assess adults with autism to have specialist training (see paragraphs 6.83–6.88 of the Guidance);
- local authorities must refer individuals to the relevant NHS body where it appears that they may be eligible for NHS continuing healthcare (regulation 7).

Guidance

8.10 Key features of the *Care and Support Statutory Guidance* (March 2016), Chapters 6 and 7 are:
- the assessment process (paragraphs 6.1–6.43);
- supported self-assessments (paragraphs 6.44–6.53);
- cases where a safeguarding issue arises (paragraphs 6.54–6.57);
- fluctuating needs and prevention (paragraphs 6.58–6.62);
- the person's strengths and capabilities (paragraphs 6.63–6.64);
- the 'whole family approach' (paragraphs 6.65–6.71);
- combined and integrated assessments (paragraphs 6.72–6.77);
- NHS continuing healthcare cases (paragraphs 6.78–6.81);
- roles, training, record-keeping and delegation (paragraphs 6.82–6.97);
- eligibility and service provision (paragraphs 6.98–6.132);
- independent advocacy (Chapter 7).

8.11 Paragraphs 6.87 of the *Care and Support Statutory Guidance* (March 2016) requires additional guidance to be taken into consideration:
- Think Autism (2014);
- Fulfilling and Rewarding Lives (2014 Update);
- the strategy for adults with autism in England.

8.12 Accordingly, before one even embarks on the substance of an assessment a number of critical questions arise:
- is the statutory threshold for an assessment met?
- is the person undertaking the assessment suitably qualified to do so? Is an expert view required?
- how are all the relevant people going to be properly involved?
- should there be a referral to the NHS?
- should there be a supported self-assessment?
- should there be an independent advocate?
- should there be a combined or integrated assessment?
- how long should the process take?

Eligibility

8.13 The Care Act 2014 sweeps away the long-standing entitlement of each local authority to determine its own local eligibility criteria, albeit, in recent years, by reference to nationally applicable banding criteria, based on 'Critical', 'Substantial', 'Moderate' and 'Low' needs, as defined. Instead, there are now fixed, nationally applicable eligibility criteria, designed to end the worst features of the 'postcode lottery' and facilitate the 'portability' of care packages by establishing a minimum level of provision.

8.14 The new national eligibility criteria are to be found in the Care and Support (Eligibility Criteria) Regulations 2015. Regulation 2 sets out the eligibility criteria for adults, regulation 3 for carers:

Needs which meet the eligibility criteria: adults who need care and support

2(1) An adult's needs meet the eligibility criteria if–
(a) the adult's needs arise from or are related to a physical or mental impairment or illness;
(b) as a result of the adult's needs the adult is unable to achieve two or more of the outcomes specified in paragraph (2); and
(c) as a consequence there is, or is likely to be, a significant impact on the adult's well-being.

(2) The specified outcomes are–
(a) managing and maintaining nutrition;
(b) maintaining personal hygiene;
(c) managing toilet needs;
(d) being appropriately clothed;
(e) being able to make use of the adult's home safely;
(f) maintaining a habitable home environment;
(g) developing and maintaining family or other personal relationships;
(h) accessing and engaging in work, training, education or volunteering;
(i) making use of necessary facilities or services in the local community including public transport, and recreational facilities or services; and
(j) carrying out any caring responsibilities the adult has for a child.

(3) For the purposes of this regulation an adult is to be regarded as being unable to achieve an outcome if the adult–
(a) is unable to achieve it without assistance;
(b) is able to achieve it without assistance but doing so causes the adult significant pain, distress or anxiety;
(c) is able to achieve it without assistance but doing so endangers or is likely to endanger the health or safety of the adult, or of others; or
(d) is able to achieve it without assistance but takes significantly longer than would normally be expected.

(4) Where the level of an adult's needs fluctuates, in determining whether the adult's needs meet the eligibility criteria, the local authority must take into account the adult's circumstances over such period as it considers necessary to establish accurately the adult's level of need.

Needs which meet the eligibility criteria: carers

3(1) A carer's needs meet the eligibility criteria if–
(a) the needs arise as a consequence of providing necessary care for an adult;
(b) the effect of the carer's needs is that any of the circumstances specified in paragraph (2) apply to the carer; and
(c) as a consequence of that fact there is, or is likely to be, a significant impact on the carer's well-being.

(2) The circumstances specified in this paragraph are as follows–
(a) the carer's physical or mental health is, or is at risk of, deteriorating;
(b) the carer is unable to achieve any of the following outcomes–
(i) carrying out any caring responsibilities the carer has for a child;

(ii) providing care to other persons for whom the carer provides care;
(iii) maintaining a habitable home environment in the carer's home (whether or not this is also the home of the adult needing care);
(iv) managing and maintaining nutrition;
(v) developing and maintaining family or other personal relationships;
(vi) engaging in work, training, education or volunteering;
(vii) making use of necessary facilities or services in the local community, including recreational facilities or services; and (viii) engaging in recreational activities.

(3) For the purposes of paragraph (2) a carer is to be regarded as being unable to achieve an outcome if the carer–
(a) is unable to achieve it without assistance;
(b) is able to achieve it without assistance but doing so causes the carer significant pain, distress or anxiety; or
(c) is able to achieve it without assistance but doing so endangers or is likely to endanger the health or safety of the carer, or of others.

(4) Where the level of a carer's needs fluctuates, in determining whether the carer's needs meet the eligibility criteria, the local authority must take into account the carer's circumstances over such period as it considers necessary to establish accurately the carer's level of need.

8.15 Advice about these provisions is to be found at Chapter 6 of the *Care and Support Statutory Guidance*. Paragraphs 6.103 and 6.104 are critical:

6.103 The second condition that authorities must consider is whether the adult is 'unable' to achieve two or more of the outcomes set out in the regulations. Authorities must also be aware that the regulations provide that 'being unable' to achieve an outcome includes any of the following circumstances, where the adult:

- is unable to achieve the outcome without assistance. This would include where an adult would be unable to do so even when assistance is provided. It also includes where the adult may need prompting for example, some adults may be physically able to wash but need reminding of the importance of personal hygiene;
- is able to achieve the outcome without assistance but doing so causes the adult significant pain, distress or anxiety. For example, an older person with severe arthritis may be able to prepare a meal, but doing so will leave them in severe pain and unable to eat the meal;
- is able to achieve the outcome without assistance, but doing so endangers or is likely to endanger the health or safety of the adult, or of others – for example, if the health or safety of another member of the family, including any child, could be endangered when an adult attempts to complete a task or an activity without relevant support;
- is able to achieve the outcome without assistance but takes significantly longer than would normally be expected. For example, an adult with a physical disability is able to dress themselves in the morning, but it takes them a long time to do this, leaves them exhausted and prevents them from achieving other outcomes.

6.104 The Eligibility Regulations set out a range of outcomes. Local authorities must consider whether the adult is unable to achieve two or more of these outcomes when making the eligibility determination. The following section of the guidance provides examples of how local authorities should consider each outcome set out in the Eligibility Regulations (which do not constitute an exhaustive list) when determining the adult's eligibility for care and support:

(a) managing and maintaining nutrition – local authorities should consider whether the adult has access to food and drink to maintain nutrition, and that the adult is able to prepare and consume the food and drink.

(b) maintaining personal hygiene – local authorities should, for example, consider the adult's ability to wash themselves and launder their clothes.

(c) managing toilet needs – local authorities should consider the adult's ability to access and use a toilet and manage their toilet needs.

(d) being appropriately clothed – local authorities should consider the adult's ability to dress themselves and to be appropriately dressed, for instance in relation to the weather to maintain their health.

(e) being able to make use of the home safely – local authorities should consider the adult's ability to move around the home safely, which could for example include getting up steps, using kitchen facilities or accessing the bathroom. This should also include the immediate environment around the home such as access to the property, for example steps leading up to the home.

(f) maintaining a habitable home environment – local authorities should consider whether the condition of the adult's home is sufficiently clean and maintained to be safe. A habitable home is safe and has essential amenities. An adult may require support to sustain their occupancy of the home and to maintain amenities, such as water, electricity and gas.

(g) developing and maintaining family or other personal relationships – local authorities should consider whether the adult is lonely or isolated, either because their needs prevent them from maintaining the personal relationships they have or because their needs prevent them from developing new relationships.

(h) accessing and engaging in work, training, education or volunteering – local authorities should consider whether the adult has an opportunity to apply themselves and contribute to society through work, training, education or volunteering, subject to their own wishes in this regard. This includes the physical access to any facility and support with the participation in the relevant activity.

(i) making use of necessary facilities or services in the local community including public transport and recreational facilities or services – local authorities should consider the adult's ability to get around in the community safely and consider their ability to use such facilities as public transport, shops or recreational facilities when considering the impact on their wellbeing. Local authorities do not have responsibility for the provision of NHS services such as patient transport, however they should consider needs for support when the adult is attending healthcare appointments.

(j) carrying out any caring responsibilities the adult has for a child – local authorities should consider any parenting or other caring responsibilities the person has. The adult may for example be a step-parent with caring responsibilities for their spouse's children.

8.16 In addition, the Social Care Institute for Excellence has published advice about decision-making on eligibility.[6]

6 www.scie.org.uk/care-act–2014/assessment-and-eligibility/eligibility/.

Different types of assessments

8.17 The Guidance sets out some of the different types of assessment process that a local authority might decide to adopt as the most appropriate/proportionate in a particular case:

> 6.3 An 'assessment' must always be appropriate and proportionate. It may come in different formats and can be carried out in various ways, including but not limited to:
>
> - A face-to-face assessment between the person and an assessor, whose professional role and qualifications may vary depending on the circumstances, but who must always be appropriately trained and have the right skills and knowledge.
> - A supported self-assessment, which should use the same assessment materials as a face-to-face assessment, but where the person completes the assessment themselves and the local authority assures itself that it is an accurate reflection of the person's needs (for example, by consulting with other relevant professionals and people who know the person with their consent).
> - An online or phone assessment, which can be a proportionate way of carrying out assessments (for example where the person's needs are less complex or where the person is already known to the local authority and it is carrying out an assessment following a change in their needs or circumstances).
> - A joint assessment, where relevant agencies work together to avoid the person undergoing multiple assessments (including assessments in a prison, where local authorities may need to put particular emphasis on cross-agency cooperation and sharing of expertise).
> - A combined assessment, where an adult's assessment is combined with a carer's assessment and/or an assessment relating to a child so that interrelated needs are properly captured and the process is as efficient as possible.

8.18 Regulation 2 of the Care and Support (Assessment) Regulations 2014 requires local authorities proposing to undertake an assessment to ascertain whether the subject wishes it to be a supported self-assessment (reg 2(2)) and, if so, the assessment must take that form, so long as the subject has the capacity to engage (reg 2(3)): supported self-assessments are addressed in the Guidance at paragraphs 6.44–6.53.

8.19 Once the person has completed the assessment, 'the local authority must ensure that it is an accurate and complete reflection of the person's needs, outcomes, and the impact of needs on their well-being' (paragraph 6.46 of the Guidance). This is consistent with the approach established under the earlier regime, under which it was clearly recognised that the ultimate responsibility for ensuring that there was an adequate needs assessment lay with the local authority.[7] See also:

> 6.47 In assuring self-assessments local authorities may consider it useful to seek the views of those who are in regular contact with the person self-assessing, such as their carer(s) or other appropriate people from their support network, and any professional involved in providing care such as a housing support officer, a GP, a treating clinician, a district nurse, a rehabilitation officer or relevant prison staff. In doing this, the local authority

7 *R (B) v Cornwall CC* [2009] EWHC 491 (Admin), (2009) 12 CCLR 381 at para 68.

should first seek the person's consent. This may be helpful in allowing local authorities to build an understanding of the individual's desires, outcomes, needs, and the impact on their wellbeing.

Other publicly available material on assessment and care planning

8.20 The Department of Health's Factsheet 3 deals with assessing needs and determining eligibility.[8]

8.21 The Social Care Institute for Excellence has published a range of resources to support local authority staff, social workers and others involved in assessment and eligibility.[9]

8.22 The Social Care Institute for Excellence has also published advice about independent advocacy.[10] There is a briefing note by the Department of Health, Association of Directors of Adult Social Care Services (ADASS) and the Local Government Association (LGA) on independent advocacy.[11]

8.23 It should also be noted that the Mental Capacity Act 2005, and access to an Independent Mental Capacity Advocate, will apply for all those who may lack capacity: see chapter 23 below.

The previous legislative scheme

8.24 The statutory basis for assessments of adults was section 47 of the National Health Service and Community Care Act 1990 which provided, inter alia, immediately before its repeal:

> **Assessment of needs for community care services**
>
> 47(1) Subject to subsections (5) and (6) below, where it appears to a local authority that any person for whom they may provide or arrange for the provision of community care services may be in need of any such services, the authority–
>
> (a) shall carry out an assessment of his needs for those services; and
>
> (b) having regard to the results of that assessment, shall then decide whether his needs call for the provision by them of any such services.

Children in transition

8.25 The statutory machinery relevant to the transition between children's and adult social care is located at:

- sections 58–66 of the Care Act 2014;
- the Care and Support (Children's Carers) Regulations 2015;
- Chapter 16 of the Care and Support Statutory Guidance.

8 www.gov.uk/government/publications/care-act–2014-part–1-factsheets/care-act-factsheets-–2#factsheet–3-assessing-needs-and-determining-eligibility).

9 www.scie.org.uk/care-act–2014/assessment-and-eligibility/).

10 www.scie.org.uk/care-act–2014/advocacy-services/commissioning-independent-advocacy/duties/independent-advocacy-care-act.asp.

11 www.local.gov.uk/documents/10180/5756320/Briefing+note+V1+for+Advocacy+providers++final_LPlogo.pdf/4f1c20ad–3933–4291-b842–558511d8836f.

8.26 The Care Act 2014 seeks to help preparation for adulthood by focussing on transitional planning for:

- 'children' (sections 58–59, 65–66);
- 'child's carers' (sections 60–62, 65–66); and
- 'young carers' (sections 63–64, 65–66).

Children

8.28 The duty to assess a child's need for care and support under the Care Act 2014 after becoming 18 is as follows:

Assessment of a child's needs for care and support

58(1) Where it appears to a local authority that a child is likely to have needs for care and support after becoming 18, the authority must, if it is satisfied that it would be of significant benefit to the child to do so and if the consent condition is met, assess–

(a) whether the child has needs for care and support and, if so, what those needs are, and

(b) whether the child is likely to have needs for care and support after becoming 18 and, if so, what those needs are likely to be.

8.29 The '*consent condition*' is met if:

- a child with capacity consents;
- or it is in the best interests of an incapacitated child; except that
- the local authority must always undertake an assessment if it considers that the child is experiencing or at risk of abuse or neglect –

(sections 58(3)–(4)).

8.30 A local authority must give written reasons for any refusal to undertake a '*child's needs assessment*' under this section at the request of a parent or carer (sections 58(5)–(8)).

8.31 It is fundamental to a '*child's needs assessment*' that the local authority does, as required by section 58(1), assess:

- whether the child currently has needs for care and support and, if so, what those needs are; and
- whether the child is likely to have needs for care and support after the child turns 18 and, if so, what those needs are likely to be.

8.32 However, a '*child's needs assessment*' requires far more than that. By virtue of section 59:

Child's needs assessment: requirements etc.

59(1) A child's needs assessment must include an assessment of–

(a) the impact on the matters specified in section 1(2) of what the child's needs for care and support are likely to be after the child becomes 18,

(b) the outcomes that the child wishes to achieve in day-to-day life, and

(c) whether, and if so to what extent, the provision of care and support could contribute to the achievement of those outcomes.

...

(3) When carrying out a child's needs assessment, a local authority must also consider whether, and if so to what extent, matters other than the provision of care and support could contribute to the achievement of the outcomes that the child wishes to achieve in day-to-day life.

(4) Having carried out a child's needs assessment, a local authority must give the child–
   (a) an indication as to whether any of the needs for care and support which it thinks the child is likely to have after becoming 18 are likely to meet the eligibility criteria (and, if so, which ones are likely to do so), and
   (b) advice and information about–
      (i) what can be done to meet or reduce the needs which it thinks the child is likely to have after becoming 18;
      (ii) what can be done to prevent or delay the development by the child of needs for care and support in the future.

8.33 In undertaking the assessment, the local authority:

- must involve the child, their parents and other relevant persons (section 59(2));
- must provide the section 59(4) advice and information to the parents when the child lacks capacity; and
- may treat the assessment as a 'needs assessment' once the child turns 18.

(section 59(6)–(7)).

Child's carers

8.34 A *'child's carer'* is an adult (including one who is a parent of the child) who provides or intends to provide care for the child, usually when that is otherwise than under a contract or as voluntary work (section 60(7)–(9)).

8.35 The duty to undertake a *'child's carer's assessment'* is found at section 60 of the Care Act 2014 and arises in similar circumstances to the duty to undertake a children's transitional assessment (see above): the question is, essentially, whether the child's carer is likely to have needs for support under the Care Act 2014 after the child becomes 18 and it would be of significant benefit to the carer to undertake an advance assessment.

8.36 It is a fundamental requirement, imposed by section 60(1), that a *'child's carer's assessment'* assesses whether the carer has needs for support and, if so, what those needs are and whether the carer is likely to have needs for support after the child becomes 18 and, if so, what those needs are likely to be.

8.37 Again, however, far more is required:

Child's carer's assessment: requirements etc.

61(1) A child's carer's assessment must include an assessment of–
   (a) whether the carer is able to provide care for the child and is likely to continue to be able to do so after the child becomes 18,
   (b) whether the carer is willing to do so and is likely to continue to be willing to do so after the child becomes 18,
   (c) the impact on the matters specified in section 1(2) of what the carer's needs for support are likely to be after the child becomes 18,
   (d) the outcomes that the carer wishes to achieve in day-to-day life, and
   (e) whether, and if so to what extent, the provision of support could contribute to the achievement of those outcomes.

(2) A local authority, in carrying out a child's carer's assessment, must have regard to–
   (a) whether the carer works or wishes to do so, and

(b) whether the carer is participating in or wishes to participate in education, training or recreation.

...

(4) When carrying out a child's carer's assessment, a local authority must also consider whether, and if so to what extent, matters other than the provision of support could contribute to the achievement of the outcomes that the carer wishes to achieve in day-to-day life.

(5) Having carried out a child's carer's assessment, a local authority must give the carer–

(a) an indication as to whether any of the needs for support which it thinks the carer is likely to have after the child becomes 18 are likely to meet the eligibility criteria (and, if so, which ones are likely to do so), and

(b) advice and information about–

(i) what can be done to meet or reduce the needs which it thinks the carer is likely to have after the child becomes 18;

(ii) what can be done to prevent or delay the development by the carer of needs for support in the future.

8.38 The process is similar to the process for '*child's needs assessments*' (see sections 61(3) and (5)–(8)) and, ultimately, the local authority has a power to meet the '*child's carer's*' needs for support (section 62).

Young carers

8.39 A '*young carer* is '*a person under 18 who provides or intends to provide care for an adult*', usually otherwise than under a contract or as voluntary work (sections 63(6)–(8)).

8.40 The duty to undertake a '*young carer's assessment'* arises when it appears that a young carer is likely to have needs for support after turning 18 and the local authority is satisfied that it would of significant benefit to the young carer to undertake an advance assessment) (section 63(1)).

8.41 The assessment is of whether the young carer is likely to have needs for support after turning 18 and, if so, what those needs are likely to be (section 63(1)). However, in addition:

Young carer's assessment: requirements etc.

64(1) A young carer's assessment must include an assessment of–

(a) whether the young carer is able to provide care for the person in question and is likely to continue to be able to do so after becoming 18,

(b) whether the young carer is willing to do so and is likely to continue to be willing to do so after becoming 18,

(c) the impact on the matters specified in section 1(2) of what the young carer's needs for support are likely to be after the young carer becomes 18,

(d) the outcomes that the young carer wishes to achieve in day-to-day life, and (e) whether, and if so to what extent, the provision of support could contribute to the achievement of those outcomes.

(2) A local authority, in carrying out a young carer's assessment, must have regard to–

(a) the extent to which the young carer works or wishes to work (or is likely to wish to do so after becoming 18),

(b) the extent to which the young carer is participating in or wishes to participate in education, training or recreation (or is likely to wish to do so after becoming 18).

...

(4) When carrying out a young carer's assessment, a local authority must also consider whether, and if so to what extent, matters other than the provision of support could contribute to the achievement of the outcomes that the young carer wishes to achieve in day-to-day life.

(5) Having carried out a young carer's assessment, a local authority must give the young carer–

(a) an indication as to whether any of the needs for support which it thinks the young carer is likely to have after becoming 18 are likely to meet the eligibility criteria (and, if so, which ones are likely to do so), and

(b) advice and information about–

(i) what can be done to meet or reduce the needs for support which it thinks the young carer is likely to have after becoming 18;

(ii) what can be done to prevent or delay the development by the young carer of needs for support in the future.

8.42 The process is similar to that for *'child's needs assessments'* and *'child's carers' assessments'* (sections 64(3) and (6)–(8)).

General

8.43 Section 65 contains provision for combining *'child's needs assessments'*, *'young carer's assessments'* and *'child's carers' assessments'* with each other and with other assessments.

8.44 Section 66 inserts section 17ZH and 17ZI at the end of section 17 of the Children Act 1989 which, in essence, requires local authorities to continue to provide services under section 17 of the Children Act 1989 in cases where they are under a duty to undertake a *'child's needs assessment'*, *'young carer's assessment'* or *'child's carers' assessment'* and certain other cases.

8.45 Section 66 also inserts section 2A into the Chronically Sick and Disabled Persons Act 1970, which requires there to be continued provision of services under section 2 of the 1970 Act to disabled children, until the completion of transitional planning under the Care Act 2014, in cases where such transitional planning is required and certain other cases.

8.46 There is detailed practical guidance in Chapter 16 of the *Care and Support Statutory Guidance*, which is particularly useful as to:

- the relationship between planning under the Care Act 2014 and planning for children with special educational needs, who will be subject to an Education, Health and Care (EHC) plan; and
- the duty of co-operation, in particular between children's and adults' professionals.

8.47 Section 23CZA, added by the Children and Families Act 2014, allows local authorities to make arrangements whereby a *'former relevant child'* may continue to live with their foster carer up to the age of 21:

- the statutory guidance in the *Children Act 1989 Regulations and Guidance, Volume 3: planning transition to adulthood for care leavers*[12] has been updated accordingly; and
- The Children's Partnership has published *Staying Put: a good practice guide.*[13]

Cases

Threshold for assessments

8.48 *R v Bristol CC ex p Penfold* (1997–8) 1 CCLR 315, QBD

The threshold for an assessment is low and the duty arises irrespective of the likelihood of resources being available to meet the need

Facts: Ms Penfold was a homeless single parent who suffered from anxiety and depression. She was no longer entitled to assistance under the Housing Acts. Bristol declined to assess Ms Penfold's needs under the National Health Service and Community Care Act 1990, on the ground that she did not appear to be a person who 'may' need services and, in any event, there was no realistic prospect of the local authority providing her with accommodation under any of the community care legislation, given its straightened resources and the applicant's accommodation history.

Judgment: Scott Baker J held (at 322E) as follows:

> It seems to me that Parliament has expressed section 47(1) in very clear terms. The opening words of the subsection, the first step in the three stage process, provide a very low threshold test. The reference is to community care services the authority *may* provide or arrange for. And the services are those of which the person *may* be in need. If that test is passed it is mandatory to carry out the assessment. The word *shall* emphasises that this is so ... As a matter of logic, it is difficult to see how the existence or otherwise of resources to meet a need can determine whether or not that need exists ... Even if there is no hope from the resources point of view of meeting any needs identified in the assessment, the assessment may serve a useful purpose in identifying for the local authority unmet needs which will help it to plan for the future ... Resource implications in my view play no part in the decision whether to carry out an assessment.

Comment: the principle has been encapsulated in the Care Act 2014 and its machinery but the case remains a useful authority as to what a low threshold means in practice.

8.49 *R v Berkshire CC ex p P* (1997–8) 1 CCLR 141, QBD

The duty to assess arises whenever there is a power to make provision

Facts: P lived in a care home in London but sought an assessment from Berkshire, where he used to live. A dispute arose as to where P was ordinarily resident and Berkshire declined to assess P's needs on the ground that he was not ordinarily resident in Berkshire.

12 www.gov.uk/government/uploads/system/uploads/attachment_data/file/397649/CA1989_Transitions_guidance.pdf.

13 www.ncb.org.uk/media/1154341/staying_put.pdf.

Judgment: Laws J held that the duty to assess arose whenever a local authority had power to provide services to a person who it appeared might need them and that, since a local authority was entitled to provide services to a person who was ordinarily resident in another area, the duty to assess had arisen.

8.50 *R (NM) v Islington LBC* [2012] EWHC 414 (Admin), (2012) 15 CCLR 563

There is no duty to assess a prisoner until the Parole Board has decided in principle they should be released, or MAPPA needs information about what care services would be available

Facts: NM had a significant learning disability and was in prison. The Parole Board had made directions about the making of MAPPA (multi agency public protection) arrangements but no such arrangements had as yet been initiated. NM sought a community care assessment from Islington, so as to inform the Parole Board as to what support would be available to him on release. Islington declined to undertake such an assessment.

Judgment: Sales J held that, since no relevant MAPPA process had as yet been undertaken, the prospect of NM's release was as yet too speculative for the duty to assess to arise. A duty would arise when the Parole Board takes a decision in principle that someone should be released and, also, when there has been a full MAPPA consideration with an indication that community care services would be likely to be required and the Parole Board needs more information about that.

Comment: nothing in the Care Act 2014 seems to displace this somewhat restrictive approach.

Urgent cases

8.51 *R (AA) v Lambeth LBC* [2001] EWHC 741 (Admin), (2002) 5 CCLR 36

The court is entitled to order a local authority to provide services pending assessment, even where the local authority does not consider that the criteria for interim provision are met

Facts: AA, a destitute asylum-seeker, got into dire straits and applied to Lambeth for urgent assistance. Lambeth submitted that, notwithstanding the terms of section 47(5) of the National Health Service and Community Care Act 1990, it had no power to provide interim assistance under section 21 of the National Assistance Act (NAA) 1948 unless and until it had completed an assessment of need: section 47 could not affect that.

Judgment: Forbes J held that Lambeth had statutory power to provide services before completing an assessment, because section 47(5) simply spelled out what had always been implicit in section 21, but, in any event, the court had jurisdiction to grant an interim injunction in the exercise of its general discretion to grant interim relief (under what is now section 37 of the Senior Courts Act 1981).

Comment: section 19(3) of the Care Act 2014 contains a wider power to provide services in urgent cases, before completing an assessment but it is still contingent on the local authority forming the view that the situation is urgent; therefore, the overarching power of the High Court to grant interim relief remains important.

8.52 *R (Alloway) v Bromley LBC* [2004] EWHC 2108 (Admin), (2005) 8 CCLR 61

Services may be provided pending completion of a re-assessment even in cases where there have been prior assessments

Facts: Mr Alloway was a 19-year-old man who was autistic and suffered from learning disabilities. Bromley's community care assessment concluded that he should be placed at Hesley Village and College. However, the Council then purported to place him at a cheaper option at Robinia Care. However, Bromley did not assert that its decision-making was affected by, or justified by, resources considerations.

Judgment: Crane J quashed this decision and said this at paragraphs 80–82:

> 80. I say in parenthesis that if any of the facilities mentioned can be urged to keep open the offers made, then that would certainly be desirable and the court's view about that can be conveyed to them.
>
> 81. I note in passing that it would be open to the defendant, if it so wished, to decide that a new assessment was required in all the circumstances, and that it needed to act on a temporary basis under section 47, subsection (5) and subsection (6). A temporary placement could be made in those circumstances. But that, is one of the matters that I simply bring to the local authority's attention.
>
> 82. It seems to me, and it is difficult to reach a conclusion about the best way ahead, so far as remedy is concerned, that the only remedy I need to grant is the quashing of the two decisions, if that is what they are, which I have mentioned. It does not seem to me, at the moment, that any declaration is required. In my view the judgment will speak for itself and, subject to counsel's submissions, I would propose merely to make an order quashing the decisions made so far and to leave the judgment to speak rather than to grant declarations. The other remedies sought I refuse.

Nature of an assessment

8.53 *R v Avon CC ex p M* (1999) 2 CCLR 185, [1994] 2 FCR 259, QBD

An assessment must also encompass psychological needs and an authority had to have strong reasons for diverging from the cogently reasoned conclusions of a complaints panel

Facts: a social services complaints review panel concluded that, as a result of his Down's Syndrome, M had developed the entrenched view that it was necessary for him to live in residential accommodation at a place called Milton Heights, such that to place him elsewhere would cause serious damage to his health; thus, he had a strong psychological need to live there. The panel recommended a placement at Milton Heights for three years, to allow for M to develop his living skills and be prepared to move elsewhere. In response, Avon concluded that whilst M had a strong personal preference to live at Milton Heights, his needs could be met at Berwick Lodge, which was substantially cheaper.

Judgment: Henry J held that Avon was under a duty to meet needs, including psychological needs of the kind that the panel held existed in this case and that Avon had not had *Wednesbury* rational reasons for disagreeing with the panel's assessment:

> Examining their reasons in detail, the following comments can be made:
>
> - The panel correctly found that in law the assessment must be based on current needs.
> - The panel correctly found that in law need is clearly capable of including psychological need. In particular, that must be so when (as it was on the evidence before them) that psychological need was contributed to by the congenital Down's Syndrome condition itself. I have recited the evidence that the panel had had as to that. That evidence was all one way once Mr Passfield had agreed that he was not an expert on Down's Syndrome.
> - Next, the panel had found that M's entrenched position was part of his psychological need. This is the crucial finding of fact. It is arrived at against the background, recited in these reasons, that M would not be forced to live anywhere against his will; that the only place he would presently consider would be Milton Heights, that that entrenched position was contributed to by the Down's Syndrome, and that his present needs included a need for a period of stability.
>
> …
>
> But the making of the final decision did not lie with the review panel. It lay with the social services committee. I would be reluctant to hold (and do not) that in no circumstances whatsoever could the social services committee have overruled the review panel's recommendation in the exercise of their legal right and duty to consider it. Caution normally requires the court not to say 'never' in any obiter dictum pronouncement. But I have no hesitation in finding that they could not overrule that decision without a substantial reason and without having given that recommendation the weight it required. It was a decision taken by a body entrusted with the basic fact-finding exercise under the complaints procedure. It was arrived at after a convincing examination of the evidence, particularly the expert evidence. The evidence before them had, as to the practicalities, been largely one way. The panel had directed themselves properly in law, and had arrived at a decision in line with the strength of the evidence before them. They had given clear reasons and they had raised the crucial factual question with the parties before arriving at their conclusion.
>
> The strength, coherence, and apparent persuasiveness of that decision had to be addressed head on if it were to be set aside and not followed. These difficulties were not faced either by the respondents' officers in their paper to the social services committee, or by the social services committee themselves. Not to face them was either unintentional perversity on their part, or showed a wrong appreciation of the legal standing of that decision. It seems to me that you do not properly reconsider a decision when, on the evidence, it does not seem that that decision was given the weight it deserved. That is, in my judgment, what the social services committee failed to do here. To neglect to do that is not a question which merely, as is suggested in one of the papers, impugns the credibility of the review panel, but instead ignores the weight to which it is prima facie entitled because of its place in

> the statutory procedure, and further, pays no attention to the scope of its hearing and clear reasons that it had given.
>
> It seems to me that anybody required, at law, to give their reasons for reconsidering and changing such a decision must have good reasons for doing so, and must show that they gave that decision sufficient weight and, in my judgment, it is that that the social services committee have here failed to do. Their decision must be quashed. As is often the case in Wednesbury quashings, it can be put in a number of ways: either unintentional perversity, or failure to take the review panel's recommendation properly into account, or an implicit error of law in not giving it sufficient weight.

8.54 *R v Bristol CC ex p Penfold* (1997–8) 1 CCLR 315, QBD

An assessment must fully explore needs

Facts: Ms Penfold was a homeless single parent who suffered from anxiety and depression. She was no longer entitled to assistance under the Housing Acts. Bristol declined to assess Ms Penfold's needs under the National Health Service and Community Care Act 1990, on the ground that she did not appear to be a person who 'may' need services and, in any event, there was no realistic prospect of the local authority providing her with accommodation under any of the community care legislation, given its straightened resources and the applicant's accommodation history.

Judgment: Scott Baker J held (at 321B) as follows:

> An assessment is something that is directed at the particular person who presents with an apparent need. One cannot be said to have been carried out unless the authority concerned has fully explored that need in relation to the services it has the power to supply. In some cases the exercise will be very simple; in others more complex.

8.55 *R v Haringey LBC ex p Norton* (1997–8) 1 CCLR 168, QBD

An assessment must explore social and recreational needs, not just social care needs

Facts: Mr Norton was severely disabled as a result of Multiple Sclerosis. Haringey reduced his care provision from 24 hours/day live-in care, to five hours a day practical assistance for budgetary reasons. There was no suggestion that Mr Norton's needs had changed. However, on re-assessment, Haringey concluded that Mr Norton had not, in reality, needed his earlier care package and that five hours a day was sufficient to meet his needs.

Judgment: Deputy High Court Judge Henderson QC held it had been unlawful only to assess Mr Norton's social care needs and not, also, his social, recreational and leisure needs:

> I consider that the Respondent misdirected itself in law. Reading the underlined sentences of the decision letter in context, the Respondent differentiated between the Applicant's social, recreational and leisure needs for which it did not believe that it needed to provide from the Applicant's personal care needs for which it recognised that it did need to provide. While the differentiation itself was not objectionable in point of law, because the Act of 1970 itemises such matters separately, it was impermissible to carry out the reassessment by putting social, recreation and leisure needs on one side and saying that 'I would be happy to provide you with details of the Winkfield Road Resource Centre.

Assessment process

8.56 *R v North Yorkshire CC ex p William Hargreaves* (1997–8) 1 CCLR 104, QBD

Account must be taken of the service user's views even where they are difficult to ascertain, for whatever reason

Facts: a dispute arose between Mr Hargreaves and North Yorkshire as to what form suitable respite care ought to take for Mr Hargreaves' intellectually impaired sister, Beryl Hargreaves. North Yorkshire had experienced great difficulty in communicating with Ms Hargreaves, exacerbated by Mr Hargreaves' overly protective actions. However, Ms Hargeaves had demonstrated an ability to express preferences and there was some evidence that her preferences were not identical to her brother's.

Judgment: paragraphs 3.15 and 3.25 of the statutory guidance at the time, the Policy Guidance, required local authorities to involve the individual service user in the assessment process and take account of their preferences. At 112H, Dyson J held that:

> ... the Respondent made its decision without taking into account the preferences of Miss Hargreaves on the issue in question. It must follow that the decision was unlawful in the sense that it was made in breach of paragraphs 3.16 and 3.25 of the Policy Guidance.

Comment: no doubt, had it been impossible or impracticable to ascertain Ms Hargreaves' preferences, North Yorkshire's failure to do so would have been lawful because it would have had a cogent reason for departure from the statutory guidance. However, under the current statutory scheme, the question would arise as to why the local authority had not appointed an independent advocate, or an IMCA, see:

- involvement/independent advocates/relevance of Mental Capacity Act 2005, above (para 7.53); and
- *R (SG) v Haringey LBC* [2015] EWHC 2579 (Admin), (2015) 18 CCLR 444 (see para 8.68 below), where an assessment was quashed owing to the local authority's failure to appoint an independent advocate, in breach of section 67 of the Care Act 2014.

8.57 *R v Islington LBC ex p Rixon* (1997–8) 1 CCLR 119, QBD

Assessments are central; they must comply in substance with statutory guidance and demonstrably have regard to relevant departmental guidance

Facts: the applicant was a severely mentally and physically disabled 24-year-old man, whose mother considered that inadequate provision had resulted in him losing skills acquired at his special needs school and failing to develop his full potential. It was common ground that Islington's assessment and care plan failed to address comprehensively the applicant's needs and failed to comply with relevant central government guidance.

Judgment: Sedley J held that Islington had acted unlawfully in failing to 'act under' statutory guidance and in failing properly to take into account non-statutory guidance:

This section, therefore, creates a positive duty to arrange for recreational and 'gateway' educational facilities for disabled persons. It is, counsel agree, a duty owed to the individual and not simply a target duty. I will come later to the question of its legal ambit and content. It introduces in turn section 7(1) of the Local Authority Social Services Act 1970:

> *Local authorities shall, in the exercise of their social services functions, including the exercise of any discretion conferred by any relevant enactment, act under the general guidance of the Secretary of State.*

(By an amendment introduced into the statute, section 7A *requires* local authorities to exercise their social services functions in accordance with any such *directions* as may be given to them by the Secretary of State.)

What is the meaning and effect of the obligation to 'act under the general guidance of the Secretary of State'? Clearly guidance is less than direction, and the word 'general' emphasises the non-prescriptive nature of what is envisaged. Mr McCarthy, for the local authority, submits that such guidance is no more than one of the many factors to which the local authority is to have regard. Miss Richards submits that, in order to give effect to the words 'shall act', a local authority must follow such guidance unless it has and can articulate a good reason for departing from it. In my judgment Parliament in enacting section 7(1) did not intend local authorities to whom ministerial guidance was given to be free, having considered it, to take it or leave it. Such a construction would put this kind of statutory guidance on a par with the many forms of non-statutory guidance issued by departments of state. While guidance and direction are semantically and legally different things, and while 'guidance does not compel any particular decision' (*Laker Airways Ltd v Department of Trade* [1967] QB 643, 714 per Roskill LJ), especially when prefaced by the word 'general', in my view Parliament by section 7(1) has required local authorities to follow the path charted by the Secretary of State's guidance, with liberty to deviate from it where the local authority judges on admissible grounds that there is good reason to do so, but without freedom to take a substantially different course.

...

A failure to comply with the statutory policy guidance is unlawful and can be corrected by means of judicial review: *R v North Yorkshire County Council ex p Hargreaves* (1997–98) 1 CCLR 104 (Dyson J, 30 September 1994). Beyond this, there will always be a variety of factors which the local authority is required on basic public law principles to take into account. Prominent among these will be any recommendations made in the particular case by a review panel: *R v Avon County Council ex p M* [1994] 2 FLR 1006 (Henry J). In contradistinction to statutory policy guidance, a failure to comply with a review panel's recommendations is not by itself a breach of the law; but the greater the departure, the greater the need for cogent articulated reasons if the court is not to infer that the panel's recommendations have been overlooked.

A second source of considerations which manifestly must be taken into account in coming to a decision is the practice guidance issued by the Department of Health. This currently takes the form of a Practitioners' Guide entitled 'Care Management and Assessment', which sets out 'a set of principles' derived from 'current views of practice'. The guidance breaks care management down into a series of stages, moving through communication and assessment to assembly of a care plan, and then on to the implementation, monitoring and periodic review of the plan.

...

> The care plan, as Mr McCarthy readily admits, does not comply either with the policy guidance or the practice guidance issued by central government. There has been a failure to comply with the guidance contained in paragraph 3.24 of the policy document to the effect that following assessment of need, the objectives of social services intervention as well as the services to be provided or arranged should be agreed in the form of a care plan. For the reasons which I have given, if this statutory guidance is to be departed from it must be with good reason, articulated in the course of some identifiable decision-making process even if not in the care plan itself. In the absence of any such considered decision, the deviation from the statutory guidance is in my judgment a breach of the law; and so *afortiori* is the reduction of the Flexiteam service from 3 hours as originally agreed, whatever the activity, to 3 hours swimming or 1 hours at home. I cannot accept Mr McCarthy's submission that the universal knowledge that no day centre care was available for Jonathan was so plainly the backdrop of the section 2 decision that there was no need to say so. It is one thing for it to have been a backdrop in the sense of a relevant factor, but another for it to have been treated as an immoveable object. The want of any visible consideration of it disables the respondent from showing that it was taken into account in the way spelt out in the *Gloucestershire* case. I do, however, accept Mr McCarthy's submission that Miss Richards' further contention that the respondent has failed to consider alternatives to day centre care for Jonathan comes so late that there has been no opportunity to file evidence about it. Further, the whole situation in relation to day centre provision is about to change, making this element marginal save perhaps by way of fallback.
>
> The care plan also fails at a number of points to comply with the practice guidance on, for example, the contents of a care plan, the specification of its objectives, the achievement of agreement on implementation on all those involved, leeway for contingencies and the identification and feeding back of assessed but still unmet need. While such guidance lacks the status accorded by section 7 of [Local Authority Social Services Act 1970], it is, as I have said, something to which regard must be had in carrying out the statutory functions. While the occasional lacuna would not furnish evidence of such a disregard, the series of lacunae which I have mentioned does, in my view, suggest that the statutory guidance has been overlooked.
>
> In such a situation I am unable to accede to Mr McCarthy's submission that the failures to follow the policy guidance and practice guidance are beyond the purview of the court. What he can, I think, legitimately complain of is the fact that both of these submissions, in their present formulation, have emerged for the first time in the presentation of the applicant's case in court and were not adumbrated earlier. While he has not suggested that the lateness of the points has prevented material evidence from being placed before the court, Mr McCarthy may be entitled to rely on it in resisting any consequential relief, and I will hear him in due course on this.

Comment: this is a generally, although not universally, accepted statement of the legal consequences of failing to 'act under' statutory guidance, or properly take into account non-statutory guidance. Sedley J's decision in relation to statutory guidance turned on the language of section 7(1) of the Local Authority Social Services Act 1970; but section 78 of the Care Act 2014 contains the same duty, to 'act under the general guidance of the Secretary of State'; and there continues to be relevant non-statutory guidance. So this decision should have continued relevance. Perhaps more questionable is whether there is such a great difference in the approach to statutory and non-statutory guidance, as is indicated by Sedley J, or whether there is a continuum which recognises that statutory guidance is inherently more likely to require a good reason for departure but that each set of guidance is to some extent different in what it requires and that a cogent reason may be required for any substantial divergence from some departmental guidance. It may also be considered that even a substantial departure from statutory guidance can, in principle, be justified by a sufficiently cogent reason.

8.58 *R v Kensington and Chelsea RLBC ex p Kujtim* (1999) 2 CCLR 340, CA

Local authorities are required to re-assess the possible needs of persons, even after their service has been terminated as a result of persistent, unequivocal misconduct, if it appears that they intend to conduct themselves properly

Facts: Kensington & Chelsea refused to continue to provide Mr Kujtim with residential accommodation after complaints about his misconduct, which continued after a written warning.

Judgment: once a local authority had assessed a person as 'needing' residential accommodation, it was under a duty to provide it as long as the need remained in existence and unless the applicant manifested a persistent and unequivocal refusal to observe reasonable requirements relating to occupation of the accommodation. Even in such cases, it was essential that the local authority carefully considered the applicant's current needs and circumstances, the causes of his conduct and the surrounding circumstances, allowing the applicant a fair opportunity of putting his case. The duty arose again, once the applicant satisfied the local authority that his needs required service provision to be made and that he will no longer persist in refusing to observe the local authority's reasonable requirements:

> *The extent of the duty under section 21 (l)(a) of the 1948 Act*
>
> 30. That being so, the question which arises is whether or not there is any limitation upon the duty to provide or continue to provide such accommodation for as long as the need, once assessed, continues. In my view the position is as follows. Once a local authority has assessed an applicant's needs as satisfying the criteria laid down in s21(1)(a), the local authority is under a duty to provide accommodation on a continuing basis so long as the need of the applicant remains as originally assessed, and if, for whatever reason, the accommodation, once provided, is withdrawn or otherwise becomes unavailable to the applicant, then (subject to any negative reassessment of the applicant's needs) the local authority has a continuing duty to provide further accommodation. That said, however, the duty of the local authority is not absolute in the sense that it has a duty willy-nilly to provide such accommodation *regardless of the applicant's willingness to take advantage of it.*
>
> 31. In this connection there are two realities to be recognised. First, the duty to provide accommodation is predicated upon the co-operation of the applicant in the sense of his willingness to occupy it on such terms and in accordance with such requirements as the local authority may reasonably impose in relation to its occupation. The second, and connected, reality is that the resources of the local authority are finite and that, in providing accommodation for the needy, save in rare cases where individual

or special accommodation may be necessary and available to meet the special needs of a particular applicant, the accommodation may, and will usually be, provided within multi-occupied premises, whether in the form of flats, or hostel or bed and breakfast accommodation, in relation to which it will be reasonable for the local authority to lay down certain requirements as to the use of such accommodation and the activities to be permitted in it, whether from a health and safety point of view, or for the purpose of preventing injury, nuisance or annoyance to fellow occupiers of the premises.

32. Thus it seems to me that, when the circumstances warrant, if an applicant assessed as in need of Part III accommodation either unreasonably refuses to accept the accommodation provided or if, following its provision, by his conduct he manifests a persistent and unequivocal refusal to observe the reasonable requirements of the local authority in relation to the occupation of such accommodation, then the local authority is entitled to treat its duty as discharged and to refuse to provide further accommodation. That will remain the position unless or until, upon some subsequent application, the applicant can satisfy the local authority that his needs remain such as to justify provision of Part III accommodation and that there is no longer reason to think that he will persist in his refusal to observe the reasonable requirements of the local authority in respect of the provision of such accommodation.

33. In formulating the right of the local authority to treat its duty as discharged by conduct as requiring manifestation of *persistent and unequivocal* refusal, rather than a single transgression, I have in mind the following matters which were urged upon us by Mr Gordon as part of his submission that the duty of providing Part III accommodation is unqualified and absolute. The provisions of section 21 of the 1948 Act as amended are 'safety net' provisions designed to assist the poorest and most needy members of society, at rock bottom as it were. For a variety of reasons of personal and social disadvantage, they may well be persons who find difficulty complying with the norms of social behaviour or self control, while falling outside the specific areas of need catered for by other provision within the Community Care Services or under housing legislation. To create a class consisting of a substantial number of persons outside the scope even of the minimum requirements of the safety net provisions cannot lightly be contemplated. To withdraw Part III accommodation in respect of persons with such needs is likely to reduce such persons to living and sleeping on the streets; not only does it tend to defeat the overall purpose of the 1948 Act as well as Community Care, but it produces the socially undesirable effect of increasing rather than alleviating deprivation and encourages return to the practice of begging in the streets

34. In the particular case of a genuine refugee who is homeless while awaiting resolution of his claim for asylum (and, as already indicated, there is no reason to doubt the genuineness of Mr Kujtim's claim) the effect of a refusal to supply Part III accommodation despite the existence of need is to remove from him basic food and shelter in a situation where, upon recognition of his claim, he would be entitled to receive the usual benefits available to British citizens in a position of hardship and unemployment; further, in the case of an applicant who is unwell, there may result damage to health, or in extreme cases threat to life, as a result of his being put out on the streets.

35. The existence of those considerations makes it essential that local authorities should reach the conclusion that their duty to supply Part III

accommodation is discharged in respect of any particular applicant only after being satisfied of his persistent and unequivocal refusal to comply with the local authority's requirements, coupled with a careful consideration of his *current* needs and circum stances. Either or both may involve consideration of any relevant medical condition or infirmity known to the local authority. Before concluding that there has been such refusal, it will plainly be desirable for a local authority to write a letter of final warning of the kind written by the respondents to the applicant in this case. As to the question of current need, the instant case provides a good example of why a re-consideration of need is essential. Had the respondents been aware, as they were not when they reached their decision, that the behaviour of the applicant in failing to observe their requirements to obey local hostel rules and to comply with the warning given to him by letter following his first expulsion, was the product of a depressive condition associated with the very ill-treatment which had driven him to seek refuge in this country, it seems unlikely that they would have treated his actions as manifesting a persistent and unequivocal refusal to comply with their requirements. However, they were entirely unaware of his medical condition and, in those circumstances, cannot be blamed for ignoring it.

8.59 *R v Birmingham CC ex p Killigrew* (2000) 3 CCLR 109, QBD

An assessment contain an explanation for its decision and take into account up-to-date medical evidence and evidence from carers

Facts: Birmingham had provided the claimant with 12 hours care each day, in the light of her severe disability. It then moved the claimant to better adapted accommodation and reduced her hours of care to three and a half hours during weekdays, with some additional care over the weekend. The decision was unreasoned. After the issue of a judicial review, Birmingham undertook an assessment, which concluded that the hours should be increased to six hours each day, and which gave as its reason that, under the existing arrangements, little direct care was provided for most of the day.

Judgment: Hooper J held that it was notable that the reduction in the hours of care coincided with a decision that two carers rather than one needed to be provided, to comply with manual handling requirements, and that it was important that the reduction in hours was not driven by the economic consequences of that decision. In any event, Birmingham's assessment was unlawful for two reasons: (1) it contained no proper analysis of why 12 hours care had been provided, why that was no longer necessary and what would be done if an emergency arose, (2) in breach of the statutory guidance, Birmingham had failed to take into account up-to-date medical evidence and the views of the GP and the claimant's carers.

8.60 *R v Newham LBC ex p Patrick* (2001) 4 CCLR 48, QBD

Referring a homeless woman with care needs to a housing charity did not amount to a discharge of the duty to assess or meet her needs

Facts: Ms Patrick, a single woman who suffered from physical and mental ill health, was evicted on the ground of neighbour nuisance and found intentionally homeless. Newham had purported to discharge its duty towards her under section 21 of the National Assistance Act 1948, by offering her accommodation provided by a charity, which she had refused. Ms Patrick then slept rough.

Judgment: Henriques J held that Newham had failed in breach of statutory duty to assess Ms Patrick's needs and had not discharged its duty under section 21:

> 27. Her solicitor in her witness statement says that she did not take up the accommodation provided by HOST because she believed she was being sent to Sunderland and not to Southwark. In any event, Southwark was a distance away from her sister and from her medical support network.
>
> 28. Since the offer of accommodation was on 28 April and the certificate of mental incapacity to handle her affairs was granted on 9 May, it requires no mental gymnastics to conclude that her decision to reject the offer of accommodation at Southwark was neither considered nor likely to have been well informed.
>
> 29. It is of particular significance that the respondent knew that solicitors were acting for the applicant as they had written on her behalf on 5 April.
>
> 30. Further, they had informed the respondent that they could obtain no clear instructions from the applicant due to her mental health and enclosed a note from her general practitioner.
>
> 31. If the respondent sought to put an end to its section 21 duties to provide accommodation, they ought in my judgment at the very least to have ensured that the applicant was legally represented when the offer was made to her to ensure not only that she understood what the offer was, both in terms of location and services offered, but also that she understood the legal consequences or potential legal consequences of refusing the offer.
>
> 32. Since she may well not have understood what was being offered and its location, I am not prepared to find that her refusal of it was unreasonable.
>
> 33. In the exercise of its duty to provide accommodation a local authority must have a concurrent duty to explain fully and to the point of comprehension any offer it may make. I am not persuaded that the local authority has discharged its duty. In my judgment the duty to provide Part III accommodation continues pursuant to section 21 of the 1948 Act.

8.61 ### *R (A and B) v East Sussex CC and the Disability Rights Commission* [2003] EWHC 167 (Admin), (2003) 6 CCLR 194

Local authorities were under a duty to assess the needs and take into account the preferences of persons even when those persons have substantial communication difficulties, including by consulting carers as to how it is best to communicate

Facts: A and B were severely disabled sisters who continued to live in the family home, owing to a dispute with Sussex over aspects of the care package, in particular, as to the extent to which Sussex could be required to instruct carers to undertake manual lifting.

Judgment: Munby J held that the Manual Handling Operations Regulations 1992 imposed a duty on Sussex to avoid or minimise the risk of injury from hazardous lifts so far as reasonably practicable. That required Sussex to balance the Article 8 rights of the sisters, and their carers. On the difficulty of assessing persons lacking capacity to participate in the process, Munby J said this:

132. I have said that the assessment must take account of the disabled person's wishes, feelings and preferences. How are these to be ascertained?

133. In a case where the disabled person is, by reason of their disability, prevented, whether completely or in part, from communicating their wishes and feelings it will be necessary for the assessors to facilitate the ascertainment of the person's wishes and feelings, so far as they may be deduced, by whatever means, including seeking and receiving advice – advice, not instructions – from appropriate interested persons such as X and Y involved in the care of the disabled person.

134. Good practice, Miss Foster suggests, would indicate, and I am inclined to agree that:

(i) A rough 'dictionary' should be drawn up, stating what the closest carers (in a case such as this, parents and family, here X and Y) understand by the various non-verbal communications, based on their intimate long term experience of the person. Thus with familiarisation and 'interpretation' the carers can accustom themselves to the variety of feelings and modes of expression and learn to recognise what is being communicated.

(ii) Where the relatives are present with the carers and an occasion of 'interpretation' arises, great weight must be accorded to the relatives' 'translation'.

(iii) As I commented in *Re S* [2003] 1 FLR 292 at 306 (para 49):

... the devoted parent who ... has spent years caring for a disabled child is likely to be much better able than any social worker, however skilled, or any judge, however compassionate, to 'read' his child, to understand his personality and to interpret the wishes and feelings which he lacks the ability to express.

(iv) That said, in the final analysis the task of deciding whether, in truth, there is a refusal or fear or other negative reaction to being lifted must, as Miss Foster properly concedes, fall on the carer, for the duty to act within the framework given by the employer falls upon the employee. Were the patient not incapacitated, there could be no suggestion that the relative's views are other than a factor to be considered. Because of the lack of capacity and the extraordinary circumstances in a case such as this, the views of the relatives are of very great importance, but they are not determinative.

Comment: see now the Mental Capacity Act 2005 and the entitlement to an IMCA and, for persons who do not lack capacity but would experience substantial difficulty, see the Care and Support (Independent Advocacy Support) (No 2) Regulations 2014. For a useful and relevant analysis in relation to un-cooperative children, see *R (J) v Caerphilly CBC*.[14]

8.62 *R (Heffernan) v Sheffield CC* [2004] EWHC 1377 (Admin), (2004) 7 CCLR 350

An assessment that was incompatible with the eligibility criteria was unlawful

Facts: Mr Heffernan was severely disabled as a result of Still's Disease. Sheffield provided him with 24½ hours care per week but, on the basis of an independent report, he claimed he needed 27–30 hours and a live-in carer.

14 [2005] EWHC 586 (Admin), (2005) 8 CCLR 255.

Judgment: Collins J held that Sheffield had failed to apply the guidance in circular LAC (2002) 13: Fair Access to Care Services. In particular, it had treated '*significant health problems*' as falling within the Substantial Band, rather than the Critical Band. Care needs resulting from significant illness, or the need to prevent significant illness, fell within the Critical Band, and had to be met:

> The practical consequences of the above interpretation may be shown by the following example. Mrs Jones cannot perform the majority of personal care or domestic routines although none are vital to her independence. At the same time her involvement in one or two support systems cannot be sustained. According to the eligibility framework of paragraph 16 of the FACS policy guidance, Mrs Jones' difficulties with personal care and domestic routine fall within the substantial risk band: while her support system difficulties fall within the low risk band. If the council's eligibility criteria include critical and substantial risks, the council is only obliged to consider meeting needs associated with personal care and domestic routines. It is not obliged to address needs associated with support systems. Furthermore, the council when determining which personal care and domestic routine difficulties to address is only obliged to address those which will ameliorate, contain or reduce the substantial risks. This means that Mrs Jones may be helped with bathing, aspects of toileting, aspects of cooking and paying bills, but may not be helped with gardening, shopping for weekly groceries (because these can be delivered by the local supermarket) and writing letters to friends.
>
> There is another way to think about needs, risks and eligibility. If among an individual's needs there are some needs which if presented by themselves would lead to risks that would be placed outside a council's eligibility criteria, the council may consider it unnecessary to address those needs. The council would do so where it was sure the needs in question did not exacerbate or otherwise worsen the other needs to be addressed.
>
> When implementing and applying FACS-based eligibility criteria, it is not generally possible to identify eligible needs directly from the risks described in eligibility framework of paragraph 16. This is because the eligibility bands are expressed as risks not needs, meaning that councils have to make sense of the risks and consider how best to tackle them. Hence, in the example above, Mrs Jones may not be helped with all the personal care and domestic routines that she can no longer do.

8.63 *R (B) v Lambeth LBC* [2006] EWHC 639 (Admin), (2006) 9 CCLR 239

The function of judicial review is to pronounce upon the lawfulness or otherwise of public decision-making, not to investigate its merits

Facts: the claimant, a 15-year-old girl, brought judicial review proceedings against Lambeth after she became homeless, alleging that Lambeth had failed adequately to assess her needs or make suitable provision. After a number of hearings, she withdrew those proceedings without permission to apply for judicial review having been granted. Lambeth applied for costs on the grounds that the judicial review grounds had failed to identify clearly any error of law and that, despite repeated requests, that had not been done until the last moment.

Judgment: Munby J held that there would be no order for costs, but practitioners should be aware that costs and/or wasted costs might well be awarded in future when a judicial review application failed properly to identify any alleged errors of law: the whole of paragraphs 26–36 of the judgment, in particular, contain salutary advice to practitioners. These passages commence thus:

> 26. This is yet another case exemplifying problems about which I have had to complain on too many occasions already. As I said in *R (P, W, F and G) v Essex County Council* [2004] EWHC 2027 (Admin) at paragraphs [30]–[31]:
>
> > '[30] The present litigation exemplifies a certain type of judicial review case which experience suggests can too often end up following a less than desirable course: I have in mind community care, housing and other cases involving either children or vulnerable adults, especially those where, as here, the first task of the local or other public authority is the preparation of an assessment.
> >
> > [31] This is not the first time that I have felt impelled to express my unease about this particular type of litigation: see *R (A, B, X and Y) v East Sussex CC (No 2)* [2003] EWHC 167 (Admin), (2003) 6 CCLR 194, at paras [156]–[166], and *CF v Secretary of State for the Home Department* [2004] EWHC 111 (Fam), [2004] 1 FCR 577, at paras [217]–[219]. There is, I think, a problem here that needs to be addressed. Too often in my experience inadequate thought is given to what precisely the court is being asked or can properly be asked to do.'
>
> 27. I then went on to set out what I referred to as a few basic principles, starting with some observations on the proper function of the court in a case such as this:
>
> > '[32] What the claimants here seek to challenge are decisions taken by the County Council in pursuance of the statutory powers and duties conferred on it by Part III of the Act. So I am here concerned with an area of decision-making where Parliament has chosen to confer the relevant power on the County Council: not on the court or anyone else. It follows that we are here within the realm of public law, not private law. It likewise follows that the primary decision maker is the County Council and not the court. The court's function in this type of dispute is essentially one of review – review of the County Council's decision, whatever it may be – rather than of primary decision making. It is not the function of the court itself to come to a decision on the merits. The court is not concerned to come to its own assessment of what is in these children's best interests. The court is concerned only to review the County Council's decisions, and that is not a review of the merits of the County Council's decisions but a review by reference to public law criteria: see *A v A Health Authority, in re J (A Child), R (S) v Secretary of State for the Home Department* [2002] EWHC 18 (Fam/Admin), [2002] Fam 213, and *CF v Secretary of State for the Home Department* [2004] EWHC 111 (Fam), [2004] 1 FCR 577, at paras [20]–[32]. Just as I pointed out in *R (A, B, X and Y) v East Sussex CC (No 2)* [2003] EWHC 167 (Admin), (2003) 6 CCLR 194, at para [161], that it was the function of the local authority and not the court to make and draw up the assessments that were there in issue, so too in the present case it is for the County Council and not the court to make the initial and core assessments of these children.
> >
> > [33] Now this has two important corollaries. Although I am, in a sense, concerned with the future welfare of very vulnerable children, I am not exercising a 'best interests' or 'welfare' jurisdiction, nor is it any part of my functions to monitor, regulate or police the performance by the County Council of its statutory functions on a continuing basis. A judge

of the Family Division exercising the wardship jurisdiction has a continuing responsibility for the day to day life and welfare of the ward, exemplified by the principle that no important or major step in the life of a ward of court can be taken without the prior consent of the court: see *Kelly v British Broadcasting Corpn* [2001] Fam 59 at p75. The function of the Administrative Court is quite different: it is, as it is put in CPR Part 54.1(2)(a), to review the lawfulness of a decision, action or failure to act in relation to the exercise of a public function. In other words, the Administrative Court exists to adjudicate upon specific challenges to discrete decisions. It does not exist to monitor and regulate the performance of public authorities: see in the context of community care *R v Mayor and Burgesses of the London Borough of Hackney ex p S* (unreported, 13 October 2000) at paras [8] and [11] and *R v Mayor and Burgesses of the London Borough of Hackney ex p S (No 2)* [2001] EWHC 228 (Admin) at para [4].

Comment: this really speaks for itself and is just as applicable to cases involving vulnerable adults as it is to cases involving children. Not only is it illegitimate to use the judicial review process to persuade the court to micro-manage a public authority's decision-making process, or to interfere with substantive decisions that are lawfully made, blatant attempts to do so may result in adverse or wasted costs orders.

8.64 *R (Ireneschild) v Lambeth LBC* [2007] EWCA Civ 234, (2007) 10 CCLR 243

It was unnecessary in the particular circumstances to allow the applicant to comment on a medical adviser's adverse report before completing the assessment; assessments are iterative and should not be too finely scrutinised

Facts: Ms Ireneschild was disabled and asserted that her current accommodation was grossly unsuitable on account of her inability to manage the stairs. An occupational therapist agreed with her but Lambeth's medical advisor visited and awarded Ms Ireneschild a high amount of moving points, but not emergency transfer status.

Judgment: the Court of Appeal (Dyson and Hallett LJJ, Sir Peter Gibson) held that the assessment did take into account all relevant matters including an earlier assessment (albeit indirectly, as it was referred to in a more recent assessment) and it had not been unfair in this case not to invite Ms Ireneschild to comment on the medical adviser's report because Ms Ireneschild had been able to discuss her needs with the medical adviser and because, under the statutory scheme, service users are entitled to comment on assessments and may then utilise the complaints procedure. Hallett LJ's judgment includes the following:

44. Mr Drabble further conceded that the Respondent, having brought the proceedings to review the assessment judicially, bore the heavy burden of establishing that the assessment was unlawful. He did not attempt to persuade this court to ignore the strictures of Lord Brightman in *Puhlhofer v Hillingdon LBC* [1986] AC 484, 518B–E put before us by Mr Béar. Lord Brightman said this:

'My Lords, I am troubled at the prolific use of judicial review for the purpose of challenging the performance by local authorities of their function under the Act of 1977. Parliament intended the local authority

> to be the judge of fact. The Act abounds with the formula when, or if, the housing authority are satisfied as to this, or that, or have reason to believe this, or that. Although the action or inaction of a local authority is clearly susceptible to judicial review where they have misconstrued the Act, or abused their powers or otherwise acted perversely, I think that great restraint should be exercised in giving leave to proceed by judicial review. The plight of the homeless is a desperate one, and the plight of the applicants in the present case commands the deepest sympathy. But it is not, in my opinion, appropriate that the remedy of judicial review, which is a discretionary remedy, should be made use of to monitor the actions of local authorities under the Act save in the exceptional case. The ground upon which the courts will review the exercise of an administrative discretion is abuse of power, eg bad faith, a mistake in construing the limits of the power, a procedural irregularity, or unreasonableness in the *Wednesbury* sense – unreasonableness verging on an absurdity: see the speech of Lord Scarman in *R v Secretary of State for the Environment ex p Nottinghamshire County Council* [1986] AC 240, 247–248. Where the existence or non-existence of a fact is left to the judgment and discretion of a public body and that fact involves a broad spectrum ranging from the obvious to the debatable to the just conceivable, it is the duty of the court to leave the decision of that fact to the public body to whom Parliament has entrusted the decision-making power save in a case where it is obvious that the public body, consciously or unconsciously, are acting perversely.'

Those remarks may have been directed at a different statutory function in a different era, but, to my mind, they are as pertinent today as they were in the 1980s.

...

52. It should not be forgotten that this assessment, upon which this court and Lloyd Jones J have spent so much time, was essentially a work in progress and Ms Ireneschild in the normal course of events would have had a proper opportunity to challenge the assessment or parts thereof. Even when an assessment was finalised, nothing was writ in stone; if the Respondent's circumstances changed she could seek another assessment.

...

57. With great respect, I disagree. I see considerable force in Mr Béar's argument that Mr Drabble's challenge to the assessment on this ground took an overly critical approach to the assessment. Again, one must always bear in mind the context of an assessment of this kind. It is an assessment prepared by a social worker for his or her employers. It is not a final determination of a legal dispute by a lawyer which may be subjected to over zealous textual analysis. Courts must be wary, in my view, of expecting so much of hard pressed social workers that we risk taking them away, unnecessarily, from their front line duties.

8.65 *R (AM) v Birmingham CC* [2009] EWHC 688 (Admin), (2009) 12 CCLR 407

A properly completed assessment also discharges the disability equality duty

Facts: AM, who was severely disabled, obtained a place at university. He sought a fully adapted toilet facility including a hoist. That provision would have been expensive and Birmingham decided that because AM was continent, it was unlikely that he would need to use such a facility during the day. Accordingly, Birmingham resolved to provide only a certain amount of additional personal care. AM sought a judicial review but was granted permission only to argue that Birmingham had failed to discharge its duty under section 49A of the Disability Discrimination Act 1995.

Judgment: Cranston J dismissed the application, holding that in substance the community care assessment process had resulted in Birmingham having due regard to the need to promote equality of opportunity in education and the other obligations owed to disabled persons.

8.66 *R (B) v Cornwall CC* [2009] EWHC 491 (Admin), (2009) 12 CCLR 381

A local authority must fully involve the service user and other relevant persons but is ultimately required to undertake its own assessment

Facts: a dispute arose as to B's liability to pay charges for his home care services.

Judgment: Hickinbottom J described the general nature of the assessment process as follows:

> 9. The Secretary of State has given directions under Section 47(4), namely the Community Care Assessment Directions 2004 which, in paragraph 2, provide:
>
> > '(1) In assessing the needs of a person under Section 47(1) of the Act a local authority must comply with Paragraphs (2) to (4).
> >
> > (2) The local authority must consult the person, consider whether the person has any carers and, where they think it appropriate, consult those carers.
> >
> > (3) The local authority must take all reasonable steps to reach agreement with the person and, where they think it appropriate, any carers of that person, on the Community Care Services which they are considering providing to him to meet his needs.
> >
> > (4) The local authority must provide information to the person and, where they think it appropriate, any carers of that person, about the amount of the payment (if any) which the person will be liable to make in respect of the Community Care Services which they are considering providing to him.'
>
> These directions set a pattern for the general scheme of community care. Decision-making rests in the responsible authority, but their powers are only to be exercised after appropriate engagement with the service user and any relevant carers (who may include for example the service user's parents or other family). Prior to coming to a concluded view on needs, they should consult: prior to coming to a decision on steps to be taken to meet that need, they should attempt to reach agreement: and in relation to the on-cost to the service user, they should provide appropriate information.
>
> ...
>
> 68. Fourth, it is for the Authority to assess eligible needs. That is their statutory duty under section 47 of the 1990 Act. Of course, if requested to do so, a service user must provide evidence that DRE has actually been expended (by the provision of receipts, bills etc), and that is the specific reference to the provision of evidence in the 2003 Guidelines (see paragraph 13(ix) above). Furthermore, it is right that the views of the service user and family carers are sought as to his needs and the steps the authority propose to take in respect of those needs. The relevant guidance requires that. The user

may of course also be able to produce evidence of a particular need. But the authority cannot avoid its obligation to assess needs etc by failing to make an appropriate assessment themselves, in favour of simply requiring the service user himself to provide evidence of his needs. In this case, so far as the August assessment is concerned, I am afraid the Authority appears to have abrogated its obligation in that way. Ms Harvey appears to have accepted that the care plan fell short. In any event, I consider the Authority acted unlawfully by disallowing expenditure as DRE on the basis that B had failed to evidence the expenditure as DRE to their satisfaction whilst they gave B (effectively Mr & Mrs B) no opportunity to make good that perceived evidential deficit. In the Authority's own guidance, it is suggested that, if evidence is not forthcoming, then the Finance Officer should ask for it to be produced at the next charges review. Whilst that appears to be concerned with evidence of expenditure (receipts, bills etc), there is no suggestion in that guidance that a failure to produce evidence should be fatal, and that no opportunity should be allowed to correct evidential deficits.

8.67 *R (F, J, Ṡ, R) v Wirral BC* [2009] EWHC 1626 (Admin), (2009) 12 CCLR 452

Minor criticisms of assessments, not likely to result in changed services, should be brought through a complaints procedure

Facts: a supported living provider, Salisbury Independent Living, funded litigation brought by residents living in accommodation it provided, essentially claiming that due to inadequate assessments, Wirral had not provided the residents with funds that would in turn reimburse SIL for the assistance it provided.

Judgment: McCombe J held that, leaving aside one potentially major point that had been raised at the hearing for the first time and which the claimants would not be permitted to rely on, the criticisms of the assessments were relatively minor and ought to be have been raised in a complaints procedure, in particular because no case had emerged where it was likely that there had been a failure to meet eligible needs; accordingly, he dismissed the application for judicial review as an abuse of process.

8.68 *R (SG) v Haringey LBC* [2015] EWHC 2579 (Admin), (2015) 18 CCLR 444

The failure to appoint an independent advocate, under section 67(2) of the Care Act 2014, for a vulnerable adult, who spoke no English and was illiterate, and who suffered from PTSD, insomnia, depression and anxiety, rendered the assessment unlawful

Facts: SG was an asylum-seeker provided with asylum support. She spoke no English and was illiterate, and suffered from post-traumatic stress disorder (PTSD), insomnia, depression and anxiety. She needed help with self-care, preparing and eating food, simple tasks and medication. Haringey declined to provide residential accommodation to SG under section 21 of the National Assistance Act 1948 and then, later, under the Care Act 2014.

Judgment: Deputy High Court Judge Bowers held that the assessment under the Care Act 2014 was unlawful because (i) Haringey failed to ensure that SG was offered an independent advocate, under section 67(2) of the Care Act 2014; and (ii) Haringey failed to ask itself the correct question as to whether accommodation was required. On the issue of the independent advocate, the Deputy High Court Judge said this:

> *(1) Absence of an independent advocate*
>
> 53. The defendant appears to accept the claimant was entitled to but did not have an independent advocate when she was assessed under the Care Act, but contends nonetheless that this did not 'lead to flawed assessment process' because referral for such an advocate was made at the time of the assessment and since then an independent advocate has been appointed in the form of Mind.
>
> 54. Section 67(2) of the Act could not be clearer:
>
>> 'The authority must ... arrange for a person who is independent of the authority (an 'independent advocate') to be available to represent and support the individual for the purpose of facilitating the individual's involvement.'
>
> 55. There are detailed criteria for being an independent advocate, as set out in the Care and Support (Independent Advocacy Support) No 2 Regulations 2014 SI No 2889, together with the manner in which they are to carry out their functions. This testifies to the importance of this protection for essentially vulnerable persons.
>
> 56. Ms Okafor points to the fact that Mind has now accepted a referral and she contends that as a result of the new Care Act 'demand currently outstrips supply.' She says the claimant's services have not been prejudiced as a result concerning the outcome of the assessment, but I agree with Mr Burton that we simply do not know that. I do accept the defendant's submission that there may be cases in which it is unlikely the presence of an independent advocate would make any difference to the outcome. This is not one of them, because this appears to me the paradigm case where such an advocate was required, as in the absence of one the claimant was in no position to influence matters. I keep particularly in mind the account given by Ms Mohr-Pietsch. I think the assessment was flawed as a result and must be redone. This is the first of only two grounds of unlawfulness which I find in this case.

CHAPTER 9

Service provision decisions

continued

9.78 *R v Lambeth LBC ex p A1 and A2* (1997–8) 1 CCLR 336, CA
Where physical resources are not available to discharge a duty to meet needs, the local authorities may have to make a sincere and determined effort to secure them

9.79 *R v Kirklees MBC ex p Daykin* (1997–8) 1 CCLR 512, QBD
Local authorities are entitled to meet needs in the most cost-effective manner

9.80 *R v Wigan MBC ex p Tammadge* (1997–8) 1 CCLR 581, QBD
Local authorities are required to meet needs that they have accepted as being eligible

9.81 *R v Kensington and Chelsea RLBC ex p Kujtim* (1999) 2 CCLR 340, CA
A local authority remains under a duty to meet eligible needs unless the applicant has manifested a persistent and unequivocal refusal to observe reasonable conditions and must be ready to re-assess where it appears that the applicant will not persist

9.82 *R v Calderdale MBC ex p Houghton* (2000) 3 CCLR 228, QBD
A care plan must be a rational response to the assessment of needs

9.83 *R v South Lanarkshire Council ex p MacGregor* (2000) 4 CCLR 188, CSOH
Some waiting lists might be lawful but this waiting list was not as it did not prioritise applicants according to their needs and was a plain attempt to avoid meeting statutory duties

9.84 *R (Khana) v Southwark LBC* [2001] EWCA Civ 999, (2001) 4 CCLR 267
Local authorities are required to meet needs under section 21 of the National Assistance Act 1948, not preferences; an offer of accommodation that meets needs discharges the duty

9.85 *R v Newham LBC ex p Patrick* (2001) 4 CCLR 48, QBD
Referring a homeless woman with care needs to a housing charity did not amount to a discharge of the duty to assess or meet her needs

9.86 *R v Islington LBC ex p Batantu* (2001) 4 CCLR 445, QBD
A local authority remained under a duty to meet assessed needs despite the service user's refusal of offered services

9.87 *R (Wahid) v Tower Hamlets LBC* [2002] EWCA Civ 287, (2002) 5 CCLR 239
Local authorities are only required to provide accommodation under social care legislation when the qualifying criteria under such legislation are met

9.88 *R (A and B) v East Sussex CC* [2002] EWHC 2771 (Admin), (2003) 6 CCLR 177
A balance was to be struck between the ECHR rights of paid carers and service users. Local authorities may make payments to user independent trusts for the provision of care services

9.89 *R (Rodriquez-Bannister) v Somerset Partnership NHS and Social Care Trust* [2003] EWHC 2184 (Admin), (2004) 7 CCLR 385
A local authority may rationally prefer the views of its own expert as to what services to provide

9.90 *R (Alloway) v Bromley LBC* [2004] EWHC 2108 (Admin), (2005) 8 CCLR 61
A local authority fetters its discretion if it rules out one service from the start on costs grounds and does not fairly compare the rival options

9.91 *R (Hughes) v Liverpool CC* [2005] EWHC 428 (Admin), (2005) 8 CCLR 243
It was unlawful to fail to meet a statutory need for residential accommodation but that did not necessarily result in a breach of ECHR rights

9.92 *Casewell v Secretary of State for Work and Pensions* [2008] EWCA Civ 524, (2008) 11 CCLR 624
Direct payments used to pay a relative to provide home care were 'earnings' in her hands, for social security purposes

9.93 *Re an application by LW (acting by her mother JB) for judicial review* [2010] NIQB 62, (2011) 14 CCLR 7
There was a duty to meet assessed needs under the Northern Ireland legislation

9.94 *R (Savva) v Kensington & Chelsea RLBC* [2010] EWCA Civ 1209, (2011) 14 CCLR 75
It is lawful to use a resource allocation scheme to provide an indicative budget provided the local authority fine-tuned that budget to ensure that it met needs and provided adequate reasons that justified its ultimate budget

9.95 *R (McDonald) v Kensington & Chelsea RLBC* [2011] UKSC 33, (2011) 14 CCLR 341
The local authority was entitled to withdraw the provision of an overnight carer who helped the appellant access the commode at night, when it assessed that the appellant's needs could be equally met by the provision of incontinence pads and absorbent sheets

9.96 *R (G) v North Somerset Council* [2011] EWHC 2232 (Admin)
North Somerset had not acted unlawfully in deciding to cut the amount of direct payments and replacing direct payments with a managed care service

9.97 *R (KM) v Cambridgeshire CC* [2012] UKSC 23, (2012) 15 CCLR 374
It is lawful to use a resource allocation system to guide assessment as to what level of personal budget to provide

9.98 *R (AJ) v Calderdale BC* [2012] EWHC 3552 (Admin), (2013) 16 CCLR 50
There is no reason in principle why service and family members could not participate in evaluation panels to select service providers

9.99 *In the matter of DM (a person under disability) acting by his next friend Kathleen McCollym, for judicial review* [2012] NIQB 98, (2013) 16 CCLR 39
It was unlawful to treat the budgetary indication provided by a resource allocation scheme as final

9.100 *In the matter of an application for judicial review by JR 47* [2013] NIQB 7, (2013) 16 CCLR 179
The relevant authorities were under a duty to assess and meet community care needs, in general, in accordance with the relevant guidance

9.101 *McDonald v United Kingdom* (2014) 17 CCLR 187, ECtHR
It was not a breach of the ECHR for the local authority to re-assess a person's needs and provide them with considerably less than previously, in this case, by providing incontinence pads and absorbent sheets in place of a night-time carer and commode

9.102 *Re MN (An Adult)* [2015] EWCA Civ 411, (2015) 18 CCLR 521
The Court of Protection has no power to require a public authority to provide different services, only to consider whether services on offer are in P's best interests, so any legal challenge to the sufficiency of services offered must be brought by way of judicial review

continued

9.103 *R (SG) v Haringey LBC* [2015] EWHC 2579 (Admin), (2015) 18 CCLR 444

A failure to provide an independent advocate under section 67(2) of the Care Act 2014 rendered the assessment unlawful. A duty only arose to provide accommodation when the need was 'accommodation-related'

9.104 *R (Collins) v Nottinghamshire CC* [2016] EWHC 996 (Admin), (2016) 19 CCLR 494

It had been rational for Nottinghamshire to suspend an organisation from its list of accredited providers of direct payment support services

Introduction and principles

9.1 By this stage, the local authority will have completed a 'needs assessment' (for an adult) and/or a 'carer's assessment' (for a carer), under sections 9–12 of the Care Act 2014. It will also have determined in writing which needs meet the eligibility criteria. In the case of an adult it will have (i) 'considered' 'what could be done to meet those needs'; (ii) 'ascertained' 'whether the adult wants to have those needs met by the local authority'; and (iii) 'established' 'whether the adult is ordinarily resident in the local authority's area' (section 13(2)). In the case of a carer, the local authority will also have (i) 'considered' 'what could be done to meet those needs'; and (ii) 'established' 'whether the adult needing care is ordinarily resident in the local authority's area' (section 13(3)).

9.2 So, the scene is set for care planning, the main purpose of which is to identify eligible and other needs and how (if at all, in the case of ineligible needs) the local authority is going to meet them. The next section considers in more detail what is required during the care planning process but, at this stage, attention is drawn to two principles.

9.3 First, it is essential to lawful care planning that the local authority involves the applicant, any carer and other relevant persons so that they can address the relevant issues. The statutory duty to involve the adult, the carer and other relevant persons in the preparation of a care and support/support plan and 'take all reasonable steps to reach agreement with the adult or carer for whom the plan is being prepared about how the authority should meet the needs in question' is at section 25(3)–(5) of the Care Act 2014. As it is put in the *Care and Support Statutory Guidance* 'The person must be genuinely involved and influential throughout the planning process...' (paragraph 10.2) and:

> 10.49 In addition to taking all reasonable steps to agree how needs are to be met, the local authority must also involve the person the plan is intended for, the carer (if there is one), and/or any other person the adult requests to be involved. Where the person lacks capacity to ask the authority to do that, the local authority must involve any person who appears to the authority to be interested in the welfare of the person and should involve any person who would be able to contribute useful information. An independent advocate must be provided if section 67 of the Act applies (see chapter 7). The person, and their carers, will have the best understanding of how the needs identified fit into the person's life as a whole and connect to their overall wellbeing (see chapter 1). They are well placed to consider and identify which care and support options would best fit into their lifestyle and help them to achieve the day to day outcomes they identified during the assessment process. In practice, local authorities should give consideration to include a prompt to the person during the initial stages of the planning process to ask whether there is anyone else that the person wishes to be involved. Where the person lacks capacity, the local authority should make a best interests decision about who else should be involved.

See further at para 9.31 onwards.

9.4 Second, a striking feature of the Care Act 2014 is that it does not, as the earlier regime did, present a list of specific services that a person may qualify for. Rather, it sets out an illustrative list of the types of provision that may be offered and an illustrative list of how provision may be made, so as to promote flexible and imaginative solutions that engage with real needs and preferences directly and not through the potentially distorting lens of what services are available: see section 8 of the Care Act 2014 (set out below at para 9.27).

9.5 Otherwise, the litigation issues that have arisen in the past, and that are likely to arise in the future, are where a local authority:

- fails to complete a care plan, at all or within a reasonable period of time, or to give it to the adult/carer (paragraph 6.29 of the Guidance states that an assessment 'should be carried out over an appropriate and reasonable timescale, taking into account the urgency of needs and a consideration of any fluctuation in those needs' and that local authorities 'should inform the individual of an indicative timescale over which their assessment will be conducted and keep the individual informed throughout the assessment process');
- fails to make immediately necessary provision pending completion of an assessment;[1]
- completes an unlawful assessment, on the basis of which inadequate services are offered, for example, by failing to involve relevant persons, failing to take into account relevant material or reaching unreasoned or irrational conclusions;[2]
- fails properly to assess the level of direct payments/budget required, or give adequate reasons.[3]

9.6 As in the case of assessments, judicial review usually only succeeds when the claimant establishes a clear breach of the legal parameters: see further chapter 27 below on judicial review. The courts tend to:

- focus on the substance of the issue, rather than on the detail of what remains, even now, a highly complex and detailed scheme that cannot always be perfectly adhered to;
- defer to professional evaluation and judgment, by adopting a relatively generous reading of the assessment material;
- manifest a strong appreciation that the function of judicial review is to correct legal errors and not to engage with factual disputes or ongoing monitoring of local authority activity, particularly bearing in mind the availability of ADR and a statutory appeal procedure – see para 7.97 above),[4] especially where the challenge is perceived to be fact-specific or focussed on relatively minor aspects of the assessment process or as being little more than a challenge to the merits of the local authority assessment (see paras 27.8–27.9 and 27.15–27.28 below). That tendency is likely to increase as a result of:
  - the enactment of section 31(2A) of the Senior Courts Act 1981, which provides that the High Court must refuse to grant relief 'if

1 See, under the previous regime, *R (AA) v Lambeth LBC* [2001] EWHC 741 (Admin), (2002) 5 CCLR 36.

2 See, again under the previous regime, *R v North Yorkshire Cc ex p William Hargreaves* (1997–8) 1 CCLR 104, QBD and *R v Islington LBC ex p Rixon* (1997–8) 1 CCLR 119, QBD.

3 *R (KM) v Cambridgeshire CC* [2012] UKSC 23, [2012] 15 CCLR 364.

4 See, in particular, *R (Ireneschild) v Lambeth LBC* [2007] EWCA Civ 243, (2007) 10 CCLR 243 and *R (F, J, S, R) v Wirral BC* [2009] EWHC 1626, (2009) 12 CCLR 452.

it appears to the court to be highly likely that the outcome for the applicant would not have been substantially different if the conduct complained of had not occurred', unless there is an 'exceptional public interest' in granting relief (see para 3.8 above and para 27.10 below); and

– the forthcoming statutory appeals procedure (see para 7.97 above).

9.7 The courts tend to involve themselves more readily on issues of interim relief, in order to hold the ring or create a situation of stability; where significant errors of law may be involved; where something appears to have gone seriously awry in the assessment process and where significant numbers of people may be involved; but again the court is likely to hold back when it perceives there to be a suitable alternative remedy and that tendency is likely to increase for the reasons set out above at para 9.6.

9.8 One of the clearest duties in this context is the duty to meet needs assessed as being 'eligible' but even this duty is not absolutely absolute; not only are local authorities entitled to meet eligible needs in a cost-effective manner,[5] where physical resources are not available (eg a suitable care home) the duty is a duty to do everything reasonably possible to locate or create such resources.[6] In addition, the flexibility inherent in the notion of needs at least opens up the possibility that, in some circumstances, a rationally arranged waiting-list could result in assessed needs being met, albeit not straight away, but still lawfully.[7]

9.9 An interesting feature of social care is, however, that a local authority cannot treat itself as having 'discharged' its duty, in the way that, for example, a housing authority can. An applicant may act unreasonably by refusing offers of assistance or by failing to adhere to reasonable conditions, resulting in the service being withdrawn, but a local authority must remain willing to provide a service for which a need continues to exist, if for example the applicant has agreed to mend their ways.[8]

Statutory machinery

9.10 The preliminary machinery is set out above in chapter 8.

9.11 What then follow are a series of duties and powers, at sections 18–23, and then a series of procedural steps revolving around the completion of a care plan, at sections 24–25.

Duty owed to adults

9.12 Local authorities **must meet** the '*eligible needs*' of adult (not being met by a carer) if, having made a determination under section 13:

i) the adult is ordinarily resident in their area, or present with no settled residence; and

5 *R v Kirklees MBC ex p Daykin* (1997–8) 1 CCLR 512.

6 *R v Islington LBC ex p Rixon* (1997–8) 1 CCLR 119; *R v Lambeth LBC ex p A1 and A2* (1997–98) 1 CCLR 336.

7 *R v South Lanarkshire Council ex p MacGregor* (2000) 4 CCLR 188.

8 *R v Kensington and Chelsea RLBC ex p Kujtim* (1999) 2 CCLR 340.

ii) there is no charge under section 14 for meeting the needs; or
iii) the adult's resources are below the '*financial limit*' ('condition 1'); or
iv) the adult's resources are above the '*financial limit*' but they ask the local authority to meet their needs ('condition 2'); or
v) the adult lacks capacity to arrange their own support and no one is authorised to do so under the Mental Capacity Act 2005 ('condition 3').
(section 18).

Power in relation to adults

9.13 Having completed a needs assessment and, if required, a financial assessment, local authorities **may meet:**

i) any needs of the adult who is ordinarily resident in their area, or present with no settled residence, providing the local authority is satisfied it is not under a duty to meet those needs, under section 18;
ii) having made a determination under section 13, the 'eligible needs' of an adult who is ordinarily resident in another area, providing they notify the other local authority and there is no charge, or conditions 1, 2 or 3 in section 18 are met (see above);
iii) urgent needs (and/or the needs of a terminally ill person) whether or not the adult is ordinarily resident in their area and without having yet completed a needs assessment or a financial assessment.
(section 19).

Duty owed to carers

9.14 Local authorities **must meet** the 'eligible needs' of a carer if:

i) the adult needing care is ordinarily resident in their area, or present with no settled residence; and
ii) (if the provision is of support to the carer) there is no charge, or conditions 1 or 2 are met; and
iii) (if the provision is of care and support to the adult, in order to meet the carer's needs) there is no charge and the adult agrees to needs being meet in that way or, if there is a charge, conditions 3 or 4 are met.

9.15 For these purposes:

i) condition 1 is that the carer's resources are at or below the 'financial limit' (see paras 11.10–11.15);
ii) condition 2 is that the carer's resources are above the 'financial limit' but they ask the local authority to meet their needs;
iii) condition 3 is that the adult's resources are at or below the 'financial limit' and the adult agrees to the authority meeting the carer's needs by providing the adult with care and support; and
iv) condition 4 is that the adult's resources are above the 'financial limit', but the adult nonetheless ask the authority to meet the carer's needs by providing the adult with care and support.
(section 20).

Power in relation to carers

9.16 Local authorities **may meet** any needs of a carer if it is not under a duty to meet a carer's needs for support under section 20:

i) providing the adult needing care consents to the provision of any care and support to them; but
ii) regardless of whether the local authority is required to meet the adult's needs for care and support under section 18.

Needs that local authorities may not meet

9.17 Local authorities **may not meet** certain needs:

i) an adult's need for care and support that has arisen solely because of destitution or the physical effects, or anticipated physical effects, of destitution (section 21);
ii) health care needs required to be met under the National Health Service Act 2006, unless meeting those needs would be merely incidental or ancillary to social care and support provision and would involve a service of a nature that a local authority could be expected to provide (but is not nursing care from a registered nurse) (section 22). As the *Care and Support Statutory Guidance* clarifies, at paragraphs 15.29–15.36, the two most common types of health care that local authorities cannot provider are nursing care from a registered nurse and services that the NHS has to provide because the individual is eligible for NHS Continuing Healthcare;
iii) housing needs required to be met under the Housing Act 1996 or any other specified enactment (section 23).

Plans and adverse decisions

9.18 The procedural machinery is set out in sections 24 and 25 and essentially requires the local authority to produce a care and support plan/support plan, or written reasons for not meeting needs, plus advice and assistance.

9.19 Section 24 starts off the process:

- where a local authority is required to meet an adult's or carers needs, or decides to exercise a power to do so, under sections 18–20, it must–
  - prepare a care and support plan for the adult;
  - tell the adult which needs, if any, may be met by direct payments; and
  - help the adult with deciding how to have the needs met

  (section 24(1));
- where a local authority is not required to meet needs and has decided not to exercise a power to do so, it must give the adult:
  - written reasons; and
  - (unless it has already done so) advice and information about what can be done to prevent or delay the development of needs for care and support, or support, in the future

  (section 24(2)).

9.20 The basic minimum content of a care plan is set out at section 25 of the Care Act 2014:

- as expanded upon in sections 9(4) and 10(5) and (6) of the Care Act 2014; and
- as explained at paragraph 10.36 of the *Care and Support Statutory Guidance.*

9.21 The statutory provisions are as follows:

Care and support plan, support plan

25(1) A care and support plan or, in the case of a carer, a support plan is a document prepared by a local authority which–
(a) specifies the needs identified by the needs assessment or carer's assessment,
(b) specifies whether, and if so to what extent, the needs meet the eligibility criteria,
(c) specifies the needs that the local authority is going to meet and how it is going to meet them,
(d) specifies to which of the matters referred to in section 9(4) the provision of care and support could be relevant or to which of the matters referred to in section 10(5) and (6) the provision of support could be relevant,
(e) includes the personal budget for the adult concerned (see section 26), and
(f) includes advice and information about–
(i) what can be done to meet or reduce the needs in question;
(ii) what can be done to prevent or delay the development of needs for care and support or of needs for support in the future.
(2) Where some or all of the needs are to be met by making direct payments, the plan must also specify–
(a) the needs which are to be so met, and
(b) the amount and frequency of the direct payments.
...
(6) In seeking to ensure that the plan is proportionate to the needs to be met, the local authority must have regard in particular–
(a) in the case of a care and support plan, to the matters referred to in section 9(4);
(b) in the case of a support plan, to the matters referred to in section 10(5) and (6).
...

Assessment of an adult's needs for care and support

9 ...
(4) A needs assessment must include an assessment of–
(a) the impact of the adult's needs for care and support on the matters specified in section 1(2),
(b) the outcomes that the adult wishes to achieve in day-to-day life, and
(c) whether, and if so to what extent, the provision of care and support could contribute to the achievement of those outcomes.
...

Assessment of a carer's needs for support

10 ...
(6) A local authority, in carrying out a carer's assessment, must have regard to–
(a) whether the carer works or wishes to do so, and
(b) whether the carer is participating in or wishes to participate in education, training or recreation.

9.22 The relevant parts of the *Care and Support Statutory Guidance* are at Chapters 6 and 10.

9.23 The Department of Health's Factsheet 3 deals with assessing needs and determining eligibility.[9]

9.24 The Social Care Institute for Excellence has published a range of resources to support local authority staff, social workers and others involved in assessment and eligibility.[10]

9.25 The Social Care Institute for Excellence has also published advice about independent advocacy.[11] There is a briefing note by the DoH, ADASS and the LGA on independent advocacy.[12]

9.26 It should also be noted that the Mental Capacity Act 2005 will apply for all those who may lack capacity: see para 7.53 above.

How needs may be met

9.27 A striking feature of the Care Act 2014 is that it does not, as the earlier regime did, present a list of specific services that a person may qualify for. Rather, it sets out an illustrative list of the types of provision that may be offered and an illustrative list of how provision may be made, so as to promote flexible and imaginative solutions that engage with real needs and preferences directly and not through the potential distorting lens of what services are available:

> **How to meet needs**
>
> 8(1) The following are examples of what may be provided to meet needs under sections 18 to 20–
> (a) accommodation in a care home or in premises of some other type;
> (b) care and support at home or in the community;
> (c) counselling and other types of social work;
> (d) goods and facilities;
> (e) information, advice and advocacy.
>
> (2) The following are examples of the ways in which a local authority may meet needs under sections 18 to 20–
> (a) by arranging for a person other than it to provide a service;
> (b) by itself providing a service;
> (c) by making direct payments.

9.28 As the *Care and Support Statutory Guidance* puts it, at paragraph 10.10 'The concept of "meeting needs" is intended to be broader than a duty to provide or arrange a particular service'. Thus, at paragraph 10.11 onwards the Guidance encourages consideration to be given to a wide range of options, including traditional services such as care homes or home care, but extending (non-exhaustively) to assistive technology, local community or voluntary groups, universal services, the use of individual service funds, the use of brokering services.

9 www.gov.uk/government/publications/care-act–2014-part–1-factsheets/care-act-factsheets-–2#factsheet–3-assessing-needs-and-determining-eligibility.

10 www.scie.org.uk/care-act–2014/assessment-and-eligibility/.

11 www.scie.org.uk/care-act–2014/advocacy-services/commissioning-independent-advocacy/duties/independent-advocacy-care-act.asp.

12 www.local.gov.uk/documents/10180/5756320/Briefing+note+V1+for+Advocacy+providers++final_LPlogo.pdf/4f1c20ad–3933–4291-b842–558511d8836f.

Relevance of carers to assessments of adults

9.29 It is implicit in the Act and spelled out in the *Care and Support Statutory Guidance* that local authorities must assess an adult's needs regardless of any care and support being provided by a carer, but can provide services that take into account such provision, so long as the carer is willing and able to continue:

> 6.15. During the assessment, local authorities must consider all of the adult's care and support needs, regardless of any support being provided by a carer. Where the adult has a carer, information on the care that they are providing can be captured during assessment, but it must not influence the eligibility determination. After the eligibility determination has been reached, if the needs are eligible or the local authority otherwise intends to meet them, the care which a carer is providing can be taken into account during the care and support planning stage. The local authority is not required to meet any needs which are being met by a carer who is willing and able to do so, but it should record where that is the case. This ensures that the entirety of the adult's needs are identified and the local authority can respond appropriately if the carer feels unable or unwilling to carry out some or all of the caring they were previously providing.
>
> ...
>
> 10.26 Local authorities are not under a duty to meet any needs that are being met by a carer. The local authority must identify, during the assessment process, those needs which are being met by a carer at that time, and determine whether those needs would be eligible. But any eligible needs met by a carer are not required to be met by the local authority, for so long as the carer continues to do so. The local authority should record in the care and support plan which needs are being met by a carer, and should consider putting in place plans to respond to any breakdown in the caring relationship.

9.30 It is consistent with this, that a carer's assessment must consider 'whether the carer is able, and is likely to continue to be able, to provide care' (section 10(1)(a)) and 'whether the carer is willing, and is likely to continue to be willing, to do so' (section 10(1)(b)), having regard to whether the carer works, or wishes to do so, or participates in education, training or recreation, or wishes to do so.

Involvement/advocacy/Mental Capacity Act 2005

9.31 Paragraph 7.53 and following above addresses the importance of involvement, independent advocacy and the Mental Capacity Act 2005. All those considerations apply equally at the care planning stage, as indicated by the duty at sections 23(3)–(5) of the Care Act 2014 to involve the adult, the carer and other relevant persons in the preparation of a care and support/support plan and 'take all reasonable steps to reach agreement with the adult or carer for whom the plan is being prepared about how the authority should meet the needs in question'. As it is put in the *Care and Support Statutory Guidance*:

> 10.2 The person must be genuinely involved and influential throughout the planning process, and should be given every opportunity to take joint ownership of the development of the plan with the local authority if they

> wish, and the local authority agrees. There should be a default assumption that the person, with support if necessary, will play a strong pro-active role in planning if they choose to. Indeed, it should be made clear that the plan 'belongs' to the person it is intended for, with the local authority role being to ensure the production and sign-off of the plan to ensure that it is appropriate to meet the identified needs.
>
> ...
>
> 10.49 In addition to taking all reasonable steps to agree how needs are to be met, the local authority must also involve the person the plan is intended for, the carer (if there is one), and/or any other person the adult requests to be involved. Where the person lacks capacity to ask the authority to do that, the local authority must involve any person who appears to the authority to be interested in the welfare of the person and should involve any person who would be able to contribute useful information. An independent advocate must be provided if section 67 of the Act applies (see chapter 7). The person, and their carers, will have the best understanding of how the needs identified fit into the person's life as a whole and connect to their overall wellbeing (see chapter 1). They are well placed to consider and identify which care and support options would best fit into their lifestyle and help them to achieve the day to day outcomes they identified during the assessment process. In practice, local authorities should give consideration to include a prompt to the person during the initial stages of the planning process to ask whether there is anyone else that the person wishes to be involved. Where the person lacks capacity, the local authority should make a best interests decision about who else should be involved.

Combined and joint assessments and plans

9.32 Section 12(5) of the Care Act 2014 provides that a local authority may, with the consent of those involved, combine a needs assessment or a carer's assessment with an assessment of another person.

9.33 In practical terms, this means (for example) that local authorities can combine its assessment of an adult and their carer; or of two adults in the same household who both need care and support; or an adult and their child carer; or of an adult and a child in the same household who both need social care.

9.34 That is followed through in section 25(11), which allows a local authority to combine care and support plans/support plans, in the same circumstances.

9.35 There is no provision for joint care and support plans/support plans (prepared jointly with other bodies) but there is provision for joint assessments at section 12(7) insofar as where another body is undertaking an assessment at the same time as a local authority, the local may carry out that other assessment on behalf of, or jointly with, that other body (or bodies).

Personal budgets

9.36 It is mandatory for a care and support plan to include 'the personal budget for the adult concerned' (section 25(1)(e)). The amount of the personal budget must be:

- arrived at co-operatively with the service user and other relevant persons;
- transparently reached and adequately reasoned;
- sufficient to meet needs.

9.37 The purpose of specifying, in a personal budget, the cost of meeting needs, is to enable the individual to choose whether to meet all or some of those meets themselves, via direct payments, or through the local authority (which will retain the personal budget), or an individual service fund (a third party provider, to whom the personal budget is transferred). Again, it is all about providing the individual with choice and control.

9.38 The level of personal budget is obviously of critical importance. Consistently with the case-law, paragraph 11.7 of the Guidance states that 'An indicative amount should be shared with the person, and anybody else involved, at the start of care and support planning, with the final amount of the personal budget confirmed through this process'. This issue is considered in detail at paragraphs 11.22–11.28, which emphasis the importance of 'transparency', 'timeliness' and 'sufficiency':

- local authorities should have a consistent and transparent methodology;
- the methodology should be flexible: it should not include arbitrary ceilings or use algorithmic-based systems such as Resource Allocation Schemes in more complex cases where they may be unsuitable;
- individuals must be informed how the budget is calculated;
- the care planning process should start with an '*indicative amount*' that can be fine-tuned as the process continues, in particular in the light of the individual's feedback;
- ultimately, the personal budget must be sufficient to meet eligible needs and the needs that the local authority has decided to meet and it must take into account the individual's reasonable preferences.

9.39 The personal budget statutory machinery is at sections 26 and 28 of the Care Act 2014, although sections 26(2)–(2)(b)(ii) and the whole of section 28 are not yet in force and are unlikely to come into force until 2020 (see 'The cap on care costs' at para 7.88 above).

9.40 A personal budget is defined in section 26(1):

26(1) A personal budget for an adult is a statement which specifies–
(a) the cost to the local authority of meeting those of the adult's needs which it is required or decides to meet as mentioned in section 24(1),
(b) the amount which, on the basis of the financial assessment, the adult must pay towards that cost, and
(c) if on that basis the local authority must itself pay towards that cost, the amount which it must pay.

(2) In the case of an adult with needs for care and support which the local authority is required to meet under section 18, the personal budget must also specify–
(a) the cost to the local authority of meeting the adult's needs under that section ...

9.41 Thus the personal budget must separately identify the cost of meeting the eligible needs that the local authority is under a duty to meet, and other needs.

9.42 The personal budget may also specify other amounts of public money available to the adult, for example, in relation to housing, health care or welfare (section 26(3)),

9.43 The Care and Support (Personal Budget: Exclusion of Costs) Regulations 2014 provides that in cases where intermediate care and re-ablement support services are provided, the costs of doing so must be excluded from the adult's personal budget if the local authority is not permitted to make a charge for providing the services by regulations made under section 14 of the Care Act 2014, or, if it is permitted to make a charge, it does not do so:

- the Care and Support (Charging and Assessment of Resources) Regulations 2014 prohibits charging for intermediate care and re-ablement for the first six weeks, so the personal budget cannot include the cost of intermediate care and re-ablement for the first six weeks;
- local authorities have a discretion whether to charge after six weeks, by virtue of section 14 of the Care Act 2014, to be exercised acting under the guidance in Chapter 8 of the *Care and Support Statutory Guidance*. Therefore, when a local authority decides to provide intermediate care or re-ablement for longer than six weeks, without making a charge, the cost of such provision may not be included in the personal budget.

9.44 Personal budgets are considered at Chapter 11 of the *Care and Support Statutory Guidance*, which provides the following overview:

> 11.3. The personal budget is the mechanism that, in conjunction with the care and support plan, or support plan, enables the person, and their advocate if they have one, to exercise greater choice and take control over how their care and support needs are met. It means:
>
> - knowing, before care and support planning begins, an estimate of how much money will be available to meet a person's assessed needs and, with the final personal budget, having clear information about the total amount of the budget, including proportion the local authority will pay, and what amount (if any) the person will pay;
> - being able to choose from a range of options for how the money is managed, including direct payments, the local authority managing the budget and a provider or third party managing the budget on the individual's behalf (an individual service fund), or a combination of these approaches;
> - having a choice over who is involved in developing the care and support plan for how the personal budget will be spent, including from family or friends;
> - having greater choice and control over the way the personal budget is used to purchase care and support, and from whom.
>
> 11.4. It is vital that the process used to establish the personal budget is transparent so that people are clear how their budget was calculated, and the method used is robust so that people have confidence that the personal budget allocation is correct and therefore sufficient to meet their care and support needs. The allocation of a clear upfront indicative (or 'ballpark') allocation at the start of the planning process will help people to develop the plan and make appropriate choices over how their needs are met.

Preferred accommodation

9.45 Local authorities must provide certain types of accommodation at the adult's preferred location, providing various conditions are met, including that the adult or a third party pays any additional cost, beyond that provided for in the adult's personal budget.

9.46 The statutory basis for preferred accommodation is section 30 of the Care Act 2014 and the Care and Support and After-care (Choice of Accommodation) Regulations 2014[13] which provide that the local authority must arrange for an adult to be accommodated in the accommodation of his choice (reg 2) when:

- it is going to meet the adult's needs under sections 18–20 of the Care Act 2014 by providing or arranging accommodation in a care home (reg 6), pursuant to the shared lives scheme (reg 7), in a supported living arrangement (reg 8) or in accommodation pursuant to after-care arrangements under section 117 of the Mental Health Act 1983 (reg 4);
- the preferred accommodation (reg 3) is the same type of accommodation as that specified in the adult's care and support plan; it is suitable to the adult's needs; it is available; the provider agrees to provide the accommodation on the local authority's usual terms and any additional cost beyond that specified in the adult's personal budget (or beyond the cost the local authority would usually expect to pay, in the case of after-care services) is going to be met in accordance with reg 5;
- a written agreement complying with the conditions in reg 5 is entered into. This entails that where the payer is the accommodation resident, either the 12-week property disregard applies or the resident enters into a deferred payment agreement. Otherwise, some other person must agree to pay the additional cost.

9.47 As one might expect, section 76(4) dis-applies section 30 in relation to prisoners and adults residing in approved premises, except for the purpose of making provision after their release.

9.48 Otherwise, this qualified right to choose where to be accommodated is a particularly clear example of placing the individual at the heart of the assessment and planning process. Annex A of the *Care and Support Statutory Guidance* explains how local authorities are expected to support this entitlement, starting with this:

> 2. The care and support planning process will have determined what type of accommodation will best suit the person's needs. This could be, for example, a care home, shared lives or extra care housing. Where the type of accommodation is one of those specified in regulations, the person will have a right to choose the particular provider or location, subject to certain conditions. Where this is the case, the following guidance should be applied and in doing so, local authorities should have regard to the following principles:
>
> - good communication of clear information and advice to ensure well informed decisions;
> - a consistent approach to ensure genuine choice;

13 SI No 2670.

- clear and transparent arrangements for choice and any 'top-up' arrangements;
- clear understanding of potential consequences should 'top-up' arrangements fail with clear exit strategies; and
- the choice is suitable to the person's needs.

3. Local authorities must also remember that the regulations and guidance on choice of accommodation and additional costs apply equally to those entering care for the first time, those who have already been placed by a local authority, and those who have been selffunders, but because of diminishing resources are on the verge of needing local authority support.

4. Local authorities should also be mindful of their duties under Section 1 of the Care Act 2014 to promote individual wellbeing. Further detail is available in Chapter 1.

9.49 As under the previous regime, local authorities must not use the preferred accommodation and top up process to avoid:

- ensuring that there is a genuine choice of quality, diverse accommodation locally;
- arranging (and paying for) accommodation that meets relatively expensive needs;
- arranging (and paying for) more expensive accommodation when that is all that is available to meet eligible needs.

9.50 Note also, that a local authority must provide written reasons for any refusal to arrange for the provision of preferred accommodation: the Care and Support and After-care (Choice of Accommodation) Regulations 2014 reg 9.

9.51 Age UK has produced a useful factsheet.[14]

9.52 See para 11.48 for more about the process of recovering top ups.

Direct payments

9.53 The overall thrust of the legislation and guidance is that, subject to safeguards, local authorities should make direct payments wherever feasible and terminate them only as a last resort.

9.54 As the *Care and Support Statutory Guidance* states:

12.2 Direct payments have been in use in adult care and support since the mid-1990s and they remain the Government's preferred mechanism for personalised care and support. They provide independence, choice and control by enabling people to commission their own care and support in order to meet their eligible needs.

12.3 Direct payments, along with personal budgets and personalised care planning, mandated for the first time in the Care Act, provide the platform with which to deliver a modern care and support system. People should be encouraged to take ownership of their care planning, and be free to choose how their needs are met, whether through local authority or third-party provision, by direct payments, or a combination of the three approaches.

14 www.ageuk.org.uk/Documents/EN-GB/Factsheets/FS60_Choice_of_accommodation_care_homes_fcs.pdf?dtrk=true.

9.55 The statutory regime is found at sections 31–33, 73(5) and 75(7) of the Care Act 2014 and the Care and Support (Direct Payments) Regulations 2014. Chapter 12 of the *Care and Support Statutory Guidance* applies.

What services direct payments may cover

9.56 Direct payments can be made so as to enable the adult to purchase any kind of service without any limit except in relation to care home accommodation: only the local authorities identified by name in Schedule 2 to the Care and Support (Direct Payments) Regulations 2014[15] can make direct payments for the provision of care home accommodation for more than four consecutive weeks in any 12-month period (reg 6).

9.57 Section 75(7) of the Care Act 2014 provides that a local authority may discharge its duty under the Mental Health Act 1983, to make after-care provision, by making direct payments. Schedule 4 to the Act amends section 31 and 32 for this purpose, by changing the language so that, when after-care services are under consideration, those sections apply to after-care services.

9.58 The Care and Support (Direct Payments) Regulations 2014 provide that:

- direct payments must be made subject to the condition that they are not used to pay specified family members except insofar as the local authority considers it necessary to direct otherwise, either in relation to care provision or in relation to the provision of administrative and management support (reg 3(1)–(3));
- the local authority is required to endeavour to harmonise its direct payments with any payments made to the adult under the National Health Service Act 2006, to minimise any administrative or other burden on the adult (reg 10);
- regulation 11 substitutes words in the other regulations where after-care services under section 117 of the Mental Health Act 1983 are under consideration.

Who may receive direct payments

9.59 Section 31 provides that direct payments must be made in cases where the adult possesses relevant capacity and where:

- the adult's personal budget specifies an amount which the authority must pay towards the cost of meeting the needs to which the personal budget relates; and
- the adult requests the local authority to meet some or all of those needs by making direct payments to the adult or a nominated person; and
- four conditions are met, namely:
  - any nominated person has agreed to receive the payments;
  - the local authority is not prohibited by the Care and Support (Direct Payments) Regulations 2014 from meeting the adult's needs by direct payments or, where the authority has a discretion not to

15 SI No 2871.

make direct payments, the local authority has not exercised that discretion;
- the local authority is satisfied that the adult or nominated person is capable of managing direct payments by themselves or with accessible help;
- the local authority is satisfied that making direct payments is an appropriate way to meet the needs in question.

9.60 Section 32 provides that direct payments must be made in cases where the adult lacks relevant capacity and where:

- the adult's personal budget specifies an amount which the authority must pay towards the cost of meeting the needs to which the personal budget relates; and
- the adult lacks capacity to do so, but an authorised person[16] requests the local authority to meet some or all of those needs by making direct payments to the authorised person; and
- five conditions are met, namely:
  - if there is a person authorised under the Mental Capacity Act 2005, they support the request;
  - the local authority is not prohibited by the Care and Support (Direct Payments) Regulations 2014 from meeting the adult's needs by direct payments or, where the authority has a discretion not to make direct payments, the local authority has not exercised that discretion;
  - the local authority is satisfied that the authorised person will act in the adult's best interests in arranging for the provision of care and support with the direct payments;
  - the local authority is satisfied that the authorised person is capable of managing direct payments by themselves or with accessible help;
  - the local authority is satisfied that making direct payments to the authorised person is an appropriate way to meet the needs in question.

9.61 Section 73(5) disapplies the direct payments provisions in the case of prisoners and adults residing in approved premises.

9.62 The Care and Support (Direct Payments) Regulations 2014 provide that:

- direct payments may not be made to persons falling within Schedule 1 (in outline, persons who abuse substances in a criminal context) (reg 2 and Sch 1);
- direct payments must be made subject to the condition that they are not used to pay specified family members except insofar as the local authority considers it necessary to direct otherwise, either in relation to care provision or in relation to the provision of administrative and management support (reg 3(1)–(3));

16 A person who is authorised under the Mental Capacity Act 2005 to make decisions about the adult's needs for care and support, or who is nominated by such a person as being suitable for this purpose or who is considered by the local authority to be suitable in the absence of any other authorised person.

- a direct payment made under section 32 of the Act must be subject to the condition that the authorised person (i) notifies the local authority if the adult no longer lacks capacity, (ii) obtains enhanced criminal record certificates for all those involved in providing care other than specified family members or friends of the adult (reg 3(4)–(5));
- a local authority may impose conditions, including that needs may not be met by a particular person (but not that they must be) and that reasonable information is provided (reg 4);
- a local authority has to take various steps before concluding that it would be appropriate for there to be direct payments, including consulting with the adult and other relevant persons, and obtaining enhanced criminal record certificates for any authorised person (reg 5);
- direct payments may be continued during a period of temporary incapacity if a person capable of managing the payments is prepared to do so (reg 8);
- local authorities may continue to make direct payments to an authorised person, despite the adult regaining capacity, where that is temporary and the direct payments are made on condition that the authorised person allows the adult to manage the direct payments for any period during which the authority is satisfied that they have the capacity to do so (reg 9).

9.63 Chapter 12 of the *Care and Support Statutory Guidance* advises that:

- local authorities should use their power to allow payments to be made to specified family members for care and, in particular, for administrative and management support (paragraphs 12.35–12.40);
- local authorities should give advice to individuals in receipt of direct payments about becoming an employer (paragraphs 12.48–12.51).

Review and termination

9.64 Where the 'conditions' cease to be met, the local authority must terminate the provision of direct payments (section 33(4)).

9.65 Otherwise, when conditions imposed under Regulations are not met, the local authority has a discretion to terminate provision and require repayments (section 33(5)).

9.66 See para 9.62 above for events that may trigger review and determination.

9.67 Chapter 12 of the *Care and Support Statutory Guidance* advises that direct payments should only be terminated 'as a last resort, or where there is clear and serious contradiction of the Regulations or where the conditions in sections 31 or 32 of the Act are no longer met (except in cases of fluctuating capacity ...)' (paras 12.67–12.84).

Portability

9.68 The statutory scheme that applies when service users move from one local authority area to another is set out in:

- sections 37–38 of the Care Act 2014;
- the Care and Support (Continuity of Care) Regulations 2014;
- Chapter 20 of the *Care and Support Statutory Guidance*.

9.69 The purpose of the scheme is to ensure that service users can move from one local authority area to another with the minimum interruption of their care. That purpose is obviously assisted by the fact that, under section 13 of the Care Act 2014 and the Care and Support (Eligibility Criteria) Regulations 2015, there are now nationally applicable minimum eligibility criteria. The portability scheme aims to make the process of moving from one local authority area to another even easier.

9.70 The machinery is triggered when section 37(1) applies (sections 37(2) and (3) are not in force):

> **Notification, assessment, etc.**
>
> **37**(1) This section applies where–
> (a) an adult's needs for care and support are being met by a local authority ('the first authority') under section 18 or 19,
> (b) the adult notifies another local authority ('the second authority') (or that authority is notified on the adult's behalf) that the adult intends to move to the area of the second authority, and
> (c) the second authority is satisfied that the adult's intention is genuine.

9.71 Thus, while the machinery is not triggered if a carer with support needs proposes to move, it is triggered when an adult in receipt of care and support services proposes to move and become ordinarily resident in the new area, whether or not the services provided meet eligible needs, but provided the second authority is satisfied that the intention to move is genuine.

9.72 The *Care and Support Statutory Guidance* suggests that:

> 20.12 To assure itself that the intention is genuine, the second authority should:
> - establish and maintain contact with the person and their carer to keep abreast of their intentions to move;
> - continue to speak with the first authority to get their view on the person's intentions;
> - ask if the person has any information or contacts that can help to establish their intention.

9.73 The machinery set in motion is as follows:

- the first authority provides the adult/carer with 'appropriate information' (section 37(4)(a))(this is to help the adult/carer reach an informed decision whether to move). The *Guidance* indicates as follows:

  > 20.13. When the second authority is satisfied that the person's intentions to move are genuine, it must provide the adult and the carer if also intending to move, with accessible information about the care and support available in its area. This should include but is not limited to, details about:

- the types of care and support available to people with similar needs, so the adult can know how they are likely to be affected by differences in the range of services available:
  - support for carers;
  - the local care market and organisations that could meet their needs;
  - the local authority's charging policy, including any charges which the person may be expected to meet for particular services in that area.
- the second authority provides the first authority with a copy of the care and support plan, of any carer's support plan where the carer will continue to provide care after the move and of any independent personal budget (section 37(4)(b));

- the first authority completes an assessment of the adult's and any carer's needs having regard to the second authority's care and support/support plans (section 37(6)–(8));
- the first authority must keep in touch with the second authority and the adult (sections 37(9)–(10));
- the second authority must provide a written explanation if its needs assessment, or the cost of meeting needs, differs from that of the first authority (sections 37(11)–(13)).

9.74 Section 38 provides, in essence, that when, on the day of the intended move, the second authority has not completed its assessment and undertaken the other steps required by section 37, then on and from that day the second authority has to meet needs whilst the first authority is no longer any duty to do so:

- the second authority must meet the needs for care and support/support being met by the first authority, until it has completed all the steps required by section 37;
- it need not meet them in the same way, but it must involve the adult, any carer and other relevant persons in the decision how to meet needs and try to reach agreement with them.

Cases

9.75 *R v Gloucestershire CC ex p Barry* (1997–8) 1 CCLR 40, HL

Resources were relevant to decisions whether to meet needs under section 2 of the Chronically Sick and Disabled Persons Act 1970

Facts: Mr Barry was a disabled 79-year-old man whom Gloucestershire had assessed as needing home care assistance including with cleaning and laundry. Gloucestershire then withdrew those services owing to a shortage of financial resources. The House of Lords decided by a 3:2 majority that Gloucestershire had been entitled to take its resources into account.

Judgment: the case turned on section 2(1) of the Chronically Sick and Disabled Persons Act 1970, which requires specified services to be provided when, inter alia, 'a local authority ... are satisfied ... that it is necessary in order to meet the needs of that person for that authority to make arrangements for all or any of the following matters ...'

Lord Nicholls held at 49E that:

> ... needs for services cannot sensibly be assessed without having some regard to the cost of providing them.

He said, at 49J, that:

> The local authority sets the standards to be applied within its area. In setting the standards, or 'eligibility criteria' as they have been called, the local authority must take into account current standards of living, with all the latitude inherent in this concept. The authority must also take into account the nature and extent of the disability. The authority will further take into 'account the manner in which, and the extent to which, quality of life would be improved by the provision of this or that service or assistance, at this

or that level: for example, by home care, once a week or more frequently. The authority should also have regard to the cost of providing this or that service, at this or that level. The cost of daily home care, or of installing a ground floor lavatory for a disabled person in his home and Q widening the doors to take a wheelchair, may be substantial. The relative cost will be balanced against the relative benefit and the relative need for that benefit.

Thus far the position is straightforward. The next step is the crucial step. In the same way as the importance to be attached to cost varies according to the benefit to be derived from the suggested expenditure, so also must the importance of cost vary according to the means of the D person called upon to pay. An amount of money may be a large sum to one person, or to one person at a particular time, but of less consequence to another person, or to the same person at a different time. Once it is accepted, as surely must be right, that cost is a relevant factor in assessing a person's needs for the services listed in section 2(1), then in deciding how much weight is to be attached to cost some evaluation or assumption £ has to be made about the impact which the cost will have upon the authority. Cost is of more or less significance depending upon whether the authority currently has more or less money. Thus, depending upon the authority's financial position, so the eligibility criteria, setting out the degree of disability which must exist before help will be provided with laundry or cleaning or whatever, may properly be more or less stringent.

Lord Clyde said:

The right given to the person by section 2(1) of the Act of 1970 was a right to have the arrangements made which the local authority was satisfied were necessary to meet his needs. The duty only arises if or when the local authority is so satisfied. But when it does arise then it is clear that a shortage of resources will not excuse a failure in the performance of the duty. However neither the fact that the section imposes the duty Q towards the individual, with the corresponding right in the individual to the enforcement of the duty, nor the fact that consideration of resources is not relevant to the question whether the duty is to be performed or not, means that a consideration of resources may not be relevant to the earlier stages of the implcmentation of the section which lead up to the stage when the satisfaction is achieved. The earlier stages envisaged by the section require to be distinguished from the emergence of the duty. And if D that distinction is kept in mind, the risk uf which counscl for Mr. Barry warned, namely the risk of the duty becoming devalued into a power, should not arise.

The words 'necessary' and 'needs' are both relative expressions, admitting in each case a considerable range of meaning. They are not defined in the Act and reference to dictionary definitions does not seem to g me to advance the construction of the subsection. In deciding whether there is a necessity to meet the needs of the individual some criteria have to be provided. Such criteria are required both to determine whether there is a necessity at all or only, for example, a desirability, and also to assess the degrcc of necessity. Counsel for Mr. Barry suggested that a criterion could be found in the values of a civilised society. But I am not persuaded that that is sufficiently precise to be of any real assistance. It is possible to F draw up categories of disabilities, reflecting the variations in the gravity of such disabilities which could be experienced. Such a classification might enable comparisons to be made between persons with differing kinds and degrees of disability. But in determining the question whether in a given case the making of particular arrangements is necessary in order to meet the needs of a given individual it seems to me that a mere list of disabling Q conditions graded

> in order of severity will still leave unanswered the question at what level of disability is the stage of necessity reached. The determination of eligibility for the purposes of the statutory provision requires guidance not only on the assessment of the severity of the condition or the seriousness of the need but also on the level at which there is to be satisfaction of the necessity to make arrangements. In the framing of the criteria to be applied it seems to me that the severity of a 'condition may have to be to be matched against the availability of resources. Such an exercise indeed accords with everyday domestic experience in relation to things which we do not have. If my resources limited I have to need the thing very much before I am satisfied that it is necessary to purchase it. It may also be observed that the range of the facilities which are listed as being the subject of possible arrangements, 'the service list,' is so extensive as to make it unlikely that Parliament intended that they might all be provided regardless of the cost involved. It is not necessary to hold that cost and resources are always an element in determining the necessity. It is enough for the purposes of the ' present case to recognise that they may be a proper consideration. I have not been persuaded that they must always and necessarily be excluded from consideration. Counsel for Mr Barry founded part of his submission on the claim that on the appellants' approach there would be an unmet need. However once it is recognised that criteria have to be devised for assessing the necessity required by the statutory provision it will be Q possible to allege that in one sense there will be an unmet need; but such an unmet need will be lawfully within what is contemplated by the statute. On a more exact analysis, whereby the necessity is measured by the appropriate criteria, what is necessary to be met will in fact be met and in the strict sense of the words no unmet need will exist.

Comment: As far as concerns disabled children, section 2 of the Chronically Sick and Disabled Persons Act 1970 remains in force and applicable as, therefore, does this case.

As far as concerns adults and carers, we now have nationally applicable eligibility criteria, by virtue of section 13 of the Care Act 2014 and the Care and Support (Eligibility Criteria) Regulations 2015. These govern the question of what needs are required to be met.

As far as concerns whether resources are relevant to the first question, whether a need exists at all, *R (KM) v Cambridgeshire CC*[17] suggests that they are not.

As far as concerns whether a lack of resources can excuse a failure to meet an eligible need, the *Barry* principle still applies and, indeed, the Care Act 2014 makes it clear that, in principle, local authorities must meet eligible needs (although they may have regard to their resources, and the relative cost of different ways of meeting eligible needs, when deciding which services to fund to meet eligible needs).

Resources will remain relevant to decisions whether to meet needs that are not eligible needs.

It may also be important to note that the *Barry* principle has never been treated as applying whatever the statutory context:

17 [2012] UKSC 23, [2012] 15 CCLR 374.

- in *R v Sefton MBC ex p Help the Aged/Blanchard,*[18] it was decided that local authority resources were only of marginal relevance in determining whether a person needed 'care and attention' for the purposes of the National Assistance Act 1948; the applicant's resources were relevant only to the extent that they exceeded a statutory threshold for means-testing;
- in *In Re T,*[19] it was held that resources were irrelevant to determining what was 'suitable education' for the purposes of section 298 of the Education Act 1993 (now section 19 of the Education Act 1996);
- in *R v Birmingham CC ex p Taj Mohammed,*[20] it was held that resources were irrelevant to determining whether to approve a disabled facilities grant under section 23(1) of the Housing Grants, Construction and Regeneration Act 1996, notwithstanding that section 24(3) precluded such approval unless the authority was 'satisfied ... that the relevant works are necessary and appropriate to meet the needs of the disabled occupant' – language very similar to that considered in *Barry*).

9.76 *R v Islington LBC ex p Rixon* (1997–8) 1 CCLR 119, QBD

Assessment and care planning must not deviate substantially from statutory guidance and must demonstrably have regard to departmental guidance. Where physical resources are unavailable to meet needs, local authorities must seek to secure the physical resources to do so

Facts: the applicant was a severely mentally and physically disabled 24-year-old man, whose mother considered that inadequate provision had resulted in him losing skills acquired at his special needs school and failing to develop his full potential. It was common ground that Islington's assessment and care plan failed to address comprehensively the applicant's needs and failed to comply with relevant central government guidance.

Judgment: Sedley J held that Islington had acted unlawfully in failing to 'act under' statutory guidance and properly to take into account non-statutory guidance (see above). He also held that Islington had acted unlawfully by providing an inadequate service because insufficient '*physical resources*' were available: it should have sought to secure such resources:

> There are two points at which, in my judgment, the respondent local authority has fallen below the requirements of the law. The first concerns the relationship of need to availability. The duty owed to the applicant personally by virtue of section 2(1) of the Chronically Sick and Disabled Persons Act 1970 includes the provision of recreational facilities outside the home to an extent which Islington accepts is greater than the care plan provides for. But the local authority has, it appears, simply taken the existing unavailability of further facilities as an insuperable obstacle to any further attempt to make provision. The lack of a day care centre has been treated, however reluctantly, as a complete answer to the question of provision for Jonathan's recreational needs. As McCowan LJ explained in the *Gloucestershire* case, the section 2(1) exercise is needs-led and not resources-led. To say this is not to ignore the existing resources either in terms of regular voluntary

18 (1997–8) 1 CCLR 57.
19 (1997–8) 1 CCLR 352.
20 (1997–8) 1 CCLR 441.

care in the home or in budgetary terms. These, however, are balancing and not blocking factors. In the considerable volume of evidence which the local authority has provided, there is no indication that in reaching its decision on provision for Jonathan the local authority undertook anything resembling the exercise described in the *Gloucestershire* case of adjusting provision to need

In relation to the importance of care planning, Sedley J said this:

> It is Miss Richards' first submission that in order to comply with the statutory duties, both personal and 'target', and to demonstrate that regard has been had to other relevant matters, the local authority must prepare a care plan which addresses the issues required by law and, where it deviates from the target, explains in legally acceptable terms why it is doing so. Mr McCarthy responds by pointing out first of all that nowhere in the legislation is a care plan, by that or any other name, required. This Miss Richards accepts, but she contends, in my judgment rightly, that she is entitled to look to the care plan (which is commended in the statutory policy guidance) as the best available evidence of whether and how the local authority has addressed Jonathan's case in the light of its statutory obligations. If, of course, further evidential material bears on this question, it too is admissible in relation to the challenge before the court. In other words, as I think Mr McCarthy accepts, his submission that a care plan is nothing more than a clerical record of what has been decided and what is planned, far from marginalising the care plan, places it at the centre of any scrutiny of the local authority's due discharge of its functions. As paragraph 3.24 of the policy guidance indicates, a care plan is the means by which the local authority assembles the relevant information and applies it to the statutory ends, and hence affords good evidence to any inquirer of the due discharge of its statutory duties. It cannot, however, be quashed as if it were a self-implementing document.
>
> ...
>
> The care plan, as Mr McCarthy readily admits, does not comply either with the policy guidance or the practice guidance issued by central government. There has been a failure to comply with the guidance contained in paragraph 3.24 of the policy document to the effect that following assessment of need, the objectives of social services intervention as well as the services to be provided or arranged should be agreed in the form of a care plan. For the reasons which I have given, if this statutory guidance is to be departed from it must be with good reason, articulated in the course of some identifiable decision-making process even if not in the care plan itself. In the absence of any such considered decision, the deviation from the statutory guidance is in my judgment a breach of the law; and so *a fortiori* is the reduction of the Flexiteam service from 3 hours as originally agreed, whatever the activity, to 3 hours swimming or 1 hours at home. I cannot accept Mr McCarthy's submission that the universal knowledge that no day centre care was available for Jonathan was so plainly the backdrop of the section 2 decision that there was no need to say so. It is one thing for it to have been a backdrop in the sense of a relevant factor, but another for it to have been treated as an immoveable object. The want of any visible consideration of it disables the respondent from showing that it was taken into account in the way spelt out in the *Gloucestershire* case. I do, however, accept Mr McCarthy's submission that Miss Richards' further contention that the respondent has failed to consider alternatives to day centre care for Jonathan comes so late that there has been no opportunity to file evidence about it. Further, the whole

situation in relation to day centre provision is about to change, making this element marginal save perhaps by way of fallback.

The care plan also fails at a number of points to comply with the practice guidance on, for example, the contents of a care plan, the specification of its objectives, the achievement of agreement on implementation on all those involved, leeway for contingencies and the identification and feeding back of assessed but still unmet need. While such guidance lacks the status accorded by section 7 of [Local Authority Social Services Act 1970], it is, as I have said, something to which regard must be had in carrying out the statutory functions. While the occasional lacuna would not furnish evidence of such a disregard, the series of lacunae which I have mentioned does, in my view, suggest that the statutory guidance has been overlooked.

In such a situation I am unable to accede to Mr McCarthy's submission that the failures to follow the policy guidance and practice guidance are beyond the purview of the court. What he can, I think, legitimately complain of is the fact that both of these submissions, in their present formulation, have emerged for the first time in the presentation of the applicant's case in court and were not adumbrated earlier. While he has not suggested that the lateness of the points has prevented material evidence from being placed before the court, Mr McCarthy may be entitled to rely on it in resisting any consequential relief, and I will hear him in due course on this.

9.77 *R v Sutton LBC ex p Tucker* (1997–8) 1 CCLR 251, QBD

Assessment and care planning must comply in substance with the statutory guidance and include effective long-term planning

Facts: the applicant's daughter, who was severely disabled and experienced substantial communication difficulties, had remained in hospital for two years after she was ready to be discharged because of Sutton's failure to complete an assessment and care plan that addressed its long-term obligations so as to enable her discharge.

Judgment: Hidden J accepted the applicant's submission that Sutton had acted unlawfully by failing to 'act under' statutory guidance. He also held that the complaints procedure would not have been an adequate alternative remedy, so as to trigger the court's discretion to refuse judicial review relief. On the care plan, he said this:

Mr Gordon submits that this is not a care plan, or if it can be regarded as a care plan, it is woefully inadequate and suffers from the same faults as were pinpointed by Sedley J in the case of *Rixon* at pages 19, 20 and 24 [(1997–8) 1 CCLR 119 at pp129–131]. Mr Gordon says there is no stated overall objective in terms of long term obligations or carers' obligations or those of the service providers. Since no objectives are recorded there is equally no criteria for the measurement of the objectives. There are no costings and no long term options as to residential care options considered. There are no recorded points of difference between the parties and there is no reference to unmet needs or the reasons therefore. There is no reference to the next date of review. Mr Gordon submits that the care plan is as far from the guidance given in the policy guidance as was the care plan in the *Rixon* case. What, he submits, it should have done was to demonstrate the efforts made by the Local Authority and show a realistic time scale for discharge of their obligations. It should have recorded the long term needs and Mrs Tucker's needs, but in fact it marks a concerted, contradictory and unyielding stance by the Local Authority to finding any long term placement.

> ...
>
> Mr Gordon submitted that Sutton had acted unlawfully in having no lawful care plan which would show exactly the points of disagreement between Mrs Tucker and Sutton which would identify unmet need and would set out clearly the objectives for Therese and the criteria for meeting such objectives. Had there been such a care plan the efforts or lack of efforts of the Local Authority would have been transparent. Again I find Mr Gordon is right in his criticisms of the document which is put forward as a care plan in that, as he correctly submits, there are no stated overall objectives in terms of long term obligations, carers' obligations or service providers, there is no criteria for the measurement of objectives because the objectives themselves are not recorded in any care plan. There are no costings, no long term options, no residential care options considered,there are no recorded points of difference, there is no reference to unmet need and there is no reference to a next date of review. I am satisfied that the criticisms that Mr Gordon makes of the care plan are valid ones.
>
> ...
>
> I accept the criticisms made by Mr Gordon of what is said to be the care plan in this case, those criticisms I have just referred to. I accept Mr Gordon's submissions that the care plan sought to be put forward in this case is as far from the policy guidelines as was that in the *Rixon* case. I find the respondent has acted unlawfully and departed without good reason from the policy guidance issued by the Secretary of State. I find that the respondent has used its undoubted discretion to make short term and interim decisions in relation to the care of the applicant. The use of such discretion cannot in my view replace the duty to make a service provision decision as to the long term future of the applicant. I therefore find the respondent has acted unlawfully in the matters and in the manner I have indicated. I would also be prepared to find that such actions were *Wednesbury* unreasonable if that were necessary. As to the relief to be granted by the court I shall listen to any submissions from counsel.

9.78 *R v Lambeth LBC ex p A1 and A2* (1997–8) 1 CCLR 336, CA

Where physical resources are not available to discharge a duty to meet needs, the local authorities may have to make a sincere and determined effort to secure them

Facts: Lambeth had undertaken a number of assessments under various enactments; they were all flawed to a greater or lesser extent but the fact remained that Lambeth was aware and accepted that this family were in dire need of urgent rehousing because of adult care and children's welfare issues.

Judgment: The Court of Appeal (Hirst and Robert Walker LJJ, Harman) held that Owen J had been right to refuse relief, notwithstanding legal flaws in the assessments, because the heart of the matter was not Lambeth's failure to assess the problem but its failure to solve it:

> As I have said, what this court has to do is determine the appeal from Owen J. There are nine grounds of appeal in the notice of appeal against the rejection of Mrs A's application. The first is that the judge was wrong to defer questions under the Children Act, the 1970 Act and the 1995 Act until the issue of rehousing is resolved. Miss Maxwell has urged on us that comprehensive assessments were needed. She has said that only comprehensive

> assessments can meet the answer. I have to say that I do not accept that at all. There have been numerous assessments in this case, to some but not all of which I have referred. It may be that some are better than others. It may be that some do not explicitly state under what statute or statutes they have been made, but judicial review is a discretionary remedy. The judge exercised his discretion properly and, if I may say so, with eminent good sense, when he said that 'What this lad needs and what his parents need is a new home.' Everyone knows the problem. What is needed is a sincere and determined resumption of the search for a solution.
>
> The second ground of appeal is connected with the first. It seems to me that any correction of a lack of formal assessment in the past would simply be a bit of tidy minded putting the files in order and would not assist the resolution of the real problem.

Comment: notwithstanding the more pragmatically focussed language, this decision appears consistent with *Rixon*: when a need is identified, but physical resources are not immediately available to meet it, the local authority must make '*a sincere and determined*' effort to find a solution.

9.79 *R v Kirklees MBC ex p Daykin* (1997–8) 1 CCLR 512, QBD

Local authorities are entitled to meet needs in the most cost-effective manner

Facts: Kirklees decided to provide adapted ground floor accommodation, rather than a stair lift in the applicants' existing accommodation, because it was significantly cheaper.

Judgment: Collins J held the applicants' need was to be able to get into and out of their dwelling, rather than for a stairlift; this was, therefore, a case about deciding how to meet need and that Kirklees had been entitled to meet the need in the most cost-effective manner:

> ... But one has to differentiate between what are needs and what are the services to meet those needs because, as the case of *Barry*, which I have already cited, makes clear, financial considerations cannot enter into the assessment of needs whereas they can enter into the question as to how those needs are to be met. Once the needs have been established, then they must be met and cost cannot be an excuse for failing to meet them. The manner in which they are met does not have to be the most expensive. The Council is perfectly entitled to look to see what is the cheapest way for them to meet the needs which are specified.
>
> In the context of section 2 of the 1970 Act, it is not always easy to differentiate between what is a need and what is merely the means by which such need can be met. I say that because if one looks at the judgments in the *Barry* case one sees that Swinton Thomas LJ at page 439 pointed out that some of the matters in section 2(1) of the 1970 Act may be regarded as themselves needs as opposed to the means of meeting the needs. For example, he says, if the need is a provision for the TV set (that is within section 2(1)(b)) that need can be met by the provision of a new or a second-hand set. It may be said that the need is a need for contact with the outside world in some form or another and that the television set provides that contact. Thus the television set is the means whereby the need is to be met. If one returns to the wording of section 2, it talks about the 'making of arrangements for all or any of the following matters in order to meet the needs of that person' which on the whole suggests that one is looking to the matters set out in (a) to (h) more in terms of the way in which the needs are to be met rather

> than the needs themselves, although that is not necessarily an entire guide. So far as the circumstances of this case are concerned, it seems to me perfectly clear that the needs that have led to the question about the provision of a stair lift are the needs for the applicants to be able to get in and out of the premises. Those are the relevant needs. They can be met, as it seems to me, either by removing them to other premises where access is possible for them, which in the context of this case, would be ground floor premises, or adapting the existing premises to provide a stair lift.
>
> It is, in my judgment, impossible to regard the provision of a stair lift at home as 'the need'. In those circumstances, it is open to the local authority to reconsider the way in which those needs can be met provided that there has been no positive decision to meet them in a particular fashion. I say 'provided there has been no positive decision', but of course such a decision itself could itself be changed upon reconsideration. One must always bear in mind that it is the duty of the authority to meet the needs and that means to meet them as soon as is reasonably practical. It does mean that the authority is entitled to sit on things and debate with itself for a substantial period of time. Once they have identified after discussion the manner in which those needs are to be met, then the Act requires that they get on with it and meet those needs. But it seems to me that they are entitled to the flexibility as to how those needs are to be met.

Comment: this decision seems to foreshadow that of *R (McDonald) v Kensington & Chelsea RLBC*[21] (see below at para 9.95).

9.80 *R v Wigan MBC ex p Tammadge* (1997–8) 1 CCLR 581, QBD

Local authorities are required to meet needs that they have accepted as being eligible

Facts: the social services complaints review panel concluded that the applicant and her family were in urgent need of re-housing for health and care reasons. Wigan accepted that and ascertained that the most cost-effective solution was to knock together two adjacent houses in its area. However, Wigan then decided not to undertake that course because 'the potential benefits ... do not justify the significant costs'.

Judgment: Forbes J held that while resources were relevant to a limited extent when determining whether and if so what needs existed for residential accommodation under section 21 of the National Assistance Act 1948, once a need has been assessed as existing, the authority is under a duty to make provision for that need. That applied in this case and Wigan was ordered to undertake the work that it had itself determined as being the most cost-effective solution:

> I have come to the firm conclusion that Mr Gordon's submissions are correct. In my view, SSCRP's finding as to Mrs Tammadge's need for larger accommodation is perfectly clear from the wording in which that particular conclusion is expressed. Moreover, that conclusion is entirely in keeping with views of Wigan's own professionally qualified staff and advisers, as expressed both before and after the hearing before the SSCRP. I am therefore satisfied that, by a date no later than 22 October 1996 (when it was acknowledged that Wigan had accepted the SSCRP finding: see above), Mrs Tammadge's need for larger accommodation was established. I reject

21 [2011] UKSC 33, (2011) 14 CCLR 341.

Miss Patterson's submissions to the contrary. As a result, from that date Wigan have been obliged to make provision of such accommodation to Mrs Tammadge and her family: see *ex p M* at pages 1009–1010. Once the duty had arisen in this way, it was not lawful of Wigan to refuse to perform that duty because of a shortage of or limits upon its financial resources or for any of the other reasons expressed in Mr Walker's letters of 30 July and 28 August 1997: see *ex p Sefton* at page 58 and also at page 671–J, where Lord Woolf said this:

> 'However, in this case it is clear from the evidence that Sefton accepted that Mrs Blanchard met its own threshold as a person in need of care and attention. What it was seeking to do was to say that because of its lack of resources notwithstanding this it was not prepared to meet the duty which was placed upon it by the section. This it was not entitled to do.'

Comment: the principle should still apply under section 18 of the Care Act 2014 and, in relation to carers, under section 20.

9.81 *R v Kensington and Chelsea RLBC ex p Kujtim* (1999) 2 CCLR 340, CA

A local authority remains under a duty to meet eligible needs unless the applicant has manifested a persistent and unequivocal refusal to observe reasonable conditions and must be ready to re-assess where it appears that the applicant will not persist

Facts: Kensington & Chelsea refused to continue to provide Mr Kujtim with residential accommodation after complaints about his misconduct, which continued after a written warning.

Judgment: the Court of Appeal (Peter Gibson and Potter LJJ, Blofeld J) held that once a local authority had assessed a person as 'needing' residential accommodation, it was under a duty to provide it as long as the need remained in existence and unless the applicant manifested a persistent and unequivocal refusal to observe reasonable requirements relating to occupation of the accommodation. Even in such cases, it was essential that the local authority carefully considered the applicant's current needs and circumstances, the causes of his conduct and the surrounding circumstances, allowing the applicant a fair opportunity of putting his case. Further, the duty revived, once the applicant satisfied the local authority that his needs required service provision to be made and that he would no longer persist in refusing to observe the local authority's reasonable requirements:

> *The Extent of The Duty Under Section 21 (l)(a) of The 1948 Act*
>
> 30. That being so, the question which arises is whether or not there is any limitation upon the duty to provide or continue to provide such accommodation for as long as the need, once assessed, continues. In my view the position is as follows. Once a local authority has assessed an applicant's needs as satisfying the criteria laid down in s21(1)(a), the local authority is under a duty to provide accommodation on a continuing basis so long as the need of the applicant remains as originally assessed, and if, for whatever reason, the accommodation, once provided, is withdrawn or otherwise becomes unavailable to the applicant, then (subject to any negative reassessment of the applicant's needs) the local authority has a continuing duty to provide further accommodation. That said, however,

the duty of the local authority is not absolute in the sense that it has a duty willy-nilly to provide such accommodation *regardless of the applicant's willingness to take advantage of it*.

31. In this connection there are two realities to be recognised. First, the duty to provide accommodation is predicated upon the co-operation of the applicant in the sense of his willingness to occupy it on such terms and in accordance with such requirements as the local authority may reasonably impose in relation to its occupation. The second, and connected, reality is that the resources of the local authority are finite and that, in providing accommodation for the needy, save in rare cases where individual or special accommodation may be necessary and available to meet the special needs of a particular applicant, the accommodation may, and will usually be, provided within multi-occupied premises, whether in the form of flats, or hostel or bed and breakfast accommodation, in relation to which it will be reasonable for the local authority to lay down certain requirements as to the use of such accommodation and the activities to be permitted in it, whether from a health and safety point of view, or for the purpose of preventing injury, nuisance or annoyance to fellow occupiers of the premises.

32. Thus it seems to me that, when the circumstances warrant, if an applicant assessed as in need of Part III accommodation either unreasonably refuses to accept the accommodation provided or if, following its provision, by his conduct he manifests a persistent and unequivocal refusal to observe the reasonable requirements of the local authority in relation to the occupation of such accommodation, then the local authority is entitled to treat its duty as discharged and to refuse to provide further accommodation. That will remain the position unless or until, upon some subsequent application, the applicant can satisfy the local authority that his needs remain such as to justify provision of Part III accommodation and that there is no longer reason to think that he will persist in his refusal to observe the reasonable requirements of the local authority in respect of the provision of such accommodation.

33. In formulating the right of the local authority to treat its duty as discharged by conduct as requiring manifestation of *persistent and unequivocal* refusal, rather than a single transgression, I have in mind the following matters which were urged upon us by Mr Gordon as part of his submission that the duty of providing Part III accommodation is unqualified and absolute. The provisions of section 21 of the 1948Act as amended are 'safety net' provisions designed to assist the poorest and most needy members of society, at rock bottom as it were. For a variety of reasons of personal and social disadvantage, they may well be persons who find difficulty complying with the norms of social behaviour or self control, while falling outside the specific areas of need catered for by other provision within the Community Care Services or under housing legislation. To create a class consisting of a substantial number of persons outside the scope even of the minimum requirements of the safety net provisions cannot lightly be contemplated. To withdraw Part III accommodation in respect of persons with such needs is likely to reduce such persons to living and sleeping on the streets; not only does it tend to defeat the overall purpose of the 1948 Act as well as Community Care, but it produces the socially undesirable effect of increasing rather than alleviating deprivation and encourages return to the practice of begging in the streets

34. In the particular case of a genuine refugee who is homeless while awaiting resolution of his claim for asylum (and, as already indicated, there is no reason to doubt the genuineness of Mr Kujtim's claim) the effect of

a refusal to supply Part III accommodation despite the existence of need is to remove from him basic food and shelter in a situation where, upon recognition of his claim, he would be entitled to receive the usual benefits available to British citizens in a position of hardship and unemployment; further, in the case of an applicant who is unwell, there may result damage to health, or in extreme cases threat to life, as a result of his being put out on the streets.

35. The existence of those considerations makes it essential that local authorities should reach the conclusion that their duty to supply Part III accommodation is discharged in respect of any particular applicant only after being satisfied of his persistent and unequivocal refusal to comply with the local authority's requirements, coupled with a careful consideration of his *current* needs and circum stances. Either or both may involve consideration of any relevant medical condition or infirmity known to the local authority. Before concluding that there has been such refusal, it will plainly be desirable for a local authority to write a letter of final warning of the kind written by the respondents to the applicant in this case. As to the question of current need, the instant case provides a good example of why a re-consideration of need is essential. Had the respondents been aware, as they were not when they reached their decision, that the behaviour of the applicant in failing to observe their requirements to obey local hostel rules and to comply with the warning given to him by letter following his first expulsion, was the product of a depressive condition associated with the very ill-treatment which had driven him to seek refuge in this country, it seems unlikely that they would have treated his actions as manifesting a persistent and unequivocal refusal to comply with their requirements. However, they were entirely unaware of his medical condition and, in those circumstances, cannot be blamed for ignoring it.

Comment: in the adult and child social care context, the question of discharge of duty is dealt with very differently than in other contexts, for example, housing: an authority must always be ready to meet the eligible needs of a person who is willing to comply with reasonable conditions.

9.82 *R v Calderdale MBC ex p Houghton* (2000) 3 CCLR 228, QBD

A care plan must be a rational response to the assessment of needs

Facts: Mrs Houghton issued an application for judicial review challenging her care plan on the basis that it was not rationally justified by the assessment of her needs.

Judgment: Smith J held that the care plan seemed to bear no relationship with the assessment of needs. Therefore, the claimant's application for judicial review would probably have succeeded and she should recover her legal costs.

9.83 *R v South Lanarkshire Council ex p MacGregor* (2000) 4 CCLR 188, CSOH

Some waiting lists might be lawful but this waiting list was not as it did not prioritise applicants according to their needs and was a plain attempt to avoid meeting statutory duties

Facts: South Lanarkshire had assessed Mr MacGregor as requiring a nursing care home and had placed him on a waiting list, informing him that he would have to wait for several months until funding was available for his placement.

Judgment: Lord Hardie held that although the use of waiting lists could be lawful, in order to help local authorities utilise their resources effectively, in this case it was unlawful as there had been no attempt to prioritise those on the waiting list in relation to their needs and it amounted to an illegitimate attempt to use a shortage of financial resources as a reason for not discharging a statutory duty.

Comment: this case turned on the provisions of the Social Work (Scotland) Act 1968, but the principle that a shortage of financial resources cannot justify delaying the discharge of a statutory duty ought to hold good in the rest of Britain.

9.84 *R (Khana) v Southwark LBC* [2001] EWCA Civ 999, (2001) 4 CCLR 267

Local authorities are required to meet needs under section 21 of the National Assistance Act 1948, not preferences; an offer of accommodation that meets needs discharges the duty

Facts: Mrs Khana was elderly and disabled. Her elderly husband was her primary carer and they lived together with their daughter in a one-bedroom flat. They wished to be re-housed under section 21 of the National Assistance Act 1948 in a two-bedroom flat, where the husband and daughter could continue to care for Mrs Khana. Southwark's assessment, however, concluded that such an arrangement would not meet Mrs Khana's needs; he needed residential accommodation (where her husband could also reside) where 24-hour care was available.

Judgment: the Court of Appeal (Henry and Mance LJJ, McKinnon J) held that Southwark had taken into account, as legislation and guidance required, the family's preferences and the need to preserve the independence of elderly people in the community for as a long as possible. It was, also, the case that Southwark had power to provide 'ordinary accommodation' under section 21 of the Nationality Assistance Act 1948. Ultimately, however, Southwark had reached a rational conclusion on the facts. This was not a case of Mrs Khana having a 'psychological need', as in *R v Avon CC ex p M* (see above para 8.53) but of insisting on her preferences. Nor was this a case of Southwark choosing an alternative way of meeting needs to conserve resources (where evidence of a resources difficulty could be required), nor was it a case of Southwark choosing between one of two alternative way of meeting needs, which could give rise to different issues: Southwark had positively concluded that the provision of larger ordinary accommodation, where the family remained Mrs Khana's primary carers, would not meet her needs, in important ways. If necessary, Southwark would be entitled to treat its duties towards Mr Khana as discharged, if she chose not to accept the offer of residential accommodation:

> 57. Further, although I do not consider that the case requires analysis in these terms, I would, if necessary, also treat Mrs K's refusal of the offer of residential home accommodation – the only course that would meet her assessed needs – as unreasonable in the sense intended by Potter LJ, when

> he was considering in ex p. Kujtim what would discharge a local authority from any further duty for so long as such refusal was maintained. Her position has, it is true, received some strong support from distinguished sources, but the local authority's assessment of her needs, the appropriateness of their offer and the inappropriateness (in terms of meeting all Mrs K's needs) of Mrs K's position are not ultimately challenged.
>
> 58. If this had been a case where Mrs K's assessed needs could be met in different ways, then, on the authorities already cited, Southwark would have been entitled to take into account its resources in deciding which way to adopt. Mrs Justice Hallett in her judgment seems at certain points to have taken the view that a question of resources did arise in this case. For my part, I would agree with Mr Drabble that any problem of resources would require to made out by evidence, and cannot be assumed to be present. There is no material enabling comparison between the cost of a two bedroom ground floor flat provided by the authority – with or without further community care services – and the costs of living in a residential home.

9.85 *R v Newham LBC ex p Patrick* (2001) 4 CCLR 48, QBD

Referring a homeless woman with care needs to a housing charity did not amount to a discharge of the duty to assess or meet her needs

Facts: Ms Patrick was a single woman who suffered from physical and mental ill health, was evicted on the ground of neighbour nuisance and found intentionally homeless. Newham had purported to discharge its duty towards her under section 21 of the National Assistance Act 1948, by offering her accommodation provided by a charity, which she had refused. Ms Patrick then slept rough.

Judgment: Henriques J held that Newham had failed in breach of statutory duty to assess Ms Patrick's needs and had not discharged its duty under section 21:

> 27. Her solicitor in her witness statement says that she did not take up the accommodation provided by HOST because she believed she was being sent to Sunderland and not to Southwark. In any event, Southwark was a distance away from her sister and from her medical support network.
>
> 28. Since the offer of accommodation was on 28 April and the certificate of mental incapacity to handle her affairs was granted on 9 May, it requires no mental gymnastics to conclude that her decision to reject the offer of accommodation at Southwark was neither considered nor likely to have been well informed.
>
> 29. It is of particular significance that the respondent knew that solicitors were acting for the applicant as they had written on her behalf on 5 April.
>
> 30. Further, they had informed the respondent that they could obtain no clear instructions from the applicant due to her mental health and enclosed a note from her general practitioner.
>
> 31. If the respondent sought to put an end to its section 21 duties to provide accommodation, they ought in my judgment at the very least to have ensured that the applicant was legally represented when the offer was made to her to ensure not only that she understood what the offer was, both in terms of location and services offered, but also that she understood the legal consequences or potential legal consequences of refusing the offer.
>
> 32. Since she may well not have understood what was being offered and its location, I am not prepared to find that her refusal of it was unreasonable.

> 33. In the exercise of its duty to provide accommodation a local authority must have a concurrent duty to explain fully and to the point of comprehension any offer it may make. I am not persuaded that the local authority has discharged its duty. In my judgment the duty to provide Part III accommodation continues pursuant to section 21 of the 1948 Act.

9.86 *R v Islington LBC ex p Batantu* (2001) 4 CCLR 445, QBD

A local authority remained under a duty to meet assessed needs despite the service user's refusal of offered services

Facts: Mr Batantu was disabled and lived in over-crowded, unsuitable accommodation with his family. Islington assessed him as needing to be re-housed to more spacious, adapted accommodation but then simply referred his case to the housing department. Mr Batantu then refused offers of accommodation. Mr Batantu sought a judicial review of Islington's failure to offer him ordinary accommodation under section 21 of the National Assistance Act 1948.

Judgment: Henriques J held that the assessment had given rise to a duty on Islington's social services department; a single refusal by Mr Batantu to contemplate private rented accommodation, and a refusal to accept a three-bedroom flat in a different area, had not absolved Islington of its duty:

> 40. A single refusal in principle to contemplate private rented accommodation, post March this year, coupled with the refusal to accept a three-bedroom flat out of the area and with a number of unsuitable steps in March of 1999, between one mile and one-and-a-half miles away from their present home, cannot conceivably, in my judgment, absolve the respondents from their continuing duty to provide accommodation. It is perfectly easy to appreciate why the applicant would have chosen to decline the offer of private sector, short-let accommodation, and the applicant has not begun to stretch the duty to the point of willy-nilly.
>
> 41. The respondent continues in argument to assert that even if there is a duty, nevertheless, the respondent can do no more. The respondent most certainly can do more and must. It is significant that upon instructions, Mr Harrop-Griffiths asserted that his clients had not considered themselves under a duty to provide accommodation pursuant to section 21 between March of this year and the present moment. That is an unfortunate, albeit frank, concession, having regard to the clarity of the judgments of both Potter LJ and Forbes J in *ex p Kujtim* and *ex p Tammadge* respectively. The respondents most certainly can do more. They can buy accommodation and let it to the applicant by way of long lease, assuming all other efforts fail.

Comment: The decision in *Kujtim* (see above para 9.81) sets out the very limited circumstances in which local authorities may terminate their social care duties.

Section 23 of the Care Act 2014 now provides that a local authority may not meet needs under sections 18–20 'by doing anything which it or another local authority is required to do under – (a) the Housing Act 1996, or (b) any other enactment specified in regulations'. However, at the time of *Batantu* and other similar cases, section 21(8) of the National Assistance Act 1948 had contained an even wider prohibition.

The primary question now, is whether an adult meets the criteria in the Care and Support (Eligibility Criteria) Regulations 2015. If the adult does, then it may be thought that ordinary accommodation may be provided, still, to meet that needs, since that it something that is not required to be done under the Housing Act 1996.

9.87 *R (Wahid) v Tower Hamlets LBC* [2002] EWCA Civ 287, (2002) 5 CCLR 239

Local authorities are only required to provide accommodation under social care legislation when the qualifying criteria under such legislation are met

Facts: Mr Wahid was mentally unwell and lived with his family in suitable accommodation. Tower Hamlets concluded that Mr Wahid had a medical and social need for better accommodation (to be met under the Housing Acts) but did not need 'care and attention', so as to trigger the duty to provide residential accommodation under section 21 of the National Assistance Act 1948.

Judgment: the Court of Appeal (Pill, Mummery and Hale LJJ) upheld Tower Hamlets' decision: whilst residential accommodation could be ordinary accommodation, it was a precondition of such a duty arising that the applicant had been assessed as needing '*care and attention*', which means more than just housing:

> 30. I agree that this appeal should be dismissed for the reasons given by Pill LJ. Some basic points may deserve emphasis given the recent expansion of litigation in this field. Under section 21(1)(a) of the National Assistance Act 1948, local social services authorities have a duty to make arrangements for providing residential accommodation for people over 18 (who are ordinarily resident in their area or in urgent need) where three inter-related conditions are fulfilled:
>
> (1) the person is in need of care and attention;
>
> (2) that need arises by reason of age, illness, disability or any other circumstances; and
>
> (3) that care and attention is not available to him otherwise than by the provision of residential accommodation under this particular power.
>
> Three further points are also relevant:
>
> (1) it is for the local social services authority to assess whether or not these conditions are fulfilled, and if so, how the need is to be met, subject to the scrutiny of the court on the ordinary principles of judicial review;
>
> (2) section 21 does not permit the local social services authority to make provision which may or must be made by them or any other authority under an enactment other than Part III of the 1948 Act (see section 21(8)); but
>
> (3) having identified a need to be met by the provision of residential accommodation under section 21, the authority have a positive duty to meet it which can be enforced in judicial review proceedings (see *R v Sefton Metropolitan Borough Council ex p Help the Aged* [1997] 4 All ER 532, CA; *R Kensington and Chelsea London Borough Council ex p Kujtim* [1999] 4 All ER 161, CA).

31. Mr Goudie's argument, skilfully and attractively though it was put, was ultimately circular. It is common ground that the 'residential accommodation' which may be provided under section 21 includes ordinary housing (see, on this point, *R v Newham London Borough Council ex p Medical Foundation for the Care of Victims of Torture* (1997–8) 1 CCLR 227; *R v Bristol City Council ex p Penfold* (1997–8) 1 CCLR 315; *R (Batantu) v Islington London Borough Council* (2001) 4 CCLR 445). I agree with Stanley Burnton J, at first instance in this case (see (2001) 4 CCLR 455, at para 27), that there are several indications in the Act that the kind of accommodation originally envisaged was in a residential home or hostel. This is the power under which local authorities provided elderly and aged people's homes or arranged accommodation in such homes run by others. However, it can no longer be assumed that a need for care and attention can only be properly met in an institutional setting. There are people who are undoubtedly in need of care and attention for whom local social services authorities wish to provide residential accommodation in ordinary housing. The most obvious examples are small groups of people with learning disabilities who are able to live in ordinary houses with intensive social services support; or single people with severe mental illnesses who will not receive the regular medication and community psychiatric nursing they need unless they have somewhere to live. Whatever the words 'residential accommodation' may have meant in 1948, therefore, they are a good example of language which is 'always speaking' and can be change its meaning in the light of changing social conditions (see the observations of this Court in *R v Westminster City Council ex p M, P, A and X* (1997–8) 1 CCLR 85 at 90). Hence Mr Knafler, in common with others who have appeared for local social services authorities, has conceded that 'residential accommodation' can mean ordinary housing without the provision of any ancillary services.

32. But it does not follow that because residential accommodation can mean ordinary housing and the claimant is in need of ordinary housing, a duty arises to provide him with that housing under section 21(1)(a). That duty is premised on an unmet need for 'care and attention' (a 'condition precedent', as this Court put it in the *Westminster* case, at p 93E). These words must be given their full weight. Their natural and ordinary meaning in this context is 'looking after': this can obviously include feeding the starving, as with the destitute asylum seekers in the *Westminster* case. Ordinary housing is not in itself 'care and attention'. It is simply the means whereby the necessary care and attention can be made available if otherwise it will not (I do not understand this Court to have rejected that part of the local authority's argument in the *Westminster* case, at p93B-D). The destitute asylum seekers in the *Westminster* case had a claim because their destitution would reduce them to a situation in which they required such care and attention and it could not be made available to them in any other way because of the restrictions placed upon their ability to seek other forms of support by the Asylum and Immigration Act 1996.

Comment: The primary question now, is whether an adult meets the criteria in the Care and Support (Eligibility Criteria) Regulations 2015. If the adult does, then it may be thought that ordinary accommodation may still be provided to meet those needs, since that is something that is not required to be done under the Housing Act 1996.

9.88 *R (A and B) v East Sussex CC* [2002] EWHC 2771 (Admin), (2003) 6 CCLR 177

A balance was to be struck between the ECHR rights of paid carers and service users. Local authorities may make payments to user independent trusts for the provision of care services

Facts: A and B were severely disabled sisters who continued to live in the family home, owing to a dispute with Sussex over aspects of the care package, in particular, as to the extent to which Sussex could be required to instruct carers to undertake manual lifting.

Judgment: Munby J held that the Manual Handling Operations Regulations 1992 required Sussex to minimise the risk of injury from hazardous lifting, as far as reasonably practicable. What was required was a balancing of the Article 8 rights of A and B, and those of the carers:

> 119. The other aspect of the matter which, in my judgment, is of considerable importance relates to what is meant by dignity in this context. Much of the debate with East Sussex County Council (ESCC) and much of the argument which has been addressed to me has proceeded on the scarcely articulated but nonetheless pervasive assumption that manual handling is dignified whereas mechanical handling is undignified, in other words that A and B's dignity interests are served by manual handling but are not served if equipment is used. This, as it seems to me, is a highly questionable, in truth a dangerous and misleading, assumption. I say so for two reasons.
>
> 120. I recognise of course that the compassion of the carer is itself a vital aspect of our humanity and dignity and that at a very deep level of our instinctive feelings e value and need the caring touch of the human hand. That no doubt is one of the reasons why the nobility of compassionate carers as different in their ways as Florence Nightingale, Leonard Cheshire and Mother Teresa resonates so strongly with us. It underlies the most savage of AWN Pugin's Contrasts, his comparison of the compassionate care of the medieval monastery and the cruel heartlessness of the early modern workhouse. Even those who do not believe in any God know that a human being is more than a machine consisting of a few rather basic chemicals operated by electric currents controlled by some animalistic equivalent of a computer located in the skull – and that, no doubt, is why we have an instinctive and intuitive preference for the touch of the human hand rather than the assistance of a machine. As disabled persons or invalids our instinctive preference is to be fed by a nurse with a spoon rather than through a naso-gastric or gastrostomy tube.
>
> 121. But, and this is the first point, insistence on the use of dignified means cannot be allowed to obstruct more important ends. On occasions our very humanity and dignity may itself demand that we be subjected to a certain amount – sometimes a very great deal – of indignity. Dignified ends may sometimes demand the use of undignified means. The immediate dignity of a person trapped in a blazing building is probably the very last thing on his mind or in the mind of the fireman who bundles him undignified out of the window to save his life. And one thinks of the gross violence and indignity of the methods necessarily used by the crash team in its desperate efforts to save life in the Accident and Emergency Department. But this does not mean that means must be allowed to triumph over ends. There is a balance to be held – and it is often a very difficult balance to strike. It is difficult enough to balance the utility or possible futility of means against the utility or possible futility of ends: it is all the more difficult when one has

to assess in addition the dignity or possible indignity of the means against the end in view. Modem medical law and ethics illustrate the excruciating difficulty we often have in achieving the right balance between using undignified means in striving to achieve dignified ends.

122. The other point is this. One must guard against jumping too readily to the conclusion that manual handling is necessarily more dignified than the use of equipment. A disabled person or invalid may prefer manual handling by a relative or friend to the use of a hoist but at the same time prefer a hoist to manual handling by a stranger or a paid carer. The independently minded but physically disabled person might prefer to hoist himself up from his bath or chair rather than to be assisted even by his devoted wife. Dignity in the narrow context in which it has been used during much of the argument in this case is in truth part of a much wider concept of dignity, part of a complicated equation including such elusive concepts as, for example, (feelings of) independence and access to the world and to others. Hoisting is not inherently undignified, let alone inherently inhuman or degrading. I agree with Ms Lang that certain forms of manual lift, for example the drag lift, may in certain circumstances be less dignified than hoisting. Hoisting can facilitate dignity, comfort, safety and independence. It all depends on the context.

The power, under section 29 of the National Assistance Act 1948, to 'make arrangements' for the provision of relevant services, permitted payments to be made to a 'user independent trust' for the provision of care services; as did section 30(1) of the NAA 1948, section 111 of the Local Government Act 1972 and section 2 of the Local Government Act 2000.

Comment: it now seems even clearer, under section 8 of the Care Act 2014, that user independent trusts can be created – and, indeed, a range of similar vehicles.

9.89 *R (Rodriquez-Bannister) v Somerset Partnership NHS and Social Care Trust* [2003] EWHC 2184 (Admin), (2004) 7 CCLR 385

A local authority may rationally prefer the views of its own expert as to what services to provide

Facts: Mr Rodriquez-Bannister was a 35-year-old man who suffered from Asperger's Syndrome. His mother and Somerset were in dispute as to whether his needs could be met in supported accommodation or only in residential care. Each had sought independent expert evidence, but the experts disagreed.

Judgment: Somerset was entitled rationally to prefer the views of the independent expert it had commissioned and to consider that the concerns of the mother's expert could be addressed. Also, it had not been not unfair to invite the mother to attend the complaints panel meeting that had considered her expert's report: she had already attended an earlier meeting and her views would not have affected the decision.

9.90 ## *R (Alloway) v Bromley LBC* [2004] EWHC 2108 (Admin), (2005) 8 CCLR 61

A local authority fetters its discretion if it rules out one service from the start on costs grounds and does not fairly compare the rival options

Facts: Mr Alloway was a 19-year-old man who was autistic and suffered from learning disabilities. Bromley's community care assessment concluded that he should be placed at Hesley Village and College. However, the Council then purported to place him at a cheaper option at Robinia Care. However, Bromley did not assert that its decision-making was affected by, or justified by, resources considerations.

Judgment: Crane J quashed this decision, holding that Bromley had fettered its discretion by ruling out Hesley from the start, on cost grounds, that Bromley had not undertaken a fair comparison of the various alternative placement options and that whilst Bromley had to consider up-to-date information, it was not required to undertake a further formal assessment (and could make provision pending completion of such assessment).

9.91 ## *R (Hughes) v Liverpool CC* [2005] EWHC 428 (Admin), (2005) 8 CCLR 243

It was unlawful to fail to meet a statutory need for residential accommodation but that did not necessarily result in a breach of ECHR rights

Facts: Mr Hughes was a young man who was severely disabled, mentally and physically. He was cared for at home by his mother, with help from outside agencies. Liverpool acknowledged, however, that his mother's accommodation was wholly unsuitable for him. An assessment concluded that he needed suitable accommodation and, also, respite care. However, none was provided.

Judgment: Mitting J held that Liverpool was in breach of section 21 and 29 of the National Assistance Act 1948, by failing to meet Mr Hughes' assessed needs. He ordered respite care to be provided each weekend, and a re-assessment of the mother's needs. He rejected, however, a claim for damages under the ECHR.

9.92 ## *Casewell v Secretary of State for Work and Pensions* [2008] EWCA Civ 524, (2008) 11 CCLR 624

Direct payments used to pay a relative to provide home care were 'earnings' in her hands, for social security purposes

Facts: the local authority paid Mr Casewell's wife £73.50 to purchase home care which, with the local authority's agreement, she purchased from her husband, Mr Casewell. However, the Social Security Commissioner held that, subject to a disregard of £20.00, this money was 'earnings' for the purposes of the social security legislation and caused his Income Support to be reduced £ for £. Mr Casewell appealed.

Judgment: the Court of Appeal (Tuckey and Rix LJJ, Sir Robin Auld) dismissed the appeal, holding that the sums concerned did not fall within the statutory definition of '*community care payments*' but did fall within the definition of '*earnings*'.

9.93 *Re an application by LW (acting by her mother JB) for judicial review* [2010] NIQB 62, (2011) 14 CCLR 7

There was a duty to meet assessed needs under the Northern Ireland legislation

Facts: the Belfast Health and Social Care Trust assessed LW, who was seriously disabled, as requiring three/four days each week and at a residential unit, spending the rest of the time at home, and in both settings receiving substantial personal care. However, several years on, neither the residential unit, nor all the personal care required, had been provided.

Judgment: McCloskey J held that the Trust was in breach of duty under section 2 of the Chronically Sick and Disabled Persons (Northern Ireland) Act 1978, whether one construed the section as giving rise to a duty to meet assessed needs, or a duty to act reasonably in meeting assessed needs. The provision of accommodation was under the power, at article 15 of the Personal Social Services (Northern Ireland) Order 1972 but once a need had been assessed, the Trust was under a duty to meet it. The Trust had been in breach of that duty for some years, whether one construed the assessment under article 15 as giving rise to a duty to meet assessed needs, or a duty to act reasonably in meeting assessed needs.

9.94 *R (Savva) v Kensington & Chelsea RLBC* [2010] EWCA Civ 1209, (2011) 14 CCLR 75

It is lawful to use a resource allocation scheme to provide an indicative budget provided the local authority fine-tuned that budget to ensure that it met needs and provided adequate reasons that justified its ultimate budget

Facts: Kensington decided to meet Ms Savva's needs by providing her with a personal budget, calculated with the assistance of its resource allocation system (RAS), which involved assessing an individual's needs in relation to the needs/budgets of others in its area. Ms Savva challenged the methodology and the absence of reasons explaining how her personal budget had been calculated.

Judgment: the Court of Appeal (Maurice Kay, Longmore and Patten LJJ) held that the methodology was lawful, in that the figure generated by the RAS was simply a starting point and Kensington never lost sight of the fact that, ultimately, the sum awarded had to be sufficient to meet Ms Savva's needs which, in fact, it was. However, Kensington's initial failure to provide adequate reasons had been unlawful.

9.95 *R (McDonald) v Kensington & Chelsea RLBC* [2011] UKSC 33, (2011) 14 CCLR 341

The local authority was entitled to withdraw the provision of an overnight carer who helped the appellant access the commode at night, when it assessed that the appellant's needs could be equally met by the provision of incontinence pads and absorbent sheets

Facts: Ms McDonald had limited mobility and a small, neurogenic bladder, which caused her to have to urinate several times a night. Kensington initially provided Ms McDonald with a commode and a night-time carer. It then assessed her need using different language, as being for incontinence pads and absorbent sheets. Ms McDonald sought a judicial review.

Judgment: the Supreme Court (Walker, Hale, Brown, Kerr and Dyson JJSC, Hale JSC dissenting) held that:

(i) Kensington had been entitled to review Ms McDonald's care needs, which included the means by which those needs were to be met, as including a need for incontinence pads and absorbent sheets rather than for a commode and a night-time carer; the process had complied with guidance and been fair;

(ii) Kensington had not interfered with Ms McDonald's rights under Article 8 ECHR because the process had respected her dignity and autonomy but, in any event, any interference would be justified by economic considerations;

(iii) the review did not amount to a 'practice, policy or procedure' for the purposes of section 21 of the Disability Discrimination Act 1995 and, in any event, even if it had done, the review had been 'a proportionate means of achieving a legitimate aim' for the purposes of section 21D(5);

(iv) it would be '*absurd*' to infer that Kensington had breached the disability equality duty at section 49A of the Disability Discrimination Act 1995 simply because it failed explicitly to refer to that duty, in a context where its whole focus was on the needs of disabled person and countervailing resources considerations.

Comment: see *McDonald v United Kingdom*, below para 9.101, which shows that the European Court of Human Rights is, if anything, even less likely to intervene in local authority judgments about what needs individuals have and how to meet them most appropriately, out of limited budgets. The approach or the ECtHR is not surprising given that its rulings of legal principle must apply throughout the Council of Europe States (of varying degrees of affluence) whilst it cannot hope to gain the detailed understanding of local economic and social factors that national institutions have.

9.96 *R (G) v North Somerset Council* [2011] EWHC 2232 (Admin)

North Somerset had not acted unlawfully in deciding to cut the amount of direct payments and replacing direct payments with a managed care service

Facts: North Somerset cut the claimants' funding by 33 per cent and replaced their direct payments with a managed care service. The claimants sought a judicial review.

Judgment: Laws J dismissed the application on the basis that, factually, whilst North Somerset had reduced the budget it was providing the same level of service and that very serious concerns had arisen about the conduct of the claimants' parents in relation to the direct payments. North Somerset had not been under a duty of consultation and any breach of the public sector equality duty (PSED) had been purely theoretical.

9.97 *R (KM) v Cambridgeshire CC* [2012] UKSC 23, (2012) 15 CCLR 374

It is lawful to use a resource allocation system to guide assessment as to what level of personal budget to provide

Facts: Cambridgeshire assessed KM as having a range of critical needs for community care services and, using a resource allocation system, and an upper banding calculator assessed his personal budget as £84,678.00. KM brought a judicial review, on the basis that this figure was too low.

Judgment: the Supreme Court (Phillips, Walker, Hale, Brown, Kerr, Dyson and Wilson JJSC) held that:

(i) when a local authority was required to decide whether it was necessary to make arrangements to meet the needs of a disabled person, for the purposes of section 2 of the Chronically Sick and Disabled Persons Act 1970 it was required to ask itself (i) what the needs of the disabled person were, (ii) whether in order to meet those needs it was necessary for the local authority to make arrangements to provide any services, and (iii) if so, what the nature and extent of those services were. At stage (ii), the local authority was required to consider whether the needs of the disabled person could reasonably be met by family, friends, other state bodies, or charities, or out of the person's own resources. At stage (ii) the availability of resources was relevant and a local authority was entitled to have regard to the scale of its resources and the weight of other demands upon it;

(ii) where, as here, a disabled person qualified for a direct payment the local authority was required to ask a further question, (iv) what the reasonable cost was of securing provision of the services identified at stage (iii);

(iii) once stage (ii) had been passed, as in this case, the duty of the local authority to make provision for needs in accordance with stages (iii) and (iv);

(iv) it was lawful for a local authority to use a resource allocation scheme and an upper banding calculator, as Cambridgeshire had done, to ascertain a starting point or indicative figure, provided that the requisite services are then costed in reasonable detail to arrive a realistic direct payment figure;

(v) in this case, Cambridgeshire had erred in not expressly stating that it did not accept the mother's assertion that KM would receive no family support and that it regarded the social worker's estimate of the cost of the claimant's needs as manifestly excessive, and it should have made a more detailed presentation to the claimant of how in its opinion he might reasonably choose to deploy the sum offered, and of its own assessment of the reasonable cost of the necessary services;

(vi) however, Cambridgeshire's reasoning had subsequently been amplified during the course of the litigation, the result of which left no real doubt about the lawfulness of the award; and that, accordingly, it would be a pointless exercise of the court's discretion to quash the determination so that the claimant's entitlement could be reconsidered.

In addition, Lord Wilson made these interesting observations, on behalf of the majority:

> 5. It is true that constraints upon its resources are a relevant consideration during one of the stages through which a local authority must pass in computing the size of a direct payment owed under section 2 of the 1970 Act. In paras 15 and 23 below I will identify four such stages; and constraints upon an authority's resources are undoubtedly relevant to the second stage. But the leading exposition of the law in this respect is to be found in the speeches of the majority of the appellate committee of the House of Lords in *R v Gloucestershire County Council ex p Barry* (1997–8) 1 CCLR 40; and, if and in so far as it was there held that constraints upon resources were also relevant to what I will describe as the first stage, there are arguable grounds for fearing that the committee fell into error: see the concerns expressed by Baroness Hale of Richmond JSC in *R (McDonald) v Kensington and Chelsea Royal London Borough Council (Age UK intervening)* [2011] UKSC 33, (2011) 14 CCLR 341, paras 69–73.
>
> ...
>
> 36. I agree with Langstaff J in *R (L) v Leeds City Council* [2010] EWHC 3324 (Admin) at [59] that in community care cases the intensity of review will depend on the profundity of the impact of the determination. By reference to that yardstick, the necessary intensity of review in a case of this sort is high. Mr Wise also validly suggests that a local authority's failure to meet eligible needs may prove to be far less visible in circumstances in which it has provided the service-user with a global sum of money than in those in which it has provided him with services in kind. That point fortifies the need for close scrutiny of the lawfulness of a monetary offer. On the other hand respect must be afforded to the distance between the functions of the decision-maker and of the reviewing court; and some regard must be had to the court's ignorance of the effect upon the ability of an authority to perform its other functions of any exacting demands made in relation to the manner of its presentation of its determination in a particular type of case. So the court has to strike a difficult, judicious, balance.

Comment: The Supreme Court has not formally decided the point, but seems to have made it clear that a lack of resources is irrelevant when deciding whether or not a person has a particular 'need'.

There may be a tension, however, between this position and the Supreme Court's position in *R (McDonald) v Kensington & Chelsea RLBC*,[22] in which the Supreme Court upheld Kensington & Chelsea's decision to re-describe Ms McDonald's needs in radically different terms, in order to save resources.

It may be possible to reconcile these decisions on the basis that *KM* means no more than that, although a local authority can re-define a need, for resources reasons, to its cheapest possible description, it cannot operate on the basis that it does not exist at all. There must however be a better solution: this does not seem satisfactory.

22 [2011] UKSC 33, (2011) 14 CCLR 341 and above at para 9.95.

9.98 *R (AJ) v Calderdale BC* [2012] EWHC 3552 (Admin), (2013) 16 CCLR 50

There is no reason in principle why service and family members could not participate in evaluation panels to select service providers

Facts: Calderdale ceased its practice of including some service users and family members on the evaluation panels selected bidders for supporting people contracts.

Judgment: Deputy High Court Judge Pelling quashed Calderdale's decision because it had been founded upon the misunderstanding that its earlier practice was incompatible with the Public Contracts Regulations 2006, or would result in the award criteria not being applied objectively; and Calderdale could not demonstrate that its decision would inevitably have been the same, without this error of law.

9.99 *In the matter of DM (a person under disability) acting by his next friend Kathleen McCollym, for judicial review* [2012] NIQB 98, (2013) 16 CCLR 39

It was unlawful to treat the budgetary indication provided by a resource allocation scheme as final

Facts: DM's needs had been met by his attendance at a day centre, paid for by joint funding. The joint funding ended and the Northern Health and Social Care Trust decided to pay DM £21 per day by way of direct payments; however, the day centre cost £47 per day. DM sought a judicial review of the Trust's decision.

Judgment: Horner J held that the Trust had failed to follow the approach set out by Lord Wilson in *R (KM) v Cambridgeshire CC*.[23] It had failed to ask at the outset what DM's needs were and appeared to have rolled up the question what services were necessary with the question what was the reasonable cost of making provision and, while it was legitimate to use a resource allocation scheme as a tool, to create a 'ball park figure', the Trust was then required to cost the services needed in reasonable detail.

9.100 *In the matter of an application for judicial review by JR 47* [2013] NIQB 7, (2013) 16 CCLR 179

The relevant authorities were under a duty to assess and meet community care needs, in general, in accordance with the relevant guidance

Facts: Mr E had a learning disability and was a long-stay hospital patient, assessed as being suitable for re-settlement in the community. However, over a period of 11 years, only two offers of accommodation in the community, both unsuitable, had been made.

Judgment: McCloskey J held that, in Northern Ireland, there was a statutory duty to assess apparent community care needs, that there was a legitimate expectation that such assessments would normally be completed in accordance with the *People First* guidance and that the relevant authorities

23 [2012] UKSC 23, (2012) 15 CCLR 375 and above at para 9.97.

were under a resource-free duty to meet assessed needs. In the case of JR 47, and others, those duties had been breached.

9.101 *McDonald v United Kingdom* (2014) 17 CCLR 187, ECtHR

It was not a breach of the ECHR for the local authority to re-assess a person's needs and provide them with considerably less than previously, in this case, by providing incontinence pads and absorbent sheets in place of a night-time carer and commode

Facts: Ms McDonald had limited mobility and a small, neurogenic bladder, which caused her to have to urinate several times a night. Kensington initially provided Ms McDonald with a commode and a night-time carer. It then assessed her need using different language, as being for incontinence pads and absorbent sheets. Ms McDonald sought a judicial review.

Judgment: the European Court of Human Rights held that Kensington & Chelsea's decision to withdraw its initial provision of night-time care amounted to an interference with Ms McDonald's private life (rather than a failure to make positive provision) and that its initial withdrawal was incompatible with Article 8 ECHR because (as the Supreme Court also held, see 9.95 above), Kensington & Chelsea had not been acting lawfully in national law, since Ms McDonald's assessment had not changed. However, once Kensington & Chelsea had re-assessed Ms McDonald's needs, its decision to provide only continence aids was compatible with Article 8 ECHR, in the light of 'the wide margin of appreciation afforded to States in issues of general policy, including social, economic and health care policies' (paragraph 54) – indeed, this aspect of the case was 'manifestly ill founded' (paragraph 58):

> 57. The Court is satisfied that the national courts adequately balanced the applicant's personal interests against the more general interest of the competent public authority in carrying out its social responsibility of provision of care to the community at large. It cannot, therefore, agree with the applicant that there has been no proper proportionality assessment at domestic level and that any reliance by it on the margin of appreciation would deprive her of such an assessment at any level of jurisdiction. In such cases, it is not for this Court to substitute its own assessment of the merits of the contested measure (including, in particular, its own assessment of the factual details of proportionality) for that of the competent national authorities (notably the courts) unless there are shown to be compelling reasons for doing so (see, for example, *X v Latvia* [GC], Application no 27853/09, para 102, ECHR 2013). The present applicant has not adduced any such compelling reasons in her pleadings before this Court.

Comment: as this case exemplifies, typically the European Court of Human Rights is reluctant to interfere with social welfare/resource allocation decisions (unless some additional element is present, such as discrimination). Its approach is inevitably coloured, to some extent, by its status as a supranational court, but in practice, courts in the UK afford public authorities just as much margin of judgment in such cases, as the decision of the Supreme Court in the *McDonald* case illustrates. The approach of the ECtHR is unsurprising given that its rulings of legal principle must apply throughout Council of Europe States (of varying degrees of affluence) whilst it cannot hope to gain the detailed understanding of local economic and social factors that national institutions have. The approach of national courts in the UK turns on how they perceive their role, constitutionally: staunch protectors of core rights, such as the right to liberty and freedom from similar, serious wrongs perpetrated by the State; but engaging only with the legal parameters of socio-economic decisions, on the basis that the substantive judgment in such cases is for elected persons to take on a political basis.

9.102 *Re MN (An Adult)* [2015] EWCA Civ 411, (2015) 18 CCLR 521

The Court of Protection has no power to require a public authority to provide different services, only to consider whether services on offer are in P's best interests, so any legal challenge to the sufficiency of services offered must be brought by way of judicial review

Facts: MN was a severely disabled young adult. It was reluctantly conceded by his parents that it was in his best interests to live in a residential placement but they disputed that the package of care on offer was in MN's best interests and asked the Court of Protection (COP) to investigate and make a declaration on that issue. The COP declined to take that course on the basis that its role was limited to determining whether care packages actually on offer were in P's best interests. MN's parents appealed.

Judgment: the Court of Appeal (Sir James Munby (President), Treacey and Gloster LJJ) dismissed the appeal, holding that that the COP had no power to require a public authority to provide a different care package, only to consider whether what was on offer was in the best interests of P; if P or some other person wanted to secure change in the care package, then they had to bring judicial review proceedings. Accordingly, it was pointless and inappropriate for the COP to embark upon an investigation on whether a different care plan would be in P's best interests:

> 11. The starting point, in my judgment, is the fundamentally important principle identified by the House of Lords in *A v Liverpool City Council* [1982] AC 363 and re-stated by the House in *In re W (A Minor) (Wardship: Jurisdiction)* [1985] AC 791. For present purposes I can go straight to the speech of Lord Scarman in the latter case. Referring to *A v Liverpool City Council*, Lord Scarman said (page 795):
>
> > 'Authoritative speeches were delivered by Lord Wilberforce and Lord Roskill which it was reasonable to hope would put an end to attempts to use the wardship jurisdiction so as to secure a review by the High Court upon the merits of decisions taken by local authorities pursuant to the duties and powers imposed and conferred upon them by the statutory code.'
>
> He continued (page 797):
>
> > 'The High Court cannot exercise its powers, however wide they may be, so as to intervene on the merits in an area of concern entrusted by Parliament to another public authority. It matters not that the chosen public authority is one which acts administratively whereas the court, if seized by the same matter, would act judicially. If Parliament in an area of concern defined by statute (the area in this case being the care of children in need or trouble) prefers power to be exercised administratively instead of judicially, so be it. The courts must be careful in that area to

> avoid assuming a supervisory role or reviewing power over the merits of decisions taken administratively by the selected public authority.'
>
> 12. Lord Scarman was not of course disputing the High Court's power of judicial review under RSC Ord 53 (now CPR Pt 54) when exercised by what is now the Administrative Court: he was disputing the High Court's powers when exercising in the Family Division the parens patriae or wardship jurisdictions. This is made clear by what he said (page 795):
>
> > 'The ground of decision in *A v Liverpool City Council* [1982] AC 363 was nothing to do with judicial discretion but was an application in this field of the profoundly important rule that where Parliament has by statute entrusted to a public authority an administrative power subject to safeguards which, however, contain no provision that the High Court is to be required to review the merits of decisions taken pursuant to the power, the High Court has no right to intervene. If there is abuse of the power, there can of course be judicial review pursuant to RSC Ord 53: but no abuse of power has been, or could be, suggested in this case.'
>
> It is important to appreciate that Lord Scarman was not referring to a rule going to the exercise of discretion; it is a rule going to jurisdiction.
>
> ...
>
> 80. The function of the Court of Protection is to take, on behalf of adults who lack capacity, the decisions which, if they had capacity, they would take themselves. The Court of Protection has no more power, just because it is acting on behalf of an adult who lacks capacity, to obtain resources or facilities from a third party, whether a private individual or a public authority, than the adult if he had capacity would be able to obtain himself. The *A v Liverpool* principle applies as much to the Court of Protection as it applies to the family court or the Family Division. The analyses in *A v A Health Authority* and in *Holmes-Moorhouse* likewise apply as much in the Court of Protection as in the family court or the Family Division. The Court of Protection is thus confined to choosing between available options, including those which there is good reason to believe will be forthcoming in the foreseeable future.
>
> 81. The Court of Protection, like the family court and the Family Division, can explore the care plan being put forward by a public authority and, where appropriate, require the authority to go away and think again. Rigorous probing, searching questions and persuasion are permissible; pressure is not. And in the final analysis the Court of Protection cannot compel a public authority to agree to a care plan which the authority is unwilling to implement.

Comment: there seems to be no reason why a complaints process, or judicial review proceedings challenging a service provision decision, cannot be run in tandem with COP proceedings or, even, why a High Court judge entitled to sit in the Administrative Court and COP should not determine both the public law and best interests issues, providing that he or she carefully separated the different functions being exercised. All that this case decides, reflecting earlier case-law, is that one cannot use the best interests jurisdiction to 'get around' the limits of judicial review.

9.103 ## *R (SG) v Haringey LBC* [2015] EWHC 2579 (Admin), (2015) 18 CCLR 444

A failure to provide an independent advocate under section 67(2) of the Care Act 2014 rendered the assessment unlawful. A duty only arose to provide accommodation when the need was 'accommodation-related'

Facts: SG was an asylum-seeker provided with asylum support. She suffered from severe mental health problems and needed help with self-care, preparing and eating food, simple tasks and medication. Haringey declined to provide residential accommodation to SG under section 21 of the National Assistance Act 1948 and then, later, under the Care Act 2014.

Judgment: Deputy High Court Judge Bowers held that the assessment under the Care Act 2014 was unlawful because (i) Haringey failed to ensure that SG was offered an independent advocate, under section 67(2) of the Care Act 2014; and (ii) Haringey failed to ask itself the correct question:

> 56. I first reiterate that the authorities already considered stand for these propositions, which I think continue to apply under the Care Act:
>
> (a) the services provided by the council must be accommodation-related for accommodation to be potentially a duty;
>
> (b) in most cases the matter is best left to the good judgment and common sense of the local authority;
>
> (c) 'accommodation-related care and attention' means care and attention of a sort which is normally provided in the home or will be 'effectively useless' if the claimant has no home.
>
> 57. Mr Burton submits there is a duty here to provide accommodation because it would be irrational not to do so in order to meet the adult's care and support needs. He has the lesser case, however, that the Council did not ask itself the correct questions. I agree with Mr Burton in the latter argument that the only suggestion that the question of whether or not the defendant was under a duty to provide accommodation was even considered by the defendant is contained in the pre-action letter. I also accept that there is no evidence that the defendant asked itself whether, even if services could have been provided in a non-home environment, they would have been rendered effectively useless if the claimant were homeless and sleeping on the street. This is so despite the fact that it was acknowledged that it was 'agreed that [the claimant] would benefit from some structured activities to minimise her PTSD symptoms but before that she needs help with the very basic practical support before she can be referred for more structured activities.' I thus think that the care plan has to be redone.

9.104 ## *R (Collins) v Nottinghamshire CC* [2016] EWHC 996 (Admin) (2016) 19 CCLR 494

It had been rational for Nottinghamshire to suspend an organisation from its list of accredited providers of direct payment support services

Facts: two former employees of a direct payment support service provider, Direct Payment Service Users Ltd ('DPSUL') raised concerns about its conduct and financial practices with Nottinghamshire. In addition, the Trading Standards Department informed Nottinghamshire that a criminal investigation into DPSUL was progressing. That investigation raised serious concerns. Having given DPSUL some opportunity of response, Nottinghamshire then suspended DPSUL from its list of accredited direct payment support service providers, which effectively prevented DPSUL from dealing with the funds of potentially vulnerable individuals and from using and administering public funds. A group of service users brought a judicial review.

Judgment: Patterson J refused permission to apply for judicial review on the basis that Nottinghamshire had acted rationally and there was nothing in the Care Act 2014 that precluded it from taking such action.

CHAPTER 10

Re-assessments, reviews and terminations of individual services

10.1 **Introduction, principles and statutory machinery**

Cases

10.10 *R v Islington LBC ex p McMillan* (1997–8) 1 CCLR 7, QBD
Reduced care provision is only justifiable on the basis of a revised assessment (at least in the context of needs assessed as having been 'eligible')

10.11 *R v Gloucestershire CC ex p RADAR* (1997–8) 1 CCLR 476, QBD
The duty to re-assess before reducing services is not discharged by sending care users a pro forma letter inviting them to seek a re-assessment

10.12 *R v Kensington and Chelsea RLBC ex p Kujtim* (1999) 2 CCLR 340, CA
A local authority remains under a duty to meet eligible needs unless the applicant has manifested a persistent and unequivocal refusal to observe reasonable conditions and must be ready to re-assess where it appears that the applicant will not persist

10.13 *R v Birmingham CC ex p Killigrew* (2000) 3 CCLR 109, QBD
The reduction in care was not justified by a sufficiently adequate assessment

10.14 *R (Khana) v Southwark LBC* (2001) 4 CCLR 267, CA
A local authority may be entitled to treat its duties as discharged if an applicant refuses an offer of services assessed as meeting their needs

10.15 *R v Newham LBC ex p Patrick* (2001) 4 CCLR 48, QBD
Referring a homeless woman with care needs to a housing charity did not amount to a discharge of the duty to assess or meet her needs

10.16 *R (S) v Leicester CC* [2004] EWHC 533 (Admin), (2004) 7 CCLR 254
A relatively formal re-assessment was required before services were terminated

10.17 *R (Goldsmith) v Wandsworth LBC* [2004] EWCA Civ 1170, (2004) 7 CCLR 472
The assessment was not sufficiently careful to justify significant service reduction

10.18 *R (Alloway) v Bromley LBC* [2004] EWHC 2108 (Admin), (2005) 8 CCLR 61
A local authority need not always undertake a further formal assessment but can take into account up-to-date information in determining what services to provide

continued

10.19 *R (G) v North Somerset Council* [2011] EWHC 2232 (Admin)
North Somerset had not acted unlawfully in deciding to cut the amount of direct payments and replacing direct payments with a managed care service

10.20 *R (W) v Croydon LBC* [2011] EWHC 696 (Admin), (2011) 14 CCLR 247
Fair consultation was required before reducing services; where the service user lacks capacity, fair consultation with parents/carers is required by section 4(7) of the Mental Capacity Act 2005

10.21 *R (McDonald) v Kensington & Chelsea RLBC* [2011] UKSC 33, (2011) 14 CCLR 341
It was lawful to re-assess the needs of a disabled person as being for incontinence pads and absorbent sheets rather than for a night-time carer to provide help getting to a commode

10.22 *R (KM) v Cambridgeshire CC* [2012] UKSC 23, [2012] 15 CCLR 374
It is lawful to use a resource allocation system to guide assessment as to what level of personal budget to provide

10.23 *McDonald v United Kingdom* (2014) 17 CCLR 187, ECtHR
It was not a breach of the ECHR for the local authority to re-assess a person's needs and provide them with considerably less than previously, in this case, by providing incontinence pads and absorbent sheets in place of a night-time carer and commode

10.24 *R (Perry Clarke) v Sutton LBC* [2015] EWHC 1081 (Admin), (2015) 18 CCLR 317
There had been a failure to understand the applicant's needs such that the reduction in his care package could not be justified

10.25 *R (OH) v Bexley LBC* [2015] EWHC 1843 (Admin)
Changes of care provision are required to be justified, with reasons, in an assessment and revised support plan

Introduction, principles and statutory machinery

10.1 Section 27 of the Care Act 2014 requires local authorities to keep under review care and support/support plans and, also, to review them on a reasonable request made by or on behalf of the adult/carer.

10.2 If the local authority is satisfied that circumstances have changed in a way that affects a care and support/support plan then it must undertake a further assessment, financial assessment and determination of eligible needs and prepare a revised care and support/support plan.

10.3 The review of care and support plans is dealt with at Chapter 13 of the *Care and Support Statutory Guidance*. The Guidance advises, at paragraph 13.32, that reviews are undertaken every 12 months (with a 'light touch' review six/eight weeks after completion of a new care and support/support plan).

10.4 Most reviews are uncontroversial – they are an obviously necessary way of fine-tuning a care and support/support package so that it keeps in step with changes of need.

10.5 Difficult cases can arise when a local authority reviews a care package because budgetary pressures have persuaded it to endeavour to reduce the cost of care packages. However:

- it is unlawful simply to reduce care provision because of budgetary pressures;
- there has to be a re-assessment that demonstrates that eligible needs will continue to be met.[1]

10.6 The new national eligibility threshold will limit local authorities' freedom of manoeuvre to some extent, in that they will no longer be able to 'review down' care packages as a result of adopting diminished eligibility criteria (unless their criteria are more generous than the national threshold).

10.7 It can be expected, however, that during times of continued budgetary pressures, local authorities will re-examine care packages to see whether (i) eligible needs can be assessed as less than before; (ii) eligible needs can be met more cost-effectively; (iii) non-eligible needs should continue to be met; and (iv) charges should apply/be increased.

10.8 In such circumstances, the potential for budgetary pressures unduly to distort the assessment process, and the suffering resulting from lost or reduced services, often results in complaints or litigation and can be expected to continue to do so.

10.9 The sense one gets from the cases, is that the courts will often bring a more intense scrutiny to bear on assessments that appear to seek to reduce care services, for budgetary reasons.[2]

1 *R v Islington LBC ex p McMillan* (1997–8) 1 CCLR 7, QBD and below at para 10.10.

2 See, for example, *R v Birmingham CC ex p Killigrew* (2000) 3 CCLR 109; *R (Goldsmith) v Wandsworth LBC* [2004] EWCA Civ 1170, (2004) 7 CCLR 472.

Cases

10.10 *R v Islington LBC ex p McMillan* (1997–8) 1 CCLR 7, QBD

Reduced care provision is only justifiable on the basis of a revised assessment (at least in the context of needs assessed as having been 'eligible')

Facts: local authorities had ceased to provide home care services, or substantially reduced provision, because their changed financial position had left them facing a deficit.

Judgment: the Divisional Court (McCowan LJ and Waller J) held that the authorities were entitled to take their financial situation in to account but, in these cases, had acted unlawfully by treating their reduced resources as the sole relevant factor and without re-assessing the needs of those concerned, weighing their needs against those of others; in addition, a shortage of resources could not rationally justify a decision that left an individual at severe physical risk:

> For these reasons I for my part have concluded that a local authority are right to take account of resources both when assessing needs and when deciding whether it is necessary to make arrangements to meet those needs. I should stress, however, that there will, in my judgment, be situations where a reasonable authority could only conclude that some arrangements were necessary to meet the needs of a particular disabled person and in which they could not reasonably conclude that a lack of resources provided an answer. Certain persons would be at severe physical risk if they were unable to have some practical assistance in their homes. In those situations, I cannot conceive that an authority would be held to have acted reasonably if they used shortage of resources as a reason for not being satisfied that some arrangement should be made to meet those persons' needs.
>
> On any view section 2(1) is needs-led by reference to the particular needs of a particular disabled person. A balancing exercise must be carried out assessing the particular needs of that person in the context of the needs of others and the resources available, but if no reasonable authority could conclude other than that *some* practical help was necessary, that would have to be their decision.
>
> Furthermore, once they have decided that it is necessary to make the arrangements, they are under an absolute duty to make them. It is a duty owed to a specific individual and not a target duty. No term is to be implied that the local authority are obliged to comply with the duty only if they have the revenue to do so. In fact, once under that duty, resources do not come into it.
>
> It would certainly have been open to the Gloucestershire County Council to reassess the individual applicants as individuals, judging their current needs and taking into account all relevant factors including the resources now available and the competing needs of other disabled persons. What they were not entitled to do, but what in my judgment they in fact did, was not to re-assess at all but simply to cut the services they were providing because their resources in turn had been cut. This amounted to treating the cut in resources as the sole factor to be taken into account, and that was, in my judgment, unlawful. Moreover, I see no reason to deny the applicants a declaration to that effect.

Comment: see the cases about care home and other service closures: it can be lawful to reach a 'macro' budgetary decision on the basis that it is not irreversible, but is subject to the completion of individual assessments in due course that ensure that eligible needs and met.

10.11 *R v Gloucestershire CC ex p RADAR* (1997–8) 1 CCLR 476, QBD

The duty to re-assess before reducing services is not discharged by sending care users a pro forma letter inviting them to seek a re-assessment

Facts: after the decision in *Islington* (above para 10.10), Gloucestershire circulated 1,000 individuals facing removal or reduction of their services, inviting them to take up the offer of a re-assessment.

Judgment: Carnwath J held this did not satisfy the duty to re-assess community care needs before removing or reducing services: where there is an 'appearance of need' the duty to assess/re-assess arises without any explicit request having been made. However, it was lawful/rational for Gloucestershire not to take a blanket decision to restore all the services that it had unlawfully withdrawn or reduced prior to the decision in *Islington*. Also, given that the case gave rise to a general issue of principle, the complaints procedure was not a reasonable alternative remedy:

> On the other hand, the court in *Mahfood* did not – and was not asked to – quash the policy decision, made in September 1994, which led to the individual reductions. The court did not lay down precisely what the authority were required to do in cases other than those specifically at issue. Services of the type here in question inevitably raise considerations of an individual and personal nature. The council could properly take the view that a blanket decision to restore the services precisely as they were in September 1994 would not be appropriate. In particular I see force in the point that it would be confusing and unsatisfactory for services to be restored for a short time, only to be withdrawn or reduced shortly afterwards following a reassessment.
>
> Thus, I do not think that RADAR were entitled reasonably to insist on a decision to restore services before the reassessments were carried out. Equally, it has to be recognised that those reassessments need to be carried out by properly trained persons and that the process will take time. It is not for the court to lay down a programme, but the arrangements outlined by Mr Davies to deal with the workload appear to achieve a reasonable balance.
>
> Where, however, I would take issue with the authority, is the suggestion that the task of reassessment following the judgment is satisfied by writing letters to those affected or potentially affected, and simply offering them reassessment. In some areas of the law that might be an adequate response, where those affected can be assumed to be capable of looking after their own interests, and where silence in response to an offer can be treated as acceptance or acquiescence. However, that approach is not valid in the present context. The obligation to make an assessment for community care services does not depend on a request, but on the 'appearance' of need. Indeed, under section 47(2) of the 1990 Act [National Health Service and Community Care Act], where it appears that a person is disabled, the authority is specifically required to make a decision as to the service he requires without waiting for a request. Of course, the authority cannot carry out an effective reassessment without some degree of co-operation from the service user or his helpers. However, that is a very different thing from

> saying that they can simply rest on having sent a letter of the type to which I have referred.
>
> In my judgment, the authority has not discharged its obligations following the judgment simply by reassessing those 273 persons who replied to the letter. By implication, all the people affected by the September 1974 decision were people who, prior to that date, 'appeared' to the authority to have need of its services. For the authority to justify the continued reduction or withdrawal of the services, it must carry out a reassessment as required by the judgment of the Divisional Court. Quite apart from the judgment, the clear scheme of section 47 is thatdecisions on services should follow assessments. As the Divisional Court recognised, that means individual assessments. There is no suggestion in the report to the Council in June 1995 that there is any practical difficulty in carrying out the reassessment of the 1,059 users. Clearly money would need to be found for it, but it is not suggested that that is impossible.
>
> To summarise, I think both parties have taken unduly extreme positions. RADAR were wrong to insist upon full reinstatement prior to reassessment. But the Council were wrong to think that merely reassessing the 273 who had replied to their letters discharged their duties.
>
> ...
>
> Next, Mr Eccles suggests that there is an alternative remedy by way of complaint, under the procedure set up pursuant to section 7B of the Local Authority Social Services Act 1970 (inserted by the 1990 Act s50). This may be relevant in particular cases, especially where individual relief is being sought. However, in relation to a general issue of principle as to the authority's obligations in law, such as I have been discussing here, I do not think that can be regarded as a suitable or alternative remedy to the procedure of Judicial Review.

Comment: it would seem to be even more clearly the case, under sections 19, 25 and 27 of the Care Act 2014, that local authorities are required to deliver the care and support plan unless and until there has been a lawful re-assessment.

10.12 *R v Kensington and Chelsea RLBC ex p Kujtim* (1999) 2 CCLR 340, CA

A local authority remains under a duty to meet eligible needs unless the applicant has manifested a persistent and unequivocal refusal to observe reasonable conditions and must be ready to re-assess where it appears that the applicant will not persist

Facts: Kensington & Chelsea refused to continue to provide Mr Kujtim with residential accommodation after complaints about his misconduct, which continued after a written warning.

Judgment: the Court of Appeal (Peter Gibson and Potter LJJ, Blofeld J) held that once a local authority had assessed a person as 'needing' residential accommodation, it was under a duty to provide it as long as the need remained in existence and unless the applicant manifested a persistent and unequivocal refusal to observe reasonable requirements relating to occupation of the accommodation. Even in such cases, it was essential that the local authority carefully considered the applicant's current needs and circumstances, the causes of his conduct and the surrounding circumstances, allowing the applicant a fair opportunity of putting his case.

Further, the duty revived, once the applicant satisfied the local authority that his needs required service provision to be made and that he would no longer persist in refusing to observe the local authority's reasonable requirements:

> *The Extent of The Duty Under Section 21 (l)(a) of The 1948 Act*
>
> 30. That being so, the question which arises is whether or not there is any limitation upon the duty to provide or continue to provide such accommodation for as long as the need, once assessed, continues. In my view the position is as follows. Once a local authority has assessed an applicant's needs as satisfying the criteria laid down in s21(1)(a), the local authority is under a duty to provide accommodation on a continuing basis so long as the need of the applicant remains as originally assessed, and if, for whatever reason, the accommodation, once provided, is withdrawn or otherwise becomes unavailable to the applicant, then (subject to any negative reassessment of the applicant's needs) the local authority has a continuing duty to provide further accommodation. That said, however, the duty of the local authority is not absolute in the sense that it has a duty willy-nilly to provide such accommodation *regardless of the applicant's willingness to take advantage of it*.
>
> 31. In this connection there are two realities to be recognised. First, the duty to provide accommodation is predicated upon the co-operation of the applicant in the sense of his willingness to occupy it on such terms and in accordance with such requirements as the local authority may reasonably impose in relation to its occupation. The second, and connected, reality is that the resources of the local authority are finite and that, in providing accommodation for the needy, save in rare cases where individual or special accommodation may be necessary and available to meet the special needs of a particular applicant, the accommodation may, and will usually be, provided within multi-occupied premises, whether in the form of flats, or hostel or bed and breakfast accommodation, in relation to which it will be reasonable for the local authority to lay down certain requirements as to the use of such accommodation and the activities to be permitted in it, whether from a health and safety point of view, or for the purpose of preventing injury, nuisance or annoyance to fellow occupiers of the premises.
>
> 32. Thus it seems to me that, when the circumstances warrant, if an applicant assessed as in need of Part III accommodation either unreasonably refuses to accept the accommodation provided or if, following its provision, by his conduct he manifests a persistent and unequivocal refusal to observe the reasonable requirements of the local authority in relation to the occupation of such accommodation, then the local authority is entitled to treat its duty as discharged and to refuse to provide further accommodation. That will remain the position unless or until, upon some subsequent application, the applicant can satisfy the local authority that his needs remain such as to justify provision of Part III accommodation and that there is no longer reason to think that he will persist in his refusal to observe the reasonable requirements of the local authority in respect of the provision of such accommodation.
>
> 33. In formulating the right of the local authority to treat its duty as discharged by conduct as requiring manifestation of *persistent and unequivocal* refusal, rather than a single transgression, I have in mind the following matters which were urged upon us by Mr Gordon as part of his submission that the duty of providing Part III accommodation is unqualified and absolute. The provisions of section 21 of the 1948 Act as amended are 'safety

net' provisions designed to assist the poorest and most needy members of society, at rock bottom as it were. For a variety of reasons of personal and social disadvantage, they may well be persons who find difficulty complying with the norms of social behaviour or self control, while falling outside the specific areas of need catered for by other provision within the Community Care Services or under housing legislation. To create a class consisting of a substantial number of persons outside the scope even of the minimum requirements of the safety net provisions cannot lightly be contemplated. To withdraw Part III accommodation in respect of persons with such needs is likely to reduce such persons to living and sleeping on the streets; not only does it tend to defeat the overall purpose of the 1948 Act as well as Community Care, but it produces the socially undesirable effect of increasing rather than alleviating deprivation and encourages return to the practice of begging in the streets

34. In the particular case of a genuine refugee who is homeless while awaiting resolution of his claim for asylum (and, as already indicated, there is no reason to doubt the genuineness of Mr Kujtim's claim) the effect of a refusal to supply Part III accommodation despite the existence of need is to remove from him basic food and shelter in a situation where, upon recognition of his claim, he would be entitled to receive the usual benefits available to British citizens in a position of hardship and unemployment; further, in the case of an applicant who is unwell, there may result damage to health, or in extreme cases threat to life, as a result of his being put out on the streets.

35. The existence of those considerations makes it essential that local authorities should reach the conclusion that their duty to supply Part III accommodation is discharged in respect of any particular applicant only after being satisfied of his persistent and unequivocal refusal to comply with the local authority's requirements, coupled with a careful consideration of his *current* needs and circum stances. Either or both may involve consideration of any relevant medical condition or infirmity known to the local authority. Before concluding that there has been such refusal, it will plainly be desirable for a local authority to write a letter of final warning of the kind written by the respondents to the applicant in this case. As to the question of current need, the instant case provides a good example of why a re-consideration of need is essential. Had the respondents been aware, as they were not when they reached their decision, that the behaviour of the applicant in failing to observe their requirements to obey local hostel rules and to comply with the warning given to him by letter following his first expulsion, was the product of a depressive condition associated with the very ill-treatment which had driven him to seek refuge in this country, it seems unlikely that they would have treated his actions as manifesting a persistent and unequivocal refusal to comply with their requirements. However, they were entirely unaware of his medical condition and, in those circumstances, cannot be blamed for ignoring it.

Comment: in the adult and child social care context, the question of discharge of duty is dealt with very differently than in other contexts, for example, housing: an authority must always be ready to meet the eligible needs of a person who is willing to comply with reasonable conditions.

10.13 *R v Birmingham CC ex p Killigrew* (2000) 3 CCLR 109, QBD

The reduction in care was not justified by a sufficiently adequate assessment

Facts: Birmingham had provided Ms Killigrew with 12 hours care each day, in the light of her severe disability. It then moved Ms Killigrew to better adapted accommodation and reduced her hours of care to three and a half hours during weekdays, with some additional care over the weekend. The decision was unreasoned. After the issue of a judicial review, Birmingham undertook an assessment, which concluded that the hours should be increased to six hours each day, and which gave as its reason that, under the existing arrangements, little direct care was provided for most of the day.

Judgment: Hooper J held that it was notable that the reduction in the hours of care coincided with a decision that two carers rather than 1 needed to be provided, to comply with manual handling requirements and it was important that the reduction in hours was not driven by the economic consequences of that decision. In any event, Birmingham's assessment was unlawful for two reasons: (1) it contained no proper analysis of why 12 hours care had been provided, why that was no longer necessary and what would be done if an emergency arose, (2) in breach of the statutory guidance, Birmingham had failed to take into account up-to-date medical evidence and the views of the GP and the claimant's carers:

> 25. Although the New Plan was then being put forward as a basis for discussion, it was adopted by the respondent.
>
> 26. What was needed was a very careful assessment of why, if that was the case, 12 hours care was no longer needed. The importance of the respondent satisfying itself that this was the case is obvious. The applicant and her husband were asking for at least the 12 hours care to continue. Her condition was inevitably and steadily deteriorating. Not continuing the 12 hours care could, it was being said, have serious consequences for the applicant, and was certainly likely to cause deep distress to the applicant (see page 17). The decision to reduce was made at a time when it had been decided that two carers were needed for lifting. It was important that the reduction to six hours care was not driven by the need to have two carers to carry out the task. On the evidence available before me, the reduction could only be justified if there was no continuing need for 12 hours care and not simply because two carers were needed when only one had sufficed earlier.
>
> 27. Do we find that careful assessment in the October Care Plan, in particular in pages 110 and 111, which I have already read? Making all allowances for the fact that this is not a legal document and should not be construed as such, I have no doubt that we do not. There is no proper analysis of why the 12-hour Care Plan had been originally adopted. What were the perceived advantages of that plan at the time of its implementation? Why are those perceived advantages no longer seen as advantages, if such be the case? The author of the plan, Meg Allot, refers to 'the flexibility which has been *requested* to allow for unpredictable care needs' (emphasis added). The use of the word "requested" shows that the author is not concentrating on the plan in place. Her argument for dismissing this flexibility is also of note. She writes that this flexibility 'has in fact led carers to undertake tasks which they were not contracted to do, and are outside the responsibility of social services department'. If, to quote the earlier plan, the 12 hours care was chosen to help with the tasks of 'supervision' and 'of appropriate

stimulation', it is likely that in the event (for example) of no emergency, other things will be done. What is important is not to assess what happens if there is no emergency, but what will happen if there is an emergency and no one is supervising her.

10.14 *R (Khana) v Southwark LBC* (2001) 4 CCLR 267, CA

A local authority may be entitled to treat its duties as discharged if an applicant refuses an offer of services assessed as meeting their needs

Facts: Mrs Khana was elderly and disabled. Her elderly husband was her primary carer and they lived together with their daughter in a one-bedroom flat. They wished to be re-housed under section 21 of the National Assistance Act 1948 in a two-bedroom flat, where the husband and daughter could continue to care for Mrs Khana. Southwark's assessment, however, concluded that such an arrangement would not meet Mrs Khana's needs; she needed residential accommodation (where her husband could also reside) where 24-hour care was available.

Judgment: the Court of Appeal (Henry and Mance LJJ, McKinnon J) held that Southwark had taken into account, as legislation and guidance required, the family's preferences and the need to preserve the independence of elderly people in the community for as a long as possible. It was, also, the case that Southwark had power to provide 'ordinary accommodation' under section 21 of the Nationality Assistance Act 1948. Ultimately, however, Southwark had reached a rational conclusion on the facts. This was not a case of Mrs Khana having a 'psychological need', as in *R v Avon CC ex p M* (at para 8.131 above) but of insisting on her preferences. Nor was this a case of Southwark choosing an alternative way of meeting needs to conserve resources (where evidence of a resources difficulty could be required), nor was it a case of Southwark choosing between one of two alternative way of meeting needs, which could give rise to different issues: Southwark had positively concluded that the provision of larger ordinary accommodation, where the family remained Mrs Khana's primary carers, would not meet her needs, in important ways. If necessary, Southwark would be entitled to treat its duties towards Mr Khana as discharged, if she chose not to accept the offer of residential accommodation:

> 57. Further, although I do not consider that the case requires analysis in these terms, I would, if necessary, also treat Mrs K's refusal of the offer of residential home accommodation – the only course that would meet her assessed needs – as unreasonable in the sense intended by Potter L.J., when he was considering in *ex p Kujtim* what would discharge a local authority from any further duty for so long as such refusal was maintained. Her position has, it is true, received some strong support from distinguished sources, but the local authority's assessment of her needs, the appropriateness of their offer and the inappropriateness (in terms of meeting all Mrs K's needs) of Mrs K's position are not ultimately challenged.
>
> 58. If this had been a case where Mrs K's assessed needs could be met in different ways, then, on the authorities already cited, Southwark would have been entitled to take into account its resources in deciding which way to adopt. Mrs Justice Hallett in her judgment seems at certain points to have taken the view that a question of resources did arise in this case. For my part, I would agree with Mr Drabble that any problem of resources

would require to made out by evidence, and cannot be assumed to be present. There is no material enabling comparison between the cost of a two bedroom ground floor flat provided by the authority – with or without further community care services – and the costs of living in a residential home.

10.15 *R v Newham LBC ex p Patrick* (2001) 4 CCLR 48, QBD

Referring a homeless woman with care needs to a housing charity did not amount to a discharge of the duty to assess or meet her needs

Facts: Ms Patrick was a single woman who suffered from physical and mental ill health, was evicted on the ground of neighbour nuisance and found intentionally homeless. Newham had purported to discharge its duty towards her under section 21 of the National Assistance Act 1948, by offering her accommodation provided by a charity, which she had refused. Ms Patrick then slept rough.

Judgment: Henriques J held that Newham had failed in breach of statutory duty to assess Ms Patrick's needs and had not discharged its duty under section 21:

> 27. Her solicitor in her witness statement says that she did not take up the accommodation provided by HOST because she believed she was being sent to Sunderland and not to Southwark. In any event, Southwark was a distance away from her sister and from her medical support network.
>
> 28. Since the offer of accommodation was on 28 April and the certificate of mental incapacity to handle her affairs was granted on 9 May, it requires no mental gymnastics to conclude that her decision to reject the offer of accommodation at Southwark was neither considered nor likely to have been well informed.
>
> 29. It is of particular significance that the respondent knew that solicitors were acting for the applicant as they had written on her behalf on 5 April.
>
> 30. Further, they had informed the respondent that they could obtain no clear instructions from the applicant due to her mental health and enclosed a note from her general practitioner.
>
> 31. If the respondent sought to put an end to its section 21 duties to provide accommodation, they ought in my judgment at the very least to have ensured that the applicant was legally represented when the offer was made to her to ensure not only that she understood what the offer was, both in terms of location and services offered, but also that she understood the legal consequences or potential legal consequences of refusing the offer.
>
> 32. Since she may well not have understood what was being offered and its location, I am not prepared to find that her refusal of it was unreasonable.
>
> 33. In the exercise of its duty to provide accommodation a local authority must have a concurrent duty to explain fully and to the point of comprehension any offer it may make. I am not persuaded that the local authority has discharged its duty. In my judgment the duty to provide Part III accommodation continues pursuant to section 21 of the 1948 Act.

10.16 ## *R (S) v Leicester CC* [2004] EWHC 533 (Admin), (2004) 7 CCLR 254

A relatively formal re-assessment was required before services were terminated

Facts: Leicester had placed S in the Newcastle on Tyne area, for reasons connected with her education, but then decided to terminate that provision (the educational course having ended) and accommodate S in residential accommodation in the Leicester area. S utilised the complaints procedure, but her complaints were rejected.

Judgment: Leveson J held that it had been unlawful for Leicester to decide to change provision without first undertaking a re-assessment with an appropriate degree of formality. The complaints process had not corrected this flaw but had added one in that it had taken into account a new factor which S had not had the opportunity to address. However, the stage 3 complaints panel had not been required to reach its own conclusions as to the facts.

10.17 ## *R (Goldsmith) v Wandsworth LBC* [2004] EWCA Civ 1170, (2004) 7 CCLR 472

The assessment was not sufficiently careful to justify significant service reduction

Facts: after she fell and required hospital treatment, Wandsworth decided that Mrs Goldsmith should be moved from her residential care home to a nursing care home. Mrs Goldsmith wished to remain where she was, with some additional support, Wandsworth and Mrs Goldsmith's daughter each secured expert evidence supporting their point of view.

Judgment: the Court of Appeal (Brooke, Chadwick and Wall LJJ) allowed Mrs Goldsmith's appeal, holding that the relevant decision-making panel had not kept minutes or disclosed its reasons or membership and it did not have before it an assessment completed by one of Wandsworth's own social workers, that indicated that the residential care home could continue to look after Mrs Goldsmith, with the additional support it was willing to provide. Its findings, therefore, were seriously vitiated; also, because of its reliance on the report of an expert instructed by Wandsworth, because of the partial manner of the instructions. Ultimately, Wandsworth had failed to take a rounded decision, having regard to all relevant matters, and to articulate that decision clearly.

10.18 ## *R (Alloway) v Bromley LBC* [2004] EWHC 2108 (Admin), (2005) 8 CCLR 61

A local authority need not always undertake a further formal assessment but can take into account up-to-date information in determining what services to provide

Facts: Mr Alloway was a 19-year-old man who was autistic and suffered from learning disabilities. Bromley's community care assessment concluded that he should be placed at Hesley Village and College. However, the Council then purported to place him at a cheaper option at Robinia Care.

However, Bromley did not assert that its decision-making was affected by, or justified by, resources considerations.

Judgment: Crane J quashed this decision, holding that Bromley had fettered its discretion by ruling out Hesley from the start, on cost grounds, that Bromley had not undertaken a fair comparison of the various alternative placement options and that whilst Bromley had to consider up-to-date information, it was not required to undertake a further formal assessment (and could make provision pending completion of such assessment).

10.19 *R (G) v North Somerset Council* [2011] EWHC 2232 (Admin)

North Somerset had not acted unlawfully in deciding to cut the amount of direct payments and replacing direct payments with a managed care service

Facts: North Somerset cut the claimants' funding by 33 per cent and replaced their direct payments with a managed care service. The claimants sought a judicial review.

Judgment: Laws J dismissed the application on the basis that, factually, whilst North Somerset had reduced the budget it was providing the same level of service and that very serious concerns had arisen about the conduct of the claimants' parents in relation to the direct payments. North Somerset had not been under a duty of consultation and any breach of the PSED had been purely theoretical.

10.20 *R (W) v Croydon LBC* [2011] EWHC 696 (Admin), (2011) 14 CCLR 247

Fair consultation was required before reducing services; where the service user lacks capacity, fair consultation with parents/carers is required by section 4(7) of the Mental Capacity Act 2005

Facts: Croydon formed the strong provisional view that W's placement was no longer suitable and completed assessments of need to that effect. Since W lacked capacity, Croydon arranged a meeting with W's parents to discuss the assessments. However, they only disclosed the assessments to the parents a short time before the meeting. The parents objected to this late disclosure and stated that they disagreed with much of the content of the assessments. A few days later, Croydon decided to move W and he/the parents brought a judicial review.

Judgment: Ouseley J held that Croydon had not made its mind up before the meeting (although it had had a firm view), but that its consultation with the parents (required by section 4(7) of the Mental Capacity Act 2005) had been inadequate, in that it had not given the parents sufficient time before the meeting to consider the assessments and formulate their response; and by the time the parents did respond, about two weeks after the meeting, the decision had already been taken.

10.21 ## *R (McDonald) v Kensington & Chelsea RLBC* [2011] UKSC 33, (2011) 14 CCLR 341

It was lawful to re-assess the needs of a disabled person as being for incontinence pads and absorbent sheets rather than for a night-time carer to provide help getting to a commode

Facts: Ms McDonald had limited mobility and a small, neurogenic bladder, which caused her to have to urinate several times a night. Kensington initially provided Ms McDonald with a commode and a night-time carer. It then assessed her need using different language, as being for incontinence pads and absorbent sheets. Ms McDonald sought a judicial review.

Judgment: the Supreme Court (Walker, Hale, Brown, Kerr and Dyson JJSC, Hale JSC dissenting) held that:

(i) Kensington had been entitled to review Ms McDonald's care needs, which included the means by which those needs were to be met, as including a need for incontinence pads and absorbent sheets rather than for a commode and a night-time carer; the process had complied with guidance and been fair;

(ii) Kensington had not interfered with Ms McDonald's rights under Article 8 ECHR because the process had respected her dignity and autonomy but, in any event, any interference would be justified by economic considerations;

(iii) the review did not amount to a 'practice, policy or procedure' for the purposes of section 21 of the Disability Discrimination Act 1995 and, in any event, even if it had done, the review had been 'a proportionate means of achieving a legitimate aim' for the purposes of section 21D(5);

(iv) it would be '*absurd*' to infer that Kensington had breached the disability equality duty at section 49A of the Disability Discrimination Act 1995 simply because it failed explicitly to refer to that duty, in a context where its whole focus was on the needs of disabled person and countervailing resources considerations.

Comment: see *McDonald v United Kingdom*, at para 10.23 below, which shows that the European Court of Human Rights (ECtHR) is, if anything, even less likely to intervene in local authority judgments about what needs individuals have and how to meet them most appropriately, out of limited budgets. The approach of the ECtHR is not surprising given that its rulings of legal principle must apply throughout Council of Europe States (of varying degrees of affluence) whilst it cannot hope to gain the detailed understanding of local economic and social factors that national institutions have.

10.22 ## *R (KM) v Cambridgeshire CC* [2012] UKSC 23, [2012] 15 CCLR 374

It is lawful to use a resource allocation system to guide assessment as to what level of personal budget to provide

Facts: Cambridgeshire assessed KM as having a range of critical needs for community care services and, using a resource allocation system (RAS), and an upper banding calculator assessed his personal budget as

£84,678.00. KM brought a judicial review, on the basis that this figure was too low.

Judgment: the Supreme Court (Phillips, Walker, Hale, Brown, Kerr, Dyson and Wilson JJSC) held that:

(i) when a local authority was required to decide whether it was necessary to make arrangements to meet the needs of a disabled person, for the purposes of section 2 of the Chronically Sick and Disabled Persons Act 1970. it was required to ask itself (i) what the needs of the disabled person were, (ii) whether in order to meet those needs it was necessary for the local authority to make arrangements to provide any services, and (iii) if so, what the nature and extent of those services were. At stage (ii), the local authority was required to consider whether the needs of the disabled person could reasonably be met by family, friends, other state bodies, or charities, or out of the person's own resources. At stage (ii) the availability of resources was relevant and a local authority was entitled to have regard to the scale of its resources and the weight of other demands upon it;

(ii) where, as here. a disabled person qualified for a direct payment the local authority was required to ask a further question, (iv) what the reasonable cost was of securing provision of the services identified at stage (iii);

(iii) once stage (ii) had been passed, as in this case, the duty of the local authority to make provision for needs in accordance with stages (iii) and (iv);

(iv) it was lawful for a local authority to use a resource allocation scheme and an upper banding calculator, as Cambridgeshire had done, to ascertain a starting point or indicative figure, provided that the requisite services are then costed in reasonable detail to arrive a realistic direct payment figure;

(v) in this case, Cambridgeshire had erred in not expressly stating that it did not accept the mother's assertion that KM would receive no family support and that it regarded the social worker's estimate of the cost of the claimant's needs as manifestly excessive, and it should have made a more detailed presentation to the claimant of how in its opinion he might reasonably choose to deploy the sum offered, and of its own assessment of the reasonable cost of the necessary services;

(vi) however, Cambridgeshire's reasoning had subsequently been amplified during the course of the litigation, the result of which left no real doubt about the lawfulness of the award; and that, accordingly, it would be a pointless exercise of the court's discretion to quash the determination so that the claimant's entitlement could be reconsidered.

In addition, Lord Wilson made these interesting observations, on behalf of the majority:

> 5. It is true that constraints upon its resources are a relevant consideration during one of the stages through which a local authority must pass in computing the size of a direct payment owed under section 2 of the 1970 Act. In paras 15 and 23 below I will identify four such stages; and constraints upon an authority's resources are undoubtedly relevant to the second stage. But the leading exposition of the law in this respect is to be found in the

speeches of the majority of the appellate committee of the House of Lords in *R v Gloucestershire County Council ex p Barry* [1997] AC 584; and, if and in so far as it was there held that constraints upon resources were also relevant to what I will describe as the first stage, there are arguable grounds for fearing that the committee fell into error: see the concerns expressed by Baroness Hale of Richmond JSC in *R (McDonald) v Kensington and Chelsea Royal London Borough Council (Age UK intervening)* [2011] UKSC 33, (2011) 14 CCLR 341, paras 69–73.

...

36. I agree with Langstaff J in *R (L) v Leeds City Council* [2010] EWHC 3324 (Admin) at [59] that in community care cases the intensity of review will depend on the profundity of the impact of the determination. By reference to that yardstick, the necessary intensity of review in a case of this sort is high. Mr Wise also validly suggests that a local authority's failure to meet eligible needs may prove to be far less visible in circumstances in which it has provided the service-user with a global sum of money than in those in which it has provided him with services in kind. That point fortifies the need for close scrutiny of the lawfulness of a monetary offer. On the other hand respect must be afforded to the distance between the functions of the decision-maker and of the reviewing court; and some regard must be had to the court's ignorance of the effect upon the ability of an authority to perform its other functions of any exacting demands made in relation to the manner of its presentation of its determination in a particular type of case. So the court has to strike a difficult, judicious, balance.

Comment: the Supreme Court has not formally decided the point, but seems to have made it clear that a lack of resources is irrelevant when deciding whether or not a person has a particular 'need'. There may be a tension, however, between this position and the Supreme Court's position in *R (McDonald) v Kensington & Chelsea RLBC*,[3] in which the Supreme Court upheld Kensington & Chelsea's decision to re-describe Ms McDonald's needs in radically different terms, in order to save resources. *KM* would then mean, at least, that although a local authority can re-define a need, for resources reasons, to its cheapest possible description, it cannot operate on the basis that it does not exist at all.

10.23 *McDonald v United Kingdom* (2014) 17 CCLR 187, ECtHR

It was not a breach of the ECHR for the local authority to re-assess a person's needs and provide them with considerably less than previously, in this case, by providing incontinence pads and absorbent sheets in place of a night-time carer and commode

Facts: Ms McDonald had limited mobility and a small, neurogenic bladder, which caused her to have to urinate several times a night. Kensington initially provided Ms McDonald with a commode and a night-time carer. It then assessed her need using different language, as being for incontinence pads and absorbent sheets. Ms McDonald sought a judicial review.

Judgment: the European Court of Human Rights held that Kensington & Chelsea's decision to withdraw its initial provision of night-time care amounted to an interference with Ms McDonald's private life (rather than

3 [2011] UKSC 33, (2011) 14 CCLR 341.

a failure to make positive provision) and that its initial withdrawal was incompatible with Article 8 ECHR because (as the Supreme Court also held, see para 10.21 above), Kensington & Chelsea had not been acting lawfully in national law, since Ms McDonald's assessment had not changed. However, once Kensington & Chelsea had re-assessed Ms McDonald's needs, its decision to provide only continence aids was compatible with Article 8 ECHR, in the light of 'the wide margin of appreciation afforded to States in issues of general policy, including social, economic and health care policies' (paragraph 54) – indeed, this aspect of the case was 'manifestly ill founded' (paragraph 58):

> 57. The Court is satisfied that the national courts adequately balanced the applicant's personal interests against the more general interest of the competent public authority in carrying out its social responsibility of provision of care to the community at large. It cannot, therefore, agree with the applicant that there has been no proper proportionality assessment at domestic level and that any reliance by it on the margin of appreciation would deprive her of such an assessment at any level of jurisdiction. In such cases, it is not for this Court to substitute its own assessment of the merits of the contested measure (including, in particular, its own assessment of the factual details of proportionality) for that of the competent national authorities (notably the courts) unless there are shown to be compelling reasons for doing so (see, for example, *X v Latvia [GC]*, Application no 27853/09, para 102, ECHR 2013). The present applicant has not adduced any such compelling reasons in her pleadings before this Court.

Comment: as this case exemplifies, typically the European Court of Human Rights is reluctant to interfere with social welfare/resource allocation decisions (unless some additional element is present, such as discrimination). Its approach is inevitably coloured, to some extent, by its status as a supranational court, but in practice, courts in the UK afford public authorities just as much margin of judgment in such cases, as the decision of the Supreme Court in the *McDonald* case illustrates. The approach of the ECtHR is unsurprising given that its rulings of legal principle must apply throughout Council of Europe States (of varying degrees of affluence) whilst it cannot hope to gain the detailed understanding of local economic and social factors that national institutions have. The approach of national courts in the UK turns on how they perceive their role, constitutionally: staunch protectors of core rights, such as the right to liberty and freedom from similar, serious wrongs perpetrated by the State; but engaging only with the legal parameters of socio-economic decisions, on the basis that the substantive judgment in such cases is for elected persons to take on a political basis.

10.24 *R (Perry Clarke) v Sutton LBC* [2015] EWHC 1081 (Admin), (2015) 18 CCLR 317

There had been a failure to understand the applicant's needs such that the reduction in his care package could not be justified

Facts: Mr Clarke suffered from severe epilepsy. For some years, he had received care form a specialist provider which included checks being made on him each night. Despite medical and care evidence that, in the absence of such checks, Mr Clarke was at a major risk of death, Sutton changed the care package, so that care would be provided by a non-specialist provider, with nightly checks on only three nights each month.

Judgment: Deputy High Court Judge Sycamore held that Sutton had simply failed to understand and address Mr Clarke's needs and so had failed to take into account relevant material; the care plan was also defective in that it failed to spell out how care and medication would be delivered; whilst requiring Mr Clarke to move to non-specialist accommodation was, in these circumstances, incompatible with Article 8 ECHR.

10.25 *R (OH) v Bexley LBC* [2015] EWHC 1843 (Admin)

Changes of care provision are required to be justified, with reasons, in an assessment and revised support plan

Facts: Bexley provided 24 hours' interim support per week, pending completion of an assessment, but then ceased to make that provision and failed to complete the assessment.

Judgment: Deputy High Court Judge Ter Haar allowed the application for judicial review on the basis that (i) Bexley had failed to re-assess OH's needs and compile a revised support plan; and (ii) whilst the situation 'cried out' for an explanation for the reduction in care, Bexley had not provided any reasons.

CHAPTER 11

Financial matters

continued

11.61 *Robertson v Fife Council* [2002] UKHL 35, (2002) 5 CCLR 543
The availability of notional capital did not negate the existence of a need that was required to be met

11.62 *R (Kelly) v Hammersmith & Fulham LBC* [2004] EWHC 325 (Admin), (2004) 7 CCLR 542
A secure tenant's right to buy discount counted as a contribution towards the purchase price, the presumption of a resulting trust applied and the local authority was entitled to place a caution on the register and levy a charge

11.63 *Derbyshire CC v Akrill* [2005] EWCA Civ 308, (2005) 8 CCLR 173
A person is in general entitled to raise public law issues in defence of a claim for care charges

11.64 *Jones v Powys Local Health Board and Neath Port Talbot Local Health Board* [2008] EWHC 2562 (Admin), (2009) 12 CCLR 68
It was an abuse of process to defend an action for the recovery of care home charges on the basis that the resident was entitled to NHS Continuing Healthcare when that issue had been adversely determined administratively and not challenged by way of judicial review

11.65 *DM v Doncaster MBC* [2012] EWHC 3652 (Admin), (2012) 15 CCLR 128
Local authorities were required to charge for care home accommodation, even where the resident was detained in such accommodation by virtue of the Mental Capacity Act 2005

11.66 *Aster Healthcare Ltd v Estate of Mohammed Shafi* [2014] EWCA Civ 1350, (2014) 17 CCLR 419
A local authority which places a person in a care home is contractually liable for the fees until an effective supervening event

Charging: other services

11.67 *Avon CC v Hooper and Bristol and District Health Authority* (1997–8) 1 CCLR 366, CA
An indemnity was a financial resource for the purposes of means-testing

11.68 *R v Powys CC ex p Hambidge (No 2)* (1999) 2 CCLR 460, QBD
There was no duty to consult before amending a charging policy

11.69 *R v Powys CC ex p Hambidge* (2000) 3 CCLR 231, CA
It is not necessarily discrimination to levy increased charges on persons in receipt of disability benefits

11.70 *R (Carton) v Coventry CC* (2001) 4 CCLR 41, QBD
Consultation on a changed charging scheme had been unfair and the resultant scheme irrational

11.71 *R (Stephenson) v Stockton-on-Tees* [2004] EWHC 2228 (Admin), (2004) 7 CCLR 459
It was not irrational to decline to treat as expenditure for means-testing purposes sums paid to a family carer

11.72 *R (Spink) v Wandsworth LBC* [2005] EWCA Civ 302, (2005) 8 CCLR 272
Local authorities were entitled to charge for service provided to disabled children under section 2 of the Chronically Sick and Disabled Persons Act 1970 and to take into account parental resources

11.73 *R (BG) v Medway Council* [2005] EWHC 1932 (Admin), (2005) 8 CCLR 448

It was lawful to provide assistance under section 2 of the Chronically Sick and Disabled Persons Act 1970 and to attach rational conditions to the loan

11.74 *R (Stephenson) v Stockton-on-Tees* [2005] EWCA Civ 960, (2005) 8 CCLR 517

It was rational in general to disregard sums paid to family carers, for means-testing, but the policy had been applied too inflexibly in this case

11.75 *R (B) v Cornwall CC* [2010] EWCA Civ 55, (2010) 13 CCLR 117

A fundamentally flawed financial assessment was liable to quashed irrespective of whether the local authority could then make a retrospective assessment (though it probably could)

Financial assessments and charges

Statutory machinery

11.1 Unlike most NHS care, social care is not in general a free service. Prior to the Care Act 2014 there was different machinery for care home charges (section 22 of the National Assistance Act 1948) and home care charges (under section 17 of the Health and Social Services and Social Security Adjudications Act 1983). That is reflected in the division of cases below, into care home and home care charging cases. Part 1 of the Care Act 2014 unifies these two charging regimes for adults into a single statutory code, while preserving the main differences between the two previous schemes. The main provisions are:

- sections 14, 17, 26, 30, 34–36 and 69–70 of the Care Act 2014;
- the Care and Support (Charging and Assessment of Resources) Regulations 2014;[1]
- the Care and Support and After-care (Choice of Accommodation) Regulations 2014;[2]
- the Care and Support (Deferred Payment) Regulations 2014;[3]
- Chapters 8 and 9, and Annexes A to F, of the *Care and Support Statutory Guidance*.

Charging policies

11.2 Within the parameters of the statutory scheme, local authorities continue to have a discretion whether to charge for care services and how to frame local charges, in particular in relation to non-residential services. Therefore, it will be necessary for local authorities to continue to review their charging policies (subject to consultation, discharge of the public sector equality duty (PSED) and publication – see paragraph 8.45 of the *Care and Support Statutory Guidance*).

11.3 In setting their charging policy, local authorities must have regard to the advice contained in the Guidance, in particular, that:

- care home residents are expected to contribute most of their income, excluding earnings (paragraph 8.35);
- in relation to non-residential charges, local authorities should not simply adopt the minimum income threshold but consider setting a maximum percentage of disposable income available for meeting charges and/or a maximum charge, based on a percentage of care home charges in the local area (paragraphs 8.46–8.55);
- charging for support to carers may be a false economy and it may be inefficient systematically to charge carers (paragraphs 8.50–8.55);
- local authorities should be alive to special circumstances in which a mechanical application of minimum income thresholds may have unreasonable effects in individual cases (paragraphs 8.45–8.64).

1 SI No 2672.
2 SI No 2670.
3 SI No 2671.

11.4 As the *Care and Support Statutory Guidance* explains, at paragraph 8.2, 'The overarching principle is that people should only be required to pay what they can afford'.

What charges may cover

11.5 By virtue of section 14(1), (2) and (4) a local authority may charge for the cost of meeting needs under sections 18–20 of the Care Act 2014, but not for the cost of putting in place arrangements for meeting those needs, except in the special cases considered below.

Charging the cost of meeting needs

11.6 This applies where a local authority:

- meets the eligible needs of adults who are ordinarily resident, or of no settled residence;
- meets the eligible needs of adults who are ordinarily resident elsewhere;
- meets an adult's non-eligible needs;
- meets the eligible needs of carers who are ordinarily resident, or of no settled residence;
- meets the non-eligible needs of carers or the eligible needs of carers who are ordinarily resident elsewhere.

Charging the cost of meeting needs and making arrangements

11.7 In special cases, by virtue of sections 14(1) and (2), and regulation 5 of the Care and Support (Charging and Assessment of Resources) Regulations 2014, a local authority may charge for the cost of meeting needs under sections 18–20 and, also, for the cost of putting in place arrangements for meeting those needs. This applies where:

- an adult's resources are above the 'financial limit' (see paras 11.10–11.15 below) but they ask the local authority nonetheless to meet their needs;
- a carer's resources are above the 'financial limit', but they ask the local authority nonetheless to meet their needs; or
- the local authority is to meet the carer's needs by providing care and support to the adult, and the adult's resources are above the '*financial limit*', but they ask the local authority nonetheless to meet their needs.

Services for which no charge may be made

11.8 Local authorities may not charge for the services referred to at paragraph 8.14 of the Guidance:

- assessments;
- community equipment and minor adaptations, intermediate care, re-ablement for up to six weeks and care for CJD sufferers (exempted by regulations 3 and 4 of the Care and Support (Charging and Assessment of Resources) Regulations 2014);

- services provided under other legislation, such as after-care services under section 117 of the Mental Health Act 1983.

11.9 In addition, local authorities may not charge carers for support provided under section 20, by way of providing care and support for the adult (section 14(3)).

Financial assessments

11.10 In essence, where a local authority's policy is to levy a charge for a particular service, it has to undertake means-testing (a 'financial assessment') to ensure that no one is required to pay more than they can afford: as the *Care and Support Statutory Guidance* explains, at paragraph 8.2, 'The overarching principle is that people should only be required to pay what they can afford'.

11.11 Where a local authority has determined that an adult or carer has needs for support that it would charge for, if it met them, then it must complete a financial assessment in accordance with the Care and Support (Charging and Assessment of Resources) Regulations 2014 and provide the adult/carer with a copy (section 17). A financial assessment is an assessment of the adult's/carer's financial resources and their ability to pay charges (section 17).

11.12 The detailed machinery of financial assessments is set out in the Care and Support (Charging and Assessment of Resources) Regulations 2014 and Annexes A to F of the *Care and Support Statutory Guidance.*

The 'financial limits' and their effect

11.13 The three critical concepts are:

- the 'financial limit' (also known as the 'upper capital limit'), which is the amount of capital a person may have, beyond which they will not be entitled to local authority provision of home care 'at cost', or local authority care home provision at all;
- the 'lower capital limit', which is the level below which a person's capital is disregarded for these purposes;
- the amount of income that all persons must be left with, after means-testing and charging.

11.14 The 'financial limit' is currently £23,250.00 (regulation 12 of the Care and Support (Charging and Assessment of Resources) Regulations 2014) whereas the 'lower capital limit' is currently £14,250.00 (*Guidance*, paragraph 8.12):

- a person whose resources fall below the 'financial limit' is entitled to means-tested services 'at cost';
- means-testing must disregard a person's capital below the 'lower capital limit'.

11.15 Where a person's capital exceeds the 'financial limit':

- the local authority has a power, but is not under a duty, to make care home arrangements, if requested to do so (see regulation 12(1) of the

Care and Support (Charging and Assessment of Resources) Regulations 2014 and the Guidance, at paragraph 8.56);

- otherwise, they are entitled to require the local authority to make arrangements to meet their needs, although the local authority may charge for both the cost of meeting the needs and the cost of making the arrangements and the person will not be entitled to any financial assistance (sections 14(1) and (2) of the Care Act 2014 and regulation 6 of the Care and Support (Charging and Assessment of Resources) Regulations 2014).

Protected income

11.16 As far as concerns income, a local authority may not charge insofar as the effect of charging would be to reduce the applicant's income below:

- £24.40 per week (for care home residents); or
- income support plus 25 per cent, plus various premiums (other cases)

(section 14(7) of the Care Act 2014 and regulations 6 and 7 of the Care and Support (Charging and Assessment of Resources) Regulations 2014).

'Deemed' and 'light touch' financial assessments

11.17 In addition to full financial assessments, provisions is made, at regulation 10 of The Care and Support (Charging and Assessment of Resources) Regulations 2014, for 'deemed' financial assessments:

- where the applicant refuses to co-operate;
- where the case is 'open and shut' and with the applicant's consent the local authority decides not to charge;
- where the case is 'open and shut' and with the applicant's consent the local authority decides to make a charge.

The last two types of care are referred to in the Guidance as 'light touch' financial assessments.

Personal injury awards

11.18 The starting point is that such awards fall to be disregarded for the purpose of means testing. Further information is provided below in chapter 13 on 'Local authorities and tortfeasors'.

Deprivations of capital

11.19 In some cases, persons try to avoid paying for care and support by depriving themselves of assets. In such cases, the local authority may (i) charge the person concerned as if they still possessed such assets; (ii) seek to recover the lost income from the person to whom such assets were transferred; and/or (iii) use its powers to recover lost income from the person concerned. What the local authority cannot do, is cease to provide a service to meet 'eligible needs'.

11.20 Regulations 17 and 22 of the Care and Support (Charging and Assessment of Resources) Regulations 2014 require local authorities to take into account income and capital of which a person has 'deprived themselves for the purpose of decreasing the amount they may be liable to pay towards the cost of meeting their needs for care and support, or their needs for support'.

11.21 The *Guidance* advises about deprivation of assets at paragraphs 8.27–8.30 and Annex E.

11.22 Paragraph 5 of Annex E reminds local authorities that 'the overall principle should be that when a person has tried to deprive themselves of assets, this should not affect the amount of local authority support they receive'.

11.23 Paragraphs 11 and 23 of Annex E then summarise the case-law relevant to the deprivation of capital as follows:

> 11. There may be many reasons for a person depriving themselves of an asset. A local authority should therefore consider the following before deciding whether deprivation for the purpose of avoiding care and support charges has occurred:
> (a) Whether avoiding the care and support charge was a significant motivation;
> (b) The timing of the disposal of the asset. At the point the capital was disposed of could the person have a reasonable expectation of the need for care and support?; and
> (c) Did the person have a reasonable expectation of needing to contribute to the cost of their eligible care needs?
>
> 12. For example, it would be unreasonable to decide that a person had disposed of an asset in order to reduce the level of charges for their care and support needs if at the time the disposal took place they were fit and healthy and could not have foreseen the need for care and support.

11.24 Paragraphs 18–23 of Annex E explain how to charge a service user who has deprived themselves of capital or income, and who is to be treated as continuing notionally to possess that capital or income, and how to recover charges from third parties.

11.25 Annex E advises local authorities more widely on the various methods of recovering debts from service users.

Financial assessments and personal budgets

11.26 Sections 25(1)(a) and 26 of the Care Act 2014 require a care and support plan for an adult to include a personal budget (see paras 9.36–9.44 above, on personal budgets). After the financial assessment concludes, the adult is given a personal budget showing the local authority's cost of meeting their needs and (separately) their eligible needs, the payments required from the adult and the payments to be made by the local authority.

Security, recovery and deferred payments

The scheme in outline

11.27 Previously, local authorities had a power, under section 22 of the Health and Social Services and Social Security Adjudications Act 1983, to place charges unilaterally against property to secure care home charges, and a discretion whether to enter into a deferred payment agreement, under section 55 of the Health and Social Care Act 2001.

11.28 These have been replaced by a duty to enter into a deferred payment agreement in many 'care home cases', and a power to enter into deferred payment agreements in other 'care home and supported living accommodation cases', with a power to take security in a range of different ways: under sections 34–36 of the Care Act 2014 and the Care and Support (Deferred Payment) Regulations 2014.

11.29 The *Care and Support Statutory Guidance* describes as 'the universal deferred payment scheme', the aim of which is that 'people should not be forced to sell their home in their lifetime to pay for their care' (paragraph 9.3).

11.30 The statutory basis of the deferred payment scheme is sections 34–36, and section 69, of the Care Act 2014, which define a 'deferred payment agreement', and make additional provision, as follows:

> **34**(2) A 'deferred payment agreement' is an agreement under which a local authority agrees not to require until the specified time either or both of the following–
> (a) the payment of the specified part of the amounts due from an adult to the authority under such provision of this Part or of regulations under this Part as is specified in regulations;
> (b) the repayment of the specified part of a loan made under the agreement by the authority to an adult for the purpose of assisting the adult to obtain the provision of care and support for the adult.
>
> (3) The care and support mentioned in subsection (2)(b) includes care and support the provision of which–
> (a) the authority does not consider to be necessary to meet the adult's needs;
> (b) is in addition to care and support which is being provided, arranged for, or paid for (in whole or in part) by the authority.
>
> **Recovery of charges, interest etc.**
>
> **69**(1) Any sum due to a local authority under this Part is recoverable by the authority as a debt due to it.
>
> (2) But subsection (1) does not apply in a case where a deferred payment agreement could, in accordance with regulations under section 34(1), be entered into, unless–
> (a) the local authority has sought to enter into such an agreement with the adult from whom the sum is due, and
> (b) the adult has refused.

11.31 Thus, by virtue of section 69(1) and (2), even though a local authority may not be under a direct duty to enter into a deferred payment agreement, in a particular case, it must offer to do so wherever it has power to do so, under the Care and Support (Deferred Payment) Regulations 2014, otherwise it will not be entitled to seek to recover any charges owing to it.

11.32 The advantage for some care home and support living residents may be that, in addition to preserving the 'family home' for emotional reasons, they may be able to continue to take advantage of any increases in its value and, also, rent it out to obtain income to defray their care charges.

The detailed scheme

11.33 The detailed scheme is found in the Care and Support (Deferred Payment) Regulations 2014.

When the local authority must enter into a deferred payment agreement

11.34 The 'duty' arises when the adult has an 'eligible need' for care home accommodation but their capital is less than £23,250.00 excluding the value of their home. By virtue of regulation 2 of the Care and Support (Deferred Payment) Regulations 2014, a local authority must enter into a deferred payment agreement when:

- an adult is able to provide adequate security (under reg 4);
- the adult agrees to the local authority's terms and conditions (under reg 11);
- the local authority is meeting the adult's eligible needs by providing them with care home accommodation, or would have done so (but the adult is making their own care home arrangements);
- the adult has assets amounting to less than £23,250.00 (excluding the value of their home); and
- the adult's home is not disregarded for means-testing purposes (eg because it is occupied by a spouse or dependent relative, as defined in the charging machinery).

When the local authority may enter into a deferred payment agreement

11.35 The power arises where an adult has an *'eligible need'* for care home or supported living accommodation and intends to retain their home, irrespective of the value of the adult's capital.

11.36 By virtue of regulation 3 of the Care and Support (Deferred Payment) Regulations 2014, a local authority may enter into a deferred payment agreement when:

- an adult is able to provide adequate security (under reg 4); and
- agrees to the local authority's terms and conditions (under reg 11); and
- the local authority has decided to meet the adult's eligible needs by providing care home or supported living accommodation and the adult intends to retain their home, or when that is the decision the local authority would have reached, had it been asked to meet the adult's needs (but the adult is making their own arrangements).

11.37 Paragraphs 9.5 and 9.8 of the *Care and Support Statutory Guidance* encourage local authorities to exercise their discretionary power generously and, as has already been seen, by virtue of section 69(1) and (2), a local authority must offer to enter into a deferred payment agreement whenever it has power to do so under the Care and Support (Deferred Payment) Regulations 2014, otherwise it will not be entitled to seek to recover the charges owing to it.

The machinery

11.38 Both the duty and the power to enter into a deferred payment agreement is contingent on the service user being able provide '*adequate security*', as defined in regulation 4 of the Care and Support (Deferred Payment) Regulations 2014, that is:

- a first legal charge; or
- such other security as the local authority considers sufficient; in both cases
- equal to the amount of the deferred charges plus any deferred interest or administration costs

11.39 Local authorities should have 'an explicit and publicly-accessible policy of what other types of security they are willing to consider in addition to a first charge, but local authorities may consider the merits of each case individually': paragraph 9.62 of the *Care and Support Statutory Guidance*, which goes on to give examples of potential alternative forms of security.

11.40 The total deferred amount is defined in regulations 5 and 6 of the Care and Support (Deferred Payment) Regulations 2014:

- the starting point is 100 per cent of the charges for care home or supported living accommodation, or of any loan made for the purpose of assisting the adult to obtain care home or supported living accommodation, plus the amount of any top-ups under section 30(2) of the Care Act 2014 which the local authority has agreed to include, up to the '*equity limit*';
- but there is then provision for adjustments to be made, most notably, that a local authority need not defer an amount where, after payment, the adult would retain at least £144.00 of their weekly income.

11.41 Time for repayment of the deferred amount is, by virtue of regulation 7, whichever is the soonest of:

- the date of sale or disposal of the land or other secured asset; or
- 90 days after the death of the adult (or some longer period allowed by the local authority).

11.42 There is further machinery as follows:

- deferred payment agreements can be terminated early by the adult on reasonable notice (reg 8);
- the local authority can charge restricted sums in interest and for administration (regs 9 and 10);
- deferred payment agreements must contain certain terms, conditions and information (reg 11).

11.43 The Department of Health has produced standard sample deferred payments legal agreements as well as other supporting material.[4]

11.44 The *Care and Support Statutory Guidance* addresses deferred payments in Chapter 9, advising in particular:

4 www.local.gov.uk/care-support-reform/-/journal_content/56/10180/6522542/ARTICLE.

- that local authorities are entitled not to include 'top up' payments in deferred payment agreements (paragraph 9.12);
- that while, in certain circumstances, local authorities may stop deferring care costs, that only means that future care charges are not deferred (paragraphs 9.14–9.18);
- that local authorities should provide information and advice (paragraphs 9.19–9.31);
- on the mechanics of deferred agreements (paragraph 9.32 onwards).

11.45 The Department of Health and the Local Government Association has produced a range of additional practical guidance.[5]

11.46 Section 36 of the Care Act 2014 makes provision for regulations that will entitle local authorities to enter into 'alternative financial arrangements of a specified description with an adult', similar to deferred payment agreements.

Remedies

11.47 Where the service user declines to enter into a deferred payment agreement, and arrears accrue, the ordinary remedies apply, pursuant to section 69 of the Care Act 2014: usually, an action to recover the debt followed by an application for a charging order under the Charging Orders Act 1979 and Part 73 of the Civil Procedure Rules 1998, protecting the charge by entry of a notice or restriction at HM Land Registry.

Top ups

11.48 In 'Preferred accommodation' at para 9.45 above, it was noted that local authorities must provide certain types of accommodation at the adult's preferred location, providing various conditions are met, including that the adult or a third party pays any additional cost, beyond that provided for in the adult's personal budget.

11.49 This section looks in a little more detail at the machinery of 'top ups'.

11.50 There has to be a written agreement committing the payer to paying the additional cost and addressing a list of specified matters and the local authority must ensure that the payer has access to sufficient information and advice to enable them to understand the agreement (regulation 5 of the Care and Support (Choice of Accommodation) Regulations 2014). The agreement must address the following matters:

> (3) The written agreement must include–
> (a) the additional cost;
> (b) the amount specified in the adult's personal budget in relation to the provision of accommodation;
> (c) the frequency of payments;
> (d) details of the person to whom the payments are to be made;
> (e) provision for review of the agreement;
> (f) provisions about the matters specified in paragraph (4).

5 www.local.gov.uk/care-support-reform/-/journal_content/56/10180/6522542/ARTICLE.

(4) The specified matters are–
(a) the consequences of ceasing to make payments;
(b) the effect of increases in charges made by the provider of the preferred accommodation;
(c) the effect of changes in the payer's financial circumstances.

11.51 As the *Care and Support Statutory Guidance* makes clear, at Annex A, if the payer ceases to make the payments due, for whatever reasons:

- the local authority may move the adult to alternative accommodation (although this will be subject to a re-assessment of needs and consideration of the adult's well-being);
- the local authority may seek to recover any outstanding debt from the payer.

11.52 Age UK has produced a useful factsheet on the choice of accommodation.[6]

Complaints/appeals about financial matters

11.53 Currently, any complaints may invoke the Local Authority Social Services and NHS Complaints (England) Regulations 2009.

11.54 As noted above, it is likely that additionally, or by way of substitution, the government will introduce an appeal procedure: it has created a power in the Care Act 2014, at section 72, to introduce an appeals procedure by way of regulations, in relation to all or many decisions made under Part 1 of the Care Act 2014 and is currently undertaking a consultation.[7]

The cap on care costs and associated means-testing

11.55 The Care Act 2014 contains provision for a lifetime cap on care costs, in sections 15 and 16, which was to be set at £72,000.00, whether those costs were incurred in care homes or by way of home care. '*Hotel costs*' associated with care provision are excluded from the cap, but were to be made subject to a separate cap of £12,000.00 per annum.

11.56 In addition, the Care Act 2014 contains provision for means testing, under section 17. The government's intention had been to raise the upper limit to £118,000 and the lower limit to £17,000, so that only those with assets worth more than £118,000.00 would have to pay the full price, whereas all those with assets of between £17,000 and £118,500 who met the eligibility criteria for care would be entitled to some financial support according to a sliding scale.

11.57 Both these changes were due to be brought into force in April 2016, but that has now been deferred until 2020.

11.58 There is a government fact sheet about these changes.[8]

6 www.ageuk.org.uk/Documents/EN-GB/Factsheets/FS60_Choice_of_accommodation_care_homes_fcs.pdf?dtrk=true.

7 www.gov.uk/government/uploads/system/uploads/attachment_data/file/400757/2903104_Care_Act_Consultation_Accessible_All.pdf.

8 www.gov.uk/government/uploads/system/uploads/attachment_data/file/268683/Factsheet_6_update__tweak_.pdf.

Cases

Charging: residential accommodation cases

11.59 *Yule v South Lanarkshire Council (No 2)* (2001) 4 CCLR 383, CSIH

A local authority had to consider whether all the circumstances justified the inference that a person had deliberately deprived themselves of an asset in order to avoid having to pay care charges and it was only necessary that the purpose of avoiding having to pay care charges was a significant part of the purpose

Facts: the Court of Session (Lords Cameron of Lochbroom, Osborne and Reed) Mrs Yule transferred her home to her granddaughter, 'in consideration of love, favour and affection', about 15 months before she went into residential accommodation. She was 78 years old at the time of the transfer and had been deteriorating gradually over the preceding six or seven years, for example, so as to develop paranoid ideas about a neighbour for several years. The family maintained that, at the time, it was not contemplated that Mrs Yule would have to go into residential care, that an unforeseen accident precipitated her admission (which was the case) and that it was always Mrs Yule's intention to transfer her home to her granddaughter, of whom she was particularly fond: there was no intention to deprive herself of capital. South Lanarkshire decided that Mrs Yule had deprived herself of capital for the purpose of decreasing the amount that she might be liable to pay for her residential accommodation, for the purposes of regulation 25 of the National Assistance (Assessment of Resources) Regulations 1992.

Judgment: the Court of Session (Lords Cameron of Lochbroom, Osborne and Reed) held that it was inappropriate to analyse the matter in terms of burden of proof. A local authority must seek information from the application and other sources and reach a rational conclusion as to whether it could be inferred that a deprivation of capital had taken place deliberately and with the intention of asserting an inability to pay. It was unnecessary for the applicant to know of the actual capital limit: it was sufficient if it was a reasonable inference from all the circumstances that the purpose of a transaction had been to avoid having to pay charges. In this case, the applicant had been an elderly woman with no substantial capital assets, the transfer had not been for monetary consideration and there was no reason why the granddaughter needed to live in that particular house. These were sufficient primary facts to found the reasonable inference that the applicant had deliberately decided to deprive herself of the house in order to avoid having to pay care home charges. These were sufficient primary facts to found the reasonable inference that at least part of the purpose of the transfer had been a deliberate decision to the applicant had deliberately decided to deprive herself of the house in order to avoid having to pay care home charges:

> 30. In the present case, it was clear that the respondents could look for information no further than the members of the family to whom they applied for information. Furthermore, it was clear that the family were indicating that they were not able to throw any further light on the purpose of the transaction by which Mrs Yule deprived herself of her capital asset in the house

beyond what was contained in the correspondence up to and including the letter of 4 February 1997. It may have been the case that the respondents only learnt some time after they made their determination that, at the same time as executing the disposition of her house, Mrs Yule had also granted a power of attorney to her son, the petitioner. However, the respondents cannot be faulted for proceeding to make their assessment on the information available to them at the time. ...

31. When regard is had to the letter in which the respondents' decision was conveyed to the family, the respondents properly set out the question which they required to ask themselves, when they said that 'in determining any application for public funding the Council is required...to consider whether the transfer of any property by the resident was carried out either in full or in part with the motive of avoiding that property being taken into account in determining his or her eligibility for public funding'...

32. In our opinion, looking to that material, a number of primary facts stand out. This was an elderly woman with no substantial capital assets other than her house. She was putting her affairs in order. She elected to dispone her house while retaining a limited interest in it, by way of a liferent, giving her the right to occupy it during her lifetime. This would protect her while she remained able to do so. The fee in the house was disponed out of her hands for no consideration, other than the love, favour and affection that she had for her granddaughter. There was nothing suggested to the respondents to the effect that the granddaughter had need at the time to succeed to any interest in the house or to live in it in the future, or that there was any prior legal obligation to that effect. The suggestion that Mrs Yule was in good health ran counter to the information that was before the respondents prior to the letter of 1 November 1996 in which they first applied to Miss Yule for information. That was a factor which, it would appear from the pleadings, was in mind at the time that the decision was taken. From what was put before the respondents in regard to all these matters, we consider that there were sufficient primary facts to entitle the respondents reasonably to conclude that Mrs Yule had deliberately determined to denude herself of her one substantial asset because, by doing so, she might thereby avoid the prospect that if she were to enter residential care in her lifetime, her house would require to be sold and the proceeds, at least in part, would require to be devoted to payment for that care, to the detriment of her family's interest in the succession to her estate on her death...

33. We agree with the Lord Ordinary that it is open to a local authority to reach a view as to the purpose of a transaction such as the present, without any specific finding as to the exact state of knowledge or intention of the applicant, so long as the primary facts are such as reasonably to lead to the inference that the purpose was at least in part that specified in reg 25(1).

Comment: regulation 25 of the 1992 regulations is reproduced, materially identically, at regulation 17 of the Care and Support (Charging and Assessment of Resources) Regulations 2014.

11.60 *R (Beeson) v Dorset CC* [2001] EWHC 981 (Admin), (2002) 5 CCLR 5, QBD

The test was a subjective one: did the applicant 'deliberately' deprive themselves of assets, 'knowing' that that they might receive care services for which they might have to pay?

Facts: Mr Beeson transferred his house to his son by deed of gift about two and a half years before he entered residential care. The son claimed that, at the time, his father was preparing to die at home, was unaware that he might go into residential accommodation and be means-tested and that his main motivation was to ensure that the son had a home. However, Dorset concluded that the father had deprived himself of capital for the purpose of decreasing the amount that he may be liable to pay for residential accommodation, in breach of regulation 25 of the National Assistance (Assessment of Resources) Regulations 1992.

Judgment: Richards J held that Dorset had been entitled to draw inferences and reject the son's evidence but it did not give any reasons for rejecting the son's evidence which, if accepted, took the case outside regulation 25: therefore, Dorset must have misdirected itself in law by applying an objective, rather than a subjective test:

> 38. The present case differs materially on its facts from *Yule v South Lanarkshire Council*, given the existence of evidence from Mr Beeson's son about his and his father's state of mind at the relevant time. This constituted input from the family of a kind that was lacking in *Yule*. True it is that the key question related to Mr Beeson's own state of mind rather than his son's state of mind and that that still had to be a matter of inference. Nonetheless his son's evidence that funding of residential care did not come into his or his father's thoughts and that the transfer took place at a time when his father intended to live in and ultimately to die in his home was evidence of central importance. If accepted as truthful and reliable evidence, it negatived the existence of a regulation 25 purpose on the correct, subjective test. Conversely, a finding that a regulation 25 purpose existed on the correct test required a rejection of his evidence and an adverse credibility finding. The surrounding circumstances provided material capable of supporting the rejection of his evidence, but any decision whether to reject or accept it required an overall assessment of that material and of the impression created by Mr Beeson's son himself in the course of stating his case and answering questions at the panel hearing.
>
> 39. Those considerations underlie my concerns about the panel's decision. If the panel was truly directing itself by reference to a subjective test when it found the existence of a regulation 25 purpose, then it had to face up to the fact that it was rejecting the evidence of Mr Beeson's son and, in order to give an adequately reasoned decision, it had to explain why it was rejecting that evidence. Yet there is nothing along those lines in the findings. It is possible that the panel thought along those lines but simply failed to state its reasons adequately. Another explanation, however, is that the absence of such reasons betokens a failure on the part of the panel to apply the correct test in the first place: the panel did not spell out the key steps in the reasoning process because it did not appreciate the true nature of the test or, therefore, the reasoning process that was required in the circumstances of the case. In view of the matters to which I have already referred, I consider

the latter explanation to be the more likely and I conclude that the panel did not direct itself correctly.

40. In my judgment that failure infects the final stage 3 decision by the Director, whose decision letter refers to the panel's finding and expresses concurrence with it. It seems to me that the panel's finding must have carried substantial weight. Indeed it would make a nonsense of the panel's role if it did not carry weight, unless of course it was appreciated that the panel had failed to apply the correct legal test. Although the Director had read the case file and correspondence, there is nothing in the letter to indicate any awareness of a problem in the panel's own decision-making process or the carrying out of a fresh analysis without regard to the panel's finding. In any event, if the panel's finding was flawed, I doubt whether the Director could have cured it by a paper exercise alone and without at least hearing oral submissions from Mr Beeson's son.

11.61 *Robertson v Fife Council* [2002] UKHL 35, (2002) 5 CCLR 543

The availability of notional capital did not negate the existence of a need that was required to be met

Facts: Fife assessed Mrs Robertson as needing nursing home accommodation but, also, as having deprived herself of capital. Consequently, it determined not to provide her with residential accommodation until the notional capital, of which she had deprived herself, fell below the capital limit, under the applicable diminishing notional capital rules. Mrs Robertson sought judicial review, seeking relief in terms that she be provided with nursing care accommodation.

Judgment: the House of Lords (Lords Slynn, Mackay, Nicholls, Hope and Hobhouse) held that the assessment of needs for community care services (which could trigger a duty to make provision) was separate from the assessment of any liability to pay. Consequently, Fife was wrong to take into account Mrs Robertson's notional capital, as a reason for declining to provide her with a service.

11.62 *R (Kelly) v Hammersmith & Fulham LBC* [2004] EWHC 325 (Admin), (2004) 7 CCLR 542

A secure tenant's right to buy discount counted as a contribution towards the purchase price, the presumption of a resulting trust applied and the local authority was entitled to place a caution on the register and levy a charge

Facts: Ms Kelly's mother exercised her '*right to buy*', purchasing her council home with a discount of £50,000.00 off the total price of £120,000.00. Ms Kelly, her daughter, was a joint purchaser and became solely responsible for paying the mortgage and other costs. There was no express declaration of trust. Ms Kelly applied for a judicial review of the decision to treat her mother as a beneficial owner of 5/12 of the home, for the purpose of assessing her liability to pay residential care charges.

Judgment: Wilson J held that the right to buy discount amounted to a contribution towards the purchase price and that, since Ms Kelly could not prove a mutual intention that her mother should not have an equitable interest, she held a proportionate share in the dwelling on trust for her mother. The local authority was entitled to take this share into account for the purpose of charging the mother and the local authority was entitled to enter a caution on the register.

11.63 *Derbyshire CC v Akrill* [2005] EWCA Civ 308, (2005) 8 CCLR 173

A person is in general entitled to raise public law issues in defence of a claim for care charges

Facts: Mr Akrill's father entered into a sale and lease-back arrangement of his home, his primary asset, shortly before entering into permanent residential care. Derbyshire initially concluded that this had not amounted to a deprivation of capital, but then decided that it had done. Mr Akrill defended proceedings brought by Derbyshire under section 423 of the Insolvency Act 1986, for the re-transfer of the house into his father's estate, in part on the basis that Derbyshire was bound by its first decision. In the county court, the judge held that it was not possible to raise a public law defence except by way of judicial review. Mr Akrill appealed.

Judgment: the Court of Appeal (Brooke, Neuberger and Latham LJJ) held that, subject to any question of abuse, a litigant was entitled to raise as a defence an alleged breach of public law, in private law proceedings, if it affects the basis of the claim against him.

11.64 *Jones v Powys Local Health Board and Neath Port Talbot Local Health Board* [2008] EWHC 2562 (Admin), (2009) 12 CCLR 68

It was an abuse of process to defend an action for the recovery of care home charges on the basis that the resident was entitled to NHS Continuing Healthcare when that issue had been adversely determined administratively and not challenged by way of judicial review

Facts: the claimant sued on his own behalf, and as administrator of the estate of his deceased wife, claiming restitution of care home fee payments, on the ground that his wife had been entitled to NHS continuing healthcare. However, the All Wales Special Review Board determined that Mrs Jones had not been entitled to NHS continuing healthcare and neither she nor Mr Jones had sought a judicial review of that decision.

Judgment: Plender J struck out the claim as being an abuse of process: the claim was in substance a public law claim (alleging that the Review Board had erred in public law), bringing a private law action deprived the public authorities concerned of the protections afforded by CPR 54 and was an abuse of process

11.65 *DM v Doncaster MBC* [2012] EWHC 3652 (Admin), (2012) 15 CCLR 128

Local authorities were required to charge for care home accommodation, even where the resident was detained in such accommodation by virtue of the Mental Capacity Act 2005

Facts: DM and her husband FM claimed the repayment of money she and her husband had paid to Doncaster for FM's accommodation in a case home when he had been detained there pursuant to the Mental Capacity Act 2005.

Judgment: Langstaff J held that FM had been accommodated under section 21 of the National Assistance Act (NAA) 1948 rather than under the Mental Capacity Act 2005 (which did not include an accommodation duty), that section 22 of the NAA 1948 required Doncaster to charge and that FM had not been discriminated against in breach of the ECHR, compared with detained mental patients and those in receipt of after-care, who were not charged.

Comment: all charging is now discretionary.

11.66 *Aster Healthcare Ltd v Estate of Mohammed Shafi* [2014] EWCA Civ 1350, (2014) 17 CCLR 419

A local authority which places a person in a care home is contractually liable for the fees until an effective supervening event

Facts: Brent placed Mr Shafi, who lacked mental capacity, at an Aster nursing home, but then indicated to the nursing home that, in its view, Mr Shafi was a self-funder. Mr Shafi's family refused to sign a contract. Aster sued the estate for substantial unpaid fees.

Judgment: the Court of Appeal (Lord Dyson MR, Beatson and Briggs LJJ) held that, on the facts, the contract remained between Aster and Brent, including having regard to the statutory context, which required Brent to continue to make arrangements until Mr Shafi had a deputy or some other person appointed to act on his behalf. It was a question of fact, for trial, whether or not Aster could recover under section 7 of the Mental Capacity Act 2005 ('s7(1): If necessary goods or services are supplied to a person who lacks capacity to contract for the supply he must pay a reasonable price for them'): on the authorities, it would depend whether Aster supplied services to Mr Shafi in circumstances in which it intended that Mr Shafi or the local authority or Mrs Shafi should pay for them.

Charging: other services

11.67 *Avon CC v Hooper and Bristol and District Health Authority* (1997–8) 1 CCLR 366, CA

An indemnity was a financial resource for the purposes of means-testing

Facts: Daniel Hooper was born severely disabled as a result of health authority negligence. His action in negligence against the health authority was compromised on terms that required the health authority to indemnify Daniel in respect of any liability he might incur to Avon for the costs of his home care, up to the date of the compromise. Avon then delivered a retrospective charge.

Judgment: The Court of Appeal (Butler-Sloss, Roch and Hobhouse LJJ) held that this was permitted under section 17 of the Health and Social Services and Social Security Adjudications Act 1983, that a service user's means fell to be assessed at the time the authority makes the decision to charge and that their means included the value of an indemnity:

> The starting point for the evaluation of these arguments is section 17 itself. It is an empowering section. It gives a local authority the power, but not the

obligation, to charge for the provision of the relevant services. It is implicit both in the language of the section and in the general law governing the activities of local authorities that the power must be exercised reasonably, that is to say, that the local authority must have relevant and reasonable grounds for choosing to exercise the power. Nothing turns upon how one construes the final words of the subsection: 'such charge (if any) for it as they consider reasonable'. As a matter of language, these words carry the implication that the charge may be waived and that the local authority need only make any charge if it considers it reasonable to do so. Thus there is an overriding criterion of reasonableness which governs the local authority's exercise of the power which is given by subsection (1).

This criterion of reasonableness provides the primary answer to the arguments of Mr Grace. If the right to charge has been waived, clearly no charge can be recovered. If the service was provided in circumstances under which it would be unreasonable for the authority subsequently to charge for it, then the authority is not entitled later to seek to recover a charge. Similarly, if, having provided a service, the local authority seeks to recover a charge it must be prepared to justify the reasonableness of doing so. The reasonableness of any conduct falls to be assessed at the time of the relevant conduct and having regard to all the relevant circumstances then existing. If the claim is first made some time after the provision of the services, the local authority must be prepared to justify the reasonableness of making the claim notwithstanding the delay. If the local authority is acting unreasonably, its claim will fail. If the local authority is acting reasonably, there is no basis in subs. (1) for the person availing himself of the service to say that the local authority should not recover.

If the local authority decides to charge and is acting reasonably in doing so, the person availing himself of the service has, in those circumstances, to satisfy the authority under subs. (3) that his means are insufficient for it to be reasonably practicable for him to pay the amount which he would otherwise be obliged to pay. It is for the recipient of the service to discharge this burden of persuasion. He must show that he has insufficient means. The time at which he has to do this is the time when the local authority is seeking to charge him for the services. If his means have been reduced, as might be the case with a business man whose business had run into difficulties after his being injured, the reduction in his means is something upon which he would be entitled to rely as making it impracticable for him to pay, even though at an earlier date he might have been better off. The consideration under subs. (3)(b) is the practical one: are his means such that it is not reasonably practicable for him to pay?

This also bears on the alternative argument of Mr Grace that only cash should be taken into account. This is too narrow a reading of subsection (3). As a matter of the ordinary use of English, the word 'means' refers to the financial resources of a person: his assets, his sources of income, his liabilities and expenses. If he has a realisable asset, that is part of his means; he has the means to pay. The subject matter of paragraph (b) is the practicability of his paying. If he has an asset which he can reasonably be expected to realise and which will (after taking into account any other relevant factor) enable him to pay, his means make it practicable for him to pay. Where the person has a right to be indemnified by another against the cost of the service, he has the means to pay. He can enforce his right and make the payment. There is nothing in any part of s17 which suggests that it is intended that subs. (3) should have the effect of relieving those liable to indemnify the recipient of the service for the cost of the service from their liability. On the contrary, it is clear that the intention of the section is to enable the local authority to recover the cost save when it is unreasonable that it should do so or impracticable for the recipient to pay. The argument of the Health Authority would, if accepted, frustrate the clear intention of the section.

Comment: there are potentially significant differences in the statutory language, but the logic of this case appears to apply charging cases arises under sections 14–17 of the Care Act 2014.

11.68 *R v Powys CC ex p Hambidge (No 2)* (1999) 2 CCLR 460, QBD

There was no duty to consult before amending a charging policy

Facts: Powys changed its charging policy and increased the charges it made for the 16 hours' home care that Mrs Hambidge received each week, from £10.50 to £32.70. It did not undertake general consultation in relation to its policy change, nor had it consulted any individual service user, including Mrs Hambidge.

Judgment: Jowitt J held that whilst guidance advised that it would be good practice to consult, but that did not give rise to a duty to do so, or create any legitimate expectation. Neither did the procedural fairness principle require consultation because Mrs Hambidge did not have any legitimate expectation that her charges would never increase and she was entitled to seek a review under section 17 of the Health and Social Services and Social Security Adjudications Act 1983, under which she could not be required to pay more than a reasonable amount, having regard to her means.

Comment: this would not appear to be authority for the proposition that local authorities need not consult persons liable to be affected by their charging policies and local authorities would be well advised to do so.

11.69 *R v Powys CC ex p Hambidge* (2000) 3 CCLR 231, CA

It is not necessarily discrimination to levy increased charges on persons in receipt of disability benefits

Facts: Powys imposed higher charges for home care services on persons in receipt of income support plus disability living allowance/attendance allowance, than on persons in receipt of income support only. Mrs Hambidge submitted, inter alia, that this amounted to discrimination in breach of section 20(1) of the Disability Discrimination Act 1995.

Judgment: the Court of Appeal (Henry, Aldous, Laws LJJ) held that there was no discrimination: the charging scheme was based on the level of resources in the hands of those in receipt of care, whether or not the presence of disability lay behind the receipt of cash in a particular case; there was no causal link between the rate charged and disability.

11.70 *R (Carton) v Coventry CC* (2001) 4 CCLR 41, QBD

Consultation on a changed charging scheme had been unfair and the resultant scheme irrational

Facts: having charged a flat rate for home care services, Coventry consulted upon then introduced a means-tested system; however, the system introduced was different from that consulted on and it took into account sums of disability living allowance, paid in respect of night-time care, as income available for means-testing in relation to day-time care.

Judgment: Sir Richard Tucker held that there were major differences between the scheme consulted on and the scheme adopted such that fairness required proper consultation on the scheme adopted; in addition, it was irrational to treat sums of disability living allowance, paid in respect of night-time care, as income available for means-testing in relation to day-time care.

11.71 *R (Stephenson) v Stockton-on-Tees* [2004] EWHC 2228 (Admin), (2004) 7 CCLR 459

It was not irrational to decline to treat as expenditure for means-testing purposes sums paid to a family carer

Facts: Mrs Stephenson was 78 and virtually house-bound on account of ill health. Stockton-on-Tees assessed her as needing 13¼ hours of care each week, in addition to the substantial amount of care already provided by her daughter. Mrs Stephenson paid her daughter £45.00 per week for this care, in part to compensate her for loss of earnings. However, when assessing what Mrs Stephenson could reasonably be expected to pay towards her care, Stockton-on-Tees declined to take into account the £45.00 as expenditure, pursuant to its policy to disregard the cost of care provided by a family member except where the assessment identified cultural issues.

Judgment: Keith J held that the Council's policy was rational because care provided by family members is normally provided voluntarily; nor was it incompatible with Article 8 ECHR or discriminatory in any way.

Comment: but see decision of the Court of Appeal below at para 11.74.

11.72 *R (Spink) v Wandsworth LBC* [2005] EWCA Civ 302, (2005) 8 CCLR 272

Local authorities were entitled to charge for service provided to disabled children under section 2 of the Chronically Sick and Disabled Persons Act 1970 and to take into account parental resources

Facts: Mr and Mrs Spink's two sons were severely disabled and a dispute arose between them and Wandsworth as to whether the financial resources of the parents were relevant, when determining whether it was necessary to provide services for the benefit of the children, under section 2 of the Chronically Sick and Disabled Persons Act 1970.

Judgment: the Court of Appeal (Lord Phillips MR, May and Rix LJJ) held that local authorities were entitled to charge for services provided to children under the age of 16, under section 2 of the Chronically Sick and

Disabled Persons Act 1970, albeit that the services were provided in the exercise of functions under the Children Act 1989. Further, the means of the parents were relevant to determining whether it was necessary to meet the needs of the children:

> 46. We would endorse the reasoning of Richards J. As a general proposition a local authority can reasonably expect that parents, who can afford the expense, will make any alterations to their home that are necessary for the care of their disabled children, if there is no alternative source of providing these. It is also reasonable to anticipate that some parents with means will not do so if they believe that this will result in the local authority making the alterations for them. (We emphasise that we are speaking in generalities and not suggesting that Mr and Mrs Spink fall into this category.) Having regard to these considerations, we agree with Richards J that a local authority can, in circumstances such as those with which we are concerned, properly decline to be satisfied that it is necessary to provide services to meet the needs of disabled children until it has been demonstrated that, having regard to their means, it is not reasonable to expect their parents to provide these.

Comment: services for disabled children are still provided under section 2 Chronically Sick and Disabled Persons Act 1970.

11.73 *R (BG) v Medway Council* [2005] EWHC 1932 (Admin), (2005) 8 CCLR 448

It was lawful to provide assistance under section 2 of the Chronically Sick and Disabled Persons Act 1970 and to attach rational conditions to the loan

Facts: BG was a very severely young child. Medway awarded his family the maximum disabled facilities grant of £25,000.00, for adaptations and extensions to the family home, a discretionary non-repayable grant of £10,000.00 and a loan of £30,000.00 secured on the home, repayable on certain conditions, including if the family moved, BG moved away or died or the home was re-possessed. The family challenged the lawfulness of the conditions.

Judgment: Richards J held that the it was lawful to provide assistance under the Chronically Sick and Disabled Persons Act 1970 by way of a loan and that the conditions imposed were rational, took into account the family's means and complied with Article 8 ECHR.

11.74 *R (Stephenson) v Stockton-on-Tees* [2005] EWCA Civ 960, (2005) 8 CCLR 517

It was rational in general to disregard sums paid to family carers, for means-testing, but the policy had been applied too inflexibly in this case

Facts: Mrs Stephenson was 78 and virtually house-bound on account of ill health. Stockton-on-Tees assessed her as needing 13¼ hours of care each week, in addition to the substantial amount of care already provided by her daughter. Mrs Stephenson paid her daughter £45.00 per week for this care, in part to compensate her for loss of earnings. However, when assessing what Mrs Stephenson could reasonably be expected to pay towards her care, Stockton-on-Tees declined to take into account the £45.00 as expenditure, pursuant to its policy to disregard the cost of care provided by a family member except where the assessment identified cultural issues.

Judgment: the Court of Appeal (Sedley and Wall LJJ, Richards J) held that it was rational for Stockton-on-Tees to have a policy of not making any allowance for expenditure on services provided by family members, as Keith J had held, but that, on the highly unusual facts of this case, the council had applied that policy with undue rigidity: the claimant was only prepared to allow her daughter to reduce her working hours, and then give up work altogether, on the basis that she was compensated financially for so doing.

11.75 *R (B) v Cornwall CC* [2010] EWCA Civ 55, (2010) 13 CCLR 117

A fundamentally flawed financial assessment was liable to quashed irrespective of whether the local authority could then make a retrospective assessment (though it probably could)

Facts: after having received NHS care for some years, B became a local authority responsibility. The judge at first instance found that Cornwall's assessment of his liability to pay changes was fundamentally unlawful, owing to failures to consult adequately, to consider the care plans or assess B's resources properly. Cornwall appealed the judge's decision to quash its decision to charge, on the basis that it would be precluded from making a retrospective charge, so the judge should have allowed it to undertake a retrospective review.

Judgment: the Court of Appeal (Waller, Hooper, Moore-Bick LJJ) held that it was not clear that Cornwall could not make a retrospective decision and, in any event, Cornwall's decision, being unlawful, was liable to be quashed. It would only be in exceptional cases that relief would not be granted where a decision was unlawful.

CHAPTER 12

Ordinary residence and local authority responsibility

continued

12.48 *R (Kent County Council) v Secretary of State for Health* [2015] EWCA Civ 81, (2015) 18 CCLR 153

Statutory deeming provisions were not retrospective

12.49 *R (Cornwall Council) v Secretary of State for Health* [2015] UKSC 46, [2015] 3 WLR 213, (2015) 18 CCLR 497

Clarifying the ordinary residence test and how it applied

12.50 *R (Tigere) v Secretary of State for Business, Innovation and Skills* [2015] UKSC 57, [2015] 1 WLR 3820

It was incompatible with Article 2 of the 1st Protocol to the ECHR and Article 14 ECHR to exclude from student loans prospective students who had not clocked up three years of lawful, ordinary residence but who had lived in the UK for most of their lives, had been educated here, could not be removed save for grave misconduct and were treated throughout as members of UK society; but the ordinary residence test was lawful

12.51 *Milton Keynes Council v Scottish Ministers* [2015] CSOH 156, 2015 SLT 843

The ordinary residence of a person lacking capacity may not change simply because they go to live elsewhere under private arrangements

Mental health

12.53 *R v Mental Health Review Tribunal, Torfaen County BC and Gwent Health Authority ex p Hall* (1999) 2 CCLR 361, QBD

The health and social care authorities responsible for after-care were those for the area where the patient had been resident before their detention or, if the patient had no ordinary residence, the responsible authorities are those for the area to where the patient is sent

12.54 *R (Hertfordshire CC) v Hammersmith & Fulham LBC* [2011] EWCA Civ 77, (2011) 14 CCLR 224

Statutory deeming provisions only applied for the purposes of the National Assistance Act 1948

12.55 *R (Sunderland CC) v South Tyneside Council, SF and Leeds CC* [2012] EWCA Civ 1232, (2012) 15 CCLR 701

A person could be ordinarily resident in a 'placement' that was, ultimately, voluntarily accepted by them

12.56 *R (Wiltshire Council) v Hertfordshire CC* [2014] EWCA Civ 712, (2014) 17 CCLR 258

A conditional discharge does not alter the ordinary residence of a person subject to a hospital order with restrictions

Introduction

12.1 While local authorities have the power, in certain circumstances, to meet the needs of adults and carers who are ordinarily resident elsewhere, they only owe duties to persons who are 'ordinarily resident' in their area, or who are of 'no settled residence' (sections 18–20 of the Care Act 2014). It is therefore important that authorities and applicants for services have a clear understanding of what 'ordinary residence' entails.

12.2 There are two types of ordinary residence for the purposes of the Care Act 2014:

- actual ordinary residence, resulting from a person's physical presence in a local authority area;
- deemed ordinary residence, resulting from the Care Act 2014 requiring a person to be treated as retaining ordinary residence in local authority area A, although they are actually resident in local authority area B pursuant to sections 39 and 76 of the Care Act 2014.

12.3 Where there is a dispute between local authorities that they are unable to resolve, the Secretary of State, or an appointed person, will determine that dispute pursuant to section 40 of the Care Act 2014.[1] That determination is susceptible to judicial review.

12.4 In addition, where local authority A provides services to a person who, it transpires, is ordinarily resident in the area of local authority B, local authority A can reclaim the cost from local authority B pursuant to section 41 of the Care Act 2014.

Meaning of ordinary residence

12.5 As the *Care and Support Statutory Guidance* states 'there is no definition of ordinary residence in the Care Act. Therefore, the term should be given its ordinary and natural meaning' (paragraph 19.12).

Adults with capacity

12.6 The ordinary residence of an adult who possesses the capacity to choose where to live is the place the person has voluntarily adopted for a settled purpose, whether for a short or long duration:[2]

- the starting point has to be a period of present or past physical residence, without which, ordinary residence cannot follow.[3] Conversely, a person will not usually retain ordinary residence in an area, if he or she

1 By virtue of article 5 of the Care Act (Transitional Provision) Order 2015, the Secretary of State will determine all ordinary residence disputes that are to be determined on or after the 1 April 2015 under section 40 of the Care Act 2014 (rather than under the predecessor legislation).

2 *R (Cornwall Council) v Secretary of State for Health* [2015] UKSC 46, [2015] 3 WLR 213, (2015) 18 CCLR 497 at paras 39–42.

3 See, by analogy, *A v A (Children)(Habitual Residence)* [2013] UKSC 60, [2014] AC 1 at para 55.

has not retained a place in that area where he or she may return to, to reside even if they have a strong connection with that area;[4]

- what is critical is where the person voluntarily eats and sleeps as a matter of fact, so that a person may be ordinarily resident in interim accommodation provided under the homelessness acts, or even in a barn at a farm where he or she is working temporarily;[5]
- a person may remain ordinarily resident in an area, notwithstanding temporary absences, whether of short or long duration;[6]
- in principle, a person may be ordinarily resident in more than one area,[7] although ultimately, for the purpose of allocating liability under the Care Act 2014, a person can only be ordinarily resident in one area so where a person has two or more places of ordinary residence it will be necessary to determine where he or she has the strongest link for the purpose of liability under the Care Act 2014;[8]
- a period of residence is voluntary, even though the person concerned may have no real choice in the matter;[9]
- however, a person cannot become ordinarily resident in an area where their presence is enforced so that, for example, prisoners do not become ordinarily resident in the area of their incarceration nor mental patients in the area where they are detained in hospital;[10]
- a person will not be able to rely on his or her residence as amounting to ordinary residence unless his or her residence is lawful;[11] in general, it will not be sufficient, either, for residence to be pursuant to a grant of temporary admission;[12]
- when the Secretary of State for Health determines an ordinary residence dispute (now, under section 40 of the Care Act 2014), his or her determination is binding unless and until it is quashed in judicial review proceedings on ordinary public law grounds;[13]
- the courts have sometimes recognised the importance of resolving disputes about local authority responsibility[14] but, also, sometimes

4 *R (Sunderland CC) v SF* [2012] EWCA Civ 1232, [2013] PTSR 549 at para 35.

5 *Mohamed v Hammersmith and Fulham LBC* [2001] UKHL 57, [2002] 1 AC 547 at para 18; *Cornwall* at para 42.

6 *Fox v Stirk* [1970] 2 QB 463 at 476E–F; *R v Barnet LBC ex p Shah* [1983] 2 AC 309 at 342A–C; *Cornwall* at paras 40–42.

7 See *Fox v Stirk* [1970] 2 QB 463 at 476E–F; *Shah* at 343F–H; *Cornwall* at paras 40–42.

8 *R (Sunderland CC) v SF* [2012] EWCA Civ 1232, (2012) 15 CCLR 701 at para 30, and the *Care and Support Statutory Guidance* at paras 19.51–19.53.

9 *R (Sunderland CC) v SF* [2012] EWCA Civ 1232, [2013] PTSR 549 at paras 32–33.

10 See *Shah*, at 343F–H; *Cornwall* at paras 40–42.

11 See *Shah*, at 343H; *R (A) v Secretary of State for Health* [2009] EWCA Civ 225, [2010] 1 WLR 279 at paras 51–62.

12 *R (A) v Secretary of State for Health* [2009] EWCA Civ 225, [2010] 1 WLR 279 at paras 60–62.

13 *R (Greenwich LBC) v Secretary of State for Health* [2006] EWHC 2576 (Admin), (2007) 10 CCLR 80 at para 20.

14 *Cornwall* at para 4 ('It is regrettable that in this way so much public expenditure has been incurred on legal proceedings. However, the amounts involved in caring for PH and others like him are substantial (some £80,000 per year, we were told). The legal issues are of general importance, and far from straightforward').

deprecated such disputes[15] – the court's approach may turn on its perception of the wider implications of the case.

12.7 The test for ascertaining the ordinary residence of adults who possess the capacity to choose where to live has been re-stated by the Supreme Court, in *R (Cornwall Council) v Secretary of State for Health.*[16]

The authorities on 'ordinary residence'

39. At the time of the 1948 Act, most prior case law on the meaning of the expression 'ordinary residence' related to income tax. Liability depended on whether a person was resident or ordinarily resident in the United Kingdom for a particular tax year. In that context it had long been established that a person could be ordinarily resident in two places. This approach was affirmed by the House of Lords in two well known cases reported in 1928: *Levene v Inland Revenue Comrs* [1928] AC 217 and *Inland Revenue Comrs v Lysaght* [1928] AC 234. In an earlier case, *Cooper v Cadwalader* (1904) 5 TC 101, an American resident in New York, who had taken a house in Scotland which he visited for two months each year, was held to be resident and ordinarily resident in the United Kingdom for tax purposes for each such year. It mattered not that for other purposes he might be treated as ordinarily resident in New York. As Viscount Sumner later observed '*Who in New York would have said of Mr Cadwalader 'his home's in the Highlands; his home is not here'?*': *Lysaght*, p244.

40. The House of Lords confirmed that approach and reached the same conclusions on the facts of the two cases in the 1928 reports. Mr Levene lived abroad, but returned each year for about five months for the purpose of obtaining medical advice, visiting relatives and other matters. Mr Lysaght lived in Ireland, but returned to England each month for business purposes, remaining for about a week and usually staying in a hotel. In both cases the special commissioners had been entitled to hold that they were resident and ordinarily resident in this country.

41 Those authorities were followed in the leading modern authority on the meaning of the expression in a statutory context. That is the speech of Lord Scarman in *R v Barnet London Borough Council ex p Nilish Shah* [1983] 2 AC 309. The question was whether four foreign students qualified for an education grant on the basis that they had been '*ordinarily resident*' in the United Kingdom '*throughout*' the three years preceding the first year of their course. The authorities had argued that their ordinary residence, in the sense of their '*real home*', was elsewhere. The House disagreed. Lord Scarman, in the leading speech, treated the tax cases as authority for the '*natural and ordinary meaning*' of the expression. In particular he cited Viscount Sumner's reference to '*ordinary*' residence as '*that part of the regular order of a man's life, adopted voluntarily and for settled purposes ...*': *Lysaght*, p 243. Lord Scarman echoed those words in his own statement of the natural and ordinary meaning of the term, at p 343G–H:

15 *R (Manchester CC) v St Helens BC* [2009] EWCA Civ 1348, (2010) 13 CCLR 48 at para 1 ('As I said in the first sentence of my judgment in litigation closely related to the appeal now before the court (see [2008] EWCA Civ 931), it is not, in my view, satisfactory when two publicly funded public authorities engage in expensive litigation to decide which of them should pay for the care in the home of a woman whose mental and psychological conditions require constant and expensive care. In the end, the money for the care and the money for the litigation is all coming out of the same purse (see also the judgment of Scott Baker LJ to the same effect in paragraph 39 of the report of that case)').

16 [2015] UKSC 46, [2015] 3 WLR 213, (2015) 18 CCLR 497.

> 'Unless, therefore, it can be shown that the statutory framework or the legal context in which the words are used requires a different meaning, I unhesitatingly subscribe to the view that 'ordinarily resident' refers to a man's abode in a particular place or country which he has adopted voluntarily and for settled purposes as part of the regular order of his life for the time being, whether of short or of long duration.'
>
> The 'mind' of the subject was relevant in two respects. First the residence must be 'voluntarily adopted', rather than for example 'enforced presence by reason of kidnapping or imprisonment'. Secondly, there must be 'a degree of settled purpose':
>
> 'This is not to say that the [subject] intends to stay where he is indefinitely; indeed his purpose, while settled, may be for a limited period ... All that is necessary is that the purpose of living where one does has a sufficient degree of continuity to be properly described as settled.': p344D.

A '*settled*' purpose did not need to be indefinite. '*Education, business or profession ... or merely love of a place*' could be enough. There was no justification for substituting a '*real home test*', as the councils had argued: p345B.

42. Although understandably this passage has been often quoted and relied on in later cases, the weight given to the concept of a '*settled purpose*' needs to be seen in context. The focus of the passage was to explain why the undoubted residence of the claimants in this country for the necessary period, albeit for the temporary purpose of education, was sufficiently settled to qualify as '*ordinary*' under the accepted meaning. It was relevant therefore to show that it was no less settled than, for example, the residence of Mr Cadwalader during his annual visit to Scotland, or that of Mr Levene on his five-month visit for medical and other reasons. Nor did it matter, it seems, that they might have had other '*ordinary*' residences in their countries of origin.

12.8 The advice given by the *Care and Support Statutory Guidance*, is:

> 19.15 ... Local authorities should in particular apply the principle that ordinary residence is the place the person has voluntarily adopted for a settled purpose, whether for a short or long duration. Ordinary residence can be acquired as soon as the person moves to an area, if their move is voluntary and for settled purposes, irrespective of whether they own, or have an interest in a property in another local authority area. There is no minimum period in which a person has to be living in a particular place for them to be considered ordinarily resident there, because it depends on the nature and quality of the connection with the new place.

Adults lacking capacity

12.9 Adults who lack capacity cannot be treated as having become ordinarily resident anywhere on the basis of the ordinary test for ordinary residence because, as a result of lacking the capacity to choose where to live, it cannot be said that such adults have 'voluntarily adopted' a place of residence.

12.10 The current test, for adult social care purposes, is in essence the test previously known as '*Vale 2*': a person lacking the capacity to choose where to live will be treated as ordinarily resident in the place where they have lived on a settled basis, as part of the regular order of their life for the time being.[17] This was made clear in the *Cornwall* case:[18]

> 45. Shortly after the Shah judgment, in *R v Waltham Forest London Borough Council ex p Vale* The Times, 25 February 1985, Taylor J had to consider a case much closer to the present, involving the application of the ordinary residence test under the 1948 Act to someone mentally incapable of forming a settled intention where to live. Judith, an English woman, had been in residential care in Ireland for over 20 years where her parents had been living. When her parents returned to England, it was decided that she should return to live near them. She stayed with them at their house in Waltham Forest for a few weeks while a suitable residential home was being found, and she was then placed in a home in Buckinghamshire. The shortfall in costs (so far as not borne by the Department of Health and Social Security) was sought from Waltham Forest on the grounds that she was '*ordinarily resident*' in the borough.
>
> 46. The case was argued and decided by reference to the *Shah* test of ordinary residence, adapted for the case of someone lacking the power to form for herself a settled intention where to live. Taylor J adopted a two-part approach suggested by counsel, but on either approach he considered that her residence with her parents could be treated as sufficiently settled to satisfy the *Shah* test. The result is unremarkable, but in view of the weight later given (particularly in the Secretary of State's guidance) to '*Vale tests 1 and 2*', it is right to quote the judge's own words. For the first approach he made reference to Lord Denning MR's concept of a child's '*base*':
>
>> 'Where the (subject) ... is so mentally handicapped as to be totally dependent upon a parent or guardian, the concept of her having an independent ordinary residence of her own which she has adopted voluntarily and for which she has a settled purpose does not arise. She is in the same position as a small child. *Her ordinary residence is that of her parents because that is her 'base'*, to use the word applied by Lord Denning in the infant case cited.' (Emphasis added.)
>
> The alternative approach, considering her as if she were a person of normal mental capacity, led to the same result:
>
>> 'I cannot accept that during the relevant month Judith should be regarded as a squatter in her parents' home. Her residence there had, in my judgment, all the attributes necessary to constitute ordinary residence within Lord Scarman's test, albeit for a short duration.'
>
> 47. There is no reason to quarrel with Taylor J's conclusion on the unusual facts of the case. In circumstances where her only previous residence had been in Ireland, there was obvious sense in treating her few weeks living with her parents as sufficiently settled to meet the *Shah* test, whether by reference to the intentions of those making decisions on her behalf, or to the '*attributes*' of the residence objectively viewed. With hindsight, it was perhaps unhelpful to elide the *Shah* test with the idea of a '*base*', used by

17 It can be relevant to whether or not the person lacking capacity has lived in a particular place on a settled basis that the person has lived there with parents, guardians or carers.

18 Although see *Milton Keynes Council v Scottish Ministers* [2015] CSOH 156, where Lord Armstrong held that an adult lacking capacity remained ordinarily resident in Milton Keynes despite having lived in a care home near Edinburgh under private arrangements for about six years, on the basis that the adult had chosen to live in Milton Keynes but had not chosen to move to Scotland, having simply been driven there by her mother.

Lord Denning MR in a different context and for a different purpose. The italicised words in the first passage quoted above cannot be read as supporting any more general proposition than that Judith's ordinary residence was to be equated with that of her parents, without reference to the period of her own actual residence with them. Nor in my view should Taylor J's two approaches be treated as separate legal tests. Rather they were complementary, common-sense approaches to the application of the *Shah* test to a person unable to make decisions for herself; that is, to the single question whether her period of actual residence with her parents was sufficiently '*settled*' to amount to ordinary residence

...

Ordinary residence in the present case

49. I agree with the Court of Appeal that the decision-maker's reasons for selecting Cornwall cannot be supported. The writer started, not from an assessment of the duration and quality of PH's actual residence in any of the competing areas, but from an attempt to ascertain his '*base*', by reference to his relationships with those concerned. Thus in deciding that the family home in Cornwall could properly be described '*as a 'base' for [PH]*' notwithstanding the infrequency of his visits, the determination stated that it was necessary to consider '*not merely the number or frequency of visits [but] ... the entirety of the relationship between [PH] and his parents ...*'. There is no suggestion that his brief periods of staying with his parents at holiday times could in themselves amount to ordinary residence.

Ordinary residence and statutory policy

12.11 In the *Cornwall* case,[19] the Supreme Court went on to decide that the policy of both the Children Act 1989 and the National Assistance Act 1948 was to leave the ordinary residence of a person provided by an authority with accommodation under the Children Act 1989 unaffected by the location of the placement, so as to prevent the authority exporting its responsibilities elsewhere, after the child turned 18 and responsibility under the Children Act 1989 ceased. Accordingly, in that case, P was treated as having remained ordinarily resident in the area of Wiltshire Council, which had placed P in South Gloucestershire under the Children Act 1989, where P had remained until he reached the age of 18, even though his parents (with whom he had lived in Wiltshire) had, in the interim, moved to live in Cornwall.

12.12 This aspect of the *Cornwall* case will continue to have effect in relation to existing cases under the previous regime and it will presumably continue to have effect in relation to new disputes about ordinary residence under the Care Act 2014 even though, as will be seen below, the Care Act 2014 sets out an even more comprehensive system of statutory disregards than before, into which it would seem even more difficult to imply additional disregards: the Supreme Court made express reference to the Care Act 2014 and was plainly aware of its provisions ie the decision cannot be said to be have been *per incuriam* the Care Act 2014. Accordingly, one should probably treat it as being implicit in the Children Act 1989 and the Care Act 2014 that a child placed by local authority A in the area of local

19 *R (Cornwall Council) v Secretary of State for Health* [2015] UKSC 46, [2015] 3 WLR 213, (2015) 18 CCLR 497.

authority B must be treated as remaining ordinarily resident in the area of local authority A for the purposes of responsibility under the Care Act 2014.

Statutory machinery

12.13 The current statutory machinery is found at:

- sections 39–41 of the Care Act 2014;
- the Care and Support (Ordinary Residence)(Specified Accommodation) Regulations 2014;
- the Care and Support (Disputes Between Local Authorities) Regulations 2014;
- articles 5 and 6 of the Care Act (Transitional Provision) Order 2015;
- the *Care and Support Statutory Guidance*, at Chapter 19 and Annex H;
- the Care and Support (Ordinary Residence) (Specified Accommodation) (Wales) Regulations 2015;
- the Care and Support (Disputes about Ordinary Residence, etc) (Wales) Regulations 2015.

12.14 It may also be useful to refer to the NHS guidance, *Who Pays: Determining responsibility for payments to providers* (August 2013).[20]

The deeming provisions

12.15 Section 39 of the Care Act 2014, read together with the Care and Support (Ordinary Residence) (Specified Accommodation) Regulations 2014,[21] sets out the statutory deeming provisions, whereby a person accommodated in the area of local authority B will be deemed to be ordinarily resident in the area of local authority A.

First deeming provision

12.16 It had been a feature of adult social care, in recent years, that after local authority A placed an adult in care home accommodation in local authority B, and that care home accommodation de-registered and became supported housing, or the adult moved out of the care home and into supported housing, or any form of housing, in the area of local authority B, responsibility shifted to local authority B.

12.17 The Care Act 2014 reverses that: responsibility in such cases, and in similar cases, will now remain with local authority A.

12.18 An adult resident in the area of local authority B must be treated for the purposes of Part 1 of the Care Act 2014 as being ordinarily resident in the area of local authority A if:

- The adult has needs for care and support which 'are only able to be met' if the adult is living in 'specified accommodation': a care home, in shared lives accommodation or in supported living accommodation;

20 www.england.nhs.uk/wp-content/uploads/2014/05/who-pays.pdf.
21 SI No 2828.

- the adult is living in such accommodation in England (or has lived in a series of such accommodations);
- he or she was ordinarily resident in local authority A immediately before going to live in 'specified accommodation', so long as he or she lives continuously in one or more kinds of 'specified accommodation';
- or, not having a settled residence, was present in local authority A immediately before going to live in 'specified accommodation', so long as he or she lives continuously in one or more kinds of 'specified accommodation':

see sections 39(1)–(3) of the Care Act 2014 and regulations 3–5 of the Care and Support (Ordinary Residence) (Specified Accommodation) Regulations 2014.

12.19 Important advice is provided by the *Care and Support Statutory Guidance*:

> 19.30 Need should be judged to be 'able to be met' or of a kind that 'can be met only' through a specified type of accommodation where the local authority has made this decision following an assessment and a care and support planning process involving the person. Decisions on how needs are to be met, made in the latter process and recorded in the care and support plan, should evidence that needs can only be met in that manner. Where the outcome of the care planning process is a decision to meet needs in one of the specified types of accommodation and it is the local authority's view it should be assumed that needs can only be met in that type of accommodation for the purposes of 'deeming' ordinary residence. This should be clearly recorded in the care and support plan. The local authority is not required to demonstrate that needs cannot be met by any other type of support. The local authority must have assessed those needs in order to make such a decision – the 'deeming' principle therefore does not apply to cases where a person arranges their own accommodation and the local authority does not meet their needs.
>
> ...
>
> 19.34 The ordinary residence 'deeming' principle applies most commonly where the local authority provides or arranges care and support in the accommodation directly. However, the principle also applies where a person takes a direct payment and arranges their own care (since the local authority is still meeting their needs). In such cases, the individual has the choice over how their needs are met, and arranges their own care and support. If the care plan stipulates that person's needs can be met only if the adult is living in one of the specified types of accommodation and the person chooses to arrange that accommodation in the area of a local authority which is not the one making the direct payments then the same principle would apply; the local authority which is meeting the person's care and support needs by making direct payments would retain responsibility. However, if the person chose accommodation that is outside what was specified in the care plan or of a type of accommodation not specified in the regulations, then the 'deeming' principle would not apply.

Second deeming provision

12.20 An adult who is being provided with accommodation as an after-care service under section 117 of the Mental Health Act 1983 must be treated for the purposes of Part 1 of the Care Act 2014 as being ordinarily resident in the area of the local authority with responsibility for providing them with after-care services: section 39(4) of the Care Act 2014.

12.21 Under section 117(3) of the Mental Health Act 1983, the local authority responsible for providing after-care services is the local authority for the area where the patient was ordinarily resident before his detention or, if he the patient had no settled residence, where the patient was present before his detention, or (if that cannot be established) the area where he is sent on discharge: see para 19.112.

Third deeming provision

12.22 An adult provided with 'NHS accommodation' must be treated for the purposes of Part 1 of the Care Act 2014 as ordinarily resident in the area where he was ordinarily resident before the accommodation was provided or, if he had no settled residence, in the area where he was present: section 39(5) of the Care Act 2014.

12.23 'NHS accommodation' is accommodation under the National Health Service Act 2006, the National Health Service (Wales) Act 2006, the National Health Service (Scotland) Act 1978 or article 5(1) of the Health and Personal Social Services (Northern Ireland) Order 1972: section 39(6) of the Care Act 2014.

Fourth deeming provision: prisoners and other persons subject to criminal law

12.24 By virtue of section 76(1)–(3) of the Care Act 2014:

- prisoners detained in prison;
- adults residing in approved premises; and
- adults residing in any other premises because of a requirement imposed as a condition of a grant of bail in criminal proceedings –

are to be treated for the purposes of Part 1 of the Care Act 2014 (all the 'care and support' provisions) as being ordinarily resident in the area of their prison/approved premises/bail accommodation.

12.25 This plainly requires prisoners (etc) to be treated as being ordinarily resident in their area of their prison (etc), so that the local authority for that area must be treated as being responsible for addressing their needs for care and support, whilst they remain so resident.

12.26 This does not entail, however, that the prisoner (etc) must be treated as continuing to be ordinarily resident in the area of their prison (etc) on release, as the *Care and Support Statutory Guidance* explains, at paragraphs 17.48–17.51. The advice given here is that:

- where the prisoner (etc) requires a type of accommodation specified under section 39 of the Care Act 2014, the presumption should be that they remain ordinarily resident in the area where they were ordinarily resident before their sentence;
- otherwise, each case must considered on an individual basis, bearing in mind that it may not be possible for some prisoners to return to their previous area of ordinary residence;
- the local authority where a prisoner (etc) with care needs intends to move should take responsibility for the assessment of need;

- there should be early involvement of all relevant agencies in release planning to minimise the scope for disagreements and ensuing difficulties.

Fifth (non-statutory) deeming provision

12.27 The Care Act 2014 does not require a person to be treated as being ordinarily resident, for the purposes of Part 1, in the area of the local authority that placed the person in local authority B under the Children Act 1989.

12.28 However, the effect of the *Cornnwall* case[22] was to create such an implied deeming provision, arising under the then statutory machinery, by way of judicial reasoning that on any view came very close to judicial legislation (and *was* judicial legislation, according to the dissenting judgment of Lord Wilson JSC). One can only imagine that the Supreme Court will stick to its guns on that issue, notwithstanding the changed legislative context, but it would certainly be convenient if legislation were to put the matter beyond doubt.

12.29 The Secretary of State is considering the policy implications of the *Cornwall* case and will publish revised statutory guidance taking it into account, in due course.[23]

Transitional provisions and the earlier regime

12.30 This is dealt with in article 6 of the Care Act 2014 (Transitional Provision) Order 2015.

12.31 Article 6(2) of the Order provides that section 39 of the Care Act 2014 does not have effect in relation to a person who was being provided with non-hospital NHS accommodation, shared lives scheme accommodation or supported living accommodation 'before the relevant date in relation to that person'. Such persons will not, therefore, be deemed to be ordinarily resident in the area of the placing authority, as a result of section 39 coming into force, but will remain ordinarily resident in the area of the receiving authority.

12.32 Article 6(1) of the Order provides that a person who was deemed to be ordinarily resident in a local authority area, by virtue of section 24(4) or (6) of the National Assistance Act 1948, 'immediately before the relevant date in relation to that person', is to be treated as being ordinarily resident in that area for the purposes of Part 1 of the Care Act 2014. Thus persons placed in 'NHS accommodation', as defined, will remain deemed to be ordinarily resident in the area where they were resident before the placement; and persons provided with residential accommodation by a local authority, with the consent of the local authority of ordinary residence, will remain deemed to be ordinarily resident in that area.

12.33 The 'relevant date' in relation to a person has to assessed using articles 1 and 2 of the Order. The 'relevant date' will be:

22 *R (Cornwall Council) v Secretary of State for Health* [2015] UKSC 46, [2015] 3 WLR 213, (2015) 18 CCLR 497.

23 www.gov.uk/government/publications/ordinary-residence-disputes-supreme-court-judgment.

- 1 April 2015, in relation to persons not in receipt of support or services, or payments towards such (articles 1 and 2(1));
- the date that the local authority has completed a review of the needs of a person who was in receipt of support or services, or payments towards such, on the 1 April 2015 (articles 1 and 2(2));
- 1 April 2016, in the case of a person who was in receipt of support or services, or payments towards such, on the 1 April 2015, but whose case was not reviewed by the 1 April 2016 (articles 1 and 2(3)).

Annex H of the *Care and Support Statutory Guidance*

12.34 Annex H contains advice and practical examples of how to apply the ordinary residence test and the deeming machinery in a number of typical situations:

- H1–7: local authorities are entitled to meet urgent needs irrespective of ordinary residence;
- H8–13: the local authority of ordinary residence is responsible for deferred payment agreements and remains responsible (despite any changes of ordinary residence) until the agreement is concluded;
- H14–20: the local authority of ordinary residence is responsible for a care home placement during the 12-week property disregard period but if, after that, the adult becomes a self-funder in a different local authority area, then his or her place of ordinary residence is likely to change;
- H21–23: those who fund and manage their own care placement will likely become ordinarily resident in the area where they choose to live but self-funders whose accommodation is arranged for them by their local authority of ordinary residence will be deemed to remain ordinarily resident in that area;
- H24–30: persons accommodated under NHS Continuing Healthcare remain ordinarily resident in the area where they were ordinarily resident before, or present (if they were not settled anywhere);
- H31–34: British citizens resuming permanent residence in England after a period abroad will usually acquire an ordinary residence straight away in the place where they are living for settled purposes and intend to remain; otherwise they may have no settled residence, or have urgent needs;
- H35–37: the same applies to veterans leaving the armed forces and their families;
- H38–39: young people in transition for children's services to adult care and support (but see now, also, the *Cornwall* case);
- H40–45: care leavers and the 1989 Act;
- H46–50: provides advice about ordinary residence disputes in the context of delayed hospital discharges;
- H51–63: provides advice about ordinary residence disputes in the context of Deprivation of Liberty Safeguards under the Mental Capacity Act 2005.

Dispute resolution

12.35 Any disputes about where an adult is ordinarily resident for the purposes of Part 1 of the Care Act 2014 are to be determined by the Secretary of State or a person appointed by the Secretary of State, subject to any review by the Secretary of State, or appointed person (undertaken within three months): section 40. By virtue of article 5 of the Care Act 2014 (Transitional Provision) Order 2015, the Secretary of State will determine all ordinary residence disputes, that are to be determined on or after the 1 April 2015, under section 40 of the Care Act 2014, even if they relate to disputes under the previous regime (usually, under section 24 of the National Assistance Act 1948).

12.36 Further detail is contained in the Care and Support (Disputes between Local Authorities) Regulations 2014:[24]

- the needs of the individual must be met by the local authority meeting needs at the time of the dispute or, if there is no such authority, the local authority where the individual is living, or present (reg 2);
- all relevant local authorities must be identified, must share information and seek to resolve the dispute and co-operate (reg 3);
- if the dispute cannot be resolved, it must be referred to the Secretary of State in accordance with a range of procedural requirements (reg 4):

Referral: disputes about ordinary residence or continuity of care

4(1) The referral must include the following documents–
(a) a letter signed by the lead authority in relation to the dispute, stating that the dispute is being referred;
(b) a statement of facts signed on behalf of each of the authorities which includes the information specified in paragraph (2); and
(c) copies of all correspondence between the authorities which relates to the dispute.

(2) The specified information is–
(a) an explanation of the nature of the dispute;
(b) a chronology of the events leading up to the referral of the dispute, including the date on which the dispute arose;
(c) details of the needs of the adult ('the relevant adult') or carer to whom the dispute relates from the beginning of the period to which the dispute relates;
(d) a statement as to which local authority has met those needs since then, how those needs have been met and the statutory provisions under which they have been met;
(e) details of the relevant adult's place of residence, and of any former places of residence which are relevant to the dispute;
(f) where the person to whom the dispute relates is a carer, details of the place of residence of the adult needing care, and of any former places of residence that are relevant to the dispute;
(g) in a case where the relevant adult's capacity to decide where to live is relevant to the dispute, either–
(i) a statement that the authorities agree that the adult has, or lacks, such capacity; or
(ii) information which appears to any of the authorities to be relevant to the question of whether the adult has, or lacks, such capacity;

24 SI No 2829.

(h) a statement as to any other steps taken by the authorities in relation to the relevant adult or carer which may be relevant to the dispute;
(i) details of the steps that the authorities have taken to resolve the dispute between themselves; and
(j) any other information which appears to any of the authorities to be relevant to the determination of the dispute.

(3) The authorities must submit any legal arguments they rely on in relation to the dispute within 14 days of the date on which the dispute is referred.
(4) If a local authority submits legal arguments, it must–
(a) send a copy of those arguments to the other authorities; and
(b) provide evidence to the appropriate person that it has done so.
(5) If the appropriate person asks any of the authorities to provide further information, the local authority to which the request is made must comply without delay.

12.37 The Secretary of State has published anonymised ordinary residence determinations on the internet, which allows one to get a feel as to how such determinations are reached and as to the matters that the Secretary of State has already decided.[25]

Financial adjustments

12.38 By virtue of section 41 of the Care Act 2014, local authority is entitled in certain circumstances to recover the cost of providing care and support, or support, from local authority B. Those circumstances are where:

- local authority A was providing care and support, or support, to X under section 18 or 20(1) of the Care Act 2014 (services provided under section 19 or 20(6) being disregarded for these purposes);
- it then transpires (whether or not because of a determination under section 40) that X was ordinarily resident in local authority B;
- local authority A agrees to assign its rights under any deferred payment agreement to local authority B.

12.39 Paragraphs 19.70–19.71 of Chapter 19 of the *Care and Support Statutory Guidance* apply.

Cross-border placements and disputes

12.40 Section 39(8), Schedule 1 to the Care Act 2014 and the Care and Support (Cross-border Placements and Business Failure: Temporary Duty)(Dispute Resolution) Regulations 2014 essentially replicate the scheme described above, so that it applies as between local authorities in England, Wales and Scotland and Health and Social Care trusts in Northern Ireland. Accordingly, in outline:

- persons placed by an English local authority in accommodation in Wales are to be treated as remaining ordinarily resident in the area of the English local authority (and so on) (Sch 1 paras 1–4) and NHS accommodation does not affect that (Sch 1 para 8);

25 www.gov.uk/government/collections/ordinary-residence-pages.

- disputes are to be determined by the relevant Secretary of State, as specified in Sch 1 para 5 and reg 2 of the Regulations), broadly in the same manner as in the case of purely English disputes (see regs 4–8);
- where an authority in one jurisdiction has provided care and support, or support, to a person whom it transpires was resident in another jurisdiction, they are entitled to reimbursement from the local authority of ordinary residence in that other jurisdiction (Sch 1 paras 6 and 7).

12.41 The *Care and Support Statutory Guidance* at Chapter 21 applies, disputes being addressed at paragraph 21.58 onwards.

12.42 Provision is made for resolving disputes about responsibility for the provision of mental health after-care between English and Welsh authorities.[26]

12.43 The Scottish government has published a suite of guidance on ordinary residence and cross-border disputes.[27]

12.44 The Welsh government has also published relevant guidance.[28]

Cases

Social care

12.45 ### *R (Greenwich LBC) v Secretary of State for Health* [2006] EWHC 2576 (Admin), (2007) 10 CCLR 80

A self-funder who moves voluntarily into care home accommodation in another area becomes ordinarily resident there

Facts: Mrs D was a self-funding care home resident in Bexley. Following an assessment by Bexley, that she needed nursing care, she moved to a nursing home in Greenwich, again on a self-funding basis. Mrs D then became entitled to local authority residential accommodation and Greenwich and Bexley disputed liability. The Secretary of State determined that Greenwich was liable, on the basis that Mrs D had been ordinarily resident in Greenwich at the time her entitlement arose, the 29 June 2002. Greenwich sought a judicial review.

Judgment: Charles J held that where a local authority had been under a duty to make a placement under section 21 of the National Assistance Act 1948 but had not done so, then for the purpose of determining ordinary residence, they would be treated as if they had done so. However, in this case, Mrs D's family had chosen to place her in Greenwich in circumstances where Bexley had not been in breach of statutory duty. Accordingly, it had been lawful for the Secretary of State to conclude that she had become ordinarily resident in Greenwich.

26 www.gov.uk/government/uploads/system/uploads/attachment_data/file/416555/MH_aftercare.pdf.

27 www.gov.scot/Topics/Health/Support-Social-Care/Financial-Help/OrdinaryResidence.

28 At http://gov.wales/topics/health/publications/socialcare/guidance1/woc4193/?lang=en and at http://gov.wales/topics/health/publicationffls/socialcare/guidance1/cross-border/?lang=en.

Comment: the logic of this decision appears to apply under the Care Act 2014 provisions, as does Charles J's two observations:

- that provided the Secretary of State/appointed decision-maker applies the right criteria, then any evaluative decision is theirs to make, subject only to *Wednesbury*, a point confirmed in the *Cornwall* case, at para 43:

  'However, it is common ground as I understand it that in the present context, once properly construed, the issue for the Secretary of State was one of factual judgement rather than executive discretion, and that his decision is 'justiciable', in the sense that it is reviewable by the courts on ordinary *Wednesbury* principles: see *Associated Provincial Picture Houses Ltd v Wednesbury Corp* [1948] 1 KB 223 ';

- if a local authority fails to make the arrangements that it ought to have made under the legislation, that would have resulted in the individual being treated as remaining ordinarily resident in its area, then deeming provisions should be applied on that basis.

12.46 *R (Mani and others) v Lambeth LBC and another* [2002] EWHC 735 (Admin), (2002) 5 CCLR 486

Residence in an area, albeit on a 'no choice' basis, could result in ordinary residence

Facts: Mr Mani and Mr Tasci had limited mobility as a result of physical disability and Mr J was seriously ill as a result of advanced HIV+: all three needed help with domestic tasks and were destitute asylum-seekers.

Judgment: Wilson H held that the claimants were entitled to residential accommodation. On the issue of where they were ordinarily resident, Wilson J held that a substantial period of residence in Lambeth, albeit pursuant to a 'no choice' placement there by the National Asylum Support Service, was sufficient to lead to ordinary residence:

> 33. The third and final question, posed in para 3 above, requires attention to the approvals and directions in LAC(93)10, referred to in para 5 above. They identify the local authority upon which in a particular case the powers and duties under section 21 are conferred and cast. The effect of the directions (which create the duties) is, insofar as is relevant, that a local authority must provide residential accommodation under section 21 to:
>
> (a) a person who is ordinarily resident in its area (paragraph 2(1)(b)); and
> (b) a person who is in urgent need thereof (paragraph 2(1)(b)); and
> (c) a person with no settled residence who is in its area and who is or has been suffering from mental disorder (paragraph 2(3)(a)).
>
> Lambeth contends that Mr Mani falls within none of those categories; he contends that, as it happens, he falls within all of them.
>
> 34. An initial issue, not fully argued, relates to the date at which Mr Mani's circumstances must satisfy one of the three criteria. Mr Giffin suggests that it is the date of Mr Mani's issue of these proceedings: with respect, that seems wholly illogical in circumstances where the focus is upon the legality of a prior decision. Mr Seddon contends that the choice is between the date of Mr Mani's application to Lambeth or the date of its rejection. Although in my view the outcome is the same, I confidently choose the latter. In *Mohamed v Hammersmith and Fulham LBC* [2001] 3 WLR 1339 Lord Slynn of Hadley, at paragraph 23, held that, when a local authority was required to consider whether an applicant for housing under the Housing Act 1996

had a local connection, it should consider the circumstances existing at the date of its decision (or later review) ...

36. In the *Mohamed* case the applicant had lived in Hammersmith for six months prior to its initial decision that he had no local connection and for a further two months prior to its review, which was to the same effect. For all but the first three months of that period he had lived in interim accommodation provided by Hammersmith pending the decision. It was held that, certainly by the time of the review and (as I infer) even by the time of the initial decision, the applicant had acquired a local connection. In paragraph 17 Lord Slynn equated normal residence with ordinary residence and cited *R v Barnet LBC ex p Shah* [1983] 2 AC 309 for the proposition, upon which Mr Giffin relies, that ordinary residence has to be an abode adopted not only voluntarily but 'for settled purposes as part of the regular order of his life for the time being, whether of short or of long duration'. Then, in paragraph 18, Lord Slynn continued:

> 'It is clear that words like 'ordinary residence' and 'normal residence' may take their precise meaning from the context of the legislation in which they appear but it seems to me that the prima facie meaning of normal residence is a place where at the relevant time the person in fact resides. That therefore is the question to be asked and it is not appropriate to consider whether in a general or abstract sense such a place would be considered an ordinary or normal residence. So long as that place where he eats and sleeps is voluntarily accepted by him, the reason why he is there rather than somewhere else does not prevent that place from being his normal residence. He may not like it, he may prefer some other place, but that place is for the relevant time the place where he normally resides. If a person, having no other accommodation, takes his few belongings and moves into a barn for a period to work on a farm that is where during that period he is normally resident, however much he might prefer some more permanent or better accommodation. In a sense it is 'shelter' but it is also where he resides. Where he is given interim accommodation by a local housing authority even more clearly is that the place where for the time being he is normally resident. The fact that it is provided subject to statutory duty does not, contrary to the appellant authority's argument, prevent it from being such.'

37. By 25 and 27 April 2001, when Lambeth interviewed him and decided to reject his application, Mr Mani had been living continuously in its area for almost six months. Mr Giffin concedes that, on Lord Slynn's analysis, his adoption of residence there was sufficiently voluntary. I hold that its purposes were also sufficiently settled, Eurotower being the compass of the regular order of his life during that period. He was ordinarily resident in Lambeth for the purpose of the first criterion.

38. Had I reached a contrary conclusion, I would have proceeded to hold that the third criterion had been satisfied in that Mr Mani had no settled residence, was in the area of Lambeth and had been suffering from mental disorder. I will say nothing about the second criterion, which raises the question whether the compulsory disregard of asylum support extends to the determination for which it calls.

Comment: it seems likely that the same result will follow under the Care Act 2014, this line of authority remaining a useful gloss on the scope of 'voluntary' residence.

12.47 *R (Manchester CC) v St Helens BC* [2009] EWCA Civ 1348, (2010) 13 CCLR 48

Having provided supported housing and care in the area of local authority A, local authority B was entitled to transfer responsibility to local authority A on it becoming clear that X had become ordinarily resident there

Facts: St Helens provided a very expensive care package to PE, within its area. PE then moved to the Manchester area and St Helens assessed PE as requiring supported housing in Manchester with, again, a very expensive, and unusual, care package which it arranged, funded and supervised. After a period of time St Helens sought to shift responsibility to Manchester. St Helens obtained a determination from the Secretary of State that PE had become ordinarily resident in Manchester and, on that basis, determined to bring its provision for PE to an end. Manchester sought a judicial review of that decision, on the basis that having set up PE's care package in the Manchester area, St Helens owed a continuing duty to make such provision for PE.

Judgment: a local authority had a power to provide services outside of its area, under section 29 of the National Assistance Act 1948, but was entitled to cease provision, subject to normal considerations of rationality, abuse of power or legitimate expectation. In this case, the Secretary of State's ordinary residence termination was a rational basis for terminating provision, including because section 29 imposed a statutory duty on Manchester. It would be an 'abuse' to 'dump' service users in other areas, but that had not occurred here.

Comment: under the new statutory scheme, this case would be decided differently, in that because of the 'first deeming provision' (see above para 12.16), St Helens would continue to be responsible. Potentially, St Helens might also now be regarded as continuing to be responsible under the *Cornwall* principle,[29] although the original placement was not under the Children Act 1989.

12.48 *R (Kent County Council) v Secretary of State for Health* [2015] EWCA Civ 81, (2015) 18 CCLR 153

Statutory deeming provisions were not retrospective

Facts: NA was living in residential accommodation in Kent, funded by the NHS, until NHS funding was withdrawn and he became entitled to provision under section 21 of the National Assistance Act (NAA) 1948. Kent accepted that NA had been ordinarily resident in its area when he became entitled to provision under section 21, but disputed the Secretary of State for Health's determination that Kent was responsible for such provision.

Judgment: the Court of Appeal (Lord Dyson MR, Tomlinson and Burnett LJJ) held that on the literal and plain meaning of section 24(5) of the NAA 1948, NA had been ordinarily resident in Kent immediately before he became entitled to provision under NAA 1948 s21, accordingly Kent was

29 *R (Cornwall Council) v Secretary of State for Health* [2015] UKSC 46, [2015] 3 WLR 213, (2015) 18 CCLR 497.

liable. It was only later that the NAA 1948 was amended so as to disregard certain periods of time spent in NHS accommodation for these purposes. If such a disregard had already been implicit in the statutory scheme, then Parliament need not have troubled to introduce it: accordingly, it had not been implicit in the statutory scheme before the scheme was expressly amended.

Comment: again, under the new statutory scheme, this case would be decided differently, in that because of the 'third deeming provision' (see above para 12.22), the local authority that had placed NA in Kent would continue to be responsible. Potentially, that authority might also now be regarded as continuing to be responsible under the *Cornwall* principle.[30]

12.49 *R (Cornwall Council) v Secretary of State for Health* [2015] UKSC 46, [2015] 3 WLR 213, (2015) 18 CCLR 497

Clarifying the ordinary residence test and how it applied

Facts: P lived in Wiltshire cared for by his parents until Wiltshire Council placed him with long-term foster carers in South Gloucestershire, under the Children Act 1989. P remained living in South Gloucestershire with his foster carers until after he reached 18, at which time he was placed in Somerset, under the National Assistance Act 1948. In the interim, P's parents had moved to Cornwall, where P occasionally visited them. The Secretary of State determined that Cornwall was responsible under the NAA 1948 because his parents' home was P's '*base*'. Cornwall appealed. The Court of Appeal held that P had become ordinarily resident in South Gloucestershire as a matter of fact and that no deeming provision required that P be treated as being ordinarily resident anywhere else.

Judgment: the Supreme Court (Hale, Carnwath, Hughes and Toulson JJSC; Wilson JSC dissenting) held that P must be treated as remaining ordinarily resident in the Wiltshire area. Although, applying the correct legal test, P might appear to have become ordinarily resident in Gloucestershire as a matter of fact, the policy of the legislation required one to deem him as remaining ordinarily resident in the area of the original placing authority, Wiltshire.

As to the correct legal test, a person with capacity to choose where to live was ordinarily resident in the place he had gone to live voluntarily, lawfully and for settled purposes as part of the regular order of his life for the time being, whether or short or long duration.

A person without the capacity to choose where to live was ordinarily resident in the place where he had gone to live lawfully and for settled purposes as part of the regular order of his life for the time being, whether or short or long duration.

30 *R (Cornwall Council) v Secretary of State for Health* [2015] UKSC 46, [2015] 3 WLR 213, (2015) 18 CCLR 497.

12.50 *R (Tigere) v Secretary of State for Business, Innovation and Skills* [2015] UKSC 57, [2015] 1 WLR 3820

It was incompatible with Article 2 of the 1st Protocol to the ECHR and Article 14 ECHR to exclude from student loans prospective students who had not clocked up three years of lawful, ordinary residence but who had lived in the UK for most of their lives, had been educated here, could not be removed save for grave misconduct and were treated throughout as members of UK society; but the ordinary residence test was lawful

Facts: Ms Tigere was excluded from a student loan because she had not clocked up three years' lawful, ordinary residence in the UK, despite the fact that she had lived in the UK for many years and been educated in England throughout her school career, had been granted leave to remain (LTR) with recourse to public funds, would qualify for indefinite leave to remain (ILR) in a few years and had obtained a university place.

Judgment: the Supreme Court (Hale, Kerr and Hughes JJSC, Sumption and Reed JJSC dissenting), held, in passing that

> 45. ...There are indeed strong public policy reasons for insisting that any period of ordinary residence required before a person becomes entitled to public services be lawful ordinary residence.

Comment: a similar approach was taken in *R (YA) v Secretary of State for Health*,[31] but a different approach was taken in the context of last-ditch support for the destitute in *R v Wandsworth LBC ex p O*.[32]

12.51 *Milton Keynes Council v Scottish Ministers* [2015] CSOH 156, 2015 SLT 843

The ordinary residence of a person lacking capacity may not change simply because they go to live elsewhere under private arrangements

Facts: Mrs R had lived in Milton Keynes for many years before a deterioration in her mental and physical health, and loss of mental capacity, caused by dementia. She needed residential care. Her daughter took her by car to Scotland and placed her in a care home near to where the daughter lived, under provide arrangements. About six years later, Mrs R was assessed under section 12A of the Social Work (Scotland) Act 1968 as needing residential accommodation with nursing and a question arose as to whether Milton Keynes or the relevant Scottish local authority, East Lothian Council, was financially responsible, The Scottish Ministers decided that Milton Keynes was responsible, on the basis that Mrs R remained ordinarily resident in Milton Keynes.

Judgment: Lord Armstrong held that the Scottish Ministers' decision was lawful: Mrs R had not voluntarily adopted her new residence in Scotland and her move to Scotland had not been decided upon by a person vested with legal authority to make decisions on her behalf, under the Mental Capacity Act 2005.

31 [2009] EWCA Civ 225, (2009) 12 CCLR 213.

32 [2000] 1 WLR 2539, (2000) 3 CCLR 237.

Mental health

12.52 See chapter 19 at 19.109–19.115 and 19.125–19.127 for the current statutory test and machinery.

12.53 ### *R v Mental Health Review Tribunal, Torfaen County BC and Gwent Health Authority ex p Hall* (1999) 2 CCLR 361

The health and social care authorities responsible for after-care were those for the area where the patient had been resident before their detention or, if the patient had no ordinary residence, the responsible authorities are those for the area to where the patient is sent

Facts: the Mental Health Review Tribunal directed that Mr Hall be released from detention under sections 37 and 41 of the Mental Health Act 1983, on condition that Mr Hall did not live in the Torfaen area, and a prescribed package of care in the community was provided. Torfaen County BC, where Mr Hall had dwelt before he was detained, declined to take responsibility. Gwent was willing to provide psychiatric supervision, but only once it was determined where Mr Hall would live.

Judgment: Scott Baker J held that the health and social care authorities responsible for after-care were those for the area where the patient had been resident before their detention or, if the patient had no ordinary residence, the responsible authorities are those for the area to where the patient is sent: Torfaen and Gwent were in breach of their duty to complete an assessment before the MHRT hearing so as to provide the MHRT with proposals or options as to where Mr Hall should live and what psychiatric supervision was available.

Comment: this case would be decided in the same way under the current machinery.

12.54 ### *R (Hertfordshire CC) v Hammersmith & Fulham LBC* [2011] EWCA Civ 77, (2011) 14 CCLR 224

Statutory deeming provisions only applied for the purposes of the National Assistance Act 1948

Facts: JM had lived in Hammersmith's area for some years but Hammersmith then placed him in Sutton's area, under section 21 of the National Assistance Act 1948. After compulsory admissions to hospital under sections 2 and 3 of the Mental Health Act (MHA) 1983, the question arose as to which authority was responsible for the provision of after-care services under MHA 1983 s117. Hertfordshire claimed that the deeming provision in section 24(5) of the NAA 1948 required JM to be treated as continuing to be ordinarily resident in Hammersmith.

Judgment: the Court of Appeal (Carnwath, Rimer and Sullivan LJJ) held that the deeming provision at NAA 1948 s24(5) only applied for the purposes of the NAA 1948 and not for the purposes of the MHA 1983. Since in actual fact JM had been ordinarily resident in Sutton prior to his sections, Sutton was responsible under MHA 1983 s117. An agreement reached between various groups of local authorities did not give rise to a legitimate expectation that Hammersmith would accept responsibility and, in any event, even if it did, that would not allow statutory responsibility to be avoided.

Comment: On the face of it, this case would be decided in the same way now, unless a purposive construction was applied by analogy with the *Cornwall* decision, so that Hammersmith was treated as continuing to hold responsibility.

12.55 *R (Sunderland CC) v South Tyneside Council, SF and Leeds CC* [2012] EWCA Civ 1232, (2012) 15 CCLR 701

A person could be ordinarily resident in a 'placement' that was, ultimately, voluntarily accepted by them

Facts: there was a dispute over which local authority was responsible for providing after-care services for SF, under section 117 of the Mental Health Act 1983. SF had lived in halls of residence at a college in Sunderland (having been placed there by Leeds) but had then moved voluntarily to reside in a hospital in the South Tyneside area before being detained in hospital.

Judgment: the Court of Appeal (Lloyd, Richards and Elias LJJ) held that South Tyneside was responsible because once Leeds terminated the college placement there was no place that could be regarded as SF's residence, other than the hospital. Ultimately, what was important was the place where a person in fact resided and if that place was, ultimately, voluntarily adopted, the reason why they were there was irrelevant.

Comment: this case would be decided in the same way under the current legislation. It emphasises that, in this context, 'voluntary' simply means 'not under compulsion' rather than 'in the exercise of a positive choice'.

12.56 *R (Wiltshire Council) v Hertfordshire CC* [2014] EWCA Civ 712, (2014) 17 CCLR 258

A conditional discharge does not alter the ordinary residence of a person subject to a hospital order with restrictions

Facts: SQ had a long history of contact with psychiatric services. He lived in the Wiltshire area until 1995 and then was made subject to a hospital order with a restriction order under sections 37 and 41 of the Mental Health Act 1983. He was conditionally discharged in 2009, one of the conditions being that he resided at a hostel in Hertfordshire. He was recalled in 2011 under section 42(3) of the MHA 1983 and detained in a hospital in Hertfordshire and then conditionally discharged again in February 2014 to the same address in Hertfordshire as before. Wiltshire and Hertfordshire disputed which of them was responsible under section 117 of the MHA 1983.

Judgment: the Court of Appeal (Moses and Kitchin LJJ, Bean J) held that Wiltshire was responsible in that SQ had continued throughout to be liable to be detained or recalled so that he had to be treated as remaining ordinarily resident in the area where he was ordinarily resident before the original hospital order.

Part III

CHAPTER 13

Local authorities and tortfeasors

Introduction and statutory machinery

13.1 One might think that any rational system would require tortfeasors (which in practice almost always means their insurers) to reimburse to public authorities the health and social care costs of their victims. However, Parliament has not legislated to this effect and, in part as a result of that, the courts have decided that no such general duty exists.[1]

13.2 One might also think that any rational system would entitle health and social care authorities to charge for the provision of health and social care to victims of torts who have recovered, as part of their damages, an award in respect of private health and social care, if the victim then seeks the same care from the public sector. The courts have not allowed this to be achieved in a direct and simple manner; but they have sanctioned victims of torts recovering the cost of private health and social care provision[2] and have provided a variety of steps aimed at ensuring that the adult victim does not then recover from public authorities free care that corresponds to the care covered by the damages award. The process could, however, be a great deal clearer and easier for public authorities to enforce.

13.3 The NHS Litigation Authority is campaigning for change.[3] Meanwhile the starting point for local authorities is that, by virtue of the Care and Support (Charging and Assessment of Resources) Regulations 2014,[4] they are required to disregard, for the purposes of means-testing, most capital (and any consequential income) that is derived from personal injury awards.[5]

Personal injury trusts and other personal injury payments

13.4 The capital and income from personal injury trusts must always be disregarded; other personal injury payments must sometimes be disregarded for a period of time. Inevitably, therefore, personal injury payments of any great size are usually structured so as to result in the creation of personal injury trusts.

13.5 Paragraphs 15 and 16 of Schedule 2 to the Care and Support (Charging and Assessment of Resources) Regulations 2014 (capital to be disregarded) provide as follows:

> 15 Any amount which would be disregarded under paragraph 12 of Schedule 10 to the *Income Support Regulations* (personal injury trusts).
>
> 16 Any amount which would be disregarded under paragraph 12A of Schedule 10 to *the Income Support Regulations* (personal injury payments) with the exception of any payment or any part of any payment that has been specifically identified by a court to deal with the cost of providing care.

1 *Islington LBC v University College Hospital Trust* [2005] EWCA Civ 596, (2005) 8 CCLR 337.

2 *Peters v East Midlands Strategic Health Authority* [2009] EWCA Civ 145, (2009) 12 CCLR 299.

3 http://www.nhsla.com/aboutus/Documents/Section%202(4)%20-%20Law%20Reform%20(Personal%20Injury)%20Act%201948%20-%20March%202013.pdf.

4 SI No 2672.

5 *Nottinghamshire CC v Bottomley* [2010] EWCA Civ 756.

13.6 Paragraphs 12 and 12A of Schedule 10 to the Income Support (General) Regulations 1987 provide for the following disregards:

12 Where the funds of a trust are derived from a payment made in consequence of any personal injury to the claimant or the claimant's partner, the value of the trust fund and the value of the right to receive any payment under that trust.

12A(1) Any payment made to the claimant or the claimant's partner in consequence of any personal injury to the claimant or, as the case may be, the claimant's partner.

(2) But sub-paragraph (1)–

(a) applies only for the period of 52 weeks beginning with the day on which the claimant first receives any payment in consequence of that personal injury;

(b) does not apply to any subsequent payment made to him in consequence of that injury (whether it is made by the same person or another);

(c) ceases to apply to the payment or any part of the payment from the day on which the claimant no longer possesses it;

(d) does not apply to any payment from a trust where the funds of the trust are derived from a payment made in consequence of any personal injury to the claimant.

(3) For the purposes of sub-paragraph (2)(c), the circumstances in which a claimant no longer possesses a payment or a part of it include where the claimant has used a payment or part of it to purchase an asset.

(4) References in sub-paragraphs (2) and (3) to the claimant are to be construed as including references to his partner (where applicable).

Court administered/controlled funds

13.7 Local authorities must always disregard personal injury awards that are administered by a relevant court or that can only be disposed of with the consent of a relevant court.

13.8 Paragraph 25 of Schedule 2 to the Care and Support (Charging and Assessment of Resources) Regulations 2014, which excludes personal injury damages that are administered by the High Court, county court or Court of Protection, or that can only be disposed of by order or direction of such court:

25 Any amount which–

(a) falls within paragraph 44(2)(a), and would be disregarded under paragraph 44(1)(a) or (b), of Schedule 10 to the Income Support Regulations; or

(b) would be disregarded under paragraph 45(a) of that Schedule.

13.9 Paragraphs 44 and 45 of the Income Support (General) Regulations 1987 provide as follows:

44(1) Any sum of capital to which sub-paragraph (2) applies and–

(a) which is administered on behalf of a person by the High Court or the county court under Rule 21.11(1) of the Civil Procedure Rules 1998 or by the Court of Protection;

(b) which can only be disposed of by order or direction of any such court; or

(c) where the person concerned is under the age of 18, which can only be disposed of by order or direction prior to that person attaining age 18.

(2) This sub-paragraph applies to a sum of capital which is derived from–

(a) an award of damages for a personal injury to that person; or

(b) compensation for the death of one or both parents where the person concerned is under the age of 18.

45\. Any sum of capital administered on behalf of a person in accordance with an order made under section 13 of the Children (Scotland) Act 1995, or under Rule 36.14 of the Ordinary Cause Rules 1993 or under Rule 128 of the Ordinary Cause Rules, where such sum derives from–

(a) an award of damages for a personal injury to that person; or

(b) compensation for the death of one or both parents where the person concerned is under the age of 18.

Income

13.10 The drafting of the Care and Support (Charging and Assessment of Resources) Regulations 2014 is unclear, however, on analysis, similar disregards apply to:

- income derived from court-administered/overseen funds, which are required to be treated as capital (and therefore disregarded by regulation 19(3) of the Care and Support (Charging and Assessment of Resources) Regulations 2014); and
- income derived from personal injury trusts/annuities (see paragraph 15 of Schedule 1 to the Care and Support (Charging and Assessment of Resources) Regulations 2014).

Protecting the local authority/health authority position

13.11 It can be expected that any claimant in line for a very substantial personal injury award will:

- recover damages on the basis that they will pay for private health and social care;
- ensure that the award is structured so that it cannot be taken into account for the purposes of social care means-testing;
- be required to enter into a mechanism that should preclude recourse to state-provided health or social care to the extent covered by the award.

13.12 In cases where local authorities have concerns, they should contact the parties and, if need be, applied to be joined to the proceedings, under CPR Part 20, as in *Peters v East Midlands Strategic Health Authority*,[6] or under CPR 19.2, as occurred and was approved in *Nottinghamshire CC v Bottomley*.[7]

6 [2009] EWCA Civ 145, [2009] 3 WLR 737, (2009) 12 CCLR 229.

7 [2010] EWCA Civ 756.

Cases

13.13 *Islington LBC v University College Hospital Trust* [2005] EWCA Civ 596, (2005) 8 CCLR 337

Tortfeasors do not owe a statutory providers of care a duty of care in negligence

Facts: Mrs J required residential accommodation under section 21 of the National Assistance Act 1948, as a result of the Trust's negligence. The damages paid to Mrs J by the Trust were held in a personal injury trust and Islington was not permitted to take them into account when assessing Mrs J's ability to contribute towards the cost of residential accommodation. Islington sued the Trust for a contribution.

Judgment: the Court of Appeal (Buxton and Clarke LJJ, Ouseley J) held that the Trust had not owed Islington a duty of care. There were strong public policy reasons why not, including the wider implications for other public bodies and the extended duties they may owe, if the Trust owed a duty in this case, and the fact that, in similar situations, Parliament had legislated to impose a duty of care where considered appropriate.

13.14 *Crofton v National Health Service Litigation Authority* [2007] EWCA Civ 71, (2007) 10 CCLR 123

Damages should be reduced where statutory care provision would be made available and where local authorities would be required to disregard damages for means-testing purposes

Facts: the NHS was responsible for severe injuries that C sustained at birth. At the time of trial, C was living in supervised accommodation where care was provided by carers paid by the local authority. The judge at first instance concluded that it was reasonable to assess damages on the basis that C would purchase private sector accommodation and care, in the future. However, he also provided for the damages to be reduced to reflect direct payments towards C's care costs that he considered that the local authority would make, in the future.

Judgment: the Court of Appeal (May, Dyson and Smith LJJ) held that when a local authority decided whether it was necessary for it to make direct payments, under section 2 of the Chronically Sick and Disabled Persons Act 1970 and/or section 29 of the National Assistance Act 1948, it was required to disregard personal injury damages administered by the Court of Protection. Unless it was very unclear whether such direct payments would be received, they should be taken into account in the assessment of damages. In this case, the issue had arisen at the last moment and important pieces of evidence were missing, as to whether the local authority would make direct payments, so the issue would be remitted.

13.15 *Peters v East Midlands Strategic Health Authority and Nottingham City Council* [2009] EWCA Civ 145, (2009) 12 CCLR 299

The victim of a tort was entitled to recover the cost of private health and social care, providing the risk of double recovery could be averted

Facts: Ms Peters was very severely disabled from birth, as a result of the negligence of her doctors. The question arose as to whether the amount of damages should be reduced to reflect Nottingham's statutory responsibility to provide Ms Peters with residential accommodation and care.

Judgment: the Court of Appeal (Sir Anthony Clarke MR, May and Dyson LJJ) held that whilst Nottingham was required to disregard all personal injury damages in determining whether it was under a statutory duty, there was no reason why Ms Peters should not recover fully for the cost of private accommodation and care, providing there was no risk of double recovery: that risk could be averted by requiring Ms Peters's deputy to give an undertaking restricting her ability to apply for public assistance.

13.16 *R (Booker) v NHS Oldham* [2010] EWHC 2593 (Admin), (2011) 14 CCLR 315

The NHS had to provide free treatment even if that treatment was covered by a personal injury award

Facts: a personal injury settlement involved a payment of damages to Ms Booker on the basis that a proportion of those damages would be used to fund private medical treatment and that further damages would become payable to the extent that necessary healthcare was not available from the NHS. Learning of this, NHS Oldham indicated that it would cease to continue to provide Ms Booker with such medical treatment as was covered by that aspect of the damages award. Ms Booker sought a judicial review of that decision.

Judgment: Deputy High Court Judge Pelling QC held that NHS Oldham had to continue to provide Ms Booker with (free) NHS treatment:

> In my judgment this reasoning does not lead to the conclusion for which the PCT contends. First, in deciding whether a service is reasonably required or is necessary to meet a reasonable requirement, the PCT is bound to have regard to the duties imposed by section 1 of the 2006 Act – see paragraph 24 to 26 of Lord Woolf's judgment in *Coughlan.* It follows that the PCT must have regard to the target duty to provide a comprehensive service free at the point of delivery. Secondly in reaching a decision the PCT is bound to have regard to the NHS Constitution for the reasons already set out above. It is therefore bound to have regard to the principle that access to NHS services is based on clinical need not on an individual's ability to pay and that a person who is otherwise eligible for treatment is entitled to receive it free of charge. Thirdly in my judgment in reaching a decision in a case such as this, the PCT is bound to have regard to and indeed to carry into effect the policy set out in the national framework document. This document established the national policy to be applied in deciding on eligibility for future healthcare. Paragraph 47 and 49 of the framework document in particular cannot support the notion that a person should not be treated as eligible by reference to the ability of the person concerned to access funding for such care from another source. Indeed, paragraph 49 of the framework

document plainly contradicts such an approach. The reality is that this claimant's need for continuing healthcare will only be removed for so long as a private package has been successfully established and implemented. Unless and until that has occurred, the principle set out in paragraph 47 of the framework document cannot apply.

13.17 *Nottinghamshire CC v Bottomley* [2010] EWCA Civ 756

It was appropriate to join the local authority to personal injury proceedings because the manner in which the award was to be structured would affect it

Facts: the claimant had obtained judgment for damages to be assessed. The local authority sought to be joined to the proceedings as a party.

Judgment: the Court of Appeal (Maurice Kay, Rix and Stanley Burnton LJJ) held that the local authority should be joined because (a) how the award of damage was structured would affect the local authority, in that it would not be able to charge for care if a lump sum award was made (rather than periodical payments); (b) it would be useful for the court to have information about all the various care options and charges; and (c) if a lump sum was awarded to cover private care, the local authority ought to be heard as to whether an undertaking ought to be given and as to its form.

13.18 *R (ZYN) v Walsall MBC* [2014] EWHC 1928 (Admin), (2015) 18 CCLR 579

Funds administered by a deputy had to be disregarded in the same way as funds administered by the Court of Protection itself

Facts: ZYN had received £550,000.00 in settlement of a personal injury claim, settled on the basis that she would not be required to contribute to the cost of her future care. Her receiver, then her deputy, was entitled to withdraw up to £50,000.00 per annum from ZYN's funds, without court approval. The local authority decided that it was entitled to take such sums into account for means-testing purposes on the basis that they were not administered by a court, for the purposes of paragraph 44 of Schedule 10 to the Income Support (General) Regulations 1987, in that the deputy administered funds on behalf of Z, not any court, and was entitled to dispose of £50,000.00 per annum without court sanction.

Judgment: Leggatt J held that the deputy was exercising powers delegated by the court, so that the disregard did apply.

CHAPTER 14

Local authorities and private providers

14.1 Old and new statutory machinery and introduction

Cases

14.17 *R v Cumbria CC ex p Professional Care Ltd* (2000) 3 CCLR 79, QBD
In judicial review proceedings, commercial operators must raise issues of law and not seek to engage in commercial litigation by other means

14.18 *Douce v Staffordshire CC* [2002] EWCA Civ 506, (2002) 5 CCLR 347
A local authority might owe a care home operator a duty of care to avoid pure economic loss

14.19 *R (Birmingham Care Consortium) v Birmingham CC* [2002] EWHC 2188 (Admin), (2002) 5 CCLR 600
Care home providers had not established that the rates on offer were unfair, especially when the local authority was able to secure adequate provision at those rates

14.20 *Hampshire CC v Supportways Community Services Ltd* [2006] EWCA Civ 1035, (2006) 9 CCLR 484
A claim for specific performance of a contract had to fail when the contract had been terminated, lawfully or unlawfully, and public law could not assist the injured party

14.21 *R (Forest Care Home Limited) v Pembrokeshire CC* [2010] EWHC 3514 (Admin), (2011) 14 CCLR 103
The local authority's methodology failed to assess local costs of providing care home accommodation in the way that it had attempted to do. However, it had been lawful for the local authority to prevent care home owners charging top ups

14.22 *Amberley (UK) Ltd v West Sussex CC* [2011] EWCA Civ 11, (2011) 14 CCLR 178
A contractual entitlement to a review of costs did not authorise a unilateral increase

14.23 *R (Broadway Care Centre Ltd) v Caerphilly CBC* [2012] EWHC 37 (Admin), (2012) 15 CCLR 82
Termination of a framework agreement for care home placements was governed solely by private law

14.24 *R (Mavalon Care Ltd) v Pembrokeshire CC* [2011] EWHC 3371 (Admin), (2012) 15 CCLR 229
An irrational failure to comply with the methodology adopted meant that the local authority had failed to have regard to the actual cost of care locally

continued

14.25 *R (Bevan & Clarke Ltd) v Neath Port Talbot CBC* [2012] EWHC 236 (Admin), (2012) 15 CCLR 294

Decisions about what standard rates to pay were, at least in Wales, public law decisions

14.26 *R (Davis) v West Sussex CC* [2012] EWHC 2152 (Admin)

A complaint about the way a local authority investigated abuse allegations involved contractual provisions but was sufficiently public to permit judicial review, in that the allegations would have been investigated irrespective of the existence of the contract

14.27 *R (South West Care Homes Ltd) v Devon CC* [2012] EWHC 1867 (Admin)

A local authority has a broad discretion when assessing the usual cost of providing care locally

14.28 *R (South West Care Homes Ltd) v Devon CC* [2012] EWHC 2967 (Admin)

A local authority deciding what standard rates to pay for care home placements had to discharge the PSED, which this authority had not done

14.29 *R (Members of the Committee of Care North East Northumberland) v Northumberland CC* [2013] EWCA Civ 1740, (2014) 17 CCLR 117

Local authorities are entitled to choose how to assess local care costs and what level of enquiry to undertake, subject to rationality

14.30 *R (Torbay Quality Care Forum Ltd) v Torbay Council* [2014] EWHC 4321 (Admin)

In this case, the Council's fee-setting had been irrational

14.31 *Abbeyfield Newcastle upon Tyne Society Ltd v Newcastle CC* [2014] EWHC 2437 (Ch), (2014) 17 CCLR 430

Where a framework agreement expired, the local authority had to pay for new placement on a quantum meruit basis, not at the old rates

14.32 *Carewatch Care Services Ltd v Focus Caring Services Ltd* [2014] EWHC 2313 (Ch)

Franchise agreements did not contain an implied term of good faith, preventing the franchisor from developing its own rival business and restrictive covenants, binding on the franchisee, were lawful at common law and did not infringe the Competition Act 1998

14.33 *Menon and Others v Herefordshire Council* [2015] EWHC 2165 (QB)

It was not appropriate to order disclosure of documents containing local authority legal advice, in an action in misfeasance against it

14.34 *R (Forge Care Homes Ltd) v Cardiff & Vale University Health Board* [2016] EWCA Civ 26, (2016) 19 CCLR 62

Local health boards were not required to pay for all the care provided by registered nurses, only for the tasks that only a registered nurse could perform

14.35 *Menon and Others v Herefordshire Council* [2016] EWHC 498 (QB)

On the facts, social workers engaged in terminating the local authority's relationship with a care home had not been guilty of misfeasance in public office

Old and new statutory machinery and introduction

14.1 The major issues that commonly arise in relation to disputes between local authorities and private sector providers are:

- is the dispute purely contractual, or is judicial review permitted? and
- in judicial review proceedings, how intensive should court scrutiny be?

14.2 Where the parties' rights in relation to the issue in dispute are set out in a contract, judicial review will not usually be permitted unless:

- the local authority is also exercising a statutory function that exists independently of the contract; or
- exceptionally, there is a case of fraud, corruption or bad faith.[1]

14.3 It can be entirely appropriate to include complex but precise formulae in contracts but in some cases private providers persuade local authorities to adopt, and in some cases local authorities choose to adopt, complex formulae to guide the discharge of their public law duties, in cases where private providers are involved (for example, to assess how much to pay private providers). Even in public law cases, private providers do sometimes then persuade the courts to embark on detailed scrutiny of how a local authority has implemented such formulae and sometimes this is justified. However, as court decisions periodically remind one, local authorities are generally accorded relatively broad powers and, providing that a local authority manages to avoid tying itself up in knots, the proper approach of a court in judicial review procedings generally is to maintain a supervisory role that accords respect to local authority judgments, and does not descend into commercial litigation by another avenue.[2]

14.4 The concern that commercial operators may abuse the judicial review system has been expressed most forcefully in planning cases, where that concern is perhaps most relevant and pressing:

- describing 'the discovery by commercial lawyers in recent years that wherever central or local government happens to have become involved, judicial review can become a way of conducting a trade war by other means';[3] and
- expressing 'dissatisfaction at the way the availability of the remedy of judicial review can be exploited – some might say abused – as a commercial weapon by rival potential developers'.[4]

14.5 The adult care context is somewhat different, in that private sector providers can be – sometimes with good reason – the only protagonists able to address unlawful decision-making, that not only affects them commercially but also harms the welfare of vulnerable individuals. So, in some cases, it might be inappropriate to apply the dicta in these planning cases to private sector providers in the care sector.

1 *Hampshire CC v Supportways Community Services Ltd* [2006] EWCA Civ 1035, (2006) 9 CCLR 484.

2 *R (Members of the Committee of Care North East Northumberland) v Northumberland CC* [2013] EWCA Civ 1740, (2014) 17 CCLR 117.

3 *R v Hammersmith & Fulham LBC ex p Burkett* [2001] Env LR 684.

4 *R (Noble Organisation) v Thanet DC* [2005] EWCA Civ 782, [2006] Env LR 185 at para 68.

14.6 A major issue in recent years has arisen in relation to the duty of local authorities to set their standard rates for care home accommodation having regard to (inter alia) the cost of providing care locally. A number of local authorities adopted relatively complex formulae to ascertain what the local cost of care was, which they then misapplied in some way[5] sometimes because they did not like the results and sometimes because the formulae were too complicated and perceived as not being realistic. More recently, the courts have upheld some decisions reached by local authorities that have adopted a broader approach, more evaluative and less mathematical, and emphasised the breadth of judgment allowed to local authorities.[6]

14.7 Under the Care Act 2014, the statutory machinery and the nomenclature will shift somewhat and the new provisions appear to possibly make such assessments less problematic for local authorities. However, it is difficult to see this area of controversy being finally resolved any time soon, in the absence of a nationally agreed approach involving all the relevant protagonists.

14.8 The first source of future problems is likely to be section 26 of the Care Act 2014, which requires local authorities to specify 'personal budgets' for adults (see, for greater detail, paras 9.36–9.44):

> **26**(1) A personal budget for an adult is a statement which specifies–
> (a) the cost to the local authority of meeting those of the adult's needs which it is required or decides to meet as mentioned in section 24(1),
> (b) the amount which, on the basis of the financial assessment, the adult must pay towards that cost, and
> (c) if on that basis the local authority must itself pay towards that cost, the amount which it must pay.
> (2) In the case of an adult with needs for care and support which the local authority is required to meet under section 18, the personal budget must also specify–
> (a) the cost to the local authority of meeting the adult's needs under that section ...

14.9 It seems easier for a local authority to specify the actual cost it would incur in meeting the adult's needs by going out into the market than, as present, to base its standard fees on an assessment, doing the best it can, of what it costs local operators to provide services.

14.10 On the other hand, it seems clear that the Care Act 2014 does not intend to permit a 'race to the bottom' in terms of fees and that, for various reasons, local authorities will have to continue to pay careful regard (albeit using such methods as they consider appropriate) to local costs given that, in reality, and in some areas more than others, the standard rates that local authorities are willing to pay can have a depressing effect on market rates that the local market may not be able to absorb while at the same time providing good quality care.

14.11 First of all, there are in the interests of service users to consider. By virtue of section 30 of the Care Act 2014 and the Care and Support and

5 *R (Mavalon Care Ltd) v Pembrokeshire CC* [2011] EWHC 3371 (Admin), (2012) 15 CCLR 229.

6 *R (Members of the Committee of Care North East Northumberland) v Northumberland CC* [2013] EWCA Civ 1740, (2014) 17 CCLR 117.

After-care (Choice of Accommodation) Regulations 2014, adults are entitled to be accommodated in the care home/shared lives/supported and after-care accommodation of their choice providing certain conditions are met, including that the adult or a third party pays any additional cost, beyond the amount provided for in the adult's personal budget (see, further, paras 11.48–11.52 on 'top-ups').

14.12 The consequence of this machinery is likely to be that, more than ever before, it will be in the interests of adults to ensure that the sum allowed for care home accommodation, in their personal budget, is sufficient to afford them a reasonable choice of good quality accommodation, without the need to resort to 'top ups'. But even if an adult is not contemplating a top up arrangement, the adult will certainly want to have a real choice of accommodation available at the standard rates in the adult's personal budget (where the case is a standard rate case). And that could well lead them, in the future, to examine very carefully the rates that local authorities are prepared to pay for different types of accommodation, just as much as care home providers have done this far.

14.13 A particular reason why that may be emerges from the advice given by the *Care and Support Statutory Guidance*:

> 11.25. The Act states the personal budget must be an amount that is the cost to the local authority of meeting the person's needs. In establishing the '*cost to the local authority*', consideration should therefore be given to local market intelligence and costs of local quality provision to ensure that the personal budget reflects local market conditions and that appropriate care that meets needs can be obtained for the amount specified in the budget. To further aid the transparency principle, these cost assumptions should be shared with the person so they are aware of how their personal budget was established. Consideration should also be given as to whether the personal budget is sufficient where needs will be met via direct payments, especially around any other costs that may be required to meet needs or ensure people are complying with legal requirements associated with becoming an employer (see Chapter 12). There may be concern that the 'cost to the local authority' results in the direct payment being a lesser amount than is required to purchase care and support from the local market due to local authority bulk purchasing and block contract arrangements. However, by basing the personal budget on the cost of quality local provision, this concern should be allayed.

14.14 Second, there is the local authority duty to promote diversity and quality provision in their local market: see para 7.79. Standard rates set too low may cause providers to be unable to improve or even maintain the quality of their service, can lead to a build-up of liabilities and, ultimately, may result in some providers becoming unable to continue in business. In any event, local authority standard rates will inevitably impact on providers' profits. Accordingly, local authorities will no doubt continue to be challenged, on the basis that their standard rates fail adequately to take into account local market intelligence and/or the costs of local provision, and fail to take into account the different rates and costs applicable to different types of accommodation in different types of areas, so as to conflict with the duty to promote well-being (at section 1) and/or the market shaping duty at section 5 (see para 7.79):

Promoting diversity and quality in provision of services

5(1) A local authority must promote the efficient and effective operation of a market in services for meeting care and support needs with a view to ensuring that any person in its area wishing to access services in the market–

(a) has a variety of providers to choose from who (taken together) provide a variety of services;

(b) has a variety of high quality services to choose from;

(c) has sufficient information to make an informed decision about how to meet the needs in question.

14.16 Paragraph 4.27 and onwards of the *Care and Support Statutory Guidance* emphasises the need to commission services having regard to cost-effectiveness and value for money, but also so as to:

- ensure that fees will enable the agreed quality of care to be provided;
- ensure that care providers' staff are properly remunerated (at 'at least' the minimum wage level) and are provided with effective training and development;
- allow for retention of staff;
- take into account guidance on minimum fee levels (as specified at paragraph 4.31 of the Guidance);
- ensure that there is a range of appropriate and high quality providers and services for people to choose from.

In principle, a local authority could abuse its dominant position as a purchaser of services so as to breach the provisions of Chapter II of the Competition Act 1998 but no case of actual abuse has ever been established.

Cases

14.17 *R v Cumbria CC ex p Professional Care Ltd* (2000) 3 CCLR 79, QBD

In judicial review proceedings, commercial operators must raise issues of law and not seek to engage in commercial litigation by other means

Facts: the applicant was an association of proprietors of private sector care homes. It brought an application for a judicial review of decisions by Cumbria (i) not to purchase respite care from them (except on a spot purchase basis, whereas it made block bookings with its own care homes); (ii) unfairly to advantage its 'in house' homes and (ii) to fail to discharge its statutory duty to provide suitable and sufficient accommodation for those in need of residential accommodation, thereby depriving its members of potential residents.

Judgment: Turner J held that Cumbria had not acted in breach of statutory duty or unlawfully in any way; the applicant had raised a plethora of factual matters, which on examination had proven incorrect:

> I would not wish to leave this case without stating that it is regrettable that scarce resources have been employed by the respondents in having to meet the claims of the applicants which I have held to be clearly inadmissible. Inappropriately these proceedings at times took on the appearance of a fiercely contested private law action.

14.18 ## *Douce v Staffordshire CC* [2002] EWCA Civ 506, (2002) 5 CCLR 347

A local authority might owe a care home operator a duty of care to avoid pure economic loss

Facts: Staffordshire had required care home proprietors to maintain staffing levels at levels that would be appropriate for fully occupied homes, even though the relevant homes were far from fully occupied for some time. The proprietors sued for pure economic loss damages, in negligence. Staffordshire applied for summary judgment.

Judgment: the Court of Appeal (Potter LJ and Sir Denis Henry) held that whilst the claimant's case was difficult, it was inappropriate to award summary judgment given that this was a developing area of law and the facts were unclear.

Comment: in the light of later authority, the care home operator in this case might be regarded as having achieved a very fortunate result.

14.19 ## *R (Birmingham Care Consortium) v Birmingham CC* [2002] EWHC 2188 (Admin), (2002) 5 CCLR 600

Care home providers had not established that the rates on offer were unfair, especially when the local authority was able to secure adequate provision at those rates

Facts: a consortium of care home owners sought a judicial review of the rates offered by Birmingham for care home provision, claiming that the rates fell short of matching the true cost of providing care.

Judgment: Stanley Burnton J held that there was evidence that Birmingham remained able to secure suitable placements at the rates offered and the claimant had not established that those rates were less than fair and would be bound to lead to a failure to provide long-term care to those in need:

> 32. Out of deference to the arguments put before me, however, I mention some general considerations. First, this case concerns the affordability of social services provided by the local authority. Absent a statutory duty compelling the expenditure in issue at the amount contended for, questions of affordability and of the allocation of resources are for the democratically elected executive and legislature, not for the courts. Secondly, affordability is in general a highly relevant consideration to be taken into account by any local authority in making its decisions on rates to be offered to service providers, subject to the local authority being able to meet its duties at the rates it offers. As Auld J said in *R v Newcastle-upon-Tyne City Council ex p Dixon* (20 October 1993, unreported but cited in the *Cleveland Care Homes Association* case):
>
>> '... where a local authority has a statutory duty to provide services and to fund them in part or in whole out of monies provided by its taxpayers it must balance two duties one against the other. On the one hand it must provide the statutory services required of it; on the other, it has a fiduciary duty to those paying for them not to waste their money. It must fairly balance those duties one against the other.'
>
> Thirdly, the court should be slow to intervene where, as in the present case, there has been a long process of consultation and the local authority and

> the service providers are, in effect, engaged in a contractual negotiation with the local authority. Lastly, the extension offered in the letter of 19 June 2002 was for a relatively short period and was expressly indicated to be an interim proposal: see the first and second bullet points on the first page, and penultimate sentence. I should have been reluctant to impeach that offer on the basis of alleged long-term effects of the rate offered for a period of nine months.

14.20 *Hampshire CC v Supportways Community Services Ltd* [2006] EWCA Civ 1035, (2006) 9 CCLR 484

A claim for specific performance of a contract had to fail when the contract had been terminated, lawfully or unlawfully, and public law could not assist the injured party

Facts: as a result of its review of Supportways' provision of Supporting People services, Hampshire declined to renew its contract at the earlier price, but offered a renewal only at a substantially lower price, which Supportways declined. Hampshire then took the view that the original contract had expired and decided not to renew it. Supportways brought a claim for judicial review and/or breach of contract on the basis that Hampshire had failed to undertake the SP review as required by public law guidance and the terms of the contract. At first instance, Mitting J accepted that the review had been deficient and ordered Hampshire to undertake a fresh review.

Judgment: the Court of Appeal (Mummery, Neuberger and Wilson LJJ) held that the case was governed by private law and an order for specific performance could not be awarded after the contract had been terminated, validly or not.

Neuberger LJ said this:

> 35. In my judgment, the basis of the Company's case was not in public law, but only in private law. The Company's complaint was that the Council had failed to comply with the Agreement, and the Company accordingly was seeking to enforce the Council's compliance. Subject to being contradicted by a closer analysis of the principles or by binding authority, such a complaint and such enforcement would appear to me respectively to involve a private law claim and a private law remedy, both of which are contractually based, albeit with common law and equitable aspects.
>
> 36. In answer to this, Mr Knafler first relied on the fact that the Council's obligations under clause 11.3 were, in reality, public law duties in that they can be traced directly to section 93 and to paragraph 71 of the 2003 Guidance. The fact that a contractual obligation is framed by reference to a statutory duty does not, in my view, render that obligation a public law duty. Of course, where the statutory duty is owed to a contracting party independently of the contractual obligation, he can normally expect to be able to seek a public law remedy by reference to the duty, as well as, or instead of, a private law remedy by reference to the obligation. However in the present case, the Council's public law duty, namely that arising under section 93, was owed to the Secretary of State in relation to the provision of grants. There was, as it seems to me, no question of that duty being owed to providers such as the Company.

37. Mr Knafler next relied on the fact that the nature of the Agreement, involving as it did the Council performing public administrative functions, was such that a claim brought under it would be a public law claim. That cannot, I think, be right. Virtually any contract entered into by a local authority, almost by definition, will involve it acting in such a way, as otherwise it would be acting *ultra vires*. Yet, it is clear that, as Mr Knafler rightly accepts, in the case of alleged breaches of many such contracts, a private law claim is the only type of claim which can be brought.

38. Thus, the mere fact that the party alleged to be in breach of contract is a public body plainly cannot, on its own, transform what would otherwise be a private law claim into a public law claim. There are, of course, circumstances where, in a contractual context, a public body is susceptible to public law remedies. However, where the claim is fundamentally contractual in nature, and involves no allegation of fraud or improper motive or the like against the public body, it would, at least in the absence of very unusual circumstances, be right, as a matter of principle, to limit a claimant to private law remedies.

39. Mr Knafler referred to a passage in the sixth (1999) edition of *de Smith, Woolf and Jowell's* Principles of Judicial Review, at paragraph 3–019, which includes the following three sentences:

> 'If a public function is being performed, and contract law does not provide an aggrieved person with an appropriate remedy, then action taken under or in pursuance of a contract should be subject to control by judicial review principles. Where a public body enters into a contract with a supplier, a dispute about the rights and duties arising out of the contract will often be determined by private law. However, the decision of a public body to enter, or not [to] enter, into a contract may be subject to judicial review.'

40. The point made in the third sentence of that passage (which is expanded in paragraph 5–035 of the book) has no application here. It is true that the result of the review of which the Company complains did result in the determination of the Agreement and in the offer of a new contract whose terms it considered objectionable. This does not mean, however, that its claim is within the scope of the third sentence in that passage. Its claim is that the 2004 review was not carried out in accordance with the Agreement, not, for instance, that the Council acted in bad faith or was guilty of an improper motive in carrying out, or in failing to carry out, the 2004 review in accordance with clause 11.3. The Company's complaints that the Agreement was not properly determined, and that it was not offered a new contract on appropriate terms, are solely based on the contention that the Council failed to comply with its (purely contractual) obligation to carry out the 2004 review in accordance with clause 11.3.

41. Mr Knafler relied on the first sentence in the passage I have quoted from *de Smith*, on the basis that, if private law could not provide a satisfactory remedy in the present case, then the Company should be entitled to resort to public law remedies. As discussed above, it does indeed appear that the Company is only entitled, in terms of private law remedies, to damages for breach of clause 11.3, and it seems likely that such damages would be very difficult to assess. Indeed, it is quite possible that they would only be nominal, as the only consequence of the breach of clause 11.3 was its reflection in the terms of the new contract offered to the Company, and, as the Judge pointed out when considering the terms of the order, the Council had no obligation to enter into a new contract with the Company.

42. However, it cannot be right that a claimant suing a public body for breach of contract, who is dissatisfied with the remedy afforded him by private law, should be able to invoke public law simply because of his dissatisfaction, understandable though it may be. If he could do so, it would place a party who contracts with a public body in an unjustifiably more privileged position than a party who contracts with anyone else, and a public body in an unjustifiably less favourable position than any other contracting party.

43. Equally importantly, it appears to me that it would be wrong in principle for a person who would otherwise be limited to a private law claim should be entitled to base his claim in public law merely because private law does not afford him a sufficiently attractive remedy. It is one thing to say that, because a contracting party is a public body, its actions are, in principle, susceptible to judicial review. It is quite another to say that, because a contracting party is a public body, the types of relief which may be available against it under a contract should include public law remedies, even where the basis of the claim is purely contractual in nature.

44. Mr Knafler relied on a number of cases relating to the circumstances in which, when making a claim in relation to a contract with a public body, the other contracting party can make a claim in public law. Two of those cases appear to me to be of some relevance to the present dispute, and, indeed, to support the conclusion that the Company cannot rely on public law in this case.

45. In *Mercury Energy Ltd v Electricity Corporation of New Zealand Ltd* [1994] 1 WLR 521, Lord Templeman, giving the judgment of the Privy Council, said this at 529B:

> 'It does not seem to me likely that a decision by a state enterprise to enter into or determine a commercial contract to supply goods or services will ever be the subject of judicial review in the absence of fraud, corruption or bad faith.'

That statement is plainly unhelpful to the Company's case: the only basis on which its claim is founded is breach of contract. Later, at 529G, Lord Templeman made the following observation, which also seems to apply to the present case:

> 'The causes of action based on breach of statutory duty, abuse of monopoly position and administrative impropriety are only relevant if the causes of action based on contract are rejected. If the causes of action based on contract are rejected, the other causes of action will only constitute attempts to obtain, by the declaration sought, specific performance of a non-existing contract. The exploitation and extension of remedies such as judicial review beyond their proper sphere should not be encouraged.'

46. In *Mercury Communications Ltd v Director-General of Telecommunications* [1996] 1 WLR 48, Lord Slynn of Hadley, (who gave the only reasoned speech) referred in a passage at 57E–G to the importance of maintaining a degree of 'flexibility as to the use of different procedures', namely public law and private law procedures. That case was concerned with the question of procedure than with that of remedy. Lord Slynn explained in the same passage that the plaintiff had properly brought private law proceedings because the dispute was 'in substance and in form ... as to the effect of the terms of the contract even if it can also be expressed as a dispute as to the terms of the licence'. In the present case, the issues which we are considering concern the meaning and effect of the Agreement.

47. In these circumstances, I conclude that the Company has no claim which it can pursue by way of judicial review, and in particular by seeking public law remedies. Since preparing this judgment, I have had the opportunity of reading the judgment of Mummery LJ which deals with this aspect of the appeal on a somewhat broader basis, and with which I agree.

Mummery LJ said this:

54. First, neither side has taken up an extreme position. Mr Knafler for the Company has not contended that judicial review is available against the Council simply because it is a public authority. Mr Straker for the Council has not argued that the mere existence of a relevant contract excludes the possibility of judicial review against a public authority.

55. Secondly, a public authority could, in principle, both be subject to claims in private law for breach of contract and to judicial review for breach of public law duties or abuse of public law powers in connection with a contract made by it.

56. Thirdly, in order to attract public law remedies, it would be necessary for the applicant for judicial review to establish, at the very least, a relevant and sufficient nexus between the aspect of the contractual situation of which complaint is made and an alleged unlawful exercise of relevant public law powers.

57. Fourthly, the respective positions of the parties on where to draw the line of the crucial private law/public law divide are helpful. Mr Knafler wants a mandatory remedy in respect of what he contends is a defective support services review conducted by the Council. He does not mind whether it is private law decree of specific performance, as was granted by the judge, or a mandatory order in public law, which was declined by the judge. He argues that the judge was right to grant specific performance, as there was a contract containing an obligation which he contended had not yet been properly performed by the Council. Alternatively, if the judge was wrong to order specific performance, he should have made a mandatory order in public law in accordance with Mr Knafler's primary case. The alternative private law remedy of damages was inadequate. The Company was entitled to have the support services review obligation properly performed in public law, as it was relevant to the grant of a new contract by the Council. There was, he contended, a sufficient public law element in the situation to attract the protection of public law. The obligation in the contract to carry out a support services review was underpinned by public law considerations derived from the 2000 Act, the Scheme, the 2003 guidance and the Council's published rules about reviews.

58. Against that Mr Straker's position is quite simply that the review was carried out by the Council under the express provisions for one, and only one, review; that, in accordance with the agreed terms, the contract expired at the end of 1 year after the review; that the judge was clearly wrong to order specific performance to require the carrying out of a further review under a contract which did not provide for one and which had, in any event, expired; and that Mr Knafler could not opt for a public law remedy to compel the performance of a private law contractual obligation on the ground that such a remedy was unavailable in private law.

59. Fifthly, I agree with Neuberger LJ that this was not a public law case. The action of the Council in conducting the support services review was not amenable to judicial review, because there was no sufficient nexus between the conduct of the review and the public law powers of the Council to make this a judicial review case. The required public law element of unlawful use

of power was missing from the support services review. The substance of the dispute between the Council and the Company was about the expiration of the Agreement after the Council had conducted the support services review under clause 11. The Council had entered into the Agreement with the Company in April 2003. The trigger provision for the expiry of the Agreement was the conduct of the support services review as contained in clauses 1.1, 2.2 and 11.2–11.3 of the Agreement. The source of the power of the Council's support services review was in the Agreement, not in the legislation or in the non-statutory 2003 Guidance and published rules. The Agreement governed the review. It spelt out the agreed consequences of a review for the life of the Agreement. Formal notice of the result of the review was given by the Council on 16 July 2004. The breach of the Agreement found by the judge did not, he held, prevent it from being a valid review for the purposes of triggering the expiration provisions. The Council declined the request of the Company to re-open the review, contending that the effect of the clause under which the support services review was conducted by it was to bring the Agreement to an end. The Company did not want the Agreement to come to an end. It sought an order quashing the review, an order requiring the Council to conduct a review 'according to law' and a declaration that, until the completion of the review, the Agreement remained extant.

60. Sixthly, although the grounds for the judicial review application use public law language of a 'decision' taken by the Council on cost-effectiveness matters in the review, of taking account of irrelevant considerations and failing to have regard to have regard to relevant considerations and of procedural unfairness in the review process, this terminology does not alter the substance of the dispute as to whether or not the Agreement had come to an end in accordance with its terms. That turns on the provision of the Agreement that that the Agreement comes to an end at the expiration of 12 months from the review. Termination of the Agreement turned on the operation of the contract according to agreed terms, not on the exercise of a statutory or common law public law power of the council which was amenable to judicial review.

61. Seventhly, it cannot be right in principle for a party to a contract with a public authority to have recourse to public law remedies simply on the ground the private law remedies, such as specific performance, are not available after the relevant contractual obligations have expired, or because they are too vague and uncertain to be specifically enforceable by the court, or because alternative private law remedies, such as damages for breach of contract, are inadequate. The relevant remedies are those available in private law for breach of contract.

14.21 *R (Forest Care Home Limited) v Pembrokeshire CC* [2010] EWHC 3514 (Admin), (2011) 14 CCLR 103

The local authority's methodology failed to assess local costs of providing care home accommodation in the way that it had attempted to do. However, it had been lawful for the local authority to prevent care home owners charging top ups

Facts: Forest challenged Pembrokeshire's methodology for assessing the cost of providing care accommodation locally, the fact that it took into account its own limited resources and the steps it took to prevent Forest seeking a contribution from residents.

Judgment: Hickinbottom J held that the local authority had mis-applied the methodology it had adopted for assessing the local capital costs of providing care and that, in other respects, its methodology had failed to capture particular aspects of local costs that it had set out to assess. However, the local authority had been entitled to include in the care home contracts provisions that prohibited care homes from seeking top up fees from residents placed by it.

Comment: a different type of approach was adopted by the local authority, and the Court of Appeal, in *R (Members of the Committee of Care North East Northumberland) v Northumberland CC.*[7]

14.22 *Amberley (UK) Ltd v West Sussex CC* [2011] EWCA Civ 11, (2011) 14 CCLR 178

A contractual entitlement to a review of costs did not authorise a unilateral increase

Facts: Amberley unilaterally increased the fees it charged for certain residents, but West Sussex refused to pay the increases. The issue was whether Amberley had been contractually entitled to increase the fees.

Judgment: the Court of Appeal (Mummery, Richards and Aikens LJJ) held that clear words in a contract would be required before a court concluded that one party was entitled to increase charges unilaterally. In this case, Amberley was not so entitled because the contract merely provided that the level of fees was subject to review if costs increased. That meant a joint review and any increases had to be agreed.

14.23 *R (Broadway Care Centre Ltd) v Caerphilly CBC* [2012] EWHC 37 (Admin), (2012) 15 CCLR 82

Termination of a framework agreement for care home placements was governed solely by private law

Facts: as a result of performance-related concerns, Caerphilly terminated its framework contract with Broadway for the provision of care home places. Broadway applied for a judicial review, on the ground that Caerphilly's decision amounted to a decision to close its care home, and so it was unlawful in public law because of a lack of prior consultation with residents and because Caerphilly failed to have regard to the welfare of residents and, also because it was in breach of the residents' rights under Article 8 ECHR and Broadway's rights under Article 1 of the 1st Protocol ECHR.

Judgment: Deputy High Court Judge Seys Llewellyn dismissed the application, holding that Caerphilly was not amenable to judicial review because it had exercised a contractual power, that Broadway did not have standing to complain about potential breaches of residents' ECHR rights, that Article 1 of the 1st Protocol was not engaged because Caerphilly had not resolved to close Broadway's care home and that, in any event, Broadway's claims were not well-founded factually.

7 [2013] EWCA Civ 1740, (2014) 17 CCLR 117.

14.24 ### *R (Mavalon Care Ltd) v Pembrokeshire CC* [2011] EWHC 3371 (Admin), (2012) 15 CCLR 229

An irrational failure to comply with the methodology adopted meant that the local authority had failed to have regard to the actual cost of care locally

Facts: Pembrokeshire agreed to set its local fees for care home accommodation by using a toolkit devised by Laing & Buisson. However, Pembrokeshire substituted the figure of six per cent for return on capital, rather than the 12 per cent used by the toolkit. Mavalon challenged the resultant rate.

Judgment: Beatson J held that Pembrokeshire had not demonstrated a rational reason for diverging from the 12 per cent rate used in the toolkit.

Comment: a different type of approach was adopted by the local authority, and the Court of Appeal, in *R (Members of the Committee of Care North East Northumberland) v Northumberland CC.*[8]

14.25 ### *R (Bevan & Clarke Ltd) v Neath Port Talbot CBC* [2012] EWHC 236 (Admin), (2012) 15 CCLR 294

Decisions about what standard rates to pay were, at least in Wales, public law decisions

Facts: the claimant care home operator challenged Neath's setting of its rate.

Judgment: Beatson J held that, contrary to Neath's submission, its decision was amenable to judicial review but that, contrary to the operator's submissions, its decision was lawful: it had not been required to use the Laing & Buisson toolkit, it had had regard to relevant considerations and, given the financial pressures to which it was subject, its decision was rational.

14.26 ### *R (Davis) v West Sussex CC* [2012] EWHC 2152 (Admin)

A complaint about the way a local authority investigated abuse allegations involved contractual provisions but was sufficiently public to permit judicial review, in that the allegations would have been investigated irrespective of the existence of the contract

Facts: West Sussex investigated abuse allegations at Mr and Mrs Davis' care home and subsequently terminated their contract with Mr and Mrs Davis on the basis of their findings. However, West Sussex only gave Mr and Mrs Davis a copy of its 22-page investigation report two days before the case conference and then held a second case conference, in the absence of Mr and Mrs Davis, to consider shortcomings in the first case conference.

Judgment: Deputy High Court Judge Mackie held that the issues in the case were not fundamentally contractual, in that West Sussex would have investigated the abuse allegations under its statutory powers even if it had not contracted with Mr and Mrs Davis, that judicial review was appropriate and that Mr and Mrs Davis' rights to procedural fairness had been violated.

8 [2013] EWCA Civ 1740, (2014) 17 CCLR 117.

14.27 *R (South West Care Homes Ltd) v Devon CC* [2012] EWHC 1867 (Admin)

A local authority has a broad discretion when assessing the usual cost of providing care locally

Facts: South West, a care home provider, sought a judicial review of Devon's decision to freeze the standard fees it would pay, inter alia, on the basis that Devon had failed to have due regard to the actual cost of providing care and had failed to consult.

Judgment: Singh J held that Devon had, unlawfully, failed to consult but that relief would not be granted on that account, owing to the passage of time. As far as concerned whether Devon had had regard to the actual cost of providing care, the manner intensity of enquiry was a matter for Devon, subject to rationality and, on the evidence. Devon had acted rationally by taking into account officers' local knowledge, the ability of care homes to function adequately on the previous standard rates and the rates paid by other local authorities.

14.28 *R (South West Care Homes Ltd) v Devon CC* [2012] EWHC 2967 (Admin)

A local authority deciding what standard rates to pay for care home placements had to discharge the PSED, which this authority had not done

Facts: South West, a care home provider, sought a judicial review of Devon's decision as to the standard fees it would pay.

Judgment: Deputy High Court Judge Milwyn Jarman held that Devon was in breach of the PSED:

> 52. Accordingly the council submits there was sufficient regard to impact on elderly and disabled residents. The Fee Structure Proposal report merely put a figure on the homes which were at risk of closure, a risk which in general terms had already been considered in the EIA. The exercise in which it was engaged did not involve the assessment of needs or the cutting of services or curtailment of choice but merely the calculation of cost.
>
> 53. In my judgment that approach fails to have due regard, in substance or with rigour or with an open mind, to the need to eliminate discrimination and to promote equality of opportunity amongst elderly or disabled residents. The council in carrying out this exercise failed to ask itself what it could do in respect of those needs. It is not good enough to say that the needs of individual residents had been or would be assessed under section 47 of the 1990 Act. In particular, even if most if not all homes identified in the Fee Structure Proposal report as at risk of closure would close in any event, there was no proper consideration of mitigation measures or proper management of such closures in setting the fees. The EIA should have been reconsidered having regard to this information. Having regard to the procedure adopted in the case of the structured closure of one home is not a sufficient regard to deal with this identified risk. Furthermore, there was no proper consideration in my judgment of the staff costs of engaging and interacting with those residents suffering from dementia.

14.29 *R (Members of the Committee of Care North East Northumberland) v Northumberland CC* [2013] EWCA Civ 1740, (2014) 17 CCLR 117

Local authorities are entitled to choose how to assess local care costs and what level of enquiry to undertake, subject to rationality

Facts: Northumberland set its standard fee rates for residential accommodation, not by an exercise of precise quantification but by exercising judgment and experience in the light of how the market functioned locally, also taking into account the fees being paid elsewhere; and around 70 per cent of local providers agreed to make provision on that basis. Others however brought a judicial review, submitting that Northumberland's methodology was flawed, with the result that it had not properly taken into account the usual cost of providing care home accommodation locally.

Judgment: the Court of Appeal (Aikens and Sullivan LJJ, Sir Stanley Burnton) held that the relevant central government guidance did not prescribe any particular methodology and, in principle, so long as a public authority took some steps to equip itself with relevant information, it was generally for the authority to decide on the manner and intensity of the inquiry to be undertaken. On the facts of this case, the judge at first instance had been plainly correct to conclude that Northumberland had regard to the cost of providing care locally. Judges at first instance had been prepared to delve into the facts to a surprising degree given that these were judicial review proceedings and such cases ought to be regarded as turning on their own facts.

Sullivan LJ said this:

> 17. The circular contains guidance. It is not to be equated with a statutory duty imposed by an enactment and as would be expected in the case of guidance, it does not prescribe any particular methodology, whether 'structured' or otherwise which local authorities must adopt in order to have had 'due regard' to the actual costs of providing care.
>
> 18. The claimants' submission, that as a matter of law a 'structured' approach (whatever that may mean, see below) is required, treats a single sentence in guidance in a circular as though it was a duty imposed by primary legislation. When we asked Ms Mountfield what the defendant had failed to do which it was under a duty to do as a matter of law, her reply was that the defendant had not focused on the question of actual cost and had failed to make a 'sufficient inquiry' contrary to the well established principle that a decision-maker must 'ask himself the right question and take reasonable steps to acquaint himself with the relevant information to enable him to answer it correctly': see *Secretary of State for Education and Science v Tameside Metropolitan Borough Council* [1977] AC 1014, 1065, per Lord Diplock.
>
> 19. The emphasis in Ms Mountfield's submissions was on the sufficiency of the defendant's inquiries. There is no dispute that the defendant took some steps to equip itself with the relevant information. The claimants' contention is that those steps were insufficient. When considering the force of this submission, it is important to remember that, provided some inquiry into the relevant factor to which due regard has to be paid is made by the decision-maker, 'it is generally for the decision-maker to decide on the manner and intensity of the inquiry to be undertaken into any relevant

factor': see per Beatson J in *R (Bevan & Clarke LLP) v Neath Port Talbot County Borough Council* [2012] LGR 728 para 56 cited in para 37 of the judgment below [2013] PTSR 1130.

20. The submission that there had been insufficient inquiry was coupled with a submission that the underlying fault in the defendant's approach was that it did not focus on ascertaining the actual cost of providing care because it never asked the correct question of the claimants, 'what are your actual costs of providing care?', and instead asked them the wrong question, 'why are you not able to provide care at the lower fee levels being paid by neighbouring local authorities in the north east?'

21. There are two answers to that submission: first, it does not accord with the judge's factual conclusions in paras 39–44 of the judgment as to what the defendant actually did, against which there was no challenge in the grounds of appeal. Secondly, in any event, the difference between the two questions is a matter of semantics rather than substance. Looking at these two answers in turn, I will not repeat the details of the judge's factual findings which can be found in paras 39–44 of his judgment. In summary, the judge found that the defendant had: (i) considered to what extent its existing rates of payment were leading to overcapacity in the market in its area; (ii) compared its own rates with those being paid by other local authorities in the region and considered whether there was anything to explain why the cost of providing care in Northumberland should be materially higher than elsewhere in the region; (iii) taken account of the position of those providers with whom it was able to reach agreement and the evidence that they had provided as to how they had determined that the proposed rates would enable them to meet the actual costs of care; (iv) sought information from the claimants and, when management accounts were provided by one of the members of CNEN, Mr McArdle, who had sought to explain why the provision of care in Northumberland costs more than elsewhere, carefully considered those accounts; (v) explained why it did not think it appropriate to accede to the claimants' request to use the PricewaterhouseCoopers ('PwC') model before calculating its 'usual costs'.

22. On the basis of those factual findings as to the steps that were taken by the defendant to acquaint itself with the relevant information, the judge's conclusion that the defendant did have 'due regard' to the actual costs of care as required by the circular was plainly correct. In reaching that conclusion the judge followed the approach adopted by Singh J in *R (South West Care Homes Ltd) v Devon County Council* [2012] EWHC 1867 (Admin): see the judgment below [2013] PTSR 1130 para 37.

14.30 *R (Torbay Quality Care Forum Ltd) v Torbay Council* [2014] EWHC 4321 (Admin)

In this case, the Council's fee-setting had been irrational

Facts: the Forum brought a challenge to the level of care home fees that Torbay determined it would pay.

Judgment: Deputy High Court Judge Lambert allowed the application for judicial review on the basis that the mathematical adopted by Torbay had been irrational and because Torbay had no justification for departing from the advice in the non-statutory guidance to disregard third party contributions when assessing the usual cost of care – it had simply disagreed with that advice:

60. *R (Bevan and Clarke) v Neath* [2012] LGR 728 contains the sage lesson that although amenable to judicial review decisions in relation to the particular statutory duty here involved are generally to be left to the decision maker and the decision maker alone is to decide on the manner and intensity of the inquiry to be undertaken into any relevant factor. The second lesson is that the weight to be given to a relevant factor is for the decision maker and not for the court in the absence of irrationality. This approach is endorsed by the Court of Appeal in *R (Members of the Committee of Care North East Northumberland) v Northumberland County Council* [2014] PTSR 758 where it is stressed that the Circular contains guidance and is not to be equated with a statutory duty and as would be expected in a case of guidance it does not prescribe any particular methodology which local authorities must adopt in order to have due regard to the actual costs of providing care. When considering the force of a submission that a local authority has taken either insufficient steps to equip itself with relevant information or has generated incorrect information for itself it is plainly important to remember as was stressed by the Court of Appeal that provided some inquiry into the relevant factor to which due regard has to be paid is made by the decision maker then 'it is generally for the decision maker to decide on the manner and intensity of the inquiry to be undertaken into the relevant factor': see per Beatson J in *R (Bevan and Clarke) v Neath* [2012] LGR 728 at paragraph 56. Previous decisions in different statutory contexts will not support the need for any particular form of analysis in the current situation. Some authorities will produce an arithmetical calculation; others may look at a number of comparables. I accept, of course, from *Northumberland* that carrying out an arithmetical calculation is but one way of having 'due regard for the actual cost of providing care' but is not the only legally permissible way. The extent to which judges in other cases have been prepared to delve in great detail into the facts is something which I approach with great caution in this case. The paradigm notion I have adopted is that of Beatson J in *Bevan and Clarke* as endorsed by Sullivan LJ and Aikens LJ in their specific comments in *Northumberland*. Borrowing further from *Bevan and Clarke* I remind myself that in judicial review the court will be particularly circumspect in engaging with the conclusions of the primary decision maker in relation to complex economic and technical questions. The normal setting of fee rates is a matter involving economic and financial assessment and a degree of expertise in how this sector operates. There is also a judgment to be made about the proper allocation of scarce resources: see Supperstone J in *R (Care North East) v Northumberland* [2013] PTSR 1130 at paragraph 58. It seems to me that this is the type of case where traditional judicial review principles in relation to administrative decisions must be honoured scrupulously. It is not the type of case where the boundaries of judicial review should be rolled back at all, particularly not by a judge at first instance. In the course of assessing the facts in this case I have tried very hard to reach a conclusion which would allow me to say that the intensity of the inquiry here being dealt with by the decision maker was a matter for them and that I should leave well alone. With regret for the consequences, but with no real hesitation as to the principle I must honour I consider that the Claimant's first ground is well made out. If the decision maker treads the path of economic modelling then it seems to me it cannot proceed with a model that is significantly flawed. I was careful to take into account the fact that one person's flawed mathematical model might be another person's best estimate. I took heavily into account the fact that the intensity and nature of the inquiry which is required of the local authority is primarily a matter for the decision maker. But if the local authority chooses to

adopt a mathematical model some scrutiny of this is available on general public law principles. Those principles require, it seems to me, that wherever possible the merits of the decision remain with the decision maker. But here the merits of the decision are so fundamentally flawed by adopting the unnecessary weighting which no-one can explain as being necessary that the decision to employ this falls fairly and squarely within the scope of judicial review as being a decision which no reasonable decision taker properly directing themselves on the facts could take. In the end no matter what epithet is used to describe the decision, whether it not adding up or being beyond the bounds of logic or all reasonableness the decision does, it seems to me, fall within that narrow band of decisions which can properly be the subject of judicial review. The deployment of the weighted average makes no sense in the first place and has no reasonable application in the model. There may, perhaps, have been some explanation for this but there is none which I can now scrutinise. The presence of an inexplicable weighting within the mathematical model shows it to be a matter of fact which no reasonable decision taker could properly take into account.

14.31 *Abbeyfield Newcastle upon Tyne Society Ltd v Newcastle CC* [2014] EWHC 2437 (Ch), (2014) 17 CCLR 430

Where a framework agreement expired, the local authority had to pay for new placement on a quantum meruit basis, not at the old rates

Facts: Abbeyfield and Newcastle operated under a Pre-Placement Agreement whereby Newcastle placed individuals in Abbeyfield care homes at rates determined under the Agreement. The Agreement expired, as a result of Abbeyfield and Newcastle being unable to agree on implementation of the price review mechanism. However, Newcastle continued to make placements. The issue was whether Newcastle was required to pay for new placements under the old rates fixed by the Agreement, before it expired, or on a *quantum meruit* basis.

Judgment: Norris J held that Newcastle was required to pay for new placements on a *quantim meruit* basis and a reasonable price would have to be paid.

14.32 *Carewatch Care Services Ltd v Focus Caring Services Ltd* [2014] EWHC 2313 (Ch)

Franchise agreements did not contain an implied term of good faith, preventing the franchisor from developing its own rival business and restrictive covenants, binding on the franchisee, were lawful at common law and did not infringe the Competition Act 1998

Facts: Carewatch sought to enforce various provisions in franchise agreements that it had entered into with Focus, its franchisee. Focus had purported to terminate its franchise agreements with Carewatch, on the basis that Carewatch had been in breach an implied duty of good faith, by setting up its own branches in competition with franchisees and ceasing to support or develop the franchise network. On Focus starting to trade outside the franchise agreement, Carewatch brought proceedings to enforce restrictive covenants against trading, that applied for 12 months following termination of the franchise agreements.

Judgment: Henderson J held that there was no implied term of 'good faith' and the restrictive covenants were all valid and enforceable at common law. Further, whilst the restrictive covenants fell within the scope of section 2(1) of the Competition Act 1998, provisions that were necessary to protect the know-how and assistance of a franchisor were not to be regarded as interfering with competition for these purposes. Carewatch was entitled to injunctive relief and damages.

14.33 *Menon and Others v Herefordshire Council* [2015] EWHC 2165 (QB)

It was not appropriate to order disclosure of documents containing local authority legal advice, in an action in misfeasance against it

Facts: owners of a residential care home claimed that local authority social workers, involved in the cessation of referrals to the home and, ultimately, the moving of all residents to other homes, were guilty of misfeasance in public office.

Judgment: Lewis J refused the owners' application for summary judgment and for disclosure of documents containing legal advice about the lawfulness of the social workers' actions, which had been provided pursuant to an order of the First-tier Tribunal (Health, Education and Social Care Chamber) in proceedings in which one of the claimants, but Herefordshire, had been a party: even in the absence of an express restriction in the order, there would have been an implied obligation or undertaking that the documents would not be used for any collateral purpose without the leave of the court or the express consent of the party disclosing or producing the document:

> 61. In my judgment, it would not be appropriate to grant permission to the claimants to use documents containing legal advice which were produced for the purposes of other proceedings. I reach that conclusion for the following reasons. First, the documents were obtained by compulsion. Secondly, they were obtained in circumstances where they were only to be used for the proceedings in the First-tier Tribunal. Thirdly, they contain legal advice and, as indicated above, there is a very high value placed upon parties being able to protect legally professionally privileged documents. Fourthly, the claimants are seeking to take advantage of an error on the part of the defendant in complying with the production order of the First-tier Tribunal without, it seems, realising that these documents contained legal advice. It is not appropriate, in my judgment, to grant permission to the claimants in these circumstances to use and rely upon the documents in these proceedings which are in their possession as a result of the production order made by the First-tier Tribunal in other proceedings.

14.34 *R (Forge Care Homes Ltd) v Cardiff & Vale University Health Board* [2016] EWCA Civ 26, (2016) 19 CCLR 62

Local health boards were not required to pay for all the care provided by registered nurses, only for the tasks that only a registered nurse could perform

Facts: In Wales, local health boards (LHBs) assessed the level of their payment for registered nursing care, in care homes, by reference to the tasks undertaken by registered nurses which only a registered nurse could perform, rather than by reference to all the tasks in fact undertaken by registered nurses, including the provision of personal care.

Judgment: the Court of Appeal (Laws and Lloyd Jones LJJ, Elias LJ dissenting) held that this approach was lawful because the language of section 49(2) of the Health and Social Care Act 2001 required a distinction to be drawn between the different services provided by nurses at a care home and indicated that the LHB was only required to pay for costs of services that only a registered nurse could perform.

14.35 *Menon and Others v Herefordshire Council* [2016] EWHC 498 (QB)

On the facts, social workers engaged in terminating the local authority's relationship with a care home had not been guilty of misfeasance in public office

Facts: owners of a residential care home claimed that local authority social workers, involved in the cessation of referrals to the home and, ultimately, the moving of all residents to other homes, were guilty of misfeasance in public office.

Judgment: Mitting J held that there had not been any misfeasance in public office: the social workers involved had suspended referrals out of concern for the residents and they had not bullied or lied to residents, who had freely chosen to leave the home.

CHAPTER 15

Status of care home and home care providers

15.1 **Introduction and statutory scheme**

Cases

15.6 *R v Servite Houses and Wandsworth LBC ex p Goldsmith and Chatting* (2000) 3 CCLR 325, QBD

A housing association was not discharging a public function for judicial review purposes when it sought possession of accommodation

15.7 *R (Heather and Callin) v The Leonard Cheshire Foundation* [2002] EWCA Civ 366, (2002) 5 CCLR 317

A charity was not performing a public function when making decisions to close one of its care homes

15.8 *R (A) v Partnerships in Care Limited* [2002] EWHC 529 (Admin), (2002) 5 CCLR 330

A private hospital exercising statutory functions in relation to detained mental patients was amenable to judicial review and liable under the Human Rights Act 1998

15.9 *Moore v Care Standards Tribunal* [2005] EWCA Civ 627, (2005) 8 CCLR 354

A home could in substance be a care home notwithstanding that occupiers had been granted assured tenancies, where in truth the establishment provided accommodation together with nursing or personal care

15.10 *R (YL) v Birmingham CC* [2007] UKHL 27, (2007) 10 CCLR 505

A privately run care home was not discharging functions of a public nature

15.11 *R (Weaver) v London and Quadrant Housing Trust* [2009] EWCA Civ 587, [2010] 1 WLR 363

On the assumption that some functions of an RSL were public functions, it was a public body for the purposes of the Human Rights Act 1998 and for the purposes of judicial review proceedings, because its termination of a social tenancy was not a private act

Introduction and statutory scheme

15.1 Section 73 of the Care Act 2014 provides that a person is to be taken as exercising a function of a public nature, for the purposes of section 6(3)(b) of the Human Rights Act (HRA) 1998 when providing care or support if:

- the care or support is arranged by an English local authority, or paid for (directly or indirectly, in whole or in part); if that is done
- under sections 2, 18, 19, 20, 38 or 48 of the Care Act 2014; and
- the care provider is registered and provides (i) care and support to an adult in the course of providing personal care in the place where the adult is residing; or (ii) residential accommodation together with nursing or personal care.

15.2 Similar provision is made in respect of Wales, Scotland and Northern Ireland: section 73(1)(b), (c) and (d) of the Care Act 2014.

15.3 It seems as though Parliament's intention was limited to imposing a public law responsibility only in the case of breaches of the ECHR.

15.4 Nonetheless, private sector providers may have other public responsibilities thrust upon them, by accident or design:

- the imposition of limited responsibility under section 73 of the Care Act 2014 may possibly be taken as a factor pointing towards a private care provider discharging public functions so as to be amenable to wider public scrutiny, through judicial review;[1]
- as discussed in more detail at para 5.17 above it seems that bodies to whom section 73 of the Care Act 2014 applies will be under the public sector equality duty (PSED);
- in addition, it seems as though registered social landlords are discharging a public function for the purposes of the Human Rights Act 1998 when they manage their social housing stock and may also be amenable to judicial review in such cases, including when they are, at the same time, providing a form of social care.[2]

15.5 Such developments seem logical: why is there a divide between public and private law? why should not any organisation that receives public money have at least some responsibility towards relevant sections of the public?

Cases

15.6 *R v Servite Houses and Wandsworth LBC ex p Goldsmith and Chatting* (2000) 3 CCLR 325, QBD

A housing association was not discharging a public function for judicial review purposes when it sought possession of accommodation

Facts: Servite Homes accommodated the applicants at May House, assuring them they could remain there for the rest of their lives. However,

1 But see *R (JL) v Birmingham CC* [2007] UKHL 27, (2007) 10 CCLR 505.

2 *R (Weaver) v London & Quadrant Housing Trust* [2009] EWCA Civ 587, [2010] 1 WLR 363.

Servite Homes then decided to close May House because it was uneconomic. The applicants sought a judicial review.

Judgment: Moses J held that Servite Homes, a housing association, was not discharging a public function so as to be amenable to judicial review.

Comment: by virtue of section 73 of the Care Act 2014, most registered care providers, providing personal care in residential or domestic settings, must be treated as exercising a function of a public nature for the purposes of section 6(3)(b) of the Human Rights Act 1998. That does not require such providers also to be treated as amenable to judicial review, but it could be a relevant factor. And, see *Weaver*, at para 15.11 below.

15.7 *R (Heather and Callin) v The Leonard Cheshire Foundation* [2002] EWCA Civ 366, (2002) 5 CCLR 317

A charity was not performing a public function when making decisions to close one of its care homes

Facts: the claimants were residents in a care home, placed there by local authorities under the National Assistance Act 1948. They applied for a judicial review of the Foundation's decision to close the home, to redevelop it, submitting that it breached their rights under Article 8 ECHR.

Judgment: the Court of Appeal (Lord Woolf LCJ, Laws and Dyson LJJ) held that the Foundation was a private body and it was not performing a public function, so as to be amenable to judicial review, or come within the HRA 1998:

> 35. The matters already referred to, can however, be put aside. In our judgment the role that Leonard Cheshire Foundation (LCF) was performing manifestly did not involve the performance of public functions. The fact that LCF is a large and flourishing organisation does not change the nature of its activities from private to public.
>
> i) It is not in issue that it is possible for LCF to perform some public functions and some private functions. In this case it is contended that this was what has been happening in regard to those residents who are privately funded and those residents who are publicly funded. But in this case except for the resources needed to fund the residents of the different occupants of Le Court, there is no material distinction between the nature of the services LCF has provided for residents funded by a local authority and those provided to residents funded privately. While the degree of public funding of the activities of an otherwise private body is certainly relevant as to the nature of the functions performed, by itself it is not determinative of whether the functions are public or private. Here we found the case of *R v HM Treasury ex p Cambridge University* [2000] 1 WLR 2514 (ECJ) at pp 2523 2534/5, relied on by Mr Henderson, an interesting illustration in relation to European Union legislation in different terms to section 6.
>
> ii) There is no other evidence of there being a public flavour to the functions of LCF or LCF itself. LCF is not standing in the shoes of the local authorities. Section 26 of the NAA provides statutory authority for the actions of the local authorities but it provides LCF with no powers. LCF is not exercising statutory powers in performing functions for the appellants.
>
> iii) In truth, all that Mr Gordon can rely upon is the fact that if LCF is not performing a public function the appellants would not be able to rely upon

> Article 8 as against LCF. However, this is a circular argument. If LCF was performing a public function, that would mean that the appellants could rely in relation to that function on Article 8, but, if the situation is otherwise, Article 8 cannot change the appropriate classification of the function. On the approach adopted in *Donoghue,* it can be said that LCF is clearly not performing any public function. Stanley Burnton J's conclusion as to this was correct.

Comment: see comment above on *Servite Homes.*

15.8 *R (A) v Partnerships in Care Limited* [2002] EWHC 529 (Admin), (2002) 5 CCLR 330

A private hospital exercising statutory functions in relation to detained mental patients was amenable to judicial review and liable under the Human Rights Act 1998

Facts: A was detained in a private psychiatric hospital and brought an application for a judicial review of a management decision by the hospital. The hospital denied that it was amenable to judicial review or liable under HRA 1998.

Judgment: Mr Justice Keith held that the hospital was amenable to judicial review and liable under HRA 1998 (the test was the same):

> 24. In my opinion, the decision of the managers of the hospital to change the focus of the ward was an act of a public nature. Decisions as to the form which treatment for a particular patient should take are clinical decisions for the psychiatrists, and the claimant is not challenging either the lawfulness of the decision to detain her in hospital, or the decision as to the type of treatment which she needs, or the decision that she is not ready to be discharged. But whether facilities can and should be provided, and adequate staff made available, to enable the treatment which the psychiatrists say should take place is another matter entirely. That is the subject of specific statutory underpinning directed at the hospital: the statutory duty imposed by regulation 12(1) of the 1984 Regulations on the hospital to provide adequate professional staff and adequate treatment facilities was cast directly on the hospital as the registered person under the Registered Homes Act 1984. The public interest in the hospital's care and treatment of its patients is apparent when one remembers that if, as a result of the lack of staff or facilities, patients detained under the Mental Health Act 1983 do not receive the care and treatment which they need, their detention may well be prolonged because they may not recover sufficiently to meet the statutory criteria for their discharge from hospital. The fact that the decision challenged is said to have been forced on the hospital by the unexpected departure of staff with the special skills needed to provide the claimant with the care and treatment which she needs goes not to whether the decision made was an act of a public nature but to whether the claim for judicial review should succeed.

15.9 ### *Moore v Care Standards Tribunal* [2005] EWCA Civ 627, (2005) 8 CCLR 354

A home could in substance be a care home notwithstanding that occupiers had been granted assured tenancies, where in truth the establishment provided accommodation together with nursing or personal care

Facts: Alternative Futures provided accommodation, board and care in a number of homes registered under the Registered Homes Act 1984. It then created a second company ('Alternative Housing') to deal with its property, which granted tenancies to the residents, with the original company continuing to provide care. The local authority refused to cancel the registration of the homes or pay housing benefit, on the basis that the registered status of the homes precluded such payments.

Judgment: the Court of Appeal (Waller and Mance LJJ, Sir William Aldous) held that a home could in substance be a care home notwithstanding that occupiers had been granted assured tenancies, where in truth the establishment provided accommodation together with nursing or personal care and, in this case, Housing and Futures, together with each house, had operated as one establishment: it was a question of act, ultimately.

15.10 ### *R (YL) v Birmingham CC* [2007] UKHL 27, (2007) 10 CCLR 505

A privately run care home was not discharging functions of a public nature

Facts: YL submitted that a privately run care home, that had given her notice to quit, had acted incompatibly with her rights under Article 8 ECHR.

Judgment: the House of Lords (Lords Bingham, Scott, Mance, Neuberger and Lady Hale, Lord Bingham and Lady Hale dissenting) held that the care home provider was not exercising functions of a public nature for the purposes of HRA 1998 s6: this was not a case where the statutory function itself had been delegated and the provision of care home accommodation was not intrinsically governmental.

Comment: now, by virtue of section 73 of the Care Act 2014, most registered care providers, providing personal care in residential or domestic settings, must be treated as exercising a function of a public nature for the purposes of HRA 1998 s6(3)(b).

15.11 ### *R (Weaver) v London and Quadrant Housing Trust* [2009] EWCA Civ 587, [2010] 1 WLR 363

On the assumption that some functions of an RSL were public functions, it was a public body for the purposes of the Human Rights Act 1998 and for the purposes of judicial review proceedings, because its termination of a social tenancy was not a private act

Facts: London and Quadrant, a registered social landlord, served a notice seeking possession on Ms Weaver, who claimed that it infringed her rights under Article 8 ECHR.

Judgment: the Court of Appeal (Lord Collins, Rix and Elias LJJ, Rix LJ dissenting) held that it conceded that some of London and Quadrant's functions were public functions, so the only question was whether the termination of a social tenancy by a social landlord was a private act: viewing all the circumstances in the round, it was not; accordingly, London and Quadrant was a public body for the purposes of the Human Rights Act 1998:

> 66. The essential question is whether the act of terminating the tenancy is a private act. When considering how to characterise the nature of the act, it is in my view important to focus on the context in which the act occurs; the act cannot be considered in isolation simply asking whether it involves the exercise of a private law power or not. As Lord Mance observed in YL's case [2008] AC 95 , both the source and nature of the activities need to be considered when deciding whether a function is public or not, and in my view the same approach is required when determining whether an act is a private act or not within the meaning of section 6(5). Indeed, the difficulty of distinguishing between acts and functions reinforces that conclusion.
>
> 67. In this case there are a number of features which in my judgment bring the act of terminating a social tenancy within the purview of the Human Rights Act 1998.
>
> 68. A useful starting point is to analyse the trust's function of allocating and managing housing with respect to the four criteria identified by Lord Nicholls in the Aston Cantlow case [2004] 1 AC 546, para 12, reproduced above at para 35(5). First, there is a significant reliance on public finance; there is a substantial public subsidy which enables the trust to achieve its objectives. This does not involve, as in YL's case, the payment of money by reference to specific services provided but significant capital payments designed to enable the trust to meet its publicly desirable objectives.
>
> 69 Second, although not directly taking the place of local government, the trust in its allocation of social housing operates in very close harmony with it, assisting it to achieve the authority's statutory duties and objectives. In this context the allocation agreements play a particularly important role and in practice severely circumscribe the freedom of the trust to allocate properties. This is not simply the exercise of choice by the RSL but is the result of a statutory duty to co-operate. That link is reinforced by the extent to which there has been a voluntary transfer of housing stock from local authorities to RSLs.
>
> 70. Third, the provision of subsidised housing, as opposed to the provision of housing itself, is, in my opinion a function which can properly be described as governmental. Almost by definition it is the antithesis of a private commercial activity. The provision of subsidy to meet the needs of the poorer section of the community is typically, although not necessarily, a function which government provides. The trust, as one of the larger RSLs, makes a valuable contribution to achieving the government's objectives of providing subsidised housing. For similar reasons it seems to me that it can properly be described as providing a public service of a nature described in the Lord Nicholls's fourth factor.
>
> 71. Furthermore, these factors, which point in favour of treating its housing functions as public functions, are reinforced by the following considerations. First, the trust is acting in the public interest and has charitable objectives. I agree with the Divisional Court that this at least places it outside the traditional area of private commercial activity. Second, the regulation to which it is subjected is not designed simply to render its activities more transparent, or to ensure proper standards of performance in the public interest. Rather the regulations over such matters as rent and eviction are

designed, at least in part, to ensure that the objectives of government policy with respect to this vulnerable group in society are achieved and that low cost housing is effectively provided to those in need of it. Moreover, it is intrusive regulation on various aspects of allocation and management, and even restricts the power to dispose of land and property.

72. None of these factors taken in isolation would suffice to make the functions of the provision of housing public functions, but I am satisfied that when considered cumulatively, they establish sufficient public flavour to bring the provision of social housing by this particular RSL within that concept. That is particularly so given that their Lordships have emphasised the need to give a broad and generous construction to the concept of a hybrid authority.

Is termination of a tenancy a private act?

73. That still leaves the central question whether the act of termination itself can none the less be treated as a private act. Can it be said that since it involves the exercise of a contractual power, it is therefore to be characterised solely as a private act? It is true that in both the Aston Cantlow case [2004] 1 AC 546 and YL's case [2008] AC 95 it is possible to find observations which appear to support an affirmative answer to that question. As I have said, in YL's case Lord Scott considered that the termination of the tenancy in that case was a private act, essentially because it involved the exercise of private rights. And in the Aston Cantlow case their Lordships focused on the private law source of the right being exercised in concluding that it was a private act.

74. Those decisions certainly lend force to the argument that the character of the act is related to and may be defined by the source of the power being exercised. Where it is essentially contractual, so the argument goes, it necessarily involves the exercise of private rights.

75. In my judgment, that would be a misreading of those decisions. The observations about private acts in the Aston Cantlow case and YL's case were in a context where it had already been determined that the function being exercised was not a public function. I do not consider that their Lordships would have reached the same conclusion if they had found that the nature of the functions in issue in those cases were public functions.

76. In my judgment, the act of termination is so bound up with the provision of social housing that once the latter is seen, in the context of this particular body, as the exercise of a public function, then acts which are necessarily involved in the regulation of the function must also be public acts. The grant of a tenancy and its subsequent termination are part and parcel of determining who should be allowed to take advantage of this public benefit. This is not an act which is purely incidental or supplementary to the principal function, such as contracting out the cleaning of the windows of the trust's properties. That could readily be seen as a private function of a kind carried on by both public and private bodies. No doubt the termination of such a contract would be a private act (unless the body were a core public authority).

77. In my opinion, if an act were necessarily a private act because it involved the exercise of rights conferred by private law, that would significantly undermine the protection which Parliament intended to afford to potential victims of hybrid authorities. Public bodies necessarily fulfil their functions by entering into contractual arrangements. It would severely limit the significance of identifying certain bodies as hybrid authorities if the fact that the act under consideration was a contractual act meant that it was a private act falling within section 6(5).

There was no warrant for applying a different approach to the question whether London and Quadrant was amenable to judicial review:

> 83. Both the *Aston Cantlow* case [2004] 1 AC 546 and *YL's* case [2008] AC 95 emphasised that it does not necessarily follow that because a body is a public body for the purposes of section 6, it is therefore subject to public law principles. The Divisional Court held, however, that in this case the two questions had to be determined the same way. Mr Arden does not now seek to contend otherwise. In my judgment, he was right not to do so.

CHAPTER 16

Care home and other service closures

continued

16.33 *R (Cowl) v Plymouth CC* [2001] EWCA Civ 1935, (2002) 5 CCLR 42
It was lawful to take a strategic decision to close a care home, subject to completion of assessments at a later date. The parties should have done far more to pursue mediation, notwithstanding the existence of some legal issues

16.34 *R (Madden) v Bury MBC* [2002] EWHC 1882 (Admin), (2002) 5 CCLR 622
The consultation process was unlawful where officers failed to communicate accurate information about the risks and benefits

16.35 *R (C, M, P, HM) v Brent, Kensington and Chelsea and Westminster Mental Health NHS Trust* [2002] EWHC 181 (Admin), (2003) 6 CCLR 335
Where disputed, the existence of a 'home for life' promise had to be clearly evidenced, especially in the context of a hospital, which is primarily a place for care and treatment

16.36 *R (Haggerty) v St Helens Council* [2003] EWHC 803 (Admin), (2003) 6 CCLR 352
The decision not to renew a contract with a private sector care home was not incompatible with the residents' ECHR rights

16.37 *Collins v United Kingdom* Application No 11909/02, (2003) 6 CCLR 388
Notwithstanding the existence of a 'home for life' promise, the decision to override that promise had been lawful in national law and compliant with the ECHR

16.38 *R (CH and MH) v Sutton and Merton PCT* [2004] EWHC 2984 (Admin), (2005) 8 CCLR 5
The court needed to consider for itself whether there was indeed an overriding public interest that justified resiling from a 'home for life' promise and whether, as was asserted, it was in the 'best interests' of residents to move

16.39 *R (Bishop) v Bromley LBC* [2006] EWHC 2148 (Admin), (2006) 9 CCLR 635
Prior assessments were only required in exceptional cases

16.40 *R (Morris) v Trafford Healthcare NHS Trust* [2006] EWHC 2334 (Admin), (2006) 9 CCLR 648
The failure to consult was unlawful but the grant of relief was not practical

16.41 *R (J) v Southend BC* [2005] EWHC 3457 (Admin), (2007) 10 CCLR 407
A local authority was entitled to assume that the needs of users of its day centre services, ordinarily resident elsewhere, would be assessed and met by the local authority of their ordinary residence

16.42 *R (Wilson) v Coventry CC, R (Thomas) v Havering LBC* [2008] EWHC 2300 (Admin), (2009) 12 CCLR 7
The decision to close care homes was not incompatible with Article 2 on account of the risks to life and was otherwise lawful

16.43 *R (Rutter) v Stockton on Tees BC* [2008] EWHC 2651 (Admin), (2009) 12 CCLR 27
Risks could be considered at Scrutiny stage and relief could be refused in all the circumstances

16.44 *R (B) v Worcestershire CC* [2009] EWHC 2915 (Admin), (2010) 13 CCLR 13
The closure decision was based on irrational premises

16.45 *R (Boyejo) v Barnet LBC* [2009] EWHC 3261 (Admin), (2010) 13 CCLR 72

The discharge of the duty to consult and the disability equality assessment had been unlawful

16.46 *Watts v United Kingdom* Application No 53586/09, (2010) 51 EHRR SE5

A carefully managed process of care home closure did not violate rights under Articles 2, 3 or 8 ECHR

16.47 *R (Broadway Care Centre Ltd) v Caerphilly CBC* [2012] EWHC 37 (Admin), (2012) 15 CCLR 82

A decision to terminate a framework contract was contractual and not amenable to judicial review, neither did it infringe ECHR rights

16.48 *R (LH) v Shropshire Council* [2014] EWCA Civ 404, (2014) 17 CCLR 216

A local authority was entitled to consult in general terms on a policy change, if it then consulted before closing individual services. Where a day centre had closed and its staff had been dispersed, no relief would be granted in relation to an unlawful disclosure process

16.49 *R (Michael Robson) v Salford CC* [2013] EWHC 3481 (Admin), (2014) 17 CCLR 474

The court summarised consultation principles and concluded that in substance consultees had been adequately informed about what was proposed and that the PSED had been lawfully discharged

16.50 *R (Michael Robson) v Salford CC* [2015] EWCA Civ 6

The consultation materials lacked clarity but overall consultees must have known what the proposal was and what the alternative were, so that the process had been fair; there may have been significant flaws in the community impact assessment but overall the PSED had been discharged

Introduction

16.1 Sometimes, local authorities close care homes, day centres and other services, and re-model local services, in a way that commands a high degree of acceptance locally. Sometimes, because of the personalities involved, the scale of the changes or the potential risks, that objective is not accomplished. However, it is in everyone's interests, including their own, that local authorities do everything they can to explain, discuss, involve, persuade and seek agreement with local voluntary groups, service users and their families: it maximises opportunities for the useful exchange of information and views, minimises the risk of expensive litigation and promotes an atmosphere of mutual understanding, fairness and respect.

16.2 There can be no doubt that, even if the service users' 'eligible needs' will still be met in other ways, as will invariably be the case, the closure of a particular service can be highly distressing and seriously damaging, in particular if a consensus has not been reached and/or the process is not well-managed. In addition to the understandable fear of change, especially among the elderly, closures are usually accompanied by highly worrying statements about budgetary cuts, creating the real prospect of a worse service even if 'eligible needs' are met, threaten the loss of important friendships and relationships with care staff at the facility targeted for closure, uncertainty, increased caring roles and visiting difficulties for family members – and so on. However, service users and their families who try to keep a service open experience a number of formidable difficulties:

- because of the way the Care Act 2014, and other primary legislation, is drafted, service users have a guarantee that their 'eligible needs' will be met, but are not usually entitled to insist on their preferred service;
- closure decisions are almost always subject to future assessments and arrangements whereby the local authority undertakes not just that 'eligible needs' will be met but that mitigating steps will be taken to minimise distress and the risks of damage, endeavour to keep friendship groups together, maintain at lest some staff continuity – and so on;
- there are usually strong budgetary or policy reasons for the change, which are the types of reasons that the court is especially cautious about supervising because these types of decisions are in principle within the constitutional remit and institutional expertise of democratically elected bodies, not the court;
- events on the ground often move on: for example, some residents opposed to the closure of a service may opt nonetheless to accept a relatively good, alternative offer, before someone else takes it up, thereby denuding the service in question of both supporters and continued viability; and
- the court may perceive that the cost and distress occasioned by correcting past procedural errors may outweigh that caused by the errors themselves and may be of little avail in terms of affecting the ultimate outcome.

16.3 However, whilst service users face an uphill struggle in this context, the courts do recognise the distress and harm that may be caused by the termination of a service, in particular when the users of that service have not been treated fairly and with respect for their situation, and it does grant remedies in appropriate cases where the process has been flawed, usually as a result of inadequate consultation or inadequate discharge of the public sector equality (PSED) (see chapters 3 and 5 above).

Homes for life

16.4 There was a period of time, when local authorities and health authorities quite often promised people that they would have a 'home for life' in a particular care home. This was usually given as an assurance to people, on the basis of which they moved without protest from some earlier accommodation where they had wanted to stay. Such promises are not made at all frequently now.

16.5 The approach of the courts has been that:

- the existence of a 'home for life' promise has to be proven, where it is disputed, by clear evidence;[1]
- a clear assurance of a 'home for life' gives rise to a legitimate expectation;[2]
- local authorities have to take into account that they have created such a legitimate expectation and must have a sufficiently cogent and proportionate reason for overriding it.[3]

Consultation

16.6 Many challenges to service closures are brought on the basis of inadequate consultation: some of the cases set out below consider such grounds of challenge and others are included in chapter 3, 'Consultation' above.

16.7 The court invariably proceeds on the basis that care home residents, day centre users and other service users have an interest that requires them to be consulted before their care service is terminated. In this context, the grounds most likely to succeed involve complaints that:

- the decision had already been taken;[4]
- inadequate time was given for considered responses;[5]
- officers failed to provide consultees and/or decision-makers with accurate information about the risks and benefits of closure;[6] and that
- the local authority failed to consult over realistic alternatives.[7]

1 *R (C, M, P, HM) v Brent, Kensington and Chelsea and Westminster Mental Health NHS Trust* [2002] EWHC 181, (2003) 6 CCLR 335.

2 *R v North and East Devon Health Authority v Coughlan* [1999] 2 WLR 622, (1999) 2 CCLR 285.

3 *R v North and East Devon Health Authority v Coughlan* [1999] 2 WLR 622, (1999) 2 CCLR 285.

4 *R (Boyejo) v Barnet LBC* [2009] EWHC 3261, (2010) 13 CCLR 72.

5 *R (Boyejo) v Barnet LBC* [2009] EWHC 3261, (2010) 13 CCLR 72.

6 *R (Madden) v Bury MBC* [2002] EWHC 1882 (Admin), (2002) 5 CCLR 622.

7 *R (Madden) v Bury MBC* [2002] EWHC 1882 (Admin), (2002) 5 CCLR 622.

16.8 It is however lawful to consult first of all on high level policy changes, which will very probably result in care home and other service closures, subject to later consultation over specific service closures.[8]

The public sector equality duty (PSED)

16.9 Broadly, the same applies to challenges brought on the basis of an alleged failure to discharge the PSED: some of the cases set out below consider such grounds of challenge and others are included in chapter 5 at paras 5.43–5.68 above.

16.10 The essential point is that decision-makers are required to read a report that:

- makes it clear, in unvarnished and robust terms, what the potential risks are of the proposed service closure, as well as what the benefits, justification, mitigating and monitoring measures are;
- advises the decision-makers clearly as to existence and content of their duty under the PSED.

16.11 The courts have made it clear that they will not quash decisions based on minor breaches of the PSED but will require local authorities to satisfy them that there has been a proper and conscientious focus on the substance of the PSED.[9]

16.12 As with consultation, it is lawful to pass a budget that is highly likely to result in service closures on the basis of a relatively general, high level discharge of the PSED, subject to later more focussed discharge of the PSED before any specific service is closed.[10]

Prior assessments

16.13 In general, local authorities are *not* required to undertake formal assessments of any of the users of a particular service before deciding in principle to terminate it. In general, it suffices for local authorities to undertake a few representative assessments, or to operate on the basis of a reasonable understanding of the levels of need of the individuals concerned and the alternative provision available to meet those needs.[11]

16.14 This approach is in line with the courts' approach to consultation and discharge of the PSED, which allows macro decisions to be made on the basis of relatively broad, high-level information, subject to more focussed consideration (with the possibility of a change of tack) in due course.[12] It is on the basis that, notwithstanding the macro service closure decision, no

8 *R (LH) v Shropshire Council* [2014] EWCA Civ 404, (2014) 17 CCLR 216 at paras 21–26.

9 *R (Michael Robson) v Salford CC* [2015] EWCA Civ 6 at paras 37–48.

10 *JG and MB v Lancashire CC* [2011] EWHC 2295 (Admin), (2011) 14 CCLR 629 at paras 43–45.

11 *R (Wilson) v Coventry CC, R (Thomas) v Havering LBC* [2008] EWHC 2300 (Admin), (2009) 12 CCLR 7.

12 *R (LH) v Shropshire Council* [2014] EWCA Civ 404, (2014) 17 CCLR 216 at paras 21–26; *JG and MB v Lancashire CC* [2011] EWHC 2295 (Admin), (2011) 14 CCLR 629 at paras 43–45.

individual will be deprived of the service in question unless and until their needs have been fully assessed and an alternative identified that meets their 'eligible needs'.

16.15 A different approach may be required, however, where statutory or non-statutory guidance advises that individual assessments should be completed before a decision is taken to close a particular service or where the circumstances strongly indicate that a failure to do so is irrational: usually, when what is contemplated is the closure of a niche or intensive service, in circumstances where it is highly questionable whether that service can be replicated elsewhere in a way that meets 'eligible needs'.[13]

Management of the closure process

16.16 Persons opposing care home closures fought long and hard, with some success, to improve the quality of closure arrangements, but were unable to establish that care home closures necessarily entailed unacceptable risks to the life or health of the residents.

16.17 The furthest the courts have gone,[14] is to accept that:

- a badly managed closure may cause distress and serious harm including personal injury or death;
- hypothetically, an irreduceable, unmanageable risk of personal injury or even death might arise, in the case of an exceptionally vulnerable individual. That could well prevent the termination of a service, no matter what stage had been reached; however,
- that risk need only be identified after an in-principle decision to close has been made, and individual assessments are being undertaken; and
- there is no reported case in which such an irreduceable risk has been recognised as existing.

16.18 In addition, the European Court of Human Rights has shown itself to be wholly unsympathetic to cases involving opposition to service closures, including care home closures: it regards such cases as prime examples of cases that involve questions of social policy that fall well within the 'margin of appreciation' of national authorities.[15]

16.19 All that notwithstanding, the courts do recognise that it is vital that local authorities have an up-to-date protocol for managing home closures and transfers and that officers advise decision-makers carefully about all the potential risks.

16.20 It is surprising that the Department of Health has still not issued nationally applicable guidance on this important subject. However:

- in Northern Ireland, the Health and Social Care Board has produced very useful guidance called *Making Choices: Meeting the current and*

13 *R (Bishop) v Bromley LBC* [2006] EWHC 2148 (Admin), (2006) 9 CCLR 635.

14 A good example, is *R (Wilson) v Coventry CC, R (Thomas) v Havering LBC* [2008] EWHC 2300 (Admin), (2009) 12 CCLR 7.

15 *Collins v United Kingdom* (2003) 6 CCLR 388; *Watts v United Kingdom* (2010) 51 EHRR SE5.

future accommodation needs of older people, Good Practice Guide – Reconfiguration of Statutory Residential Homes (November 2013);[16]
- the Personal Social Services Research Unit (PSSRU) has produced an interesting and useful review of local authority guidelines and protocols, called *Guidelines for the closure of care homes for older people: prevalence and content of local government protocols*;[17]
- there is also general guidance produced by Birmingham City Council, the Association of Directors of Adult Social Services and the Social Care Institute for Excellence called *Achieving Closure: Good practice in supporting older people during residential care closures*.[18]

Mediation and Alternative Dispute Resolution

16.21 Local authorities are often under time constraints, as well as budgetary constraints, but if there was one area of adult social care where mediation and alternative dispute resolution (ADR) ought to be used more often, in everyone's interests, this is surely it.

16.22 *R (Cowl) v Plymouth CC* (see below at para 16.33)[19] is an example of the Court of Appeal taking this point very strongly. The subsequent ADR process, convened before an extraordinary complaints panel, did in fact result in Plymouth changing its position and keeping open Granby Way, re-named Frank Cowl House in honour of Mr Cowl, who sadly died during the ADR process.

16.23 It is fair to point out, however, that the Panel's Report did itself uncover a number of serious defects in the ADR process and advised, inter alia, that it was important, to correct imbalances of power and that public funding was available to assist residents and their families in such complaints/mediation proceedings. Accordingly, local authorities desirous of promoting ADR need to consider how to address such disadvantages, for example, by the use of advocates.

Private services

16.24 The reported cases involve challenges to the closure of local authority homes and the termination of local authority services.

16.25 It is harder to imagine a challenge to the closure of a private sector home succeeding, not least because, in most cases, such closures are dictated by insolvency or enforcement activity triggered by grossly inadequate care.

16.26 However, in principle, such a case could be brought, either on contractual grounds or, more likely, on the basis of section 73 of the Care Act 2014. This legislates that a private or social sector provider is exercising a function of a public nature if, on the basis of payments or arrangements

16 www.hscboard.hscni.net/consult/Previous%20Consultations/2013–14%20Consultation-Statutory_Residential_Care_Homes/Good%20Practice%20Guide%20Statutory%20Homes.pdf.

17 www.pssru.ac.uk/pdf/dp1861_2.pdf.

18 www.birmingham.ac.uk/Documents/news/BirminghamBrief/AchievingClosureReport.pdf.

19 [2001] EWCA Civ 1935, (2002) 2 CCLR 42.

made by a local authority, it provides care and support to an adult, or support to a carer, in the course of providing i) personal care where the adult is living, or ii) residential accommodation together with nursing or personal care.

Cases

16.27 ### *R v North and East Devon Health Authority ex p Coughlan* [2001] QB 213, (1999) 2 CCLR 285, CA

In the absence of special circumstances a health authority was not required to assess the needs of patients before deciding to close a facility. The clear promise of a 'home for life' created a legitimate expectation that had not been fully taken into account, nor demonstrated to be overridden by a public interest

Facts: Ms Coughlan was rendered very severely disabled by a road traffic accident. After a period of treatment at Newcourt Hospital, which the health authority then wished to close, she and seven other patients were moved to Mardon House hospital, with an assurance that it would be their 'home for life'. However, the health authority then resolved to close Mardon House. In addition, it determined that Ms Coughlan no longer met the criteria for NHS continuing healthcare, so that she had to resort to local authority residential accommodation. Ms Coughlan submitted that it was beyond the powers of a local authority to provide her with the nursing care she needed and that it was unlawful for the health authority to resile from its 'home for life' promise; and a breach of Article 8 ECHR.

Judgment: the NHS was entitled to close Mardon House in stages and it was not necessary that it fully assessed the needs of the Mardon House residents, and decided upon alternative service provision, before reaching a decision in principle to effect closure:

> 103. The concerns of the Health Authority about the practical implications of the judge's decision on these two points are well understood. In the absence of special circumstances, normally we would expect it to be unrealistic and unreasonable, on grounds of prematurity alone, for the Health Authority in all cases to make assessments of patients and to take decisions on the details of placement ahead of a decision on closure. Neither the statutory provisions nor the Guidance issued expressly require assessments to be made or decisions on alternative placements to be taken before a decision to close can be lawfully made.

In this case, the 'home for life' promise had created legitimate expectations that North and East Devon had failed fully to take into account and had not demonstrated any overriding public interest that justified resiling from that promise:

> 89. We have no hesitation in concluding that the decision to move Miss Coughlan against her will and in breach of the Health Authority's own promise was in the circumstances unfair. It was unfair because it frustrated her legitimate expectation of having a home for life in Mardon House. There was no overriding public interest which justified it. In drawing the balance of conflicting interests the court will not only accept the policy change without demur but will pay the closest attention to the assessment

made by the public body itself. Here, however, as we have already indicated, the Health Authority failed to weigh the conflicting interests correctly. Furthermore, we do not know (for reasons we will explain later) the quality of the alternative accommodation and services which will be offered to Miss Coughlan. We cannot prejudge what would be the result if there was on offer accommodation which could be said to be reasonably equivalent to Mardon House and the Health Authority made a properly considered decision in favour of closure in the light of that offer. However, absent such an offer, here there was unfairness amounting to an abuse of power by the Health Authority.

16.28 *R v Merton, Sutton and Wandsworth Health Authority ex p Perry, Andrew and Harman* (2000) 3 CCLR 378

A closure decision was unlawful where the health authority disregarded a 'home for life' promise and failed, contrary to guidance, to undertake prior assessments

Facts: the health authority decided to close Orchard Hill, a long-stay hospital for people with profound learning disabilities, on economic grounds, despite having promised residents a 'home for life'.

Judgment: Jackson J held that the health authority's decision-making process was unlawful for two reasons: (1) it failed to take into account its promises of a 'home for life' (notwithstanding the failure of consultees to raise this matter), (2) inconsistently with the non-statutory guidance, on page 2 of HSG (92)42, it had failed to undertake individual assessments of the residents as to their future care needs.

16.29 *R v Barking and Dagenham LBC ex p Lloyd* (2001) 4 CCLR 5, QBD

On the facts, there had not been any 'home for life' promise

Facts: residents of care home accommodation submitted that the temporary closure and redevelopment of their home breached their legitimate expectations in a number of respects, including in relation to 'home for life' promises.

Judgment: Keene J held that, whilst statements by local authority officers fell to be construed objectively, rather than by reference to what the officers had subjectively intended to say, on the facts, construing the statements made in context, there had not been any 'home for life' promises.

16.30 *R v Barking and Dagenham LBC ex p Lloyd* (2001) 4 CCLR 27, CA

Parties in care home closure proceedings should mediate

Facts: residents of care home accommodation submitted that the temporary closure and redevelopment of their home breached their legitimate expectations in a number of respects, including in relation to 'home for life' promises.

Judgment: the Court of Appeal (Ward and Sedley LJJ) refused to grant permission to appeal on the 'home for life' point whilst granting permission to appeal on other grounds, on the proviso that the parties were to endeavour to mediate.

16.31 *R v Barking and Dagenham LBC ex p Lloyd* (2001) 4 CCLR 196, CA

On analysis, redevelopment plans would not breach any 'home for life' promise whilst detailed criticisms of the process should be pursued through a complaints procedure

Facts: residents of care home accommodation submitted that the temporary closure and redevelopment of their home breached their legitimate expectations in a number of respects, including in relation to 'home for life' promises.

Judgment: the Court of Appeal (Schiemann, Sedley and Arden LJJ) dismissed the appeal, holding that, on the facts, the redevelopment plans would not necessarily involve a breach of any promises and that the assessments and care plans were adequate as provisional documents. Further, in general, a complaint that an assessment or care plan was inadequate should be pursued by way of a complaints procedure:

> 27. It seems to us however that, leaving aside for the moment any undertakings to the court, the court is not the appropriate organ to be prescriptive as to the degree of detail which should go into a care plan or as to the amount of consultation to be carried out with Ms Lloyd's advisers. In practice these are matters for the council, and if necessary its complaints procedure. If the council has failed to follow the Secretary of State's guidance and is arguably in breach of its statutory duties in relation to the way it carries out its assessment and what it puts into its care plans then aggrieved persons should in an appropriate case turn first to the Secretary of State. Where there is room for differences of judgment the Secretary of State and his advisers may have a useful input. The court is here as a last resort where there is illegality. Here there is not – it is right to say these matters have not been fully canvassed in argument.

16.32 *R (Bodimeade) v Camden LBC* (2001) 4 CCLR 246

A closure decision was unlawful where the local authority had disregarded a clear 'home for life' promise and failed to undertake prior assessment

Facts: Camden decided to close an old people's care home, notwithstanding that the Resident's Handbook, and a letter to residents' had contained a 'home for life' promise, and without a prior assessment of the residents' needs.

Judgment: Turner J held that, on the facts, there had been a 'home for life' promise, which had given rise to legitimate expectations that Camden would not close the home. Camden's decision to close the home had been unlawful because it had failed to take into account the promise it had made and the expectations it had created. In addition, since the decision to close the home had been final, rather than provisional, it had been an unjustified departure from statutory guidance not to assess the residents' needs: because it meant that the services to be provided were not 'needs led'.

16.33 *R (Cowl) v Plymouth CC* [2001] EWCA Civ 1935, (2002) 5 CCLR 42

It was lawful to take a strategic decision to close a care home, subject to completion of assessments at a later date. The parties should have done far more to pursue mediation, notwithstanding the existence of some legal issues

Facts: the claimants challenged the proposed closure of their care home on the basis of inadequate consultation, lack of proper assessments and breaches of 'home for life' promises; they rejected the offer of the complaints procedure, with Plymouth's assurance that it would pay very careful regard to the views of the social services complaints panel.

Judgment: the Court of Appeal (Woolf LCJ, Mummery and Buxton LJJ) dismissed the claimants appeal on the basis that the parties could have, and should still, engage in alternative dispute resolution, notwithstanding the fact that the claimants' case involved submissions that errors of law had been made. The Court of Appeal did, however, also make it clear, that Plymouth had been entitled to reach a 'decision in principle' to close the care home (based on a limited assessment of the residents' needs), to be followed by detailed assessments later on, before moving any individual resident:

> 22. We understand the reason why the claimants attach such importance to the assessment being carried out before the decision to close. They do not want an assessment as to the propriety of moving the individual claimants to be taken against a decision that the home is to be closed as that could, they fear, prejudge the outcome. This is why they submit that the full assessment should take place before the decision to close the home is taken. The position of Plymouth now, whatever may have been the position in the past, is clearly to regard the decision to close as merely a decision in principle; that is, to close Granby Way subject to the full assessment of the impact upon the residents of their having to move. This approach on the part of Plymouth is understandable. Plymouth needed to make financial savings. The closure of Granby Way and another home would produce the required financial saving. From Plymouth's point of view therefore the first step was to consider whether closure would be a viable option. For this purpose they needed a limited assessment of the impact on the residents and of the practicality of their being re-housed, but no more than this. This exercise was carried out. The decision was made to proceed with this option. Detailed examination of what is involved in re-housing was then required so that a final decision could be made. The final decision would only be made after the full assessment of the impact upon the residents. Such an approach could be beneficial to the residents because, if the closure option was not viable, there was no need to subject them to the stress which would be involved in determining what would happen to them if they had to move.
>
> …
>
> 24. Nonetheless the decision which was taken did not have the technicality the claimants attached to it. There was nothing wrong with Plymouth adopting a two-stage process, with the detailed assessment being part of the second process. However, if this was what they were doing, it is regrettable that far from explaining it they obscured the fact that this was their intention. On the other hand, those who were acting on behalf of the claimants adopted a far too technical approach. Their treatment in their skeleton argument of the authorities on which they rely make this abundantly clear.

25. We do not single out either side's lawyers for particular criticism. What followed was due to the unfortunate culture in litigation of this nature of overjudicialising the processes which are involved. It is indeed unfortunate that, that process having started, instead of the parties focussing on the future they insisted on arguing about what had occurred in the past. So far as the claimants were concerned, that was of no value since Plymouth were prepared, as they ultimately made clear was their position, to reconsider the whole issue. Without the need for the vast costs which must have been incurred in this case already being incurred, the parties should have been able to come to a sensible conclusion as to how to dispose the issues which divided them. If they could not do this without help, then an independent mediator should have been recruited to assist. That would have been a far cheaper course to adopt. Today sufficient should be known about ADR to make the failure to adopt it, in particular when public money is involved, indefensible.

26. The disadvantages of what happened instead were apparent to the trial judge. They were also apparent to this court. At the opening of the hearing we therefore insisted on the parties focussing on what mattered, which was the future wellbeing of the claimants. Having made clear our views, building on the proposal which had been made in the 23 May letter, the parties had no difficulty in coming to a sensible agreement in the terms which are annexed to this judgment and will form part of the order of the court. The terms go beyond what Plymouth was required to do under the statutory complaint procedure. This does not however, matter because it is always open to the parties to agree to go beyond their statutory obligations. For example, sensibly the claimants are to have the benefit of representatives to appear on their behalf, who may well be non-lawyers who can be extremely experienced in handling issues of the nature of those which are involved. We trust that the parties will now draw a line under what has happened in the past and focus instead on what should happen in the future.

27. This case will have served some purpose if it makes it clear that the lawyers acting on both sides of a dispute of this sort are under a heavy obligation to resort to litigation only if it is really unavoidable. If they cannot resolve the whole of the dispute by the use of the complaints procedure they should resolve the dispute so far as is practicable without involving litigation. At least in this way some of the expense and delay will be avoided. We hope that the highly skilled and caring practitioners who practise in this area will learn from what we regard as the very unfortunate history of this case.

16.34 *R (Madden) v Bury MBC* [2002] EWHC 1882 (Admin), (2002) 5 CCLR 622

The consultation process was unlawful where officers failed to communicate accurate information about the risks and benefits

Facts: Bury provisionally decided to close two residential care homes. It gave notice of its proposal to residents and held a series of meetings, where residents and their families were able to make their views known, before it reached its final decision. The reasons advanced publicly by Bury for closure, were that one home had a structural fault in its foundations whilst the other did not meet registration standards, and that remedying these problems would be uneconomic.

Judgment: Richards J held that the consultation had been unlawful because of Bury's failure to convey accurate information: the structural fault was very minor and Bury had failed (despite requests) to disclose the relevant survey report or even to show that report to councillors that made the closure decision; in relation to the other home there had been no examination of possible alternative courses that could have resulted in that home remaining open and the reasons given had been misleading. The process had also been incompatible with Article 8 ECHR:

> 58. Of far greater concern, in my judgment, is the concern of that exercise. In my view, the initial letter of 21 May did not give an adequate summary of the true reasons for the proposed closures. References to the policy considerations that favoured a reduction in the amount of residential service provision were very brief. The specific reasons expressed for the closure, or for the proposals to close the two individuals homes, were incorrect or misleading. In the case of Warthfield, the reason was put solely on the basis of health and safety reasons arising out of a structural fault concerning the foundations. Yet the detailed survey report not only fails to support that, but shows that what was said was simply wrong. The survey report goes out of its way to emphasise the very limited nature of the problem with the building, which it is said expressly should not be taken out of context. Yet, in my view, it was taken out of context and was presented misleadingly, whether deliberately or not does not matter. Moreover, the extended timeframe of 12 years envisaged in the survey report for dealing with the problem was not mentioned, and there was no explanation of the costs of remedying the problem on the alternative basis put forward in the report.
>
> 59. In the case of Whittaker, the bare statement that closure was proposed because the home does not meet the required standards of registration under the Care Standards Regime was also inadequate, if not again misleading, even though it was thought at the time that the care standards would be legal requirements. Any proper understanding of the true reasons for the proposed closure would require at the least a comparison with the other home that the council thought it preferable to retain instead of Whittaker. The bald statement of reasons expressed in the letter was not a proper basis for consultation.
>
> 60. Indeed, in neither case was there any indication of possible alternatives, including in particular some explanation of why the closure of these two homes was favoured over the closure of others. There was no indication that this was something on which residents could make representations. What was said about future consultation was expressed to relate to the details of the proposals rather than to the principle. There was nothing to suggest that the principle of closure was being raised for consideration and comment.
>
> 61. Thus, although views were invited, too little was said by way of background and reasons to enable meaningful consultation process to take place. In that connection it is also important that the letter did not fall to be read against the background of some previously published policy review. In the circumstances, and given the relatively short timescale, I regard it as important that clear and accurate reasons for the proposal to close the homes were given, albeit briefly. The possibility that residents could influence the decision by their representation should have been made clear.
>
> 62. I bear in mind that the requirements of consultation as laid down and applied in *ex p Baker* are not particularly onerous. But what was done here was not sufficient to meet those requirements. It was not sufficient to

ensure fairness. I am not satisfied that what was said at the subsequent meetings – whether meetings with residents and relatives in the homes themselves or council meetings – was sufficient in terms of content or specificity to cure those problems and to put the consultation process onto a proper basis.

16.35 *R (C, M, P, HM) v Brent, Kensington and Chelsea and Westminster Mental Health NHS Trust* [2002] EWHC 181 (Admin), (2003) 6 CCLR 335

Where disputed, the existence of a 'home for life' promise had to be clearly evidenced, especially in the context of a hospital, which is primarily a place for care and treatment

Facts: the claimants were long-term mental health patients, who opposed the closure of their long-stay hospital on the ground that, when they moved there (as the result of the closure of their previous long-stay hospital home) they had been promised a 'home for life'.

Judgment: Newman J dismissed the application for judicial review, holding that hospitals were primarily places for care and treatment. A claimant who asserted that he had been promised a 'home for life' needed to prove it with proper evidence (first hand evidence, setting out clear who said what and in what context).

16.36 *R (Haggerty) v St Helens Council* [2003] EWHC 803 (Admin), (2003) 6 CCLR 352

The decision not to renew a contract with a private sector care home was not incompatible with the residents' ECHR rights

Facts: St Helens declined to renew its contract with a private care home, when it concluded that the price increase required by the care home was unjustifiable and the residents could be moved safely and in a planned manner. Some residents sought a judicial review of St Helens' decision not to enter into a new contract with the home.

Judgment: Mr Justice Silber held that St Helens' decision did not interfere with the residents' rights under the ECHR:

52. I have already set out the evidence concerning the likely effect of the move on the claimants. The evidence of the medical practitioners does not show that the effect of the move would come anywhere near the high threshold for the engagement of Article 3, namely of constituting 'intense mental and physical suffering'. In any event, their evidence does not comment on or take into account the precautions outlined by Mr Stoker. Professor Jolley's evidence was that the effect on the claimants of the move to another home would depend on the precautionary steps taken by the Council to ensure that any suffering was ameliorated. As the report of Age Concern produced by Professor Jolley shows, these precautions can entirely or at least very substantially obviate the adverse consequences to elderly residents of such a move. This is particularly relevant because the evidence of Mr Stoker shows that the substantial lengths to which the Council is going to ensure that the claimants do not have to suffer unnecessarily. Thus, my first reason for rejecting the Article 3 challenge is that in absence of comments by anybody medically qualified on the effect on those claimants of

moves to other homes in the light of Mr Stoker's precautions, the claimants' evidence does not show suffering up to the requisite high threshold for Article 3 to be engaged. My second reason is that the Council have as I have stated in paragraph 49 agreed to liaise with the claimant's expert on the psychiatry of the old aged on the best way of moving the claimants so as to reduce any risk to them. ...

58. I consider that the claim in respect of Article 8 fails for three reasons. First, there is no cogent evidence of disruption of home or family life or interference with the right to physical integrity. Professor Jolley and the general practitioners of the claimants do not deal in their evidence with the proposed or actual arrangements as outlined by Mr Stoker, which show that Article 8 rights are not engaged.

59. The way in which the moves are and have been planned, as described by Mr Stoker in his evidence and which is not contradicted, indicate that a great deal is being done to ensure that the move is as undisruptive to the claimants as it could possibly be. No cogent criticism has been made by Mr Skilbeck of the proposed arrangements. It is particularly noteworthy that the Council intends to do all that is necessary to preserve friendship groups and thus shows respect for what would be covered under Article 8(1) as 'family life'. The other measures that Mr Stoker outlines, show the claimants' rights to physical integrity and respect for home and family life have been safeguarded and are not infringed. As I have explained, Mr Stoker has said that the individual assessments of all residents have been carried out. I have explained in paragraph 49 above the way in which the Council has agreed to liaise with the claimants' expert consultant psychiatrist on the best ways of moving the claimants so as to reduce any risk to them.

60. Second, the financial resources of the Council is an important element to be considered to the balancing exercise required in the application of Article 8(2). Thus, in *R (F) v Oxfordshire Mental Health Care NHS Trust* [2001] EWHC 535 (Admin), Sullivan J held that it was highly relevant to the balancing exercise required by Article 8(2) that by making expensive provisions to one individual item in the Council budget, this would deprive others of services and this would thereby adversely effect their rights. As I have explained, the Council considered that the fees sought by Southern Cross were disproportionate and that if it was to agree to pay them, an improper burden would be placed on the social services budget with the result that other patients in other homes would be adversely effected. Similarly, in *R (Birmingham Care Consortium) v Birmingham CC* [2002] EWHC 2188 (Admin), Stanley Burnton J said 'affordability is in general a highly relevant consideration to be taken into account by any local authority in making a decision on rates to be offered to service providers, subject to a local authority being able to meet its duties at the rates it offers' [para 32]. This would enable the Council to justify its decision. Another way of reaching that conclusion is that, as I have explained in paragraphs 10 and 14 above, a local authority is obliged by statute and entitled to take into consideration resources when deciding how to meet individual needs.

61. A third reason why this claim based on Article 8 must fail is that the Council is entitled to a substantial degree of deference relating to the way in which it allocates its resources and provides services. This is relevant as Article 8(2) requires a balancing exercise. These are matters very much within the expertise of a local authority and with which a court should only interfere where the evidence is very clear, but this is, as I have explained, not such a case. For all those reasons, the Article 8 claim and all aspects of the ECHR challenge fail.

16.37 ## *Collins v United Kingdom* Application No 11909/02, (2003) 6 CCLR 388

Notwithstanding the existence of a 'home for life' promise, the decision to override that promise had been lawful in national law and compliant with the ECHR

Facts: Ms Collins had been promised a 'home for life' at a bungalow in the hospital grounds, where she was a long-term resident. She sought to resist a proposal to re-locate her in a community setting on the ground that it was incompatible with her rights under Article 8 ECHR.

Judgment: the application was declared inadmissible: the local authority decision had been lawful as a matter of national law and, also, proportionate:

> As regards the necessity of the decision, the court observes that the applicant's principal objections to the decision are that it runs counter to her own wishes to remain where she is and to the promise made by the local health authority (LHA) that Long Leys would be a 'home for life'. Though the applicant's family sought to argue that a move would be harmful as the applicant disliked and reacted badly to a change in routine, the consultant psychiatrist who gave evidence to the court and who had experience of such moves took the view that the impact on the residents of the move would be beneficial in a wide range of areas. While it was noted that residents and their carers could often be resistant to change for understandable reasons, it was envisaged that with proper care and support the applicant would be able to cope with the move.
>
> The court further notes that in reaching the decision to move the applicant and the other residents the LHA consulted the concerned parties and was careful to obtain legal advice as to the status of the promise of a 'home for life'. It cannot therefore be said that the LHA did not give weight to the applicant's wishes or the assurance given many years before. The propriety of the decision-making procedure was, in addition, subject to the scrutiny of the High Court which found that the LHA had acted with due regard to all the relevant factors.
>
> Though the court considers that it was highly regrettable that a promise was apparently made that misled the applicant and her family into the belief that she would be able to remain at Long Leys indefinitely, this assurance was not, in the event, found to amount to a legally binding obligation on the LHA to comply with the applicant's personal preferences. The Court does not find that this an unreasonable or arbitrary conclusion, since, given the vagaries of future circumstances, a statement made in 1990 could not realistically have been expected to guarantee the continued suitability of Long Leys as a placement for the applicant, whether for practical, medical or other reasons.
>
> In conclusion, the court finds that the decision to move the applicant from Long Leys into alternative social care was not disproportionate, gave proper consideration to her interests and was supported by relevant and sufficient reasons relative to her welfare. It may therefore be regarded as 'necessary in a democratic society' in the pursuit of protecting her rights.
>
> It follows that the application must be rejected as manifestly ill-founded pursuant to Article 35(3) and (4) of the Convention.
>
> For these reasons, the court unanimously declares the application inadmissible.

16.38 *R (CH and MH) v Sutton and Merton PCT* [2004] EWHC 2984 (Admin), (2005) 8 CCLR 5

The court needed to consider for itself whether there was indeed an overriding public interest that justified resiling from a 'home for life' promise and whether, as was asserted, it was in the 'best interests' of residents to move

Facts: the PCT decided to close a long-stay hospital for incapacitated adults with severe learning disabilities, ultimately, having taken into account '*home for life*' promises, but having decided that it was in the best interests of those concerned to live in small groups in the community. The claimants brought judicial review proceedings and also best interests proceedings in the Family Division for a declaration as to what their best interests truly were. The PCT sought to stay the best interests proceedings whilst the claimants sought an order that those proceedings and the judicial review should be heard together.

Judgment: Wilson J acceded to the claimants' application, holding that:

1) The task of the court is to identify the nature and extent of the inquiry which the court is required to conduct in order to despatch the claims in a way that is proper and lawful. It has been already established that where a court accepts that a promise of a home for life has been made such that it can only permit the public authority to close the home if there is an overriding public interest, the question as to whether there is an over- riding public interest is one for the court. This issue needs to be actively resolved rather than measured from a distance.

2) Since the defendant's justification for closing the hospital and extricating itself from the home for life promise was an assertion that it was in the patients' best interests, the patients were entitled to challenge that. This is an area of dispute that the court must determine for itself on evidence and that meant almost certainly oral evidence. Any less intrusive inquiry into the validity of the defendant's assertion as to their best interests would be inadequate.

16.39 *R (Bishop) v Bromley LBC* [2006] EWHC 2148 (Admin), (2006) 9 CCLR 635

Prior assessments were only required in exceptional cases

Facts: Bromley decided to close a day care facility attached to a care home, subject to alternative day services being made available for current service users. The claimant, a daughter of one of the service users, contended that the decision was irrational and undertaken without first assessing her mother's needs.

Judgment: Deputy High Court Judge Parker refused permission to apply for judicial review, on the basis that Bromley had rational reasons for wanting to close this day care facility (cost and over-capacity) and this was not the exceptional type of case which require Bromley to fully assess all the service users' needs before reaching its decision (applying *R v North and East Devon Health Authority ex p Coughlan*[20] (see above para 16.27). Further, the likely impact was not such as to meet the Article 8 ECHR threshold.

20 [2001] QB 213, (1999) 2 CCLR 285.

16.40 *R (Morris) v Trafford Healthcare NHS Trust* [2006] EWHC 2334 (Admin), (2006) 9 CCLR 648

The failure to consult was unlawful but the grant of relief was not practical

Facts: Trafford decided to close inpatient wards at a local hospital.

Judgment: Hodge J held that the decision would be quashed because Trafford had not undertaken prior consultation, as required by section 11 of the Health and Social Care Act 2001. However, the court did not grant a mandatory order requiring Trafford to re-open the wards, in the light of an assurance from Trafford that it would very shortly undertake public consultation, which might lead to their re-opening.

16.41 *R (J) v Southend BC* [2005] EWHC 3457 (Admin), (2007) 10 CCLR 407

A local authority was entitled to assume that the needs of users of its day centre services, ordinarily resident elsewhere, would be assessed and met by the local authority of their ordinary residence

Facts: as a result of a re-organisation of its services, Southend decided to close one of its day centres for those ordinarily resident in adjacent authorities, subject to the provision of support services to enable friendship groups to be maintained. J and others (who were ordinarily resident in Essex) sought a judicial review on the ground that Southend had failed to undertake community care assessments, and that the decision would breach Article 8 ECHR.

Judgment: Newman J held Southend was entitled to proceed on the basis that Essex would assess the needs of persons ordinarily resident in Essex and that Essex would meet the needs of those persons; any interference with Article 8 rights was justified by the policy purpose of enhancing the autonomy of service users and by the mitigating steps proposed and, in any event, there had been undue delay in applying for judicial review.

16.42 *R (Wilson) v Coventry CC, R (Thomas) v Havering LBC* [2008] EWHC 2300 (Admin), (2009) 12 CCLR 7

The decision to close care homes was not incompatible with Article 2 on account of the risks to life and was otherwise lawful

Facts: Coventry and Havering resolved to close a number of care homes, occupied by elderly residents who suffered from dementia or were physically disabled. The claimants sought a judicial review on the basis that officers had failed adequately to communicate to decision-makers the risk of serious injury or death resulting from such closures, failed to undertake adequate assessments of individual residents prior to the decisions to close, (in the case of Havering) failed to communicate to decision-makers a fair assessment of the financial implications. The claimants also submitted that the decisions were incompatible with Article 2 ECHR.

Judgment: Deputy High Court Judge Pelling QC held that there was no requirement to undertake individual assessments before deciding to close a care home, that officers had fairly communicated to decision-makers the risks involved and the financial implications and that, having regard to the broad measure of judgment accorded to public authorities, there had not been any breach of Article 2 ECHR.

16.43 *R (Rutter) v Stockton on Tees BC* [2008] EWHC 2651 (Admin), (2009) 12 CCLR 27

Risks could be considered at Scrutiny stage and relief could be refused in all the circumstances

Facts: Stockton on Tees resolved to close a care home. Its report to Cabinet failed properly to draw attention to the risks involved, to the health and lives of residents, but those risks were then drawn to the attention of the Scrutiny committee. By the time of the hearing, only the claimant remained in residence, at substantial cost to the authority, and there was medical evidence that it was in her best interests to move elsewhere.

Judgment: Wilkie J dismissed the claimant's application for a judicial review of the closure decision, on the basis that the risks entailed by moving elsewhere had been considered by the authority, albeit belatedly and that, in any event, he would have refused relief in the light of the substantial cost to the authority of keeping the home open, the very small risk to the claimant's health which could be minimised by careful transfer arrangements and the existence of medical evidence that it was in the claimant's best interests to move.

16.44 *R (B) v Worcestershire CC* [2009] EWHC 2915 (Admin), (2010) 13 CCLR 13

The closure decision was based on irrational premises

Facts: Worcestershire decided to close a day centre for adults with severe physical and learning disabilities, on the basis that their needs could be met significantly more cheaply elsewhere.

Judgment: Stadlen J held that Worcestershire's decision was irrational because it was not based on a detailed analysis or evidence necessary to support a reasoned and rational decision that the claimants' needs could be met more cheaply elsewhere: the community care assessments did not sufficiently define the level of support needed, including what staff ratio was required.

16.45 *R (Boyejo) v Barnet LBC* [2009] EWHC 3261 (Admin), (2010) 13 CCLR 72

The discharge of the duty to consult and the disability equality assessment had been unlawful

Facts: Barnet and Portsmouth both separately decided to terminate certain on-site, live-in services for sheltered tenants, substituting a mobile night-service, with an alarm call system.

Judgment: Deputy High Court Judge Milwyn Jarman held that Portsmouth's consultation had been inadequate in that its consultation document spoke in terms of a decision already having been made, did not canvass alternative and failed sufficiently to involved disabled persons; also, the time afforded for representations was too short and Portsmouth failed to take proper account of the representations made. Additionally, neither Barnet nor Portsmouth had done sufficient to draw decision-makers' attention to the duty at section 49A of the Disability Discrimination Act 1995, nor to have specific regard to the impact on those residents with a disability (cf the residents in general) nor to take account that it might be necessary to treat such persons more favourably. Further, both authorities' conclusions, in their equalities impact assessments, that there would not be any adverse impact on residents, were *Wednesbury* unreasonable.

16.46 *Watts v United Kingdom* Application No 53586/09, (2010) 51 EHRR SE5

A carefully managed process of care home closure did not violate rights under Articles 2, 3 or 8 ECHR

Facts: Wolverhampton decided to close the local authority care home in which Ms Watts resided, because it did not make cost-effective provision. Ms Watts was not successful in opposing her move to alternative residential accommodation in the UK courts so applied to the European Court of Human Rights.

Judgment: the European Court of Human Rights declared the application inadmissible on the basis that i) while Article 2 ECHR was applicable, because a badly managed transfer of an elderly care home resident could well have a negative impact on their life expectancy, on the facts of this case, including the care planning undertaken by Wolverhampton, the authorities had plainly discharged their positive obligation under Article 2 to safeguard individuals from a real and immediate risk to life; ii) while the court was content to proceed on the basis that the transfer another care home interfered with Ms Watt's private life, that interference had plainly been justified and proportionate in that there had been extensive consultation and consideration of safe management procedures, so as to minimise the adverse effects of any move, whilst there were reasons for closure based on resource allocation which required a wide margin of appreciation to be afforded.

16.47 *R (Broadway Care Centre Ltd) v Caerphilly CBC* [2012] EWHC 37 (Admin), (2012) 15 CCLR 82

A decision to terminate a framework contract was contractual and not amenable to judicial review, neither did it infringe ECHR rights

Facts: as a result of performance-related concerns, Caerphilly terminated its framework contract with Broadway for the provision of care home places. Broadway applied for a judicial review, on the ground that Caerphilly's decision amounted to a decision to close its care home, and so it was unlawful in public law because of a lack of prior consultation with residents and because Caerphilly failed to have regard to the welfare of residents and, also because it was in breach of the residents' rights under Article 8 ECHR and Broadway's rights under Article 1 of the 1st Protocol ECHR.

Judgment: Deputy High Court Judge Seys Llewellyn dismissed the application, holding that Caerphilly was not amenable to judicial review because it had exercised a contractual power, that Broadway did not have standing to complain about potential breaches of residents' ECHR rights, that Article 1 of the 1st Protocol ECHR was not engaged because Caerphilly had not resolved to close Broadway's care home and that, in any event, Broadway's claims were not well-founded factually.

16.48 *R (LH) v Shropshire Council* [2014] EWCA Civ 404, (2014) 17 CCLR 216

A local authority was entitled to consult in general terms on a policy change, if it then consulted before closing individual services. Where a day centre had closed and its staff had been dispersed, no relief would be granted in relation to an unlawful closure process

Facts: Shropshire consulted widely on a policy change, that would lead away from the provision of day centres and focus on individualised budgets, in order to make necessary budgetary savings and, also, to promote central government policy. Afterwards, Shropshire identified a number of day centres that would actually have to close.

Judgment: the Court of Appeal (Longmore, McFarlane and Lewison LJJ) held that Shropshire had been under a common law duty to consult, by reason of its duty to act fairly. The consultation it had undertaken was amply sufficient to justify its policy change, but fairness also required there to be consultation before making a decision to close an individual day centre and that had not occurred. However, given the closure of the day centre and the dispersal of its staff, the only relief granted would be declaratory.

16.49 *R (Michael Robson) v Salford CC* [2013] EWHC 3481 (Admin), (2014) 17 CCLR 474

The court summarised consultation principles and concluded that in substance consultees had been adequately informed about what was proposed and that the PSED had been lawfully discharged

Facts: Salford decided to cease direct provision of transport services in order to achieve budgetary savings. In future, it would make individual transport arrangements for each eligible adult through a variety of different means, such as a 'ring and ride' service, taxis and motability vehicles. The claimants, who were both severely disabled, challenged this decision by way of judicial review.

Judgment: Deputy High Court Judge Stephen Davies dismissed the application for judicial review, holding that there was no evidence that the result of Salford's decision would be that Salford would fail to meet eligible needs for transport and the consultation duty and PSED had been discharged. Deputy High Court Judge Davies said this about consultation:

> 53. The claimants contend that the defendant was obliged at common law to undertake a proper consultation with those affected before taking the decision to withdraw the PTU service and replace it with individualised transport arrangements. The claimants contend that this duty is an aspect

of the overarching common law duty to act in a procedurally fair manner. They rely on the decision of the Court of Appeal in *R v Devon CC ex p Baker* [1995] 1 All ER 73 in support of that proposition. They also draw my attention to the observations of Lord Reed JSC in *Osborn v Parole Board* [2013] 3 WLR 1020 at paragraphs 64–72 to emphasise first that fairness is for the court and not for the decision-maker to decide, and second his explanation of the benefits to be gained from procedurally fair decision-making. As to what is required in terms of consultation, they refer me to the well known statement of Lord Woolf MR, in *R v North & East Devon HA ex p Coughlan* [2001] QB 213 at paragraph 108, where he said that:

> *It is common ground that whether or not consultation of interested parties and the public is a legal requirement, if it is embarked upon it must be carried out properly. To be proper, consultation must be undertaken at a time when proposals are still at a formative stage; it must include sufficient reasons for particular proposals to allow those consulted to give intelligent consideration and an intelligent response; adequate time must be given for this purpose; and the product of consultation must be conscientiously taken into account when the ultimate decision is taken:* R v Brent LBC ex p Gunning *(1985) 84 LGR 168.*

54. They also refer me to the analysis of the Court of Appeal, given by Arden LJ, in *R (Royal Brompton & Harefield NHS Foundation Trust) v Joint Committee of Primary Care Trusts* [2012] EWCA Civ 472 at paragraphs 8–14. In particular they emphasise the requirement that the consultation document must present the issues in a way that facilitates an effective response, and in a way which is clear to the general body of consultees, the requirement that the available information must be presented fairly and not inaccurately, and that the unfairness need only be shown to affect a group of those affected by the consultation, as opposed to all of them.

55. Mr Greatorex in his submissions did not quarrel with the above as statements of principle. He also however emphasised paragraph 13 of the judgment in *Royal Brompton*, where Arden LJ referred to the observations of Sullivan J (as he then was) in the *Greenpeace* case, to the effect that clear unfairness must be shown, and that the error must show that there has been no proper consultation, and that something has gone clearly and radically wrong with the consultation process. He also referred me to the very recent decision of the Court of Appeal in *Rusal v London Metal Exchange* [2014] EWCA Civ 1271, where Arden LJ again summarised the law relating to consultation, and also stated (at paras 51–53) that the court should not ignore information which on the evidence was well known to the consultees anyway, even if not expressly referred to in the consultation document.

...

62. I was taken by Mr Wise QC and Mr Suterwalla to section 149, who emphasised:

> (1) the mandatory nature of the obligation imposed by the section; (2) the specific obligation to have due regard to the need to take steps to meet the different needs of (in this case) disabled adults from non-disabled adults and, in particular, to take steps which take account of disabled adults' disabilities. As to point (2), they submitted that this was far from being a vague or a general exhortation, but a hard edged requirement to have regard to the need to identify how the needs of disabled adults differed from those of non-disabled adults and to ascertain what steps could and should be undertaken to meet those needs.

63. I was also referred by them to the decision of the Divisional Court in *Brown v Secretary of State for Work & Pensions* [2008] EWHC 3158 (Admin), where Aikens LJ: (a) held that the obligation to have 'due regard' meant to have proper and appropriate regard for the goals set out in the (predecessor) section (para 82); (b) held that in order to comply with that obligation it was necessary to have due regard to the need to gather relevant information (para 85); (c) identified a number of relevant principles as to how that duty should be fulfilled in practice, including a duty to exercise the duty in substance, as opposed to box ticking, with rigour and with an open mind (paras 90–96).

64. I was also referred by Mr Wise QC and Mr Suterwalla to the decision of the Court of Appeal in *R (Bracking) v Secretary of State for Work & Pensions* [2013] EWCA Civ 1345 and, in particular, the 8 relevant principles identified by McCombe LJ at paragraph 26 of his judgment. The claimants particularly emphasised: (a) principle 4, the need to assess the risk and extent of any adverse impact and means of elimination before adopting the policy and not as a rearguard action; (b) principle 6, the need to have specific conscious, as opposed to merely general, regard; (c) principle 8, the need for a proper and conscientious focus on the statutory criteria, and the need to make inquiry.

65. Mr Greatorex did not contest these principles. He did however remind me, by reference to these authorities, that it is a duty to have regard, not a duty to achieve a particular result, and that weight was a matter for the decision maker and not the court. He also referred me to the decision of the Court of Appeal in *Bailey v Brent LBC* [2011] EWCA Civ 1586, to the effect that: (a) the decision is a fact-sensitive one (para 83); (b) section 149 does not require the decision maker to speculate, investigate or explore *ad infinitum*, or to apply the degree of forensic analysis which a QC would deploy in court (para 102). He also submitted that, although recommended as advisable, there was no positive obligation to undertake or to record the result of a formal equality impact assessment, so that I should have regard to the totality of the process, and not limit myself to conducting a forensic analysis of the words used in the impact assessment.

66. Mr Greatorex also submitted that in a case such as the present, which was concerned exclusively with disabled persons, it could not possibly be said that the defendant had overlooked its duty to have due regard to the impact of its decision on disabled persons. Mr Wise QC and Mr Suterwalla countered by submitting that this illustrated the danger of adopting a general approach, as opposed to the focussed rigorous approach which was required, particularly by reference to the need to have due regard to the need to take mitigating steps.

Comment: the Court of Appeal dismissed the appeal (see below para 16.50).

16.50 *R (Michael Robson) v Salford CC* [2015] EWCA Civ 6

The consultation materials lacked clarity but overall consultees must have known what the proposal was and what the alternative were, so that the process had been fair; there may have been significant flaws in the community impact assessment but overall the PSED had been discharged

Facts: Salford decided to cease direct provision of transport services in order to achieve budgetary savings. In future, it would make individual transport arrangements for each eligible adult through a variety of different means, such as a 'ring and ride' service, taxis and motability vehicles.

The claimants, who were both severely disabled, challenged this decision by way of judicial review.

Judgment: the Court of Appeal (Richards and Treacey LJJ, Newey J) dismissed the claimants' appeal from the decision of Deputy High Court Judge Stephen Davies. They held that the consultation had been fair in that any sensible reader of the consultation booklet would have understood that the proposal involved the withdrawal of local authority transport services from those who were assessed as able to use alternative transport arrangements so that that issue had been fairly before the consultees:

> 32. I have not found it easy to reach a decision on this issue. The lack of clarity in the Council's internal documentation (see eg the description of the proposal in the report to Cabinet on 11 March 2014, quoted at paragraph 9 above) seems to have been carried over into the documentation prepared for the consultation. The consultation material presented an incomplete picture by concentrating on the proposed assessment of users of the PTU services to see if alternative transport options could be used, without a clear statement that it was proposed to close the PTU itself. In consequence, Mr Wise's submission that the Council failed to consult on the closure proposal and/or that the consultation material was misleading has considerable attraction to it. In the end, however, I have reached the conclusion that that is too formalistic an analysis and that the judge was right to concentrate on the proposed change of approach to transport arrangements for existing users and to find that the consultation process as a whole was not unfair.
>
> 33. What was important for users and their carers was not the continued existence of the PTU as such – as I have said in the context of the assessment issue, it was possible to provide the same service by other means – but the type of transport arrangements made in their case. They can have been left in no doubt that the purpose of the proposed assessments was to see if the existing service through the PTU could be replaced in each individual case by alternative arrangements. It was implicit that the PTU service would be withdrawn from those who were assessed as able to use alternative modes of transport. The reality of all this was brought home by the information that almost one half of users of the existing service were already being helped to get alternative transport to meet their needs.
>
> 34. In order to determine whether consultees were misled or were not consulted about the actual proposal, it is also necessary to have regard to the wider picture. In my view the judge was entitled to find that Mr Clemmett's witness statement was 'not sufficient to establish that those who conducted the personal visits to make the assessments were specifically tasked with making it clear to the users and their carers that the proposal *would* involve the closure of the PTU ...'. That finding did not involve the rejection of Mr Clemmett's evidence, which was unchallenged. It was simply a finding that his evidence was insufficiently detailed and specific to make good such a conclusion. Mr Clemmett's evidence taken as a whole (including the exhibited slides and media articles) does, however, provide some support for the view that consultees were aware that the proposal included closure of the PTU. The absence of any substantial evidence on behalf of the appellants that consultees were in fact misled is also highly material.
>
> 35. In *Moseley* the consultation material conveyed a positively misleading impression that other options were irrelevant. There is nothing equivalent to that in this case. In *Moseley* it was wrong to place reliance on consultees' assumed knowledge of other options for the same reason, that the message conveyed by the local authority was that other options were irrelevant.

Again there is no equivalent in this case, and in my view it was open to the judge to make the finding he did that any sensible reader of the consultation booklet would have understood that the proposal involved the withdrawal of the PTU service from those who were assessed as able to use alternative transport arrangements. More generally, there is nothing in *Moseley* to cast doubt on the correctness of the legal principles by reference to which the judge directed himself in this case. The judge's conclusion on the fundamental question, that the consultation was fair, was in my view a proper one for him to reach.

...

44. Mr Wise submits that the judge was wrong to reject the claimants' case on this issue. He took us through various passages of the Community Impact Assessment in order to illustrate his criticisms of it, covering the ground considered by the judge in the passages I have quoted from his judgment. For example, in Section A it is stated: 'We have helped users and their families to decide how users can best reach their destinations. Full travel assessments identify any risks and the support needed to remove or mitigate them ...'. Mr Wise submits that the actual assessments do *not* identify risks or the support needed to remove or mitigate them. He submits that Section C3, concerning the information from the consultation exercise, is hopelessly inadequate. For example, rather than containing an analysis of solutions, it refers to the need to take up points individually with people, should the proposal be agreed, 'to see if there are adequate solutions in place to meet the required need'; and instead of setting out support plans, it states that individual support plans 'would need to be in place for the 40 people concerned' should the proposal be agreed. He submits that Section D does not analyse the negative impact on people with a disability, or how it will be reduced or eliminated, and he criticises the lack of an evidence base for the assertion that people 'will have more choice, control and independence'; he also takes issue with the claimed absence of a negative outcome or impact for people on a low income. In relation to Section E he complains that it focuses on a reduction in the number of people needing specialist transport services where alternatives can be used, but it contains no analysis of negative impacts and in particular of circumstances where alternatives cannot be used.

45. In relation to the judge's reasoning in the paragraphs of his judgment quoted above, Mr Wise submits that the action plan referred to in paragraph 67 was not the gathering of necessary information; and the consultation exercise to which the judge refers did not gather all the necessary information because it was about the wrong thing. He submits that Section C was merely a statistical exercise and does not show that the Council conducted a careful analysis of the results of the consultation exercise, as the judge states in paragraph 68. The judge's reference to the process operating "at a relatively high level" is said to misunderstand the section 149 duty, which requires the matter to be approached with rigour. Mr Wise acknowledges that the case under section 149 does not call for a merits review but he stresses the nature of the procedural obligation under that section. He submits that, for reasons already touched on, the Council was *not* aware of the adverse impacts on disabled service users and could not therefore take steps to eliminate or mitigate them. For those and other reasons he argues that the judge was wrong to find that the Council complied with its section 149 duty.

46. For the Council, Mr Oldham makes the point that the case so advanced by Mr Wise goes significantly wider than the relevant ground of appeal,

which asserts simply that the errors in relation to the assessment issue and the consultation issue 'fundamentally undermined the Judge's approach to whether the Respondent had lawfully discharged its PSED because the Respondent was not properly informed about the potential consequences of its decision'. He submits that the Council did enough to gather relevant information; there was no duty in law to carry out an impact assessment at all (see *Brown*), but in any event the Community Impact Assessment was sufficient and it was not necessary to consider all the individual assessments at this stage of decision-making. Even if the points about inadequacy of analysis are open to the appellants, there is no reason why the degree of analysis contended for should be necessary. The judge's reasoning on this and on the PSED issue as a whole was correct.

47. I accept Mr Oldham's submissions. In my judgment the Council did have due regard to the matters identified in section 149 in relation to the disabled adults potentially affected by the decision to close the PTU. That largely follows from the conclusions I have reached on the assessment issue and the consultation issue. Through the carrying out of individual transport assessments and a lawful consultation exercise, it had obtained sufficient information to discharge the duty of inquiry for the purposes of section 149. The information obtained was analysed in the Community Impact Assessment. It may be that the imperfections of that document went even further than was acknowledged by the judge, but in my view he was entitled to find on the basis of the document taken as a whole that the Council had proper regard to the section 149 matters. I do not accept the submission that a greater degree of analysis was required. The judge was also right to look at the matter more widely, as he did in paragraph 71 of his judgment, and to find that in its decision-making process as a whole the Council was evidently aware of the potential adverse impacts on disabled adult service users and was actively considering steps to meet the needs of such persons and to eliminate, reduce or mitigate those impacts. It seems to me that everything the Council did to ensure the discharge of its duty towards those persons under section 2 of the Chronically Sick and Disabled Persons Act 1970 1970 also helped to ensure the discharge of its public sector equality duty towards them. The case advanced by Mr Wise does appear to me to go wider than the relevant ground of appeal but even if the full width of the case is entertained it should in my judgment fail.

Part IV

CHAPTER 17

Local authority general powers

17.1 **Introduction and statutory machinery**

Cases

17.11 *R (J) v Enfield LBC* [2002] EWHC 432 (Admin), (2002) 5 CCLR 434
Local authorities are under a duty to provide support under section 2 of the LGA 2000 in cases where, otherwise, the applicant's ECHR rights would be violated

17.12 *R (Theophilus) v Lewisham LBC* [2002] EWHC 1371 (Admin), [2002] ELR 719
An LEA could use section 2 of the LGA 2000 to provide student support where it lacked the power to do so under the relevant regulations

17.13 *R (W) v Lambeth LBC* [2002] EWCA Civ 613, (2002) 5 CCLR 203
A local social services authority could provide family accommodation under section 2 of the LGA 2000

17.14 *R (A and B) v East Sussex CC* [2002] EWHC 2771 (Admin), (2003) 6 CCLR 177
A local authority could use its power under section 2 of the LGA 2000 to make payments to a user independent trust

17.15 *R (Khan) v Oxfordshire CC* [2004] EWCA Civ 309, (2004) 7 CCLR 215
Unless there would otherwise be a breach of ECHR rights, a local authority could not provide accommodation under section 2 of the LGA 2000 to a person excluded from such accommodation by other legislation

17.16 *R (PB) v Haringey LBC* [2006] EWHC 2255 (Admin), (2007) 10 CCLR 99
A local social services authority could not use section 2 of the LGA 2000 to provide ordinary accommodation to a person to whom it was prohibited from providing accommodation under the Housing Acts

17.17 *R (Morris) v Westminster CC* [2005] EWCA Civ 1184, [2006] 1 WLR 505
Section 2 of the LGA 2000 could be used to provide accommodation that could not be provided under other legislation, so long as it was not used simply to circumvent that other legislation

17.18 *R (MK) v Barking and Dagenham LBC* [2013] EWHC 3486 (Admin)
Section 1 of the Localism Act 2011 could not be used to provide accommodation and support to a destitute individual, without children or care needs

17.19 *R (GS) v Camden LBC* [2016] EWHC 1762 (Admin), (2016) 19 CCLR 398
Section 1 of the Localism Act 2006 could be used to provide accommodation to a person not entitled to accommodation under the Care Act 2014 and had to be so used insofar as necessary to avoid the breach of a person's ECHR rights

Introduction and statutory machinery

17.1 The starting point is that local authorities have the power to do anything that is calculated to facilitate or that is conducive or incidental to the discharge of any of their functions, bestowed by section 111(1) of the Local Government Act 1972 ('the ancillary power').

17.2 Local authorities additionally had a 'general well-being power' ('GWP') under sections 2–4 of the Local Government Act (LGA) 2000, which is now retained for Welsh local authorities only.

17.3 English local authorities now have a 'general power of competence' ('GPC') under sections 1–8 of the Localism Act 2011, in addition to the ancillary power and instead of the GWP.

17.4 Sections 3 and 4 of the Localism Act 2011 contain provisions relating to charging, and the setting up of companies to enable local authorities to do things for commercial purposes, which are outside the scope of this book, which focuses on the provision of services to meet needs. As far as that is concerned, the position now is that a local authority can provide almost any type of care or welfare service, under section 1 of the Localism Act 2011, providing that what it does is not inconsistent with a 'prohibition, restriction or limitation' on its statutory powers, found elsewhere.

17.5 Thus:

- where there is a statutory lacuna, a local authority can exercise its GWP (in Wales) or GPC (in England) to provide a service;[1]
- that remains the position where, although there is no lacuna, existing functions only go so far, but no further: this is not the type of case generally considered to be one where statutory powers are subject to a 'limitation' but simply where they stop at a certain point[2] and, in any event, the GPC (or the GWP) is only excluded by an express limitation;[3]
- beyond that, however, the GWP and GPC are not intended to allow local authorities to take action that would frustrate a clear Parliamentary intent that such action should not be taken, evidenced by the existence of a statutory 'prohibition, restriction or limitation';[4]
- where there is no relevant 'prohibition, restriction or limitation' a local authority is required to exercise its GWP or GPC to avoid a breach of ECHR rights;[5]
- where there is a relevant 'prohibition, restriction or limitation' case-law has cast doubt on the power to use the GWP and GPC to avoid a breach of ECHR rights;[6]
- there is, however, an important distinction to be drawn between the GWP and the GPC in that a 'post commencement limitation' will only prevent the exercise of the GPC in cases where Parliament has explicitly stipulated that it must do so:

1 *R (Theophilus) v Lewisham LBC* [2002] EWHC 1371 (Admin), [2002] ELR 710.
2 *R (W) v Lambeth LBC* [2002] EWCA Civ 613, (2002) 5 CCLR 203.
3 See the terms of section 2(4) of the Localism Act 2011.
4 *R (Khan) v Oxfordshire CC* [2004] EWCA Civ 309, (2004) 7 CCLR 215.
5 *R (J) v Enfield LBC* [2002] EWHC 432 Admin, (2002) 5 CCLR 434.
6 *R (MK) v Barking and Dagenham LBC* [2013] EWHC 3486 (Admin).

- a 'post commencement limitation' only prevents the exercise of the GPC if it is 'expressly imposed' (section 2(4) of the Localism Act 2011); and
- a 'post commencement limitation' only prevents the exercise of the GPC if it is 'expressed to apply – (i) to the general power, (ii) to all of the authority's powers, or (iii) to all of the authority's powers but with exceptions that do not include the general power' (section 2(2) of the Localism Act.[7]

17.6 The principal relevant provisions of the LGA 2000 (applicable in Wales and, prior to the Localism Act 2011, in England) are as follows:

Promotion of well-being

2(1) Every local authority in Wales are to have power to do anything which they consider is likely to achieve any one or more of the following objects–

(a) the promotion or improvement of the economic well-being of their area,

(b) the promotion or improvement of the social well-being of their area, and

(c) the promotion or improvement of the environmental well-being of their area.

(2) The power under subsection (1) may be exercised in relation to or for the benefit of–

(a) the whole or any part of a local authority's area, or

(b) all or any persons resident or present in a local authority's area.

(3B) In determining whether or how to exercise the power under subsection (1), a local authority in Wales must have regard to the community strategy for its area published under section 39(4) of the Local Government (Wales) Measure 2009 or, where the strategy has been amended following a review under section 41 of that Measure, the strategy most recently published under section 41(6).

(3C) The community strategy for the area of a community council is the strategy referred to in subsection (3B) that is published by the county council or county borough council in whose area lies the community or communities for which the community council is established.

(4) The power under subsection (1) includes power for a local authority to–

(a) incur expenditure,

(b) give financial assistance to any person,

(c) enter into arrangements or agreements with any person,

(d) co-operate with, or facilitate or co-ordinate the activities of, any person,

(e) exercise on behalf of any person any functions of that person, and

(f) provide staff, goods, services or accommodation to any person.

(5) The power under subsection (1) includes power for a local authority to do anything in relation to, or for the benefit of, any person or area situated outside their area if they consider that it is likely to achieve any one or more of the objects in that subsection.

(6) Nothing in subsection (4) or (5) affects the generality of the power under subsection (1).

7 As noted in *R (GS) v Camden LBC* [2016] EWHC 1762 (Admin), (2016) 19 CCLR 398.

Limits on power to promote well-being

3(1) The power under section 2(1) does not enable a local authority to do anything which they are unable to do by virtue of any prohibition, restriction or limitation on their powers which is contained in any enactment (whenever passed or made).

(2) The power under section 2(1) does not enable a local authority to raise money (whether by precepts, borrowing or otherwise).

(3) The Welsh Ministers may by order make provision preventing local authorities from doing, by virtue of section 2(1), anything which is specified, or is of a description specified, in the order.

(3A) The power under subsection (3) may be exercised in relation to–

(a) all local authorities,

(b) particular local authorities, or

(c) particular descriptions of local authority.

(4) Subject to subsection (4A), before making an order under subsection (3), the Welsh Ministers must consult such representatives of local government and such other persons (if any) as he considers appropriate.

(4A) Subsection (4) does not apply to an order under this section which is made only for the purpose of amending an earlier order under this section–

(a) so as to extend the earlier order, or any provision of the earlier order, to a particular authority or to authorities of a particular description, or

(b) so that the earlier order, or any provision of the earlier order, ceases to apply to a particular authority or to authorities of a particular description.

(5) Before exercising the power under section 2(1), a local authority must have regard to any guidance for the time being issued by the Welsh Ministers about the exercise of that power.

(6) Before issuing any guidance under subsection (5), the Welsh Ministers must consult such representatives of local government and such other persons (if any) as he considers appropriate.

[...]

(8) In this section 'enactment' includes an enactment comprised in subordinate legislation (within the meaning of the Interpretation Act 1978).

17.8 The principal relevant provisions of the Localism Act 2011 are as follows:

Local authority's general power of competence

1(1) A local authority has power to do anything that individuals generally may do.

(2) Subsection (1) applies to things that an individual may do even though they are in nature, extent or otherwise–

(a) unlike anything the authority may do apart from subsection (1), or

(b) unlike anything that other public bodies may do.

(3) In this section *'individual'* means an individual with full capacity.

(4) Where subsection (1) confers power on the authority to do something, it confers power (subject to sections 2 to 4) to do it in any way whatever, including–

(a) power to do it anywhere in the United Kingdom or elsewhere,

(b) power to do it for a commercial purpose or otherwise for a charge, or without charge, and

(c) power to do it for, or otherwise than for, the benefit of the authority, its area or persons resident or present in its area.

(5) The generality of the power conferred by subsection (1) ('the general power') is not limited by the existence of any other power of the authority which (to any extent) overlaps the general power.

(6) Any such other power is not limited by the existence of the general power (but see section 5(2)).
(7) Schedule 1 (consequential amendments) has effect.

Boundaries of the general power

2(1) If exercise of a pre-commencement power of a local authority is subject to restrictions, those restrictions apply also to exercise of the general power so far as it is overlapped by the pre-commencement power.
(2) The general power does not enable a local authority to do–
(a) anything which the authority is unable to do by virtue of a pre-commencement limitation, or
(b) anything which the authority is unable to do by virtue of a post commencement limitation which is expressed to apply–
(i) to the general power,
(ii) to all of the authority's powers, or
(iii) to all of the authority's powers but with exceptions that do not include the general power.
(3) The general power does not confer power to–
(a) make or alter arrangements of a kind which may be made under Part 6 of the Local Government Act 1972 (arrangements for discharge of authority's functions by committees, joint committees, officers etc);
(b) make or alter arrangements of a kind which are made, or may be made, by or under Part 1A of the Local Government Act 2000(arrangements for local authority governance in England);
(c) make or alter any contracting-out arrangements, or other arrangements within neither of paragraphs (a) and (b), that authorise a person to exercise a function of a local authority.
(4) In this section–
'post-commencement limitation' means a prohibition, restriction or other limitation expressly imposed by a statutory provision that–
(a) is contained in an Act passed after the end of the Session in which this Act is passed, or
(b) is contained in an instrument made under an Act and comes into force on or after the commencement of section 1;
'pre-commencement limitation' means a prohibition, restriction or other limitation expressly imposed by a statutory provision that–
(a) is contained in this Act, or in any other Act passed no later than the end of the Session in which this Act is passed, or
(b) is contained in an instrument made under an Act and comes into force before the commencement of section 1;
'pre-commencement power' means power conferred by a statutory provision that–
(a) is contained in this Act, or in any other Act passed no later than the end of the Session in which this Act is passed, or
(b) is contained in an instrument made under an Act and comes into force before the commencement of section 1.

17.9 The limits of the GPC are explained in the Explanatory Note[8] to the legislation[9] at paragraphs 11 and 12 and there is a useful Parliamentary Briefing Note.[10]

8 Explanatory Notes are admissible aids to the construction of legislation: see *R v Montila* [2004] UKHL 50, [2001] 1 WLR 3141 at paras 32–36.
9 www.legislation.gov.uk/ukpga/2011/20/notes/contents.
10 http://ukbriefingpapers.co.uk/BriefingPaper/SN05687.

17.10 The Department of Communities and Local Government has published *A plain English guide to the Localism Act* (November 2011).[11] The Local Government Association has also published useful guidance.[12]

Cases

17.11 ***R (J) v Enfield LBC*** **[2002] EWHC 432 (Admin), (2002) 5 CCLR 434**

Local authorities are under a duty to provide support under section 2 of the LGA 2000 in cases where, otherwise, the applicant's ECHR rights would be violated

Facts: J was a destitute person from abroad, with a daughter, who was excluded from mainstream benefits but who had an outstanding application with the Secretary of State for the Home Department for leave to remain (LTR) (not invoking Article 3 ECHR). A feature of the case was that the Court of Appeal had determined (in a decision later over-turned) that section 17 of the Children Act 1989 did not empower local authorities to provide accommodation or assistance with accommodation – so it was necessary to identify an alternative source of housing.

Judgment: Elias J held that J was owed the duty in section 21 of the National Assistance Act (NAA) 1948 and that it had not been open to Enfield to conclude that her need for assistance was not 'imminent'. He also held, however, that the general 'well-being' power in section 2 of the LGA 2000 entitled Enfield to provide financial assistance to J and her child, to secure accommodation and support and if, as in this case, a failure to exercise the power would infringe ECHR rights, there was a duty to exercise it:

> 72. In my judgment the authority has not properly exercised its powers under section 21 of the NAA 1948. Its determination on that issue should be quashed and the matter should be reconsidered by it. Even if the authority concludes that it is not open to it to exercise its section 21 powers, it is able to provide the necessary financial support by way of a deposit and the payment towards the rent by invoking its powers under section 2 of the LGA 2000. If that is the only way in which it could avoid a breach of the claimant's Article 8 rights, then in my view it would be obliged to exercise its statutory discretion in that way. In the event, it is not in my view necessary to invoke either sections 3 or 4 of the HRA 1998.

17.12 ***R (Theophilus) v Lewisham LBC*** **[2002] EWHC 1371 (Admin), [2002] ELR 719**

An LEA could use section 2 of the LGA 2000 to provide student support where it lacked the power to do so under the relevant regulations

Facts: Lewisham assured Ms Theophilus that she qualified for student financial support to study for law degree at Griffith College, a privately funded institution, in Dublin. Ms Theophilus began the course and Lewisham started to pay her fees, but then stopped when it appreciated that the Education (Student Support) Regulations 2001 only permitted it to provide support for courses of study in the UK.

11 www.gov.uk/government/uploads/system/uploads/attachment_data/file/5959/1896534.pdf.

12 www.local.gov.uk/localism/localism-act.

Judgment: Silber J held that Lewisham had created a legitimate expectation on which Ms Theophilus had relied, that it would provide her with student support at Griffith College, and that Lewisham had acted unlawfully by ceasing to make provision without even considering the fact that it was in breach of a promise or the fact that, as was the case, Lewisham had the power to provide financial assistance akin to student support under section 2 of the LGA 2000.

17.13 *R (W) v Lambeth LBC* [2002] EWCA Civ 613, (2002) 5 CCLR 203

A local social services authority could provide family accommodation under section 2 of the LGA 2000

Facts: the issue was whether local authorities had power under section 17 of the Children Act 1989 to provide accommodation for intentionally homeless families.

Judgment: the Court of Appeal (Brooke, Laws and Keene LJ) held that local authorities did have such power but that, if that was wrong, local authorities had power under section 2 of the LGA 2000:

> 75. Because of the view we take of the meaning of section 17 of the 1989 Act it is unnecessary for us to consider, as Elias J felt obliged to, the appropriateness of section 2 as a vehicle for the powers W seeks to invoke, particularly where a local authority like Lambeth has not yet finalised their community strategy. Mr Goudie argued, however, that the power under section 2(1) would not be available to his clients because they would be unable to provide accommodation to W and her family because of the 'prohibition, restriction or limitation on their powers' (see section 3(1)), which is contained in sections 190(3) and 185 of the Housing Act 1996. The language of those provisions is, however, strikingly different from the language of section 122(5) of the IAA 1999 (see paragraph 68 above). Section 190(3), for example, merely provides that a local housing authority has a more limited duty in cases where an applicant is not found to have a priority need. It does not constitute a prohibition, restriction or limitation on their powers. In any event, even if a local housing authority's powers were indeed limited in the ways suggested by Mr Goudie, these provisions say nothing about the powers of social service authorities, and we can see nothing in section 3(1) to preclude a social service authority from providing financial help, or temporary accommodation, to the family of a child in need if they think fit.

17.14 *R (A and B) v East Sussex CC* [2002] EWHC 2771 (Admin), (2003) 6 CCLR 177

A local authority could use its power under section 2 of the LGA 2000 to make payments to a user independent trust

Facts: A and B were severely disabled sisters who continued to live in the family home, owing to a dispute with Sussex over aspects of the care package, in particular, as to the extent to which Sussex could be required to instruct carers to undertake manual lifting.

Judgment: Munby J held that the power, under section 29 of the National Assistance Act (NAA) 1948, to 'make arrangements' for the provision of relevant services, permitted payments to be made to a 'user independent trust' for the provision of care services; as did section 30(1) of the NAA 1948, section 111 of the LGA 1972 and section 2 of the LGA 2000.

17.15 *R (Khan) v Oxfordshire CC* [2004] EWCA Civ 309, (2004) 7 CCLR 215

Unless there would otherwise be a breach of ECHR rights, a local authority could not provide accommodation under section 2 of the LGA 2000 to a person excluded from such accommodation by other legislation

Facts: Ms Khan, a Pakistani national, had left her husband because of his domestic violence. Excluded from mainstream benefits, she sought local authority support under the NAA 1948, or section 2 of the LGA 2000.

Judgment: the Court of Appeal (Ward and Dyson LJJ, Sir Christopher Staughton) held that the local authority had concluded lawfully that Ms Khan did not have a need for 'care and attention' for the purposes of section 21 of the NAA 1948. However, whilst section 2 of the LGA 2000 did not allow the Council to provide or make payments for accommodation, because of the express bar on making such provision for Ms Khan in section 21(1A) of the NAA 1948, that did not preclude it providing assistance with essential living needs not related to accommodation, such as clothing:

> 16. By virtue of section 3(1):
>
> > 'The power under section 2(1) does not enable a local authority to do anything which they are unable to do by virtue of any prohibition, restriction or limitation on their powers which is contained in any enactment (whenever passed or made).'
>
> …
>
> 30. It is common ground that there is a distinction between the definition of the scope of a power and the imposition of a prohibition, restriction or limitation on the exercise of a power. This distinction was articulated by Mr Philip Sales and apparently accepted by Elias J in *R(J) v Enfield LBC* [2002] LGR 390 at paras 53–57. As Mr Lewis points out in his skeleton argument, statutes frequently confer power on authorities to do specific acts in respect of specific categories of persons. The definition of the scope of a power by reference to particular criteria does not involve the imposition of a prohibition, restriction or limitation on the doing of an act in respect of person outside the scope of the criteria. Rather, the fact that the authority cannot do the act in such circumstances reflects the fact that it has not been given the power to act, and not that it has been prohibited from doing so, or subjected to any limitation or restriction.
>
> …
>
> 41. The effect of section 3(1) is to prohibit the doing of 'anything' which a local authority is unable to do by virtue of any prohibition on its powers contained in any enactment. In the present context, the "thing" which is under consideration is the provision of residential accommodation to persons who, but for the prohibition in section 21(1A), would be entitled to accommodation under section 21(1)(a). It is that 'thing' which the local authority is prohibited from providing by section 21(1A), and which it cannot provide under any other statutory power, unless it can do so under section 2. But the very reason why section 3(1) was enacted was to prevent section 2 being used to do that which is prohibited by another statute. If Mr Jay were right, it would seem that no statutory prohibition would trump

section 2 of the LGA unless it stated expressly that it was a prohibition for the purposes of section 3 of the LGA. An example of such a provision is to be found in para 1(2) to Schedule 3 to the Nationality and Asylum Act 2002. This provides that 'a power or duty under a provision referred to in subparagraph (1) may not be exercised or performed in respect of a person to whom this paragraph applies'. One of the provisions referred to in subparagraph (1) is section 2 of the LGA.

...

46. It is difficult to believe that Parliament intended to prohibit the direct provision of accommodation to persons like Mrs Khan, but not to prohibit its indirect provision by the giving of financial assistance for the securing of such accommodation. Mr Jay has not suggested that Parliament would have had any rational basis for drawing such a distinction, and no material has been place before the court to suggest that this is what Parliament in fact wanted to do. His point is quite simply that there is no power in section 21(1)(a) to give financial assistance, and the prohibition in section 21(1A) cannot apply to an activity which section 21(1)(a) does not empower.

The Court of Appeal did, however, point out that if Ms Khan or some other applicant was able to establish that a failure to provide accommodation and support would violate their rights under the ECHR, then the underlying legislation would have to be construed differently, so that it did not impose a bar on provision.

17.16 *R (PB) v Haringey LBC* [2006] EWHC 2255 (Admin), (2007) 10 CCLR 99

A local social services authority could not use section 2 of the LGA 2000 to provide ordinary accommodation to a person to whom it was prohibited from providing accommodation under the Housing Acts

Facts: Ms PB was an unlawful overstayer, with an outstanding application for LTR under a child concession policy: she had five children and, although one lived with the father and four were in foster care and subject to care proceedings, she had regular contact with them all. Ms PB was destitute but Haringey refused to provide her with accommodation under section 21 of the NAA 1948, in part on the ground that the sole cause of her need for 'care and attention' was destitution and/or its physical effects.

Judgment: Deputy High Court Judge Nicol allowed the application for judicial review on the basis that Haringey's refusal of accommodation under section 21 of the NAA 1948 was legally flawed. However, he also held that, given the express prohibitions on the provision of accommodation under section 21 of the Housing Act 1985 and Parts 6 and 7 of the Housing Act 1996, Haringey could not have provided Ms PB with housing or housing assistance under section 2 of the LGA 2000.

17.17 *R (Morris) v Westminster CC* [2005] EWCA Civ 1184, [2006] 1 WLR 505

Section 2 of the LGA 2000 could be used to provide accommodation that could not be provided under other legislation, so long as it was not used simply to circumvent that other legislation

Facts: Ms Morris was a British citizen but, because her daughter was not, they were excluded from housing assistance when homeless, under the provisions of Part 7 of the Housing Act 1996.

Judgment: the Court of Appeal (Auld, Sedley and Jonathan Parker LJJ, Jonathan Parker LJ dissenting) held that the exclusion was a violation of rights under Articles 8 and 14 ECHR. Pending the government amending that legislation, alternative provision could be used, potentially:

> 68. In *R (Hooper) v Secretary of State for Work and Pensions* [2005] 1 WLR 1681 the House of Lords had to consider, among other things, whether admittedly unjustified sex discrimination in the statutory provision for payment of certain benefits was prevented by section 6(2)from being cured by the making of equivalent ex gratia payments. The House unanimously held that the common law power of the Crown to make such payments was shielded by section 6(2), so as to afford the Crown a defence to a claim under sections 6(1) and 7(1) for failing to make such payments. Lord Hoffmann pointed out, at para 49, that unlike section 6(2)(a), which protects acts which are necessary in order to give effect to legislation, section 6(2)(b) 'assumes that the public authority could have acted differently but nevertheless excludes liability if it was giving effect to a statutory provision which cannot be read as Convention-compliant'. Lord Hoffmann went on to explain, at para 51:
>
> > 'If legislation cannot be read compatibly with Convention rights, a public authority is not obliged to subvert the intention of Parliament by treating itself as under a duty to neutralise the effect of the legislation.'
>
> 69. The description Lord Hoffmann gave to the effect of section 6(2)(b) on the decision not to pay ex gratia was that it 'immunised' the decision against a section 6(1) challenge- not that it, any more than section 6(2)(a), either forbade or demanded such a decision. Lord Hope, agreeing, approached section 6(2) as creating two exceptions to the general rule set out in section 6(1), both designed to protect Parliamentary sovereignty where interpretation in accordance with section cannot produce compliance. He recognised that paragraph (b) was addressed to the exercise of discretions, whether founded in statute or common law. He focused on exercises of discretion which are designed to give effect to non-compatible provisions of primary legislation (see paras 72, 73), whereas the present argument is about exercises of discretion designed to compensate for such non-compatible provisions. Nevertheless, what Lord Hope said at para 73 is of general application:
>
> > 'If the defence was not there the authority would have no alternative but to exercise its discretion in a way that was compatible with the Convention rights. The power would become a duty to act compatibly with the Convention, even if to do so was plainly in conflict with the intention of Parliament.'
>
> 70. Neither this decision of their Lordships, nor their contemporaneous decision in *R (Wilkinson) v Inland Revenue Comrs* [2005] 1 WLR 1718, supports Mr Bhose's strong argument that a public authority is precluded by the Human Rights Act 1998 or by the common law from using one of its statutory powers to assist a person whom it has been obliged to refuse under another of its statutory powers or duties. (We have not heard argument on the possibility, rejected by Elias J in *R (J) v Enfield London Borough Council* [2002] LGR 390, that section 3 of the Local Government Act 2000 does forbid such a use of section 2.) It would take a great deal to persuade me that this was right: it would mean, among other things, taking away a range of discretions which Parliament itself has given to public authorities,

and turning every application for help into a once-for-all gamble, dependant upon which power the applicant has decided to invoke. It is also an argument which has nothing logically to do with Convention-compatibility. What *Hooper's* case [2005] 1 WLR 1681 does in my respectful view establish is that a power to make alternative provision does not become a duty simply because the principal power is subject to statutory restrictions which are incompatible with Convention rights.

71. By parity of reasoning, all such powers remain in being. But is it then open to the public authority in whom they are vested, if minded to do so, to use them for the purpose of circumventing or replacing the non-compliant one? Once the purpose of section 6(2) is recognised as being the preservation of Parliamentary sovereignty, the answer must be no. Such a use of power would have an illicit purpose. Thus a local authority which resolved to use section 17(6) of the Children Act 1989 in all cases which fell foul of section 185(4) of the Housing Act 1996 would in my judgment be abusing its powers.

72. It is therefore in the triangle formed by these three points that the lawful exercise of powers such as those cited by Mr McGuire lies. The local authority (a) is not obliged but (b) is permitted to use its alternative powers, so long as (c) it does not exercise them with the object simply of circumventing restrictions- even restrictions which are incompatible with Convention rights- built into the impugned power. Once in this space, the exercise of each discretion will be subject to the familiar requirements of public law, but that is all.

73. One of these- the requirement to take all relevant matters into account- will, however, in Mr McGuire's submission, require the authority in considering whether to exercise each of the alternative powers he relies on to have in mind and give weight to the fact that the condition which has shut the applicant out of priority need status is non compliant with the Convention. I do not think this is right. What the authority needs to have regard to is the obligation under section to interpret its alternative powers, so far as possible, compatibly with the Convention rights, and its duty under section 6(1) not to exercise those alternative powers incompatibly with the Convention rights. These powers are by definition different from the provision which has been declared incompatible. If in exercising them the authority is not entitled, short of being required to do so by statute, to hold against Mr Badu his child's immigration status, that will be because of section 6(1), not section 4, of the Human Rights Act 1998. In other words the incompatibility of section 185(4) with the Convention rights will not be legally relevant to the potential use of the surrogate powers.

17.18 *R (MK) v Barking and Dagenham LBC* [2013] EWHC 3486 (Admin)

Section 1 of the Localism Act 2011 could not be used to provide accommodation and support to a destitute individual, without children or care needs

Facts: Ms MK was an unlawful overstayer, who had become homeless. She sought accommodation and support under section 17 of the Children Act 1989, or under section 1 of the Localism Act 2011. However, she was not a child, or a former relevant child, nor did she care for a child. Barking and Dagenham refused to provide her with support.

Judgment: Deputy High Court Judge Bidder dismissed Ms MK's application for judicial review, on the basis that she did not fall within section 17 and on the basis that section 1 of the Localism Act 2011 did not enable

Barking and Dagenham to provide support because there was a pre-commencement restriction or limitation on its powers, found in section 17 of the Children Act 1989 (in that support under that provision had to be for the purpose of safeguarding and promoting the welfare of children), and also in section 21 of the NAA 1948 and section 185 of the Housing Act 1985. He also held that neither *Limbuela*[13] nor *Clue*[14] imposed a free-standing duty to provide support.

Comment: it seems questionable whether this decision would have survived an appeal to the Court of Appeal. In any event, this decision now seems marginalised by the next judgment, at least in cases not involving the Care Act 2014, rather than the Children Act 1989.

17.19 *R (GS) v Camden LBC* [2016] EWHC 1762 (Admin), (2016) 19 CCLR 398

Section 1 of the Localism Act 2011 could be used to provide accommodation to a person not entitled to accommodation under the Care Act 2014 and had to be so used insofar as necessary to avoid the breach of a person's ECHR rights

Facts: GS was a Swiss national of Afghan origin who suffered from a number of fairly severe physical and mental health problems and had become homeless and without the means to support herself but unable to bring herself to return to Switzerland. She was excluded from all forms of mainstream benefits apart from Personal Independence Payments, which she received.

Judgment: Mr Peter Marquand sitting as a Deputy High Court Judge held that, on the particular facts, it had been lawful for Camden to conclude that GS had not required 'care and support' for the purposes of the Care Act 2014 and that a need simply for accommodation did not amount to a need for 'care and support' (applying *R (SG) v Haringey LBC* [2015] EWHC 2579 (Admin), (2015) 18 CCLR 444). However, the Judge went on to hold that section 1 of the Localism Act 2011 empowered Camden to provide GS with accommodation and that it was, on the facts, required to do so to avoid a breach of her rights under the ECHR resulting from her homelessness and lack of sufficient means to support herself. In particular, the Judge distinguished *R (MK) v Barking and Dagenham LBC* [2003] EWHC 3486 (Admin), on the basis that because the Care Act 2014 post-dated the Localism Act 2011, the very broad power in section 1 of the Localism Act 2011 was not excluded because the Care Act 2014 did not include a 'post commencement limitation', as defined in section 2(2) and (4) of the Localism Act 2011, that is, 'a prohibition, restriction or other limitation expressly imposed by a statutory provision' that is 'expressed to apply – (i) to the general power, (ii) to all of the authority's powers, or (iii) to all of the authority's powers but with exceptions that do not include the [illegible] power'.

…*imbuela) v Secretary of State for the Home Department* [2005] UKHL 66, [2006] 1 … 396, (2006) 9 CCLR 30.

…*mingham City Council v Clue* [2010] EWCA Civ 460, (2010) 13 CCLR 276.

CHAPTER 18

National Health Service provision

continued

18.31 *Sentges v The Netherlands* Application no 27677/02, (2004) 7 CCLR 400

The margin of appreciation was so wide in medical cases, especially in relation to the allocation of scarce healthcare resources, that it could not be said that the refusal to supply a robotic arm, in the context of the provision of other services, was incompatible with Article 8 ECHR

18.32 *Glass v United Kingdom* Application no 61827/00, (2005) 8 CCLR 16

The imposition of treatment on a child in defiance of his mother's interests and without seeking Court relief was incompatible with Article 8 ECHR

18.33 *van Kuck v Germany* Application no 35968/97, (2005) 8 CCLR 121

It was incompatible with Articles 6 and 8 ECHR to decline to fund gender re-assignment surgery on the basis of an incorrect understanding of the medical evidence

18.34 *Pentiacova v Moldova* Application no 14462/03, (2005) 40 EHRR SE23

It was not a breach of the ECHR radically to reduce haemodialysis provision, notwithstanding the suffering occasioned

18.35 *R (Watts) v Bedford PCT* [2006] QB 667

Faced with unacceptable delay a patient was entitled to recover the cost of speedier medical treatment in another member state

18.36 *R (Gunter) v South Western Staffordshire PCT* [2005] EWHC 1894 (Admin), (2006) 9 CCLR 121

The NHS decision to refuse services was vitiated by its failure to appreciate that it could fund a user independent trust and the importance of the patient's home life

18.37 *R (Ann Marie Rogers) v Swindon NHS PCT* [2006] EWCA Civ 392, (2006) 9 CCLR 451

Unless resources were problematic, it was irrational to accord patients different entitlement on any other than clinical grounds

18.38 *Tysiac v Poland* Application no 5410/03, (2007) 45 EHRR 42

The absence of clear procedures for determining eligibility for an abortion and resolving disputes was incompatible with Article 8 ECHR

18.39 *R (Otley) v Barking and Dagenham NHS PCT* [2007] EWHC 1927 (Admin), (2007) 10 CCLR 628

The reasons for declining to fund cancer treatment, in this case, were irrational

18.40 *R (Colin Ross) v West Sussex PCT* [2008] NLJR 1297, (2008) 11 CCLR 767

The reasons for declining cancer treatment manifested a failure properly to understand relevant matters

18.41 *R (Harrison and Garnham) v Secretary of State for Health* [2009] EWHC 574 (Admin), (2009) 12 CCLR 355

The NHS was not entitled to make direct payments

18.42 *R (Booker) v NHS Oldham* [2010] EWHC 2593 (Admin), (2011) 14 CCLR 315

The NHS was required to provide healthcare even for treatment covered by a personal injury award of damages designed to enable private healthcare to be purchased

18.43 *MAK and RK v United Kingdom* Application nos 45901/05 and 40146/06, (2010) 13 CCLR 241

Disproportionate actions by a hospital doctor, resulting in his erroneously concluding that parents had abused their daughter, were incompatible with Article 8 ECHR

18.44 *R (Condliff) v North Staffordshire PCT* [2011] EWCA Civ 910, (2011) 14 CCLR 656

The PCT was entitled to take into account only clinical factors and to disregard the social factors said to justify exceptional treatment

18.45 *Rabone v Pennine Care NHS Foundation Trust* [2012] UKSC 2, (2012) 15 CCLR 13

Hospitals are under a duty imposed by Article 2 ECHR to protect both detained and voluntary mental patients against a real and immediate risk of suicide

18.46 *R (JF) v NHS Sheffield Clinical Commissioning Group* [2014] EWHC 1345 (Admin)

It had not been unlawful to provide ward monitoring and supervision to a person who received 1:1 supervision 24 hours a day whilst at home, under NHS continuing healthcare

18.47 *R (Whapples) v Birmingham Crosscity Clinical Commissioning Group* [2015] EWCA Civ 435, (2015) 18 CCLR 300

The NHS continuing healthcare framework did not in general contemplate payment of housing costs associated with the patient's own home, even when the patient received treatment there

18.48 *Daniel v St George's Healthcare NHS Trust, London Ambulance Service* [2016] EWHC 23 (QB)

Medical practitioners and prison staff were required by the ECHR to do all that could reasonably be expected of them to avoid a real and immediate risk to life of which they have or ought to have knowledge

18.49 *R (Dyer) v Welsh Ministers and others* [2015] EWHC 3712 (Admin), (2016) 19 CCLR 84

The NHS in Wales had not been in breach of duty under section 3 of the National Health Service (Wales) Act 2006, by providing hospital accommodation for a woman with a complex mental health condition in England because of the lack of appropriate accommodation in Wales

18.50 *S (A Child) v NHS England* [2016] EWHC 1395 (Admin), (2016) 19 CCLR 336

On the facts, the decision not to fund narcolepsy treatment for a 17-year-old child had disregarded relevant considerations and applied too stringent a test of exceptionality

Social care and NHS continuing healthcare: cases and complaints

18.51 *R v North and East Devon Health Authority ex p Coughlan* (1999) 2 CCLR 285

Local authorities were only empowered to provide nursing services to adults that were merely incidental or ancillary to the provision of residential accommodation and that were of a nature that a social services authority can be expected to provide

continued

18.52 The Health Service Ombudsman's Report on NHS funding for long term care (13 February 2003)
NHS bodies had wrongly been declining to provide NHS continuing healthcare and needed to review their policies and redress the hardship caused

18.53 Complaint No E22/03 against the former Cambridgeshire Health Authority and South Cambridgeshire Primary Care Trust (The *Pointon* Case) (November 2003)
Mr Pointon had wrongly been refused NHS continuing healthcare because the NHS focussed unduly and inappropriately on the fact that he was receiving care at home and on physical problems, rather than psychological problems and the special skills needed to cater for them

18.54 The Health Service Ombudsman's NHS funding for long term care: follow up report (HC 144) (16 December 2004)
More needed to be done to revise eligibility criteria and provide redress

18.55 *R (T) v Haringey LBC* [2005] EWHC 2235 (Admin), (2006) 9 CCLR 58
Local authorities were not empowered to provide healthcare services to children

NHS continuing healthcare: cases and complaints

18.56 *R v North and East Devon Health Authority ex p Coughlan* [2001] QB 213, (1999) 2 CCLR 285, CA
Local authorities were only empowered to provide nursing services to adults that were merely incidental or ancillary to the provision of residential accommodation and that were of a nature that a social services authority can be expected to provide

18.57 *R (Gunter) v South Western Staffordshire PCT* [2005] EWHC 1894 (Admin), (2006) 9 CCLR 121
The NHS decision to refuse services was vitiated by its failure to appreciate that it could fund a user independent trust and the importance of the patient's home life

18.58 *R (Grogan) v Bexley NHS Care Trust* [2006] EWHC 44 (Admin), (2006) 9 CCLR 188
A person may be entitled to NHS continuing healthcare notwithstanding that their needs could be met in local authority residential accommodation if the services of a registered nurse were provided by the NHS

18.59 *R (St Helens BC) v Manchester PCT* [2008] EWCA Civ 931, (2008) 11 CCLR 774
Decisions as to whether a person was entitled to NHS continuing healthcare or local authority social care were to be made by the NHS bodies and any judicial review by a local authority would be on a conventional and not a merits basis

18.60 *R (Green) v South West Strategic Health Authority* [2008] EWHC 2576 (Admin), (2009) 12 CCLR 93
On their proper construction, the health authority's policy guidance did correctly incorporate the 'primary health need' test, which it properly applied

18.61 *Secretary of State for Work and Pensions v Slavin* [2011] EWCA Civ 1515, (2012) 15 CCLR 354
Although in receipt of NHS continuing healthcare, the patient was not receiving 'treatment' and so was entitled to retain the mobility component of his DLA

18.62 *R (Dennison) v Bradford Clinical Commissioning Group* [2014] EWHC 2552 (Admin)

The CCG had been wrong to refuse to review a nursing home resident's eligibility for NHS continuing healthcare during a period covered by two flawed assessments

18.63 *R (JF) v NHS Sheffield Clinical Commissioning Group* [2014] EWHC 1345 (Admin)

It had not been unlawful to provide ward monitoring and supervision to a person who received 1:1 supervision 24 hours a day while at home, under NHS continuing healthcare

18.64 *R (Whapples) v Birmingham Crosscity Clinical Commissioning Group* [2015] EWCA Civ 435, (2015) 18 CCLR 300

The NHS continuing healthcare framework did not in general contemplate payment of housing costs associated with the patient's own home, even when the patient received treatment there

18.65 *National Aids Trust v National Health Service Commissioning Board (NHS England)* [2016] EWHC 2005 Admin, (2016) 19 CCLR 459

NHS England had the power to commission and anti-retroviral drug to be used on a preventative basis for those at high risk of contracting HIV

Health care and persons subject to immigration control

18.66 *R v Hammersmith Hospitals NHS Trust ex p Reffell* (2001) 4 CCLR 371, CA

The Trust had been required to make a charge and rationally required an up-front deposit, since Mr Reffell was not prevented from securing treatment in his country of origin

18.67 *R (YA) v Secretary of State for Health* [2009] EWCA Civ 225, (2009) 12 CCLR 213

It was not lawful to require up-front deposits from failed asylum-seekers who were unable to pay for medical treatment and who needed timeous treatment but were unable to leave the UK

18.68 *R (W, X, Y, Z) v Secretary of State for Health, Secretary of State for the Home Department* [2015] EWCA Civ 1034

It was lawful for the NHS to inform the Secretary of State for the Home Department about unpaid NHS debts of overseas visitors

18.1 The National Health Service Act (NHSA) 2006 and the National Health Service (Wales) Act (NHS(W)A) 2006 are the two principal Acts. They have, however, been hugely amended and supplemented by the Health and Social Care Act 2012.

NHS bodies and their roles

18.2 The Secretary of State for Health has overall responsibility for the NHS and plays a key strategic role, particularly by setting the annual NHS Mandate for England.

18.3 NHS England is the operational name of the National Health Service Commissioning Board, which was created by section 9 of the Health and Social Care Act 2012. It licenses and to some extent manages Clinical Commissioning Groups. It also commissions a range of specialist NHS services, pursuant to NHSA 2006 ss1H and 3A including:

i) primary care (from GPs, which are almost entirely private sector businesses);
ii) dental services (which are almost entirely private sector businesses);
iii) prison health services;
iv) medical services for the armed forces;
v) services for patients with rare conditions; and
vi) a range of specialised, tertiary acute services (eg high security psychiatric services).

18.4 Clinical Commissioning Groups are corporate bodies created by section 10 of the Health and Social Care Act 2012, comprised of local GPs who hold NHS commissioning contracts with NHS England, whose function is to commission a range of acute and community NHS services for patients within its area of responsibility, other than the primary care, dental and specialist services commissioned by NHS England. Provision is largely made by NHS Trusts and NHS Foundation Trusts (which are intended shortly wholly to replace NHS Trusts).

18.5 Local authorities (unitary authorities or county councils) became responsible for public health commissioning, by virtue of sections 29-31 of the Health and Social Care Act 2012.

18.6 There are also numerous regulatory bodies:

- the Care Quality Commission[1] oversees the provision of safe, effective, compassionate and high quality care in hospitals, care homes, dental and GP surgeries and all other care services in England;
- NHS Improvement[2] brings together Monitor, the NHS Trust Development Agency and the Patient Safety elements operated by NHS England and aims to protect and promote the interests of patients by ensuring that the whole health sector works for their benefit – in effect it regulates competition within the NHS and manages performance generally;

1 www.cqc.org.uk/.
2 https://improvement.nhs.uk/.

- NHS England[3] licenses and regulates Clinical Commissioning Groups;
- Healthwatch England and Local Healthwatch organisations[4] are founded by Chapter 1 of Part 5 of the Health and Social Care Act 2012 and are designed to feed the voice of the patient into the NHS and to champion their interests (there are now 152 Local Healthwatch groups);
- Health Overview and Scrutiny Committees, set up by Chapter 3 of Part 12 of the NHSA 2006, are comprised of members of the local social services authority. They may review and scrutinise any matter relating to the planning, provision and operation of the health services in their area and are entitled to be consulted about any substantial development of the health service in their area and to refer any objection on their part to the Secretary of State for Health (see Part 4 of the Local Authority (Public Health, Health and Wellbeing Boards and Health Scrutiny) Regulations 2013);
- Health and Wellbeing Boards[5] were established by Chapter 1 of Part 5 of the Health and Social Care Act 2012, as committees of the local authority, as a forum where key leaders from the health and social care system work together to improve the health and wellbeing of their local population, in particular by promoting better joint working.

How health care needs are assessed and met

18.7 The Secretary of State for Health is under a general or 'target' duty to 'promote' a 'comprehensive health service' (section 1). The function of this, and other similar duties imposed on the Secretary of State for Health, seems to be to remind him to ensure that the NHS is as comprehensive as budgets and other resources permit.[6]

18.8 As noted above, the main commissioners of NHS services are now:

- NHS England (primary and dental care and specialist services);
- Clinical Commissioning Groups ('CCG')(a wide range of acute and community NHS services other than those commissioned by NHS England); and
- Local authorities (public health services).

18.9 The commissioning duty imposed on CCG is limited in the sense that that the duty of a CCG is to arrange for the provision of services for patients 'to such extent as it considers necessary to meet the reasonable requirements of the persons for whom it has responsibility' (section 3 of the NHSA 2006). Many of the duties imposed on NHS England are similarly constrained (see section 3B of the NHSA 2006) and the same applies to local authorities (section 2B of the NHSA 2006).

3 www.england.nhs.uk/.

4 www.healthwatch.co.uk/.

5 See the views of the LGA and the King's Fund at www.local.gov.uk/health/-/journal_content/56/10180/3510973/ARTICLE and www.kingsfund.org.uk/projects/new-nhs/health-and-wellbeing-boards.

6 *R v North and East Devon Health Authority ex p Coughlan* [2001] QB 213 at paras 24–25.

NHS issues

18.10 Three issues arise, in the main:

- whether the NHS has made a lawful decision not to provide a particular service;
- whether an individual is entitled to health or social care and, in particular, whether an individual is entitled to NHS continuing healthcare (which is in general free), rather than social care (which is usually chargeable); and
- on what basis, if at all, health care is to be provided to persons from abroad.

Service provision

18.11 As far as concerns service provision CCG have very broad decision-making powers. In practice, in England, the courts supervise the exercise of these broad powers by requiring CCG and NHS England:

- properly to understand and have regard to the NHS Constitution (issued under Chapter 1 of the Health Act 2009), central government directions (issued under NHSA 2006 s8) and the 'mandate' (issued under NHSA 2006 s13A);
- properly to understand and take into account guidance;[7]
- to operate rational policies and properly to understand and rationally to implement those policies.[8]

In addition, NHS England and CCG are now subject to a whole raft of duties at section 13C and section 14P onwards – to promote the NHS Constitution, to discharge their functions efficiently – and so on.

The public law tools available to the courts enable them to exercise a flexible albeit limited supervisory role; limited in the sense that it is very rare indeed for the courts to hold that a decision not to fund particular treatment is irrational.[9] By contrast, whilst the ECtHR does occasionally pry into the logical of national decision-making,[10] in general, in this context, the ECHR has shown itself to be relatively blunt and ineffectual,[11] except where the real issue is not service provision but treating individuals with respect along the way.[12]

7 *R v North Derbyshire HA ex p Fisher* (1997–8 1 CCLR 150.

8 *R v North West Lancashire HA ex p A, D and G* (1999) 2 CCLR 419.

9 *R v Cambridgeshire DHA ex p B* [1995] 1 WLR 898; for the exception that proves the rule, see *R (Otley) v Barking and Dagenham NHS PCT* [2007] EWHC 1927, (2007) 10 CCLR 628.

10 *Van Kuck v Germany* (2005) 8 CCLR 121.

11 The nadir probably being *Pentiacova v Moldova* (2005) 40 EHRR SE23.

12 *Glass v UK* (2005) 8 CCLR 16; *Tysiac v Poland* (2007) 45 EHRR 42.

Charging, NHS continuing healthcare and persons subject to immigration control

18.12 A key feature of NHS care is that, in general, it is free at the point of delivery (see section 1(4) and Part 9 of the NHSA 2006) whereas, in general, social care is chargeable.

In particular, it is notorious that charges for care home provision can wipe out the value of the resident's home and savings, leaving nothing to be inherited. The new deferred payment regime at para 11.27 will be of little assistance until the cost cap (currently deferred until 2020) is implemented; so it remains important for individuals that an adult entitled to NHS continuing healthcare is assessed as being such. It is also highly relevant to local authority budgets, eg in cases where they are unable to recover the cost of provision through charging. Accordingly, there is considerable, detailed machinery relating to establishing whether a person is entitled to NHS continuing healthcare (the question is, essentially, whether they have a 'primary healthcare need') and dispute resolution: see para 18.19 below.

Most persons from abroad are chargeable for NHS care but not all (eg EU workers are not and neither are asylum-seekers): see para 18.26.

The real issue, in the case of persons subject to immigration control (PSIC), is the extent to which the NHS can require payment up-front and the circumstances in which it must provide chargeable treatment in cases where, realistically, there is no chance of collecting the charge later on. Those cases are, essentially, cases where the individual concerned needs timeous treatment and for some very good reason cannot be expected to leave the UK to secure it.[13]

The core NHS provisions

18.13 The core provisions are found at sections 1–3 of the NHSA 2006 and extracts are set out as follows (the NHS(W)A 2006 is identical, save for reference to 'the Welsh Ministers' and 'Wales'):

Secretary of State's duty to promote comprehensive health service

1(1) The Secretary of State must continue the promotion in England of a comprehensive health service designed to secure improvement–
(a) in the physical and mental health of the people of England, and
(b) in the prevention, diagnosis and treatment of physical and mental illness.

(2) For that purpose, the Secretary of State must exercise the functions conferred by this Act so as to secure that services are provided in accordance with this Act.

(3) The Secretary of State retains ministerial responsibility to Parliament for the provision of the health service in England.

(4) The services provided as part of the health service in England must be free of charge except in so far as the making and recovery of charges is expressly provided for by or under any enactment, whenever passed.

13 *R (YA) v Secretary of State for Health* [2009] EWCA Civ 225, (2009) 12 CCLR 213.

Duty as to improvement in quality of services

1A(1) The Secretary of State must exercise the functions of the Secretary of State in relation to the health service with a view to securing continuous improvement in the quality of services provided to individuals for or in connection with–

(a) the prevention, diagnosis or treatment of illness, or

(b) the protection or improvement of public health.

(2) In discharging the duty under subsection (1) the Secretary of State must, in particular, act with a view to securing continuous improvement in the outcomes that are achieved from the provision of the services.

(3) The outcomes relevant for the purposes of subsection (2) include, in particular, outcomes which show–

(a) the effectiveness of the services,

(b) the safety of the services, and

(c) the quality of the experience undergone by patients.

(4) In discharging the duty under subsection (1), the Secretary of State must have regard to the quality standards prepared by NICE under section 234 of the Health and Social Care Act 2012.

Duty as to the NHS Constitution

1B(1) In exercising functions in relation to the health service, the Secretary of State must have regard to the NHS Constitution.

(2) In this Act, 'NHS Constitution' has the same meaning as in Chapter 1 of Part 1 of the Health Act 2009 (see section 1 of that Act) ...

General power

2 The Secretary of State, the Board or a clinical commissioning group may do anything which is calculated to facilitate, or is conducive or incidental to, the discharge of any function conferred on that person by this Act ...

Duties of clinical commissioning groups as to commissioning certain health services

3(1) A clinical commissioning group must arrange for the provision of the following to such extent as it considers necessary to meet the reasonable requirements of the persons for whom it has responsibility–

(a) hospital accommodation,

(b) other accommodation for the purpose of any service provided under this Act,

(c) medical, dental, ophthalmic, nursing and ambulance services,

(d) such other services or facilities for the care of pregnant women, women who are breastfeeding and young children as the group considers are appropriate as part of the health service,

(e) such other services or facilities for the prevention of illness, the care of persons suffering from illness and the after-care of persons who have suffered from illness as the group considers are appropriate as part of the health service,

(f) such other services or facilities as are required for the diagnosis and treatment of illness.

(1A) For the purposes of this section, a clinical commissioning group has responsibility for–

(a) persons who are provided with primary medical services by a member of the group, and

(b) persons who usually reside in the group's area and are not provided with primary medical services by a member of any clinical commissioning group.

(1B) Regulations may provide that for the purposes of this section a clinical commissioning group also has responsibility (whether generally or in relation to a prescribed service or facility) for persons who–
(a) were provided with primary medical services by a person who is or was a member of the group, or
(b) have a prescribed connection with the group's area.

(1C) The power conferred by subsection (1B)(b) must be exercised so as to provide that, in relation to the provision of services or facilities for emergency care, a clinical commissioning group has responsibility for every person present in its area.

(1D) Regulations may provide that subsection (1A) does not apply–
(a) in relation to persons of a prescribed description (which may include a description framed by reference to the primary medical services with which the persons are provided);
(b) in prescribed circumstances.

(1E) The duty in subsection (1) does not apply in relation to a service or facility if the Board has a duty to arrange for its provision.

(1F) In exercising its functions under this section and section 3A, a clinical commissioning group must act consistently with–
(a) the discharge by the Secretary of State and the Board of their duty under section 1(1) (duty to promote a comprehensive health service), and
(b) the objectives and requirements for the time being specified in the mandate published under section 13A ...

English NHS Constitution/NHS Wales Core Principles

18.14 The NHS Constitution (27 July 2015) 'establishes the principles and values of the NHS in England' and sets out patients, public and staffs' rights and responsibilities.[14]

18.15 The government has also issued *The Handbook to the NHS Constitution* (27 July 2015) which provides more detail about the rights and pledges in the constitution.[15]

18.16 These relate to England only and are issued under Chapter 1 of the Health Act 2009, which also imposes various duties on the Secretary of State for Health, CCG and other health bodies in relation to the Constitution and Handbook. The Secretary of State for Health is required to take the NHS Constitution into account (section 1B) and CCG are required to promote the NHS Constitution (section 14P).

18.17 In Wales, there are 'Core Principles'.[16]

Responsibility disputes

18.18 There is guidance called *Who Pays: Determining responsibility for payments to providers* (August 2013).[17]

14 www.gov.uk/government/uploads/system/uploads/attachment_data/file/480482/NHS_Constitution_WEB.pdf.

15 www.gov.uk/government/uploads/system/uploads/attachment_data/file/474450/NHS_Constitution_Handbook_v2.pdf.

16 www.wales.nhs.uk/nhswalesaboutus/thecoreprinciplesofnhswales.

17 www.england.nhs.uk/wp-content/uploads/2014/05/who-pays.pdf.

Framework for NHS continuing healthcare

18.19 One issue that commonly arises in the community care context, is whether an individual is entitled to NHS continuing healthcare, for which in general no charge is made, rather than local authority care and support, for which a charge usually is made.

18.20 Essentially, an individual is entitled to NHS continuing healthcare when he or she has a 'primary healthcare need', defined in the *National Framework for NHS continuing healthcare and NHS funded Nursing Care*[18] as follows:

> **Primary Health Need**
>
> 33. To assist in deciding which treatment and other health services it is appropriate for the NHS to provide under the 2006 Act, and to distinguish between those and the services that LAs may provide under section 21 of the National Assistance Act 1948, the Secretary of State has developed the concept of a 'primary health need'. Where a person has been assessed to have a 'primary health need', they are eligible for NHS continuing healthcare. Deciding whether this is the case involves looking at the totality of the relevant needs. Where an individual has a primary health need and is therefore eligible for NHS continuing healthcare, the NHS is responsible for providing all of that individual's assessed health and social care needs – including accommodation, if that is part of the overall need.
>
> 34. There should be no gap in the provision of care. People should not find themselves in a situation where neither the NHS nor the relevant LA (subject to the person meeting the relevant means test and having needs that fall within their eligibility criteria for adult social care[19]) will fund care, either separately or together. Therefore, the 'primary health need' test should be applied, so that a decision of ineligibility for NHS continuing healthcare is only possible where, taken as a whole, the nursing or other health services required by the individual:
>
> a) are no more than incidental or ancillary to the provision of accommodation which LA social services are, or would be but for a person's means, under a duty to provide; and
>
> b) are not of a nature beyond which an LA whose primary responsibility it is to provide social services could be expected to provide
>
> 35. There are certain limitations to this test, which was originally indicated in *Coughlan*: neither the CCG, nor the LA can dictate what the other agency should provide. Instead, a practical approach to eligibility is required – one that will apply to a range of different circumstances, including situations in which the 'incidental or ancillary' test is not applicable because, for example, the person is to be cared for in their own home. Certain characteristics of need – and their impact on the care required to manage them – may help determine whether the 'quality' or 'quantity' of care required is more than the limits of an LA's responsibilities, as outlined in *Coughlan*:
>
> **Nature**: This describes the particular characteristics of an individual's needs (which can include physical, mental health or psychological needs) and the type of those needs. This also describes the overall effect of those needs on

18 www.gov.uk/government/uploads/system/uploads/attachment_data/file/213137/National-Framework-for-NHS-CHC-NHS-FNC-Nov–2012.pdf.

19 See *Prioritising need in the context of Putting People First: A whole system approach to eligibility for social care. Guidance on Eligibility Criteria for Adult Social Care*, England 2010.

the individual, including the type ('quality') of interventions required to manage them.

Intensity: This relates both to the extent ('quantity') and severity ('degree') of the needs and to the support required to meet them, including the need for sustained/ongoing care ('continuity').

Complexity: This is concerned with how the needs present and interact to increase the skill required to monitor the symptoms, treat the condition(s) and/or manage the care. This may arise with a single condition, or it could include the presence of multiple conditions or the interaction between two or more conditions. It may also include situations where an individual's response to their own condition has an impact on their overall needs, such as where a physical health need results in the individual developing a mental health need.

Unpredictability: This describes the degree to which needs fluctuate and thereby create challenges in managing them. It also relates to the level of risk to the person's health if adequate and timely care is not provided. Someone with an unpredictable healthcare need is likely to have either a fluctuating, unstable or rapidly deteriorating condition.

36. Each of these characteristics may, alone or in combination, demonstrate a primary health need, because of the quality and/or quantity of care that is required to meet the individual's needs. The totality of the overall needs and the effects of the interaction of needs should be carefully considered.

37. There will be some circumstances where the quantity or the quality of the individual's overall general nursing care needs will indicate a primary health need, and thus eligibility for NHS continuing healthcare. CCGs and LAs should be mindful of the extent and nature of NHS-funded nursing care, as set out in the NHS-funded Nursing Care Practice Guide 2012.[20]

38. It is also important that deterioration is taken into account when considering eligibility, including circumstances where deterioration might reasonably be regarded as likely in the near future. This can be reflected in several ways:

- Where it is considered that deterioration can reasonably be anticipated to occur before the next planned review, this should be documented and taken into account. This could result in immediate eligibility for NHS continuing healthcare (i.e. before the deterioration has actually occurred). The anticipated deterioration could be indicative of complex or unpredictable needs.

- Where eligibility is not established at the present time, the likely deterioration could be reflected in a recommendation for an early review, in order to establish whether the individual then satisfies the eligibility criteria.

- If an individual has a rapidly deteriorating condition that may be entering a terminal phase, they may need NHS continuing healthcare funding to enable their needs to be met urgently (eg to allow them to go home to die or appropriate end of life support to be put in place). This would be a primary health need because of the rate of deterioration. In all cases where an individual has such needs, consideration should be given to use of the Fast Track Pathway Tool, as set out in paragraphs 97–107.

20 www.gov.uk/government/publications/national-framework-for-nhs-continuing-healthcare-and-nhs-funded-nursing-care.

- Even when an individual does not satisfy the criteria for use of the Fast Track Pathway Tool, one or more of the characteristics listed in paragraph 35 may well apply to those people approaching the end of their lives, and eligibility should always be considered.

39. Good practice in end of life care is currently supported through the National End of Life Care Programme,[21] which works with health and social care services across all sectors in England to improve end of life care for adults by implementing the Department of Health's End of Life Care Strategy.[22] The principles of the Strategy should be reflected in all NHS continuing healthcare cases that involve individuals with an end of life condition.

40. To minimise variation in interpretation of these principles, and to inform consistent decision-making, we have, in conjunction with stakeholders, developed the national Decision Support Tool (DST). The DST supports practitioners in identifying the individual's needs, which, combined with the practitioners' skills, knowledge and professional judgement, should enable them to apply the primary health need test in practice, in a way that is consistent with the limits on what can lawfully be provided by an LA, in accordance with the Coughlan and the Grogan judgements.

41. Further details about the DST and its application are set out below (paragraphs 77–89) and in the notes accompanying the tool. Before using the DST, practitioners should ensure that they have obtained evidence from all the necessary assessments (comprehensive and specialist), in line with the core values and principles outlined below.

18.21 The current criteria for entitlement to NHS continuing healthcare came into force on the 1 April 2013 and are now found set out in:

- National Framework for NHS continuing healthcare and NHS funded Nursing Care (revised 2012, last updated 1 November 2013);[23]
- NHS continuing healthcare Checklist;[24]
- Decision Support Tool for NHS continuing healthcare;[25] and
- Fast Track Pathway Tool for NHS continuing healthcare.[26]

18.22 This material is underpinned by the NHS Commissioning Board and Clinical Commissioning Groups (Responsibilities and Standing Rules) Regulations 2012, as amended.

Age UK has published a useful factsheet[27] and the NHS has produced a public information leaflet.[28]

21 Website archived at http://webarchive.nationalarchives.gov.uk/20130718121128/http:/endoflifecare.nhs.uk.

22 www.gov.uk/government/publications/end-of-life-care-strategy-promoting-high-quality-care-for-adults-at-the-end-of-their-life.

23 www.gov.uk/government/uploads/system/uploads/attachment_data/file/213137/National-Framework-for-NHS-CHC-NHS-FNC-Nov–2012.pdf.

24 www.gov.uk/government/uploads/system/uploads/attachment_data/file/213138/NHS-CHC-Checklist-FINAL.pdf.

25 www.gov.uk/government/uploads/system/uploads/attachment_data/file/213139/Decision-Support-Tool-for-NHS-Continuing-Healthcare.pdf.

26 www.gov.uk/government/uploads/system/uploads/attachment_data/file/213140/NHS-CHC-Fast-Track-Pathway-tool.pdf.

27 www.ageuk.org.uk/documents/en-gb/factsheets/fs20_nhs_continuing_healthcare_and_nhs-funded_nursing_care_fcs.pdf?dtrk=true.

28 www.gov.uk/government/uploads/system/uploads/attachment_data/file/193700/NHS_CHC_Public_Information_Leaflet_Final.pdf.

Health care and persons subject to immigration control

18.23 The current statutory machinery can be found here:

- section 175 of the National Health Service Act 2006;
- The National Health Service (Charges to Overseas Visitors) Regulations 2015;
- *Guidance on implementing the overseas visitor hospital charging regulations 2015*.[29]

18.24 The Executive Summary of the Guidance provides a useful overview and, in particular, identifies the fundamental principle based on ordinary residence as follows:

> 1. A person will be 'ordinarily resident of a trust' in the UK when that residence is lawful, adopted, voluntary, and for settled purposes as part of the regular order of their life for the time being, whether of short or long duration. Nationals of countries outside the European Economic Area (EEA) must also have indefinite leave to remain in the UK in order to be ordinarily resident here. A person who is ordinarily resident in the UK must not be charged for NHS hospital services.
>
> 2. The Charging Regulations place a legal obligation on NHS trusts, NHS foundation trusts and Local Authorities in the exercise of public health functions1 in England, to establish whether a person is an overseas visitor to whom charges apply, or whether they are exempt from charges. When charges apply, a relevant NHS body must make and recover charges from the person liable to pay for the NHS services provided to the overseas visitor. A list of exempt services and exempt categories of overseas visitor is provided in Chapter 1, with a more detailed list of exempt services at Chapter 4.

18.25 Certain NHS services and certain categories of individual are exempt from the charging regime, as explained in the Guidance as follows:

> **Chapter 1 Exempt services and individuals**
>
> This chapter sets out details of all services which are free of charge to patients, and of all individuals who are entitled to receive healthcare on the same basis as an ordinarily resident person
>
> 1.1 The following services are free at the point of use for all patients. A charge cannot be made or recovered from any overseas visitor for:
>
> - accident and emergency (A&E) services, this includes all A&E services provided at an NHS hospital, e.g. those provided at an accident & emergency department, walk-in centre or urgent healthcare centre. This does not include those emergency services provided after the overseas visitor has been accepted as an inpatient, or at a follow-up outpatient appointment, for which charges must be levied unless the overseas visitor is exempt from charge in their own right;
> - services provided outside an NHS hospital, unless the staff providing the services are employed by, or working under the direction of, an NHS hospital;
> - family planning services (does not include termination of pregnancy);

29 www.gov.uk/government/uploads/system/uploads/attachment_data/file/418634/Implementing_overseas_charging_regulations_2015.pdf.

- diagnosis and treatment of specified infectious diseases (listed at chapter 4);
- diagnosis and treatment of sexually transmitted infections;
- treatment required for a physical or mental condition caused by:
  - torture;
  - female genital mutilation;
  - domestic violence; or
  - sexual violence,

except where the overseas visitor has travelled to the UK for the purpose of seeking that treatment.

Exempt categories of person

1.1 The following categories of overseas visitor are exempt from charge:

Those who have paid the health surcharge or are covered by transitional arrangements

- Non-EEA nationals, who are subject to immigration control, are exempt from charge if one of the following applies to them while their leave to enter/remain is valid:
  - they have paid the surcharge; or
  - they are exempt from payment of the surcharge[30] or have had the requirement waived or reduced, or have had part (but not all) of the surcharge refunded to them; or
  - they would have been covered under one of the above, but for the fact that they applied for leave to enter or remain in the UK before the start of the surcharge (this will include some people already resident here without indefinite leave to remain, and a small number of people arriving after 6 April 2015 who applied for leave before that date).
- A child born in the UK to an above mentioned exempt person is also exempt from charge up to the age of three months provided that the child has not left the UK since birth.

Those with an enforceable EU right to free healthcare

- Anyone insured for healthcare in another EEA member state and who, for medically necessary treatment, presents either an EHIC from that member state or a PRC (see Introduction for definitions), or, if coming to the UK specifically for treatment, presents an S2 form for that treatment (see chapter 9 for more details).
- Anyone who has a UK-issued S1 form registered in another EEA member state or Switzerland except for family members of frontier workers.
- The spouse/civil partner and children under 18 of the above are also exempt when lawfully visiting the UK with them, unless they have an enforceable EU right in their own right.[31]

Vulnerable patients and those detained

- Refugees (those granted asylum, humanitarian protection or temporary protection under the immigration rules).
- Asylum seekers (those applying for asylum, humanitarian protection or temporary protection whose claims, including appeals, have not yet been determined).
- Individuals receiving support under section 95 of the Immigration and Asylum Act 1999 (the 1999 Act) from the Home Office.

30 Except when the exemption is because they have a visitor visa under Part 2 of the Immigration Rules or because they are visiting for six months or less.

31 That is, the exemption only applies where EU law does not provide them with a right to an EHIC or PRC of their own – in practice this is likely to be only when their same-sex marriage or civil partnership is not recognised by the insuring member state.

- Failed asylum seekers receiving support under section 4(2) of the 1999 Act from the Home Office or those receiving support under section 21 of the National Assistance Act 1948 or Part 1 of the Care Act 2014 from a local authority to provide accommodation.
- Children who are looked after by a local authority.
- Victims, and suspected victims, of modern slavery,[32] as determined by a designated competent authority, such as the UK Human Trafficking Centre or the Home Office. This includes their spouse/civil partner and any children under 18, provided they are lawfully present in the UK.
- An overseas visitor who has been granted leave to enter the UK outside the immigration rules, in whose case the Secretary of State for Health determines there to be exceptional humanitarian reasons to provide a free course of treatment. This exemption will also apply to their child and/or companion who is authorised to travel with them, for whom the exemption is limited to treatment, the need for which arose during the visit, and cannot await their return home.
- Anyone receiving compulsory treatment under a court order or who is detained in an NHS hospital or deprived of their liberty (e.g. under the Mental Health Act 1983 or the Mental Capacity Act 2005) is exempt from charge for all treatment provided, in accordance with the court order, or for the duration of the detention.
- Prisoners and immigration detainees.

UK Government employees and war pensioners

- UK armed forces members, plus their spouse/civil partner and children under 18 provided they are lawfully present in the UK (even if they are on a visit visa).
- UK Crown servants who are in the UK in the course of their employment, or who were ordinarily resident prior to being posted overseas, plus their spouse/civil partner and children under 18 provided they are lawfully present in the UK.
- Employees of the British Council or Commonwealth War Graves Commission who are in the UK in the course of their employment, or who were ordinarily resident in the UK prior to being posted overseas, plus their spouse/civil partner and children under 18 provided they are lawfully present in the UK.
- Those working or volunteering in employment overseas that is financed in part by the UK Government who are in the UK in the course of their employment, or who were ordinarily resident in the UK prior to being posted overseas, plus their spouse/civil partner and children under 18 provided they are lawfully present in the UK.
- Those receiving war pensions, war widows' pensions or armed forces compensation scheme payments, plus their spouse/civil partner and children under 18 when these family members are lawfully visiting the UK with the recipient of this pension/payment.

Those covered by reciprocal healthcare agreements, other international obligations and employees on UK-registered ships

- Anyone entitled to free healthcare in the UK under the terms of a reciprocal healthcare agreement with a country outside the EEA (usually limited to immediate medical treatment); see Chapter 10 for more details.
- Nationals of states that are contracting parties to the European Convention on Social and Medical Assistance or the European Social Charter and

32 Modern slavery includes human trafficking, as well as slavery, servitude or forced or compulsory labour.

who are lawfully present here and without sufficient resources to pay. Free treatment is limited only to that which cannot wait until the overseas visitor can return home and provided the person did not come to the UK for the purpose of seeking treatment.

- NATO personnel, when the services required cannot readily be provided by armed forces medical services, plus their spouse/civil partner and children under 18 provided they are lawfully present in the UK.
- Employees on ships registered in the UK where their normal place of work is on board a ship (even if they are here on a visit visa).

18.26 The Executive Summary of the Guidance summarise the approach to be taken in cases where NHS treatment is immediately necessary or urgent but the patient is unable to pay:

> 12. A relevant NHS body also has human rights obligations, so chargeable treatment which is considered by clinicians to be immediately necessary must never be withheld from an overseas visitor, even when that overseas visitor has indicated that they cannot pay. This does not mean that the treatment should be provided free of charge. Charges will still apply, and, if not yet recovered, should be pursued after the treatment is provided. Treatment which is not immediately necessary, but is nevertheless classed as urgent by clinicians, as it cannot wait until the overseas visitor can return home, should also be provided regardless of the patient's ability to pay. Every effort should be made to obtain payment or a deposit in the period before treatment starts. Non-urgent, or elective, treatment should not begin until full payment has been received. See Chapters 11 and 13 for more important information about how and when to ask for payment from chargeable overseas visitors.

Cases

Health care provision

18.27 *R v Cambridge DHA ex p B* [1995] 1 WLR 898, CA

A court cannot realistically quash an NHS resource-allocation decision head-on, on rationality grounds, no matter how tragic the case

Facts: B, a girl born in 1984, was diagnosed in 1990 as suffering from highly invasive cancer. Her doctors concluded that a third course of chemotherapy and a second bone marrow transplant would not be in her best interests and the hospital concluded that an experimental method of delivering such treatment would not be cost effective.

Judgment: the Court of Appeal (Sir Thomas Bingham MR, Sir Stephen Brown P and Simon Brown LJ) dismissed the father's application for a judicial review. Sir Thomas Bingham MR said this:

> I have no doubt that in a perfect world any treatment which a patient, or a patient's family, sought would be provided if doctors were willing to give it, no matter how much it cost, particularly when a life was potentially at stake. It would however, in my view, be shutting one's eyes to the real world if the court were to proceed on the basis that we do live in such a world. It is common knowledge that health authorities of all kinds are constantly pressed to make ends meet. They cannot pay their nurses as much as they would like; they cannot provide all the treatments they would like; they cannot

purchase all the extremely expensive medical equipment they would like; they cannot carry out all the research they would like; they cannot build all the hospitals and specialist units they would like. Difficult and agonising judgments have to be made as to how a limited budget is best allocated to the maximum advantage of the maximum number of patients. That is not a judgment which the court can make. In my judgment, it is not something that a health authority such as this authority can be fairly criticised for not advancing before the court.

Mr McIntyre went so far as to say that, if the authority has money in the bank which it has not spent, then it would be acting in plain breach of its statutory duty if it did not procure this treatment. I am bound to say that I regard that submission as manifestly incorrect. Unless the health authority had sufficient money to purchase everything which in the interests of patients it would wish to do, then that situation would never ever be reached. I venture to say that no real evidence is needed to satisfy the court that no health authority is in that position.

I furthermore think, differing I regret from the judge, that it would be totally unrealistic to require the authority to come to the court with its accounts and seek to demonstrate that if this treatment were provided for B. then there would be a patient C who would have to go without treatment. No major authority could run its financial affairs in a way which would permit such a demonstration ...

Such is my sympathy with the father and B herself that I have been tempted, although disagreeing with the judge's reasoning, to leave the order which he made in being and invite the authority to reconsider the matter in the light of the judge's conclusions. I have, however, concluded that that would be a cruel deception since I would be bound to make clear that, in my judgment, the authority could, on a proper review of all the relevant material, reach the same decision that it had already reached and I would feel obliged, expressly, to dissociate myself from the judge's opinion that it would be hard to imagine a proper basis upon which this treatment, at least its initial stage, could reasonably be withheld. In my judgment, it would be open to the authority readily to reach that decision since it is, as I think, the decision it has already reached.

While I have, as I hope is clear, every possible sympathy with B, I feel bound to regard this as an attempt, wholly understandable but none the less misguided, to involve the court in a field of activity where it is not fitted to make any decision favourable to the patient.

Comment: as later cases demonstrate, this starting point (and finishing point) does not prevent the success of many a more finely-tuned public challenge to NHS decisions about the provision of services.

18.28 *R v North Derbyshire Health Authority ex p Fisher* (1997–8) 1 CCLR 150, QBD

Acting contrary to guidance because of a simple disagreement with the guidance is tantamount to failing to take it into account

Facts: North Derbyshire adopted practices which, on analysis, were designed to defer making additional funding available for the prescription of Beta-Interferon (for the treatment of Multiple Sclerosis), despite the fact that the NHS executive had issued guidance advising all NHS purchasing bodies to do so.

Judgment: Dyson J held:

> In my judgment Mr Elvin and Mr Seys Llewellyn are right. If the Circular provided no more than guidance, albeit in strong terms, then the only duty placed upon health authorities would be to take it into account in the discharge of their functions. They would be susceptible to challenge only on Wednesbury principles if they failed to consider the Circular, or they misconstrued or misapplied it whether deliberately or negligently: see *Grandsden & Co Ltd and Another v Secretary of State for the Environment and Another* (1985) 54 P&CR 86, 93–94.
>
> …
>
> Mr Seys Llewellyn emphasised two points. First the respondents were under a statutory duty not to overspend: see section 97(1)(a) of the 1977 Act and the Department of Health Circular HC(91)25. Secondly, clinical decisions must always be taken with due regard to the resources available: see, for example, *R v Cambridge Health Authority* [1995] 1 WLR 898. I unreservedly accept both propositions as correct. But on the facts of this case, they do not assist the respondents. The respondents had funds available, but chose not to allocate them. As for clinical decisions, they were not for the respondents to take, and it is no part of the applicant's case to suggest that they were.
>
> I conclude therefore that the policy was unlawful because it was not a proper application of the guidance contained in the Circular, and the respondents did not properly take into account the essential requirements of the Circular in adopting and maintaining their policy. In my judgment, the respondents were aware from an early stage that they were not properly applying or taking account of the Circular. They knew that their own policy amounted to a blanket ban on Beta-Interferon treatment. A blanket ban was the very antithesis of national policy, the aim of which was to target the drug appropriately at patients who were most likely to benefit from treatment. They knew from as early as 12 January 1996 that, if there was no imminent prospect of a trial, it might be difficult to 'hold the line'. Most revealingly of all, the note of the meeting of that date spoke about the possibility of 'creative constraints'. This is surprising language to find in the context of health care.
>
> What they had in mind at this early stage was using the possibility of a trial as a creative means of avoiding the implementation of national policy. The reason was plainly that the respondents disagreed with that policy. I fear that 'creative' is a euphemism for 'disingenuous'. The prospect of a trial served its purpose as a creative constraint until that prospect disappeared. Thereafter the respondents resorted to other unacceptable and inconsistent excuses in seeking to hold the line, and hang on to their unsustainable position. My conclusion on this issue, based on the reasons that I have given, is sufficient to dispose of this application, subject to questions of relief.

18.29 *Passannante v Italy* (1998) Application no 32647/96, (2002) 5 CCLR 340

A delay in providing healthcare to which a person was entitled by virtue of contributions might raise an issue under Article 8 ECHR if there was a serious risk to health

Facts: Ms Passannate was told she would have to wait five months to see a consultant at public expense but could see him in four days on a private paying basis. She declined to see the consultant at all and claimed that her rights under Article 8 ECHR had been breached.

Judgment: the Commission declared the complaint inadmissible but held the door ajar for stronger cases:

> The Commission recalls that, while the essential object of Article 8 is to protect the individual against arbitrary interference by the public authorities, it does not merely compel the State to abstain from such interference: in addition to this negative undertaking, there may be positive obligations inherent in effective respect for private life (see ECtHR, *Stjerna v Finland* judgment of 25 November 1994, Series A No 299-B, p 61, para 38 and ECtHR, *Botta* judgment of 24 February 1998, para 33, cited above).
>
> The Commission notes the Italian public health service is based on compulsory contributions which entitle those who pay them to certain services, among which medical examinations within public hospitals. Therefore, the Commission considers that, in such circumstances where the State has an obligation to provide medical care, an excessive delay of the public health service in providing a medical service to which the patient is entitled and the fact that such delay has, or is likely to have, a serious impact on the patient's health could raise an issue under Article 8 para 1 of the Convention.
>
> The Commission notes the absence under domestic law of time-limits within which a person should be granted the required medical service. However, although the applicant submits that she had to wait five months in order merely to book the medical examination, she did not prove nor even allege that the above delay had a serious impact on her physical or psychological conditions.
>
> The Commission further notes that the applicant, after the telephone conversation with the hospital's operator, apparently renounced from seeing the doctor which indicates, in the Commission's opinion, that she did not consider the medical visit crucial for her health.
>
> Therefore the Commission considers that the circumstances of the present case are not such as to warrant the conclusion that the delay of the public authorities raises a serious issue under Article 8 of the Convention and that the present application is manifestly ill-founded within the meaning of Article 27 para 2 of the Convention.
>
> For these reasons, the Commission, unanimously, declares the application inadmissible.

18.30 *R v North West Lancashire Health Authority ex p A, D and G* (1999) 2 CCLR 419, CA

A refusal to provide a healthcare service was unlawful where the health authority had proceeded on a basis that was contrary to its own policy

Facts: A, D and G suffered from gender identity dysphoria, commonly known as transsexualism, and had been diagnosed by a specialist consultant as having a clinical need for gender reassignment surgery. The health authority refused to fund this treatment, on the basis of a policy that categorised gender reassignment surgery as a form of treatment that had not been tested by carefully conducted scientific research and where it was uncertain whether the interventions would be effective, ineffective or harmful, so that treatment would only be funded where there was evidence of overriding clinical need, or exceptional circumstances.

Judgment: the Court of Appeal (Auld, Buxton and May LJJ) held that, although the health authority had acknowledged to the court that transsexualism was an illness, reading the health authority's policy, together with the evidence that it had filed in the proceedings, it was apparent that the health authority had proceeded on the basis that transsexualism was not an illness. Therefore, the health authority's policy and its decision-making in this case were flawed by its failure to take into account the fact that, as it itself accepted, transsexualism was an illness. The criteria of '*overriding clinical need*' or '*exceptional circumstances*' failed to rescue the policy, or its application, because the starting point – that transsexualism was not an illness – was flawed. Further in effect, on the facts, the health authority operated a '*blanket policy*' not to fund gender reassignment surgery.

18.31 *Sentges v The Netherlands* Application no 27677/02, (2004) 7 CCLR 400

The margin of appreciation was so wide in medical cases, especially in relation to the allocation of scarce healthcare resources, that it could not be said that the refusal to supply a robotic arm, in the context of the provision of other services, was incompatible with Article 8 ECHR

Facts: Mr Sentges suffered from Duchenne Muscular Dystrophy, which left him unable to stand, walk or lift his arms and with minimal manual or digital function. He had an electric wheelchair with an adapted joystick and he applied to the Dutch health insurance fund for a robotic arm that would enable him to perform many tasks unassisted (he was otherwise entirely dependent on others for every act of day-to-day living).

Judgment: the ECtHR held that the refusal to provide a robotic arm was not incompatible with Article 8 ECHR:

> In the instant case the applicant complained in substance not of action but of a lack of action by the State. While the essential object of Article 8 is to protect the individual against arbitrary interference by the public authorities, it does not merely compel the State to abstain from such interference: in addition to this negative undertaking, there may be positive obligations inherent in effective respect for private or family life. These obligations may involve the adoption of measures designed to secure respect for private life even in the sphere of the relations of individuals between themselves (see, *inter alia, X and Y v The Netherlands*, cited above, para 23), *Stubbings and Others v The United Kingdom*, judgment of 22 October 1996, *Reports* 1996-IV, p1505, para 62).
>
> The court has held that Article 8 may impose such positive obligations on a State where there is a direct and immediate link between the measures sought by an applicant and the latter's private life (see *Botta v Italy*, cited above, para 34). However, Article 8 does not apply to situations concerning interpersonal relations of such broad and indeterminate scope that there can be no conceivable link between the measures the State is urged to take and an individual's private life (see *Botta*, cited above, para 35). The court has also held that Article 8 cannot be considered applicable each time an individual's everyday life is disrupted, but only in the exceptional cases where the State's failure to adopt measures interferes with that individual's right to personal development and his or her right to establish and maintain relations with other human beings and the outside world. It is

incumbent on the individual concerned to demonstrate the existence of a special link between the situation complained of and the particular needs of his or her private life (see *Zehnalovà and Zehnal v The Czech Republic* (dec.), Application no 38621/97, ECHR 2002-V).

Even assuming that in the present case such a special link indeed exists – as was accepted by the Central Appeals Tribunal –, regard must be had to the fair balance that has to be struck between the competing interests of the individual and of the community as a whole and to the wide margin of appreciation enjoyed by States in this respect in determining the steps to be taken to ensure compliance with the Convention (see *Zehnalovà and Zehnal*, cited above).

This margin of appreciation is even wider when, as in the present case, the issues involve an assessment of the priorities in the context of the allocation of limited State resources (see, *mutatis mutandis, Osman v the United Kingdom*, judgment of 28 October 1998, *Reports* 1998-VIII, p. 3159, § 116, *O'Reilly and Others v Ireland* (dec.), Application no 54725/00, 28 February 2002, unreported). In view of their familiarity with the demands made on the health care system as well as with the funds available to meet those demands, the national authorities are in a better position to carry out this assessment than an international court. In addition, the court should also be mindful of the fact that, while it will apply the Convention to the concrete facts of this particular case in accordance with Article 34, a decision issued in an individual case will nevertheless at least to some extent establish a precedent (see *Pretty*, cited above, para 75), valid for all Contracting States.

In the present case the court notes that the applicant has access to the standard of health care offered to all persons insured under the Health Insurance Act and the Exceptional Medical Expenses Act (see *Nitecki v Poland* (dec.), Application no 65653/01, 21 March 2002, unreported). It thus appears that he has been provided with an electric wheelchair with an adapted joystick. The court by no means wishes to underestimate the difficulties encountered by the applicant and appreciates the very real improvement which a robotic arm would entail for his personal autonomy and his ability to establish and develop relationships with other human beings of his choice. Nevertheless the court is of the opinion that in the circumstances of the present case it cannot be said that the respondent State exceeded the margin of appreciation afforded to it.

18.32 *Glass v United Kingdom* Application no 61827/00, (2005) 8 CCLR 16

The imposition of treatment on a child in defiance of his mother's interests and without seeking court relief was incompatible with Article 8 ECHR

Facts: hospital staff concluded that Mrs Glass's child, who was severely disabled, was dying, that further intrusive treatment was not in his best interests and that if he suffered further respiratory failure he should not be resuscitated, but that morphine should be administered, to ease his suffering. Mrs Glass and her family strongly disagreed but the hospital proceeded as it had planned in any event.

Judgment: the ECtHR held that imposing treatment on the child in defiance of his mother's objections amounted to an interference with his right to respect for his private life and physical integrity. On the facts, the situation was not so urgent that the hospital could not have applied to court for a best interests declaration and its failure to do so meant that its interference had not been 'necessary', so it was in breach of Article 8(2) ECHR. Damages of £10,000.00 were awarded to reflect the stress and anxiety suffered by the mother, as well as her feelings of powerlessness and frustration.

18.33 ### *van Kuck v Germany* Application no 35968/97, (2005) 8 CCLR 121

It was incompatible with Articles 6 and 8 ECHR to decline to fund gender re-assignment surgery on the basis of an incorrect understanding of the medical evidence

Facts: Ms van Kuck was a transsexual, who had been born male but had changed her forename to a woman's name and received hormone treatment; she now applied for funding for gender re-assignment surgery, from her insurance company, which refused to pay. The German courts heard expert evidence, which recommended surgery, but had nonetheless concluded that she had a disease which it was appropriate to endeavour to cure through psychotherapy.

Judgment: the German courts had failed to properly understand and taken into account the medical evidence, rendering the trial incompatible with Article 6 ECHR and the refusal to surgery incompatible with Article 8 ECHR, in that a fair balance had not been struck between the interests of Ms van Kuck and the German insurance company.

18.34 ### *Pentiacova v Moldova* Application no 14462/03, (2005) 40 EHRR SE23

It was not a breach of the ECHR radically to reduce haemodialysis provision, notwithstanding the suffering occasioned

Facts: for a period of years, for budgetary reasons, Moldova significantly reduced the amount of publicly-funded haemodialysis that it provided to patients with chronic renal failure, and the level of ancillary medication provided, resulting in many patients suffering a range of distressing symptoms.

Judgment: the European Court of Human Rights dismissed the application as being 'manifestly unfounded', both under Article 8 and 2 ECHR:

> Although the object of Article 8 is essentially that of protecting the individual against arbitrary interference by the public authorities, it does not merely compel the State to abstain from such interference since it may also give rise to positive obligations inherent in effective 'respect' for private and family life. While the boundaries between the State's positive and negative obligations under this provision do not always lend themselves to precise definition, the applicable principles are similar. In both contexts regard must be had to the fair balance that has to be struck between the competing interests of the individual and the community as a whole, and in both contexts the State enjoys a certain margin of appreciation (Application No 38621/97, *Zehnalová and Zehnal v Czech Republic*, Decision 14 May 2002).
>
> The court has previously held that private life includes a person's physical and psychological integrity (*Niemietz v Germany* (1993) 16 EHRR 97 at [29]). While the Convention does not guarantee as such a right to free medical care, in a number of cases the court has held that Article 8 is relevant to complaints about public funding to facilitate the mobility and quality

of life of disabled applicants (see, *Zehnalová and Zehnal,* cited above, and Application No 27677/02, *Sentges v Netherlands,* Decision 8 May 2003). The court is therefore prepared to assume for the purposes of this application, that Article 8 is applicable to the applicants' complaints about lack of sufficient funding of their treatment.

The margin of appreciation referred to above is even wider when, as in the present case, the issues involve an assessment of the priorities in the context of the allocation of limited State resources (see, mutatis mutandis, *Osman v United Kingdom* (2000) 29 EHRR 245 at [116], Application no 54725/00, *O'Reilly v Ireland,* Decision 28 February 2002). In view of their familiarity with the demands made on the health care system as well as with the funds available to meet those demands, the national authorities are in a better position to carry out this assessment than an international court. In addition, the court should also be mindful of the fact that, while it will apply the Convention to the concrete facts of this particular case in accordance with Article 34, a decision issued in an individual case will nevertheless at least to some extent establish a precedent, valid for all Contracting States (*Sentges v Netherlands,* cited above).

The court considers that the core problem in the present case reflected in the numerous complaints is the alleged insufficient public funding for the treatment of their disease. In support of their claims the applicants compare the amount of public expenditure on renal failure treatment in Moldova to that in some industrialised countries like the United States of America, the United Kingdom, Australia and Israel. The court sees no reason to question the applicants' assertion that they have no means to pay for the cost of the medication not provided free by the State and that the medication and in some cases a third haemodialysis session per week is of great importance for their fight with the disease. However, it notes that the applicants' claim amounts to a call on public funds which, in view of the scarce resources, would have to be directed from other worthy needs funded by the taxpayer.

While it is clearly desirable that everyone has access to a full range of medical treatment, including life-saving medical procedures and drugs, the lack of resources means that there are, unfortunately, in the Contracting States many individuals who do not enjoy them, especially in cases of permanent and expensive treatment.

In the present case the court notes that the applicants had access to the standard of health care offered to the general public both before the implementation of the medical care system reform, and after the implementation thereof. It thus appears that they were provided with basic medical care and basic medication before January 1, 2004, and have been provided with almost full medical care after that date. The court by no means wishes to underestimate the difficulties apparently encountered by the applicants and appreciates the very real improvement which a total haemodialysis coverage would entail for their private and family lives. Nevertheless, the court is of the opinion that in the circumstances of the present case it cannot be said that the respondent State failed to strike a fair balance between the competing interests of the applicants and the community as a whole.

Bearing in mind the medical treatment and the facilities provided to the applicants and the fact that the applicants' situation has considerably improved after the implementation of the medical care system reform in January 2004, the court considers that the respondent State cannot be said, in the special circumstances of the present case, to have failed to discharge its positive obligations under Article 8 of the Convention. As to the problem concerning the non-reimbursement of all the transportation expenses, the court, assuming that the applicants exhausted domestic remedies, notes that the Government produced copies of payment rolls recording the payment of those expenses to all the applicants and that the applicants failed to make any comment on them. Moreover, the applicants sent the court a copy of a judgment of the Briceni District Court, by which Eduard Pritula was awarded money for his travel expenses, to be paid by the local authorities.

It follows that the complaint under Article 8 of the Convention is manifestly ill-founded and must be rejected in accordance with Article 35(3) and (4) of the Convention.

C. Alleged violation of Article 2 of the Convention

The applicants complain that the failure of the State to cover the cost of all the medication necessary for their haemodialysis, and the poor financing of the haemodialysis section of the SCR, violated their right to life guaranteed by Article 2 of the Convention.

The court recalls that the first sentence of Article 2 enjoins the State not only to refrain from the intentional and unlawful taking of life, but also to take appropriate steps to safeguard the lives of those within its jurisdiction (see *LCB v United Kingdom* (1999) 27 EHRR 212 at [36]). It cannot be excluded that the acts and omissions of the authorities in the field of health care policy may in certain circumstances engage their responsibility under Article 2 (see *Powell v United Kingdom* (2000) 30 EHRR CD 362).

Moreover, an issue may arise under Article 2 where it is shown that the authorities of a Contracting State put an individual's life at risk through the denial of health care which they have undertaken to make available to the population generally (see *Cyprus v Turkey* [GC] (2002) 35 EHRR 30 at [219]; App No 65653/01, *Nitecki v Poland*, Decision 21 March 2002).

Turning to the facts of the instant case, the court notes that the applicants have failed to adduce any evidence that their lives have been put at risk. They claim that a few patients have died in recent years and rely on the example of Gheorghe Lungu, but they have not adduced any evidence that the cause of death was the lack of any specific drug or the lack of appropriate medical care. The court notes that chronic renal failure is a very serious progressive disease with a high rate of mortality, not only in Moldova but throughout the world. The fact that a person has died of this disease is not, therefore, proof in itself that the death was caused by shortcomings in the medical care system.

In any event, as regards the issue of the State's positive obligations, the court has examined the issue under Article 8 of the Convention and sees no reason to reach any different conclusion under Article 2 of the Convention.

Accordingly, the court concludes that the complaint under Article 2 of the Convention is manifestly ill-founded within the meaning of Article 35(3) of the Convention.

18.35 *R (Watts) v Bedford PCT* [2006] QB 667

Faced with unacceptable delay a patient was entitled to recover the cost of speedier medical treatment in another member state

Facts: Ms Watts had to wait for one year for hip replacement surgery in England, subsequently reduced to three to four months. Consequently, Ms Watts secured treatment in France and claimed reimbursement of the cost under Council Regulation 1408/71.

Judgment: the European Court of Justice held that a patient could, pursuant to Article 22 of Council Regulation 1408/71, go to another member state to receive medical treatment and be reimbursed the cost where there would, on an objective medical assessment of his medical circumstances, be an unacceptable delay before treatment could be provided in the UK by reason of waiting lists intended to enable the supply of hospital care to be planned and managed on the basis of predetermined clinical priorities, and where there had been no such objective medical assessment of the patient's condition.

18.36 *R (Gunter) v South Western Staffordshire PCT* [2005] EWHC 1894 (Admin), (2006) 9 CCLR 121

The NHS decision to refuse services was vitiated by its failure to appreciate that it could fund a user independent trust and the importance of the patient's home life

Facts: Ms Gunter was a 21-year-old woman, who lived with her parents, but required 24-hour nursing care. A point had been reached where the PCT wanted to provide Ms Gunter with residential care. The parents wanted care at home, provided by a user independent trust, with the parents available in a supportive/emergency role.

Judgment: Collins J held that the PCT had power to fund a user independent trust and was required to at least explore that option, to see if care at home could be provided more cheaply, so as to avoid the need of Ms Gunter to have to leave her home.

18.37 *R (Ann Marie Rogers) v Swindon NHS PCT* [2006] EWCA Civ 392, (2006) 9 CCLR 451

Unless resources were problematic, it was irrational to accord patients different entitlement on any other than clinical grounds

Facts: Herceptin had not been approved by NICE, although the National Cancer Research Institute recommended its use for women fitting certain criteria ('*the eligible group*'). The PCT's policy was to fund Herceptin treatment for breast cancer in exceptional cases only (but not to take its resources into account).

Judgment: the Court of Appeal (Sir Anthony Clarke MR, Brooke and Buxton LJJ) held that it was rational in principle to have an '*exceptional cases*' policy, but once resources were treated as irrelevant the only relevant considerations could be clinical (rather than social) need and there was no rational basis for treating some women who fell within the eligible group differently than others, in terms of their clinical need.

18.38 *Tysiac v Poland* Application no 5410/03, (2007) 45 EHRR 42

The absence of clear procedures for determining eligibility for an abortion and resolving disputes was incompatible with Article 8 ECHR

Facts: the state hospital refused Ms Tysiac an abortion, notwithstanding medical evidence that otherwise her health was at risk (the criteria for a legal abortion in Poland).

Judgment: the European Court of Human Rights held that whilst it was not its task to examine whether the ECHR guarantees the right to have an abortion, the regulation of pregnancy touched upon the sphere of private life such that the authorities were under a positive duty to secure to their citizens their right to effective respect for their physical and psychological integrity and, relevant to the present case, that required clear procedures for determining eligibility and resolving disputes, which had been absent in the present case.

18.39 *R (Otley) v Barking and Dagenham NHS PCT* [2007] EWHC 1927 (Admin), (2007) 10 CCLR 628

The reasons for declining to fund cancer treatment, in this case, were irrational

Facts: Ms Otley suffered from metastatic colorectal cancer and sought treatment with Avastin, supported by her consultant Barking and Dagenham's panel declined to make provision, on the basis that it had not been recommended by NICE and the circumstances were not exceptional.

Judgment: Mitting J held that while Barking and Dagenham's policy had been rational, its decision-making had not been:

> 26. I approach my task on a very conventional basis. The question which I have to ask is whether or not the reasoning and decision of the Panel was rational and so lawful on *Wednesbury* grounds. I have identified already respects in which in my view the decision of this panel was not rational. I summarise them in headline form. First, Dr Sharma's query about the ratio in which Avastin had been prescribed by comparison with other components of the cocktail was an irrelevant query. Secondly, there were no other treatments in practice available to Ms Otley amongst those that could be prescribed within normal National Health Service standards which were likely to have any benefit for her. Thirdly, the Panel did not take into account the slim but important chance that treatment including Avastin could prolong Ms Otley's life by more than a few months. Fourthly, on any fair minded view of the exceptionality criteria identified in the critical analysis document, her case was exceptional.

18.40 *R (Colin Ross) v West Sussex PCT* [2008] NLJR 1297, (2008) 11 CCLR 767

The reasons for declining cancer treatment manifested a failure properly to understand relevant matters

Facts: Mr Ross applied for exceptional funding to be treated with the cancer drug Lenalidomide, having become unable to tolerate any other form of treatment. The PCT applied its 'exceptional cases' policy (since Lenalidomide was not a drug on its list of drugs routinely provided, on grounds of clinical and cost effectiveness) and decided that an exceptional case had not been made out, notwithstanding powerful evidence from an expert on behalf of Mr Ross. Mr Ross sought a judicial review.

Judgment: Deputy High Court Judge Grenfell allowed the application for judicial review essentially on the basis that the PCT had misunderstood relevant matters, in particular studies that demonstrated that Lenalidomide was clinically effective in cases where other relevant drugs could no longer be tolerated:

i) The original Review Panel failed to appreciate the clear need for expert advice from a specialist in the field of oncology such as Professor Sikora. His report highlighted its failure to understand the studies which made a clear case of clinical efficacy of Lenalidomide for patients who could not tolerate Thalidomide, and, as regards the question of cost effectiveness, the report pointed out that the Panels had not taken into account the savings in not providing the other life prolonging drugs to which the Claimant had become intolerant.

ii) The PCT's policy was unlawful in that it stated that an application 'must' be refused where a patient was 'representative of a group of patients'. This was not a policy for exceptional cases but one that required the patient to show that he was unique. The Review and Appeal Panels erred, as they clearly thought that, because other patients could find themselves in the Claimant's position, the Claimant could not be exceptional.

iii) In any event, the Panels misdirected themselves that it was not exceptional to suffer unpleasant side effects to Thalidomide and therefore failed to appreciate the vital distinction that it was the Claimant's intolerance to the peripheral neuropathy which made him an exception. For these reasons the decision to refuse funding on the ground of exceptionality was logically flawed and on the evidence before the Panel the application ought to have been upheld on an ordinary reading of the term 'exceptional'.

iv) Once exceptional circumstances were established clinical efficacy and cost effectiveness should not be ignored. However, once an exceptional case was made out, particularly where matters of extending life were concerned, a PCT should take a less restrictive approach to cost effectiveness than when considering the case for funding a drug as part of its Operational Plan.

v) As regards clinical efficacy, the Panels failed to understand the strength of the evidence in favour of treating a patient such as the Claimant with Lenalidomide, as they had fundamentally misunderstood the results of the randomised control studies. They ought to have upheld the clear case on clinical efficacy presented to them.

vi) The Panels' decisions on cost-effectiveness were such that no reasonable authority could reach because they misunderstood the clinical effectiveness of Lenalidomide; they failed to understand that the actual sums sought were for 4 cycles, and if the Claimant did not respond, treatment would probably be discontinued; they misunderstood the median survival advantage figure; account was taken of those patients who would not have a response of one year's additional life, when logically, any additional cost would only arise in the event that the Claimant was responding to the treatment which would make it both clinically and cost effective; and they failed to take account of the saving to the PCT of not having to provide the expensive life prolonging treatment which had been given to the Claimant within the Operational Plan before he developed his intolerance to that treatment.

vii) The decision of the PCT was one which no reasonable authority could have made on the application before it and should be quashed.

18.41 *R (Harrison and Garnham) v Secretary of State for Health* [2009] EWHC 574 (Admin), (2009) 12 CCLR 355

The NHS was not entitled to make direct payments

Facts: the disabled claimants had been in receipt of direct payments from local authorities but became entitled to NHS continuing healthcare. Their local PCTs declined to continue to make direct payments on the ground that they lacked the power to do so. The claimants then sought a judicial review of the Secretary of State's policy guidance, on which the PCTs had relied.

Judgment: Silber J held that on a proper construction of the NHSA 2006, the NHS was not entitled to make cash payments to enable patients to purchase services and that whilst Article 8 ECHR was engaged, the differences between those in receipt of social care, and those in receipt of healthcare, justified a different approach to the provision of direct payments.

Comment: the position has now been mitigated, see:

- the National Health Service (Direct Payments) Regulations 2013; and
- the Guidance on Direct Payments for Healthcare: Understanding the Regulations.[33]

18.42 *R (Booker) v NHS Oldham* [2010] EWHC 2593 (Admin), (2011) 14 CCLR 315

The NHS was required to provide healthcare even for treatment covered by a personal injury award of damages designed to enable private healthcare to be purchased

Facts: a personal injury settlement involved a payment of damages to Ms Booker on the basis that a proportion of those damages would be used to fund private medical treatment and that further damages would become payable to the extent that necessary healthcare was not available from the NHS. Learning of this, NHS Oldham indicated that it would cease to continue to provide Ms Booker with such medical treatment as was covered by that aspect of the damages award. Ms Booker sought a judicial review of that decision.

Judgment: Deputy High Court Judge Pelling QC held that NHS Oldham had to continue to provide Ms Booker with (free) NHS treatment:

> In my judgment this reasoning does not lead to the conclusion for which the PCT contends. First, in deciding whether a service is reasonably required or is necessary to meet a reasonable requirement, the PCT is bound to have regard to the duties imposed by section 1 of the 2006 Act – see paragraph 24 to 26 of Lord Woolf's judgment in *Coughlan*. It follows that the PCT must have regard to the target duty to provide a comprehensive service free at the point of delivery. Secondly in reaching a decision the PCT is bound to have regard to the NHS Constitution for the reasons already set out above. It is therefore bound to have regard to the principle that access to NHS services is based on clinical need not on an individual's ability to pay and that a person who is otherwise eligible for treatment is entitled to receive it free of charge. Thirdly in my judgment in reaching a decision in a case such as this, the PCT is bound to have regard to and indeed to carry into effect the policy set out in the national framework document. This document established the national policy to be applied in deciding on eligibility for future healthcare. Paragraph 47 and 49 of the framework document in particular cannot support the notion that a person should not be treated as eligible

33 www.personalhealthbudgets.england.nhs.uk/_library/Resources/Personalhealthbudgets/2014/Guidance_on_Direct_Payments_for_Healthcare_Understanding_the_Regulations_March_2014.pdf.

by reference to the ability of the person concerned to access funding for such care from another source. Indeed, paragraph 49 of the framework document plainly contradicts such an approach. The reality is that this claimant's need for continuing healthcare will only be removed for so long as a private package has been successfully established and implemented. Unless and until that has occurred, the principle set out in paragraph 47 of the framework document cannot apply.

18.43 *MAK and RK v United Kingdom* Application nos 45901/05 and 40146/06, (2010) 13 CCLR 241

Disproportionate actions by a hospital doctor, resulting in his erroneously concluding that parents had abused their daughter, were incompatible with Article 8 ECHR

Facts: a hospital doctor negligently concluded that the daughter had been abused, resulting in the parents' access to their doctor being blocked, then impeded, for about a week. The English Court of Appeal struck out the parents' action in negligence.[34]

Judgment: the European Court of Human Rights held that whilst mistaken judgments or assessments by professionals do not in themselves render protection measures incompatible with Article 8 ECHR, in this case, the doctor's actions had been disproportionate: there had been a breach of Article 8 ECHR and, because the Human Rights Act 1998 had not been in force at the relevant time, of Article 13 ECHR.

18.44 *R (Condliff) v North Staffordshire PCT* [2011] EWCA Civ 910, (2011) 14 CCLR 656

The PCT was entitled to take into account only clinical factors and to disregard the social factors said to justify exceptional treatment

Facts: Mr Condliff sought bariatric surgery but the PCT refused to provide it because, under its policy, it only provided such treatment for patients whose body mass exceeded 50kg per square metre, which Mr Condliff's did not, unless there were exceptional clinical factors; Mr Condliff relied on exceptional social factors, but the PCT excluded them from consideration. Mr Condliff sought a judicial review.

Judgment: the Court of Appeal (Maurice Kay, Toulson LJJ) held that the PCT was entitled only to take into account clinical factors: nothing in any case-law supported the argument that Article 8 ECHR imposed a positive duty on health bodies to prioritise some patients on the basis of social factors whereas to take into account clinical factors only, when allocating scarce healthcare resources, was non-discriminatory and in keeping with a PCT's statutory duty.

18.45 *Rabone v Pennine Care NHS Foundation Trust* [2012] UKSC 2, (2012) 15 CCLR 13

Hospitals are under a duty imposed by Article 2 ECHR to protect both detained and voluntary mental patients against a real and immediate risk of suicide

34 *JD v East Berkshire Community Health NHS Trust* [2005] 2 AC 373, (2005) 8 CCLR 185.

Facts: M had a long history of psychiatric treatment and attempted suicide. She was in hospital on a voluntary basis, although staff had noted that, if she attempted to leave, consideration should be given to detaining her. The hospital then allowed M home leave and, after a day, she hanged herself. The hospital admitted liability in negligence but disputed liability under Article 2 ECHR.

Judgment: the Supreme Court (Walker, Hale, Brown, Mance and Dyson JJSC) held that the hospital had been liable under Article 2 ECHR; it owed her an operational duty to take reasonable steps to protect her from a real and immediate risk of suicide because she had been admitted to hospital as a real suicide risk and was extremely vulnerable, the hospital had assumed responsibility for her and she was under its control. The Court of Appeal's award of £5,000 to each parent seemed low but had not been appealed.

Comment: another example of the Court's willingness to intervene in cases of health and social care when a core right under the ECHR in engaged, in this case, the right to life under Article 2 ECHR.

18.46 *R (JF) v NHS Sheffield Clinical Commissioning Group* [2014] EWHC 1345 (Admin)

It had not been unlawful to provide ward monitoring and supervision to a person who received 1:1 supervision 24 hours a day whilst at home, under NHS continuing healthcare

Facts: JF received NHS continuing healthcare in her own home, including 1:1 supervision 24 hours a day. From time to time, JF received in-patient treatment however the CCG assessed her as needing only monitoring and supervision on the ward, on such occasions, not 1:1 supervision 24 hours a day. The hospital later undertook a detailed risk assessment, which concluded that 1:1 supervision was required, because of the unpredictability of JF's needs. JF nonetheless challenged the CCG's earlier decision.

Judgment: Stuart-Smith J held that the CCG's earlier decision had been lawful in public law and had not breached JF's rights under Articles 2 or 3 ECHR

18.47 *R (Whapples) v Birmingham Crosscity Clinical Commissioning Group* [2015] EWCA Civ 435, (2015) 18 CCLR 300

The NHS continuing healthcare framework did not in general contemplate payment of housing costs associated with the patient's own home, even when the patient received treatment there

Facts: Ms Whapples was functionally quadriplegic and also suffered from PTSD because of which she was unable to live in a care home. The CCG accepted that Ms Whapples was entitled to NHS continuing healthcare and that it had power to fund private accommodation but decided not to exercise it, as accommodation would be available through the relevant housing authority. Ms Whapples sought a judicial review.

Judgment: the Court of Appeal (Underhill, Vos and Burnett LJJ) held that in general the NHS continuing healthcare framework did not contemplate that the NHS would be responsible for funding accommodation costs where a person was receiving healthcare in their own home. To the extent that ordinary accommodation was needed, which the patient could not arrange and fund themselves, the distribution of responsibility placed a duty on local authorities rather than the NHS and the CCG's decision had been lawful in public law.

18.48 *Daniel v St George's Healthcare NHS Trust, London Ambulance Service* [2016] EWHC 23 (QB)

Medical practitioners and prison staff were required by the ECHR to do all that could reasonably be expected of them to avoid a real and immediate risk to life of which they have or ought to have knowledge

Facts: Mr James Best died in prison of a heart attack. His foster mother and biological son brought proceedings alleging that doctors and nurses had provided inadequate treatment at the scene and failed promptly to request an ambulance, and that the ambulance service had delayed unreasonably in dispatching an ambulance.

Judgment: Lang J held that medical practitioners and prison officers were both under the duty, at Article 2 ECHR, to do all that could reasonably be expected of them to avoid a real and immediate risk to life of which they have or ought to have knowledge. However, on the facts of this case, that duty had been discharged. In addition, on the facts, there had not been any unreasonable delay in calling, or dispatching an ambulance and its earlier arrival would not, in any event, have made any difference to the outcome; so there had also not been any breach of Article 3 ECHR. The first claimant, who had been Mr Best's foster mother for three years, was an *'indirect victim'* for the purposes of Article 34 ECHR and had standing to bring proceedings. The second claimant, whose relationship with Mr Best had never been formally recognised, as not.

18.49 *R (Dyer) v Welsh Ministers and others* [2015] EWHC 3712 (Admin), (2016) 19 CCLR 84

The NHS in Wales had not been in breach of duty under section 3 of the National Health Service (Wales) Act 2006, by providing hospital accommodation for a woman with a complex mental health condition in England because of the lack of appropriate accommodation in Wales

Facts: Mrs Dyer had a complex mental health condition, including an autistic spectrum disorder and a learning disability, which required her to be detained in hospital from time to time. Due to the lack of appropriate secure hospital accommodation for her in Wales, the Welsh NHS accommodated her in England. Mrs Dyer complained that the Welsh NHS had failed to assess and plan to meet the 'reasonable requirements' of women in Wales with mental disorders such as hers.

Judgment: Hickinbottom J held that the Welsh NHS had been under a duty to assess the 'reasonable requirements' of the Welsh population for hospital accommodation but the Welsh NHS had a considerable margin of judgment as to what information to collate and could not be criticised for failing to collate data on women with the particular subset of mental health conditions that afflicted Mrs Dyer, or to make a specific decision in relation to her and their needs:

> 103. As a principle, it seems to me to be self-evident that, if a public body is under an obligation to provide accommodation and other services to meet a statutory requirement, the public body must ascertain the requirement it is obliged to meet, before deciding how it should be met.
>
> ...
>
> 105. Section 3(1) is a general duty (see paragraph 17 above); and, as the authorities emphasise, the 'obligation is limited to providing the services identified to the extent that [the relevant authority] considers that they are necessary to meet all reasonable requirements' (*Coughlan* at [23] per Lord Woolf MR, in relation to the similarly worded provision in the 1977 Act: emphasis in the original). This necessarily places considerable discretion – or judgment as, in this context, it is perhaps better described – in the hands of the authority.
>
> ...
>
> 107. However, the exercise of judgment is not restricted to the substantive scope of the reasonable requirements, and the services the relevant authority considers necessary to meet those requirements. The authority also has a substantial degree of flexibility as to how it goes about its task. That principle is derived from cases such as *CREEDNZ Inc v Governor General of New Zealand* [1981] 1 NZLR 172 and *In re Findlay* [1985] AC 318, and described by Laws LJ in *R (Khatun) v London Borough of Newham* [2004] EWCA Civ 55; [2005] QB 37 at [35].
>
> 108. The principle bears upon this case in two ways.
>
> 109. First, before making an assessment of reasonable requirements or necessary services to meet them, the authority must consider whether the information it has is sufficient for it to make a properly informed decision; but that in itself requires an exercise of judgment with which this court will only interfere on public law grounds.
>
> 110. Second, Mr Wise submits that the various authorities here – notably the UHB and the WHSS Committee – erred in not focusing upon a category of patient which he has defined for the purpose and into which the Claimant falls, namely women with ASD and LD who require or may require in-patient mental healthcare (see, eg paragraph 1 of his skeleton argument). They erred, he says, in not collecting information and data about that group, and in not making a distinct discrete decision with regard to commissioning and financing (or not) of further secure accommodation in Wales for that group.
>
> 111. However, that, in my respectful view, is a somewhat simplistic view of the relevant decision-making, which misunderstands the nature of the relevant decisions. Mr Wise criticises the UHB and the WHSS Committee for not collating data in respect of a group he defines – ie women who require secure accommodation because of behaviour stemming from ASD and LD – and, thereafter, for not considering and making decisions concerning the requirements of the individuals in that group. But:
>
> > i) It is for the relevant authorities (the LHBs and the WHSS Committee in this case) to consider the criteria for the scope relevant clinical areas in respect of which, in their considered view, planning can best be made. The authorities have a wide margin of discretion in respect of the criteria they chose, and how they apply them. This assessment too

requires judgment with which, for the reasons I have given, the courts will not lightly interfere.

ii) It is in any event, in my view, arguably artificial to create a cohort by reference to the primary criterion lit upon by Mr Wise, i.e. a diagnosis of both ASD and LD, coupled with or uncoupled from the secondary criterion of a potential need for secure placement. A cohort is a group of people with a characteristic in common; and, in this context, that characteristic must be such that the individuals in the cohort have at least some common 'reasonable requirements'. However, as Mr Williams submitted, individuals with complex diagnoses including (but often, as in the Claimant's case, not restricted to) ASD and LD have varying degrees of mental health and often physical health disabilities, with different consequential behaviours and care and treatment needs, which (as again the Claimant illustrates) themselves can vary greatly over time. This is particularly so with behavioural conditions such as LD which, as I understand it, are not curable, treatment going to the goal of enabling individuals to cope with the disability. That inevitably requires a particularly subjective approach. As the Claimant's mother emphasises in her statement of 2 November 2015, such patients may at times need particularly specialised assessment, treatment and care, tailored to his or her particular condition and behaviour. Even if patients need secure provision, the nature of the required facilities will vary. Such individuals are clinically idiosyncratic, and may not have any or sufficient commonality in their 'reasonable requirements' to classify as a 'cohort' (see, eg, paragraphs 11–12 of Mr Andrew's statement dated 16 September 2015). That is particularly so if, as here, they are small in number.

iii) However, even if they can be properly categorised as Mr Wise suggests, the decision to be made about their reasonable requirements and how they might be met does not concern simply them. Such decisions cannot be made in a vacuum, or (as Mr Williams put it) in isolation from the competing needs and priorities of other cohorts of patients. To consider reasonableness of their requirements means assessing them in the context of the needs of a multiplicity of other patients and potential patients, and the many other calls on public resources allocated to NHS Wales. It is unrealistic to impose upon the relevant authority an obligation discretely to consider every possible group and subgroup of patients and potential patient, no matter how narrowly defined, who may wish to use the services of NHS Wales; and to make a discrete decision as what their precise requirements will be and whether to prioritise their needs or otherwise favour them over others with different health requirements. The relevant decision-making process is therefore particularly sophisticated. It can sensibly be done – and, perhaps, only sensibly done – in the context of a scheme whereby the requirements of all patients and potential patients are taken into account somewhere along the line.

iv) NHS Wales has such a scheme. It is described in paragraphs 59–60 above. The scheme, on a bottom up basis, is designed to identify and consider the requirements of all patients and potential patients; and the prioritisation of those requirements for the purposes of planning, including planning capital and other public expenditure. That scheme is not challenged in these proceedings.

18.50 *S (A Child) v NHS England* [2016] EWHC 1395 (Admin), (2016) 19 CCLR 336

On the facts, the decision not to fund narcolepsy treatment for a 17-year-old child had disregarded relevant considerations and applied too stringent a test of exceptionality

Facts: S was a 17-year-old girl who several years earlier succumbed to narcolepsy and cataplexy. She was academically very bright and good at sport but her affliction was seriously impact on her potential and she had ceased to respond well to existing treatment; she needed more expensive treatment but NHS England refused to fund that because, not being subject to a NICE recommendation or a general policy to fund, there had to be an Individual Funding Request, which would only be granted in two exceptional clinical circumstances.

Judgment: Collins J held as follows:

> 31. For obvious reasons, there has been emphasis placed on the claiamnt's academic expectations and her need to do as well as possible in her current A level examinations. But every child will need to do their best since otherwise their future life will be severely blighted. This is however a non-clinical factor. Ms Richards relies on the decision of the Court of Appeal in *R (Condliff) v North Staffordshire PCT* [2012] PTSR 460. The case concerned the criteria set for determining exceptionality because of the difficult ethical and practical questions in deciding, as between patients competing for limited resources, what circumstances should be taken into account as potentially exceptional. Toulson LJ, who gave the only reserved judgment, referred to and cited extensively from a paper published in 2008 by Dr Daphne Austin, a consultant in public health with many years experience. The approach to be adopted must be to ask 'on what grounds can the PCT justify funding this patient when others from the same patient group are not being funded?' The ratio of the decision in the case was that it was lawful to adopt a policy that IFR's should be considered and determined exclusively by reference to clinical factors.
>
> 32. I recognise, as Ms Richards has submitted based on the evidence of the Head of Clinical Effectiveness for Specialised Services for the defendant, that the defendant has finite resources and, as the courts have recognised (see for example *R v North Devon HA ex p Coughlan* [2001] QB 213), cannot fund every treatment for every patient. It has to make decisions, which may sometimes seem extremely harsh for individual patients, to ensure the best possible outcome for all patients. The defendant's official policy makes the point that 'there should not be a parallel system operating which allows individual treatments on patients to bypass prioritisation.' The policy states:
>
>> 'A Commissioner should not give preferential treatment to an individual patient who is one of a group of patients with the same clinical needs. Either a treatment or service is funded in order to create the opportunity for all patients with equal needs to be treated or, if this cannot be afforded, it should not be commissioned as part of NHS treatment for any patients. The NHS CB considers that if funding for treatment cannot be justified as an investment for all patients in a particular cohort, the treatment should not be offered to only some of the patients unless it is possible to differentiate between groups of patients on clinical grounds. A decision to treat some patients but not others has the potential to be unfair, arbitrary and possibly discriminatory.'

33. While accepting that the approach of the defendant is not unlawful, it must be borne in mind that there is an IFR policy which must be given some effect. Equally, I am conscious that it is not for me to strike down the decision in this case because I believe that it was too harsh and I have, as anyone would, enormous sympathy for the claimant. Mr Wise has contended that the cohort to be considered should be all those suffering from narcolepsy and cataplexy. Ms Richards submits that that cannot be right since all for whom the usual treatment is not effective would be regarded as exceptional. This would be contrary to the policy of the defendant and would in any event widen to an excessive extent the test for exceptionality. I am inclined to agree with Ms Richards but in any event I think I should regard the appropriate cohort as those who do not respond to the usual treatment.

34. The key evidence in this case is that of Dr Elphick emphasised in her letter of 18 March 2016. The claimant is not only not responding to the usual treatment but is deteriorating. This shows that she is suffering from a particularly severe form of her condition. Her condition is rare, and her failure to respond to the usual treatment is also rare. But she is in a very rare situation in that she suffers from a particularly rare form of the condition. This aspect is not dealt with in the response of the defendant's panel or screening group. Since exceptional cannot mean unique, it is in my view difficult if not impossible to see that the claimant should not be considered to meet the exceptionality test. If she is not exceptional, who is? I should add that in her case there is clear evidence that her mental and physical health is suffering and will get worse. Thus she will benefit from the treatment with sodium oxybate to a greater extent than others who are not receptive to the usual treatment. This means that, as Dr Elphick said, there is cost effectiveness in that she will not be likely to need medical care to the extent she will if not treated with sodium oxybate.

35. As I have said, I must not substitute my own judgment for that of the panel. But I have not done this since, as I have set out, there were in my view failures by the defendant to have regard to all the matters raised by Dr Elphick and an altogether too restrictive application of exceptionality. The claimant qualified within the IFR policy referred to in paragraph 13 above.

36. Normally in cases such as this, as the defendant's solicitors stated, the remedy would be to quash the decision and to require reconsideration in accordance with the judgment given. But I am satisfied that this case is indeed exceptional to the extent that a decision to refuse the treatment could not be supportable. Accordingly, I took the unusual step of making an interim order that the defendant should fund the provision of sodium oxybate to the claimant for a three month trial period to be administered under the control of Dr Elphick.

37. I have no doubt that anyone reading the circumstances of this case would be surprised that sodium oxybate is not available for children generally and for the claimant in particular. But I recognise the constraints under which those responsible in the defendant have to act. I wish to make it clear that there is no suggestion that any of those involved in the decisions lacked compassion or knowingly refused treatment they should have permitted. The difficulties facing them cannot be underestimated and I am sure that they regret the need to make decisions which result in suffering by individual patients. Nonetheless, I am satisfied that this is a very rare case in which the decision making has gone wrong.

Social care and NHS continuing healthcare: cases and complaints

18.51 *R v North and East Devon Health Authority ex p Coughlan* (1999) 2 CCLR 285

Local authorities were only empowered to provide nursing services to adults that were merely incidental or ancillary to the provision of residential accommodation and that were of a nature that a social services authority can be expected to provide

Facts: Ms Coughlan was rendered very severely disabled by a road traffic accident. After a period of treatment at Newcourt Hospital, which the health authority then wished to close, she and seven other patients were moved to Mardon House hospital, with an assurance that it would be their 'home for life'. However, the health authority then resolved to close Mardon House. In addition, it determined that Ms Coughlan no longer met the criteria for NHS continuing healthcare, so that she had to resort to local authority residential accommodation. Ms Coughlan submitted that it was beyond the powers of a local authority to provide her with the nursing care she needed and that it was unlawful for the health authority to resile from its 'home for life' promise; and a breach of Article 8 ECHR.

Judgment: local authorities were only empowered to provide nursing services that were merely incidental or ancillary to the provision of residential accommodation and that were of a nature that a social services authority can be expected to provide and the health authority's approach as to the nursing care that it was required to provide was too restrictive; in addition, its 'home for life' promise had created a legitimate expectation that, on the facts of this case, could not justifiably be frustrated:

> 30. The result of the detailed examination of the three sections can be summarised as follows:
>
> (a) The Secretary of State can exclude some nursing services from the services provided by the NHS. Such services can then be provided as a social or care service rather than as a health service.
>
> (b) The nursing services which can be so provided as part of the care services are limited to those which can legitimately be regarded as being provided in connection with accommodation which is being provided to the classes of persons referred to in section 21 of the Care Act who are in need of care and attention; in other words as part of a social services care package.
>
> (c) The fact that the nursing services are to be provided as part of social services care and will have to be paid for by the person concerned, unless that person's resources mean that he or she will be exempt from having to pay for those services, does not prohibit the Secretary of State from deciding not to provide those services. The nursing services are part of the social services and are subject to the same regime for payment as other social services. Mr Gordon submitted that this is unfair. He pointed out that if a person receives comparable nursing care in a hospital or in a community setting, such as his or her home, it is free. The Royal Commission on Long Term Care, in its report, With Respect to Old Age, (March 1999 chapter 6 pages 62 et seq. Cm 4192–1) not surprisingly agrees with this assessment and makes recommendations

to improve the situation. However, as long as the nursing care services are capable of being properly classified as part of the social services' responsibilities, then, under the present legislation, that unfairness is part of the statutory scheme.

(d) The fact that some nursing services can be properly regarded as part of social services' care, to be provided by the local authority, does not mean that all nursing services provided to those in the care of the local authority can be treated in this way. The scale and type of nursing required in an individual case may mean that it would not be appropriate to regard all or part of the nursing as being part of "the package of care" which can be provided by a local authority. There can be no precise legal line drawn between those nursing services which are and those which are not capable of being treated as included in such a package of care services.

(e) The distinction between those services which can and cannot be so provided is one of degree which in a borderline case will depend on a careful appraisal of the facts of the individual case. However, as a very general indication as to where the line is to be drawn, it can be said that if the nursing services are (i) merely incidental or ancillary to the provision of the accommodation which a local authority is under a duty to provide to the category of persons to whom section 21 refers and (ii) of a nature which it can be expected that an authority whose primary responsibility is to provide social services can be expected to provide, then they can be provided under section 21. It will be appreciated that the first part of the test is focusing on the overall quantity of the services and the second part on the quality of the services provided.

(f) The fact that care services are provided on a means tested contribution basis does not prevent the Secretary of State declining to provide the nursing part of those services on the NHS. However, he can only decline if he has formed a judgment which is tenable that consistent with his long term general duty to continue to promote a comprehensive free health service that it is not necessary to provide the services. He cannot decline simply because social services will fill the gap.

43. The fact that there is this background of possible confusion makes it important that any eligibility criteria should be drawn up with particular care. They need to identify at least two categories of persons who, although receiving nursing care while in a nursing home, are still entitled to receive the care at the expense of the NHS. First, there are those who, because of the scale of their health needs, should be regarded as wholly the responsibility of a health authority. Secondly, there are those whose nursing services in general can be regarded as being the responsibility of the local authority, but whose additional requirements are the responsibility of the NHS.

48. It is for the Health Authority to decide what should be the eligibility criteria in its area in the co-operative framework envisaged by the circulars. In doing so it can take account of conditions in its area. We do not accept the argument that there cannot be variations between the services provided by the NHS in different areas. However the eligibility criteria cannot place a responsibility on the local authority which goes beyond the terms of section 21. This is what these criteria do. Cases where the health care element goes far beyond what the section permits were being placed upon the local authority as a result of the rigorous limits placed on what services can be considered to be NHS care services. That this is the position is confirmed by the result of the assessment of Miss Coughlan and her fellow occupants. Their disabilities are of a scale which are beyond the scope of local authority services.

18.52 The Health Service Ombudsman's Report on NHS funding for long term care (13 February 2003)

NHS bodies had wrongly been declining to provide NHS continuing healthcare and needed to review their policies and redress the hardship caused

The Report[35] annexes four separate investigation reports and concludes that, owing to unduly restrictive policies operated by local authorities and the Department of Health, persons entitled to NHS continuing healthcare were being denied it. The Ombudsman made a number of important recommendations:

> 38. The findings in the cases reported today and the themes emerging from those still under investigation lead me to conclude that:
>
> - The Department of Health's guidance and support to date has not provided the secure foundation needed to enable a fair and transparent system of eligibility for funding for long term care to be operated across the country;
> - What guidance there is has been mis-interpreted and mis-applied by some health authorities when developing and reviewing their own eligibility criteria;
> - Further problems have arisen in the application of local criteria to individuals;
> - The effect has been to cause injustice and hardship to some people.
>
> 39. I therefore recommend that strategic health authorities and primary care trusts should:
>
> - Review the criteria used by their predecessor bodies, and the way those criteria were applied, since 1996. They will need to take into account the Coughlan judgment, guidance issued by the Department of Health and my findings;
> - Make efforts to remedy any consequent financial injustice to patients, where the criteria, or the way they were applied, were not clearly appropriate or fair. This will include attempting to identify any patients in their area who may wrongly have been made to pay for their care in a home and making appropriate recompense to them or their estates.
>
> 40. I also recommend that the Department of Health should:
>
> - Consider how they can support and monitor the performance of authorities and primary care trusts in this work. That might involve the Department assessing whether, from 1996 to date, criteria being used were in line with the law and guidance. Where they were not, the Department might need to co-ordinate effort to remedy any financial injustice to patients affected;
> - Review the national guidance on eligibility for continuing NHS health care, making it much clearer in new guidance the situations when the NHS must provide funding and those where it is left to the discretion of NHS bodies locally. This guidance may need to include detailed definitions of terms used and case examples of patterns of need likely to mean NHS funding should be provided;
> - Consider being more proactive in checking that criteria used in the future follow that guidance;
> - Consider how to link assessment of eligibility for continuing NHS health care into the single assessment process and whether the Department

35 www.ombudsman.org.uk/__data/assets/pdf_file/0013/1075/NHS-funding-for-long-term-care.pdf.

should provide further support to the development of reliable assessment methods.

18.53 Complaint No E22/03 against the former Cambridgeshire Health Authority and South Cambridgeshire Primary Care Trust (The *Pointon* Case) (November 2003)[36]

Mr Pointon had wrongly been refused NHS continuing healthcare because the NHS focussed unduly and inappropriately on the fact that he was receiving care at home and on physical problems, rather than psychological problems and the special skills needed to cater for them

Mr Pointon suffered from Alzheimer's disease and was receiving nursing care at home from his wife and a team of local authority carers. The Parliamentary and Health Service Ombudsman found that the PCT had got distracted from recognising Mr Pointon's need for NHS continuing healthcare by focussing unduly on the fact that Mr Pointon was being cared for at home, and on physical needs rather than psychological problems and the special skills needed to cater for them:

> 44. I turn now to the actions of the PCT who took over the responsibility for continuing care cases in April 2002. They also took over the Health Authority's eligibility criteria. Mrs Pointon had complained in January 2002 to the Health Authority about their decision not to fund an extra carer every five weeks to maintain the pattern of respite care. She had also complained to this Office. The incoming PCT agreed with Mrs Pointon that a further assessment of her husband's condition should be carried out on 15 April. It was completed by a member of the District Nursing Team and was headed 'Health Needs Assessment'. Once again this assessment followed the pattern of assessing purely physical and nursing needs against very specific criteria (paragraphs 17 and 18) that it would be very difficult to provide in the home setting. The Consultant Psychiatrist was consulted by the Manager, but once again was asked very specific questions about the type and frequency of professional input that Mr Pointon needed at that time and gave no recognition, either to Mr Pointon's psychological needs, or to the unusually high standard of care that Mrs Pointon and her team were providing.
>
> 45. The Assessor criticised the range of this assessment and confirmed that the questioning rendered funding for respite care at home practically impossible. The PCT and Social Services decided that Mr Pointon's health needs were being met, that the respite care was purely social and refused funding in May.
>
> 46. In subsequent discussions the clinicians and the nurses agreed that Mrs Pointon was giving highly personalised care with a high level of skill. This was later described by the independent Consultant as nursing care equal if not superior to that that Mr Pointon would receive in a dementia ward.
>
> 47. In September 2002 the independent Consultant commissioned by Mrs Pointon, produced a report which confirmed that Mr Pointon's symptoms stemmed solely from a health condition that was severe, complex and unpredictable, needing 24-hour care and frequent interventions to prevent him harming himself. After the Consultant Psychiatrist and the Consultant Geriatrician had confirmed the independent Consultant's opinion that Mr Pointon did meet the eligibility criteria for NHS continuing care, a package

36 www.ombudsman.org.uk/__data/assets/pdf_file/0007/1105/The-Pointon-case.pdf.

of care was agreed with Social Services whereby the NHS would fund the cost of an additional carer every fifth week. The PCT have explained that they can only make Direct Payments within a package of payments with Social Services. However, they have also agreed that should Mr Pointon require in-patient care at a future date, then he would be admitted to an in-patient facility agreed by Mrs Pointon. It is sad to reflect that this solution is the one that Mrs Pointon suggested in January 2002. Whilst I am pleased that agreement was reached eventually, I agree with the Assessor's opinion that the PCT assessed Mr Pointon against the wrong criteria, once again focusing on physical needs and also failing to recognise that the standard of care provided by Mrs Pointon was equal to that that a nurse could provide. I uphold the complaint.

48. In May 2003 in the light of the Ombudsman's report (paragraph 14), the Department of Health issued guidance to Strategic Health Authorities and PCTs on the procedure to use when reviewing continuing care cases dating back to April 1996. It is my opinion that they should also review the eligibility criteria to ensure that the criteria for funding care at home, and the recognition of patients' psychological as well as physical needs, are clearly defined. While I am aware that the continuity of her husband's care is one of Mrs Pointon's main concerns, I recommend that the PCT discuss with Mrs Pointon, in the light of the Department of Health guidance, the provision of Mr Pointon's current funding, and determine whether any retrospective payments are indicated.

18.54 The Health Service Ombudsman's NHS funding for long term care: follow up report (HC 144) (16 December 2004)[37]

More needed to be done to revise eligibility criteria and provide redress

In the follow up report, the Health Service Ombudsman focuses on guiding local authorities and PCTs in relation to revising eligibility criteria, undertaking reviews of cases and providing financial redress. This was itself followed up by the Health Service Ombudsman's Memorandum to the Health Select Committee inquiry into NHS continuing healthcare, Retrospective Continuing Care Funding and Redress (HC 386, 2006–7).[38]

18.55 *R (T) v Haringey LBC* [2005] EWHC 2235 (Admin), (2006) 9 CCLR 58

Local authorities were not empowered to provide healthcare services to children

Facts: D was a 3-year-old child with a tracheostomy (tube in her throat), which was expected to remain for several years. She was to be looked after at home, on account of multiple medical conditions, but the main area of care involved the careful management of the tracheostomy, which required very careful cleaning and monitoring, if D was to avoid serious injury. D's mother, B, undertook those tasks but needed respite care. Haringey assessed her as needing at least 10 hours more per week than was provided by the PCT. The PCT's view was that such provision was unnecessary. B claimed that, if the PCT was not liable to make such provision, then Haringey was.

37 www.ombudsman.org.uk/__data/assets/pdf_file/0014/1076/NHS-funding-for-long-term-care-follow-up-report.pdf.

38 www.gov.uk/government/uploads/system/uploads/attachment_data/file/231360/0386.pdf.

Judgment: Ouseley J held that Haringey was not liable to provide this type of respite care, under the provisions of the Children Act 1989 (or section 2 of the Chronically Sick and Disabled Persons Act 1970), because it amounted to health care, rather than social care, and was implicitly excluded. The PCT was in principle responsible but had lawfully concluded that, in its view, such provision was not reasonably necessary and its conclusion did not amount to a violation of the family's ECHR rights.

NHS continuing healthcare: cases and complaints

18.56 *R v North and East Devon Health Authority ex p Coughlan* [2001] QB 213, (1999) 2 CCLR 285, CA

Local authorities were only empowered to provide nursing services to adults that were merely incidental or ancillary to the provision of residential accommodation and that were of a nature that a social services authority can be expected to provide

Facts: Ms Coughlan was rendered very severely disabled by a road traffic accident. After a period of treatment at Newcourt Hospital, which the health authority then wished to close, she and seven other patients were moved to Mardon House hospital, with an assurance that it would be their 'home for life'. However, the health authority then resolved to close Mardon House. In addition, it determined that Ms Coughlan no longer met the criteria for NHS continuing healthcare, so that she had to resort to local authority residential accommodation. Ms Coughlan submitted that it was beyond the powers of a local authority to provide her with the nursing care she needed and that it was unlawful for the health authority to resile from its 'home for life' promise; and a breach of Article 8 ECHR.

Judgment: local authorities were only empowered to provide nursing services that were merely incidental or ancillary to the provision of residential accommodation and that were of a nature that a social services authority can be expected to provide and the health authority's approach as to the nursing care that it was required to provide was too restrictive; in addition, its 'home for life' promise had created a legitimate expectation that, on the facts of this case, could not justifiably be frustrated:

> 30. The result of the detailed examination of the three sections can be summarised as follows:
>
> (a) The Secretary of State can exclude some nursing services from the services provided by the NHS. Such services can then be provided as a social or care service rather than as a health service.
>
> (b) The nursing services which can be so provided as part of the care services are limited to those which can legitimately be regarded as being provided in connection with accommodation which is being provided to the classes of persons referred to in section 21 of the Care Act who are in need of care and attention; in other words as part of a social services care package.
>
> (c) The fact that the nursing services are to be provided as part of social services care and will have to be paid for by the person concerned, unless that person's resources mean that he or she will be exempt from having to pay for those services, does not prohibit the Secretary of State

from deciding not to provide those services. The nursing services are part of the social services and are subject to the same regime for payment as other social services. Mr Gordon submitted that this is unfair. He pointed out that if a person receives comparable nursing care in a hospital or in a community setting, such as his or her home, it is free. The Royal Commission on Long Term Care, in its report, With Respect to Old Age, (March 1999 chapter 6 pages 62 et seq. Cm 4192–1) not surprisingly agrees with this assessment and makes recommendations to improve the situation. However, as long as the nursing care services are capable of being properly classified as part of the social services' responsibilities, then, under the present legislation, that unfairness is part of the statutory scheme.

(d) The fact that some nursing services can be properly regarded as part of social services' care, to be provided by the local authority, does not mean that all nursing services provided to those in the care of the local authority can be treated in this way. The scale and type of nursing required in an individual case may mean that it would not be appropriate to regard all or part of the nursing as being part of "the package of care" which can be provided by a local authority. There can be no precise legal line drawn between those nursing services which are and those which are not capable of being treated as included in such a package of care services.

(e) The distinction between those services which can and cannot be so provided is one of degree which in a borderline case will depend on a careful appraisal of the facts of the individual case. However, as a very general indication as to where the line is to be drawn, it can be said that if the nursing services are (i) merely incidental or ancillary to the provision of the accommodation which a local authority is under a duty to provide to the category of persons to whom section 21 refers and (ii) of a nature which it can be expected that an authority whose primary responsibility is to provide social services can be expected to provide, then they can be provided under section 21. It will be appreciated that the first part of the test is focusing on the overall quantity of the services and the second part on the quality of the services provided.

(f) The fact that care services are provided on a means tested contribution basis does not prevent the Secretary of State declining to provide the nursing part of those services on the NHS. However, he can only decline if he has formed a judgment which is tenable that consistent with his long term general duty to continue to promote a comprehensive free health services that it is not necessary to provide the services. He cannot decline simply because social services will fill the gap.

43. The fact that there is this background of possible confusion makes it important that any eligibility criteria should be drawn up with particular care. They need to identify at least two categories of persons who, although receiving nursing care while in a nursing home, are still entitled to receive the care at the expense of the NHS. First, there are those who, because of the scale of their health needs, should be regarded as wholly the responsibility of a health authority. Secondly, there are those whose nursing services in general can be regarded as being the responsibility of the local authority, but whose additional requirements are the responsibility of the NHS.

48. It is for the Health Authority to decide what should be the eligibility criteria in its area in the co-operative framework envisaged by the circulars. In doing so it can take account of conditions in its area. We do not accept the argument that there cannot be variations between the services provided

by the NHS in different areas. However the eligibility criteria cannot place a responsibility on the local authority which goes beyond the terms of section 21. This is what these criteria do. Cases where the health care element goes far beyond what the section permits were being placed upon the local authority as a result of the rigorous limits placed on what services can be considered to be NHS care services. That this is the position is confirmed by the result of the assessment of Miss Coughlan and her fellow occupants. Their disabilities are of a scale which are beyond the scope of local authority services.

18.57 *R (Gunter) v South Western Staffordshire PCT* [2005] EWHC 1894 (Admin), (2006) 9 CCLR 121

The NHS decision to refuse services was vitiated by its failure to appreciate that it could fund a user independent trust and the importance of the patient's home life

Facts: Ms Gunter was a 21-year-old woman, who lived with her parents, but required 24-hour nursing care. A point had been reached where the PCT wanted to provide Ms Gunter with residential care. The parents wanted care at home, provided by a user independent trust, with the parents available in a supportive/emergency role.

Judgment: Collins J held that the PCT had power to use a voluntary organisation, such as a user independent trust, to provide services to a patient. In this case, the PCT needed to reconsider its position, as it had failed properly to take into account the importance to Ms Gunter of her home life, her expressed views and the benefits that living at home had occasioned.

18.58 *R (Grogan) v Bexley NHS Care Trust* [2006] EWHC 44 (Admin), (2006) 9 CCLR 188

A person may be entitled to NHS continuing healthcare notwithstanding that their needs could be met in local authority residential accommodation if the services of a registered nurse were provided by the NHS

Facts: Ms Grogan required regular supervision by a registered nurse and other nursing care services but was refused NHS continuing healthcare on the ground that the local authority was required to provide her with residential accommodation, whilst the NHS would provide ancillary nursing care, as required by section 49 of the Health and Social Care Act (HSCA) 2001.

Judgment: Charles J held that the Secretary of State for Health's guidance, and the local eligibility criteria for NHS continuing healthcare, were unlawful in that they suggested that a person would not qualify for NHS continuing healthcare where their healthcare needs could be met by a RNCC (registered nursing care contribution) under the HSCA 2001, including under a medium or high band, unless they had other healthcare needs that caused them to qualify. It was necessary to determine, first of all, whether a person's need for healthcare, in the round, entitled them to NHS continuing healthcare (because their primary need was for healthcare); only if not, did the RNCC become relevant.

18.59 *R (St Helens BC) v Manchester PCT* [2008] EWCA Civ 931, (2008) 11 CCLR 774

Decisions as to whether a person was entitled to NHS continuing healthcare or local authority social care were to be made by the NHS bodies and any judicial review by a local authority would be on a conventional and not a merits basis

Facts: the PCT assessed PE's needs as not being primarily healthcare needs, so that she was ineligible for NHS continuing healthcare. St Helens, the local authority on whom the social care costs then fell, sought a judicial review. Beatson J refused permission to apply for judicial review and St Helens appealed.

Judgment: the Court of Appeal (May and Scott Baker LJJ, Sir Peter Gibson) dismissed the appeal, holding that the critical statutory was that imposed on the Secretary of State for Health, under sections 1–3 of NHSA 2006; it was that legislation that was the dominant legislation in the sense that decisions under it were determinative of whether a person had a 'primary healthcare need', the local authority's function being residual. Accordingly it was for the NHS to determine whether a person was entitled to NHS continuing healthcare and, if a local authority challenged that decision, the usual judicial review principles would apply and there would not be a merits based review by the court, even though the consequence of the NHS decision was that the local authority had to shoulder a burden it considered to be ultra vires its powers.

18.60 *R (Green) v South West Strategic Health Authority* [2008] EWHC 2576 (Admin), (2009) 12 CCLR 93

On their proper construction, the health authority's policy guidance did correctly incorporate the 'primary health need' test, which it properly applied

Facts: Ms Green, who suffered from Alzheimer's disease, and lived in care home accommodation, sought a judicial review of the health authority's decision that she was not entitled to NHS continuing healthcare: she contended that the health authority's eligibility criteria were flawed.

Judgment: Wyn Williams J dismissed the application for judicial review, on the ground that, read as a whole including together with a supplementary document, the eligibility criteria were lawful:

> 44. That being so, this case is different from *Grogan*. In *Grogan*, to repeat, Charles J decided that the published criteria did not sufficiently identify the Primary Health Care Needs Test. It was in that context that he held that the phrase 'the nature or complexity or intensity or unpredictability of an individual's health needs' was insufficient guidance. Had there been an identification of the Primary Health Care Needs Test and an exposition of its content in *Grogan* I doubt whether Charles J would have considered the criteria before him to have been unlawful.

18.61 *Secretary of State for Work and Pensions v Slavin* [2011] EWCA Civ 1515, (2012) 15 CCLR 354

Although in receipt of NHS continuing healthcare, the patient was not receiving 'treatment' and so was entitled to retain the mobility component of his DLA

Facts: Mr Slavin suffered from, inter alia, a severe learning disability. After he went to stay at a care home, under NHS continuing healthcare, the Secretary of State terminated payment of the mobility component of his disability living allowance, on the basis that he was being maintained free of charge whilst undergoing medical or other treatment in a hospital or other institution.

Judgment: the Court of Appeal (Pills, Richards and Davis LJJ) held that although Mr Slavin suffered from a disability of the mind amounting to an illness, he was not receiving nursing care requiring the possession of a professional nursing qualification or training, so he was not undergoing 'treatment', accordingly, he was not disentitled to the mobility component of disability living allowance.

18.62 *R (Dennison) v Bradford Clinical Commissioning Group* [2014] EWHC 2552 (Admin)

The CCG had been wrong to refuse to review a nursing home resident's eligibility for NHS continuing healthcare during a period covered by two flawed assessments

Facts: Mr Dennison's mother had funded her nursing home accommodation prior to her death, after which her son asked the CCG to review whether his mother should have received NHS continuing healthcare throughout her period of residence. The CCG refused to undertake a review for periods of time where it had already completed assessments of the mother's entitlement to CHC.

Judgment: William Davis J held that two of the assessments in question were flawed in that the CCG had failed properly to consider whether the mother had had a primary health need and CCG would have to review those assessments.

18.63 *R (JF) v NHS Sheffield Clinical Commissioning Group* [2014] EWHC 1345 (Admin)

It had not been unlawful to provide ward monitoring and supervision to a person who received 1:1 supervision 24 hours a day while at home, under NHS continuing healthcare

Facts: JF received NHS continuing healthcare in her own home, including 1:1 supervision 24 hours a day. From time to time, JF received in-patient treatment however the CCG assessed her as needing only monitoring and supervision on the ward, on such occasions, not 1:1 supervision 24 hours a day. The hospital later undertook a detailed risk assessment, which concluded that 1:1 supervision was required, because of the unpredictability of JF's needs. JF nonetheless challenged the CCG's earlier decision.

Judgment: Stuart-Smith J held that the CCG's earlier decision had been lawful in public law and had not breached JF's rights under Articles 2 or 3 ECHR.

18.64 *R (Whapples) v Birmingham Crosscity Clinical Commissioning Group* [2015] EWCA Civ 435, (2015) 18 CCLR 300

The NHS continuing healthcare framework did not in general contemplate payment of housing costs associated with the patient's own home, even when the patient received treatment there

Facts: Ms Whapples was functionally quadriplegic and also suffered from PTSD because of which she was unable to live in a care home. The CCG accepted that Ms Whapples was entitled to NHS continuing healthcare and that it had power to fund private accommodation but decided not to exercise it, as accommodation would be available through the relevant housing authority. Ms Whapples sought a judicial review.

Judgment: the Court of Appeal (Underhill, Vos and Burnett LJJ) held that in general the NHS continuing healthcare framework did not contemplate that the NHS would be responsible for funding accommodation costs where a person was receiving healthcare in their own home. To the extent that ordinary accommodation was needed, which the patient could not arrange and fund themselves, the distribution of responsibility placed a duty on local authorities rather than the NHS and the CCG's decision had been lawful in public law.

18.65 *National Aids Trust v National Health Service Commissioning Board (NHS England)* [2016] EWHC 2005 Admin, (2016) 19 CCLR 459

NHS England had the power to commission and anti-retroviral drug to be used on a preventative basis for those at high risk of contracting HIV

Facts: NHS England claimed that it had no power to commission preventative medication because that was a 'public health function' and also medication designed to prevent sexually transmitted diseases, both of which were the responsibility of local authorities.

Judgment: Green J held that NHS England did have the power, in the light of the relevant provision of the National Health Service Act 2006, construed in the light of the purposes of that Act:

> 61. In my judgment when the NHSA 2006 is considered both as a whole but also by reference to its specific provisions it has the following broad characteristics and purposes; First, it imposes broad duties and powers on NHS England to secure the provision of health services to the entirety of the population and nation wide; second, the duty includes all aspects of preventative medicine; third it exercises its powers and duties concurrently with other providers of services which includes the Secretary of State, CCGs and local authorities; fourth these services are to be provided comprehensively and in an integrated manner; fifth, the service is to be provided efficiently and so as to avoid inequalities of provision or outcome.

Health care and persons subject to immigration control

18.66 *R v Hammersmith Hospitals NHS Trust ex p Reffell* (2001) 4 CCLR 371, CA

The Trust had been required to make a charge and rationally required an up-front deposit, since Mr Reffell was not prevented from securing treatment in his country of origin

Facts: Mr Reffell was a Nigerian national, whose medical treatment for renal failure had initially been paid for by his father's employer. That funding ceased and the applicant was unable to pay for continued treatment. The Trust refused to provide further treatment unless Mr Reffell paid in advance or provided a guarantee – except for such treatment as was required to enable Mr Reffell safely to return to Nigeria.

Judgment: the Court of Appeal (Simon Brown, Waller and Tuckey LJJ) held that the Trust was required to charge Mr Reffell, by the National Health Service (Charges to Overseas Visitors) Regulations 1989. It was implicit in the power to charge, that there was a power to require a deposit. It had been rational to require a deposit in this case because, unlike the case of an asylum-seeker, there was nothing to prevent Mr Reffell from seeking treatment in his country of origin.

18.67 *R (YA) v Secretary of State for Health* [2009] EWCA Civ 225, (2009) 12 CCLR 213

It was not lawful to require up-front deposits from failed asylum-seekers who were unable to pay for medical treatment and who needed timeous treatment but were unable to leave the UK

Facts: YA was a failed Palestinian asylum-seeker who, however, was unable to return to Palestine because it was impossible to obtain a travel document that permitted that. He was seriously ill with liver disease, received NHS treatment and was then billed for about £9,000.00. The hospital then agreed to withdraw then bill and provide further treatment without charge. YA then substituted the Secretary of State for Health as defendant and challenged the lawfulness of the Secretary of State's guidance to health authorities.

Judgment: the Court of Appeal (Ward, Lloyd and Rimer LJJ) held that where a person's residence was unlawful (as in this case, albeit that YA had 'temporary admission' to the UK) they cannot be ordinarily resident, or lawfully resident, so the Secretary of State was correct that the charging provisions under section 175 of the National Health Service Act 2006 and the National Health Service (Charges to Overseas Visitors) Regulations 1989 applied. However, trusts had a discretion to treat those who cannot or will not pay and the Secretary of State's guidance was unlawful, in that it failed to identify how that discretion was to be exercised in relation to different categories of treatment, in particular in the case of failed asylum-seekers unable to leave the UK:

> 74. The Guidance divides treatment into three categories. The first is 'immediately necessary treatment', referred to at paragraph 3.1 but further defined in paragraph 9 which makes it clear:

> 'trusts need to treat patients in need of immediately necessary care regardless of their ability to pay. This may be because their condition is life-threatening, or because if treatment is not given immediately it will become life-threatening, or because permanent serious damage will be caused by any delay ... Where immediately necessary treatment takes place and the Trust knows that payment is unlikely, treatment should be limited to that which is clinically necessary to enable the patient to return to their own country. This should not normally include routine treatment unless it is necessary to prevent a life-threatening situation. Any charge for such treatment will stand, but if it proves to be irrecoverable, then it should be written off.'

This is clear enough in so far as it advises that certain treatment should be given irrespective of the ability to pay for it but it leaves unclear what, if any, investigation should be made as to when the patient is likely to return to his own country so as to be able to decide what limits should be placed on the treatment.

75. The second category is 'urgent treatment' which is treatment which is not immediately necessary but cannot wait until the patient returns home. The advice that is given by the Guidance is that when the patient is chargeable the Trust should 'wherever possible' seek deposits equivalent to the estimated full cost of the treatment in advance of providing any treatment. The problem here is that the Guidance is silent on what should happen when it is not possible to provide that deposit. No help is given in the case of those who cannot return home before the treatment does become necessary. What is to happen to the patient who cannot wait? In those respects the guidance is not clear and unambiguous and in so far as it purports to be dealing with a category of patients like those before us, the failed asylum seekers who cannot be returned, it is seriously misleading.

76. As for non-urgent treatment, namely 'routine elective treatment which could in fact wait until the patient returned home', the advice given is that where the patient is chargeable, the Trust should not initiate treatment processes (even by putting the patient on a waiting list) until a full deposit has been obtained. The assumption has to be that the patient can return home before that routine elective treatment becomes necessary. Again, it is not clear what should be done for those who have no prospect of returning within a medically acceptable time. There is no suggestion that it may be necessary to treat in those circumstances or even that it may be necessary to investigate the likelihood and length of any undue delay. Once again the Guidance is not clear enough.

18.68 *R (W, X, Y, Z) v Secretary of State for Health, Secretary of State for the Home Department* [2015] EWCA Civ 1034

It was lawful for the NHS to inform the Secretary of State for the Home Department about unpaid NHS debts of overseas visitors

Facts: the appellants sought a judicial review of the immigration sanction regime for those seeking leave to enter or remain in the UK who had unpaid NHS debts, on the basis that disclosure of information relating to their unpaid NHS debts, by the NHS to the Secretary of State for the Home Department, breached their right to confidentiality, and under Article 8 ECHR, and was not an action that the NHS had power to undertake.

Judgment: the Court of Appeal (Lord Dyson MR, Briggs and Bean LJJ) held that the information provided was inherently private but that overseas patients were informed at the outset that, if they failed to pay, the information might be passed to the Secretary of State for the Home Department, so they could not have any reasonable expectation that the information would not be used in this way. Provision of the information was lawful at common law and proportionate under the ECHR. The Secretaries of State had power to obtain and transmit the information to each other, under section 2 of the NHSA 2006, and in order to facilitate the discharge of the function under section 2.

CHAPTER 19

Mental health

continued

19.18 *R (K) v West London Mental Health NHS Trust* [2006] EWCA Civ 118, (2006) 9 CCLR 319

The NHS is not required to make the provision recommended by clinicians as it could take into account cost and other views

19.19 *R (TF) v Secretary of State for Justice* [2008] EWCA Civ 1457, (2009) 12 CCLR 245

Where a transfer order was flawed the detention was unlawful and the court could not make it lawful on the basis that the Secretary of State could have achieved detention lawfully

19.20 *TTM (by his litigation friend TM) v Hackney LBC* [2011] EWCA Civ 4, (2011) 14 CCLR 154

While a hospital acts lawfully by detaining a patient on the basis of an application that appears valid, if the application is not valid, the detention is still unlawful and action lies against the AMHP

19.21 *MS v United Kingdom* Application no 24527/08, (2012) 15 CCLR 549

In the particular circumstances, it had been incompatible with Article 3 ECHR to detain a severely mentally ill man in police custody for four days before transferring him to a MSU

19.22 *Bostridge v Oxleas NHS Foundation Trust* [2015] EWCA Civ 79, (2015) 18 CCLR 144

Although a period of detention was unlawful, only nominal damages were awarded because the illegality had been immaterial, in the sense that had the Trust appreciated its error it would have done things differently with exactly the same result as far as concerned the detention

19.23 *Lee-Hirons v Secretary of State for Justice* [2016] UKSC 46

A conditionally discharged patient recalled to hospital was not entitled to written reasons at the time of his recall; he was entitled to an oral explanation at the time and written reasons within 72 hours but the failure to provide such reasons did not render his detention unlawful or found a claim for damages

19.24 *WD v Belgium* Application no 73548/13, 6 September 2016

The lengthy detention of a mentally disordered sex offender without suitable treatment was in breach of the ECHR

19.25 Nearest relatives

19.41 *R v Central London CC ex p Ax London* (1999) 2 CCLR 256, CA

A nearest relative can be displaced on an interim basis but unless there are cogent reasons a final displacement decision should be made prior to detention under section 3 of the MHA 1983

19.42 *Barnet LBC ex p Robin* (1999) 2 CCLR 454, CA

A nearest relative could be displaced not because of what she had done in the past but because what the evidence showed she was likely to do in the future; the appeal to the Court of Appeal was probably in relation to facts as well as law

19.43 *Dewen v Barnet Healthcare Trust and Barnet LBC* (2001) 4 CCLR 239
Approved mental health professionals are under a duty of honesty, not of reasonable enquiry

19.45 *Lewis v Gibson and MH* [2005] EWCA Civ 587, (2005) 8 CCLR 399
It was unnecessary to seek a best interests declaration but the court ought to joint the patient as a party in displacement applications

19.46 *R (H) v Secretary of State for Health* [2005] UKHL 60, [2006] 1 AC 441
The machinery for detaining persons under section 2 of the MHA 1983 during displacement proceeds was ECHR compliant

19.47 *GD v Hospital Managers Edgware Community Hospital* [2008] EWHC 3572 (Admin), [2008] MHLR 282
GD's detention had been unlawful because there had not been more than a 'nod in the direction of consultation' which seriously inhibited the chances of the nearest relative having any effective input into the process or any proper opportunity to object: habeas corpus was granted

19.48 *MH v United Kingdom* Application no 11577/06, [2013] ECHR 1008
MS's rights under Article 5 ECHR had been breached during a period of detention under section 2 of the MHA 1983 when she had been unable to apply to the tribunal to be discharged, because of her lack of the mental capacity to do so, and no one else was entitled or required to make the application on her behalf

19.49 *R (Holloway) v Oxfordshire CC* [2007] EWHC 776 (Admin), (2007) 10 CCLR 264
An interim displacement order and the ensuing detention were both lawful despite failure to notify the nearest relative of the displacement hearing, but that had been very poor practice

19.50 *R (M) v Homerton University Hospital* [2008] EWCA Civ 197
It is desirable but not legally necessary for displacement proceedings to be concluded before the patient is detained under section 3 of the MHA 1983

19.51 *R (V) v South London and Maudsley NHS Foundation Trust* [2010] EWHC 742 (Admin), (2010) 13 CCLR 181
Habeas corpus was granted when the approved mental health professional knew full well that the patient had a nearest relative who could be contacted, but had not done so

19.52 *TW v Enfield LBC* [2013] EWCA Civ 362, (2014) 17 CCLR 264
An AMHP need not consult a nearest relative when the patient objects, providing the AMHP balances the patient's right to privacy (against the nearest relative) under Article 8 ECHR, with the patient's right to liberty (which the nearest relative could support) under Article 5

continued

19.102 *MH v United Kingdom* Application no 11577/06, [2013] ECHR 1008, (2014) 58 EHRR 35

Special safeguards were required to ensure that patients who lacked capacity were able to apply for discharge from detention under section 2 of the MHA 1983 within the initial period of detention of 28 days; if detention under section 2 is then extended because of proceedings to displace a nearest relative, Article 5(4) ECHR may be satisfied by the Secretary of State referring the case to the tribunal

19.103 *Kolanis v United Kingdom* Application no 517/02, (2006) 9 CCLR 297

It was lawful to continue to detain a patient who suffered from a mental disorder warranting treatment in hospital and detention even though the patient could be discharged if services were available in the community if such services were not available; however, there would be a breach of Article 5(4) ECHR unless there continued to be regular court review

19.104 *R (SH) v Mental Health Review Tribunal* [2007] EWHC 884 (Admin), (2007) 10 CCLR 306

Discharge on condition that the patient took specified medication did not amount to compulsory treatment, merely a condition which, if broken, would justify recall

19.105 *Rayner and Marsh v Secretary of State for the Home Department* [2007] EWHC 1028 (Admin), (2007) 10 CCLR 464

Recalled conditionally discharged patients were entitled to an immediate referral of their case to the tribunal

19.106 *R (TF) v Secretary of State for Justice* [2008] EWCA Civ 1457, (2009) 12 CCLR 245

The absence of adequate reasons in medical recommendations meant that the detention had been unlawful and the fact that, later, other doctors were found who did provide adequate reasons justifying detention did not make the earlier detention lawful

19.107 *Secretary of State for Justice v RB* [2011] EWCA Civ 1608, [2012] 1 WLR 2043, [2012] MHLR 131

It is not lawful to discharge a patient to a facility which is not a hospital and where he or she will be detained otherwise than for the purposes of treatment

19.108 *DC v Nottinghamshire Healthcare NHS Trust* [2012] UKUT 92 (AAC), (2012) 15 CCLR 537

The tribunal was entitled to adjourn proceedings for evidence to be adduced as to what conditions might be appropriate to attach to a conditional discharge

19.109 *R (South Staffordshire & Shropshire Healthcare NHS Foundation Trust) v St George's Hospital Managers* [2016] EWHC 1196 (Admin), (2016) 19 CCLR 253

The decision of an independent panel exercising the function of hospital discharge was amenable to judicial review but such panels are not required to take into account decisions about discharge by the First-tier Tribunal

19.110 After-care services

19.110 Introduction

continued

Cases

19.116 *Clunis v Camden and Islington Health Authority* (1997–8) 1 CCLR 214, CA

Health and social services authorities do not owe a duty of care to patients, to discharge their duty to provide after-care services in a reasonably careful manner and, in any event, a patient who, in consequence, killed a man knowing that was wrong, would not be permitted to sue because of the ex turpi causa principle

19.117 *R v Camden and Islington Health Authority ex p K* (2001) 4 CCLR 170, CA

A patient remains lawfully detained where she continues to suffer from a mental disorder that warrants hospital detention and treatment unless psychiatric supervision in the community can be provided and, despite the authorities using reasonable endeavours, psychiatric supervision in the community cannot be provided because no psychiatrist can be found willing to provide it

19.118 *R v Manchester CC ex p Stennett* [2002] UKHL 34, (2002) 5 CCLR 500

It was not lawful to charge for after-care services

19.119 *R (W) v Doncaster MBC* [2004] EWCA Civ 378, [2004] MHLR 201

Local authorities were not under a duty to make arrangements for after-care services before the tribunal directed discharge and, when the tribunal ordered conditional discharge, were not under an absolute duty but a duty to make reasonable endeavours to make provision to satisfy the conditions: meanwhile, the patient's continued detention was lawful

19.120 *R (H) v Secretary of State for the Home Department* [2003] UKHL 59, (2004) 7 CCLR 147

Tribunals must keep deferred conditional discharges under review so as to comply with Article 5(4) ECHR but a patient remained lawfully detained where the patient suffered from a mental disorder that warranted compulsory treatment in hospital unless community services were available and it had not been possible to arrange for those services despite using reasonable endeavours

19.121 *R (B) v Camden LBC* [2005] EWHC 1366 (Admin), (2005) 8 CCLR 422

Local authorities were entitled to carry out preparatory steps but were not under a duty to monitor patients to consider the exercise of this discretion. They came under a duty to exercise reasonable endeavours to make arrangements for after-care services when a tribunal has provisionally determined that a conditional discharge is appropriate. They are entitled to explore funding issue. In this case, the authority's ineffective action had not been causative of B's continued detention but, even if it had done, B would not have been entitled to damages under Article 5 ECHR

19.122 *R (B) v Lambeth LBC* [2006] EWHC 2363 (Admin), (2007) 10 CCLR 84

A local authority is under a duty to secure alternative accommodation under section 117 of the MHA 1983 straightaway when it has assessed the need as existing

19.123 *R (Mwanza) v Greenwich LBC* [2010] EWHC 1462 (Admin), (2010) 13 CCLR 454

After-care services must address needs arising from a patient's mental disorder and may not address other needs that patient might have

19.124 *R (Afework) v Camden LBC* [2013] EWHC 1637 (Admin)

Accommodation need only be provided as an after-care service when the patient is required to occupy specialised accommodation to meet needs arising out of the condition that led to his or her detention

19.125 *Richards v Worcestershire CC* [2016] EWHC 1954 (Ch)
A patient could be entitled to bring private law proceedings in restitution, to reclaim money spent by him on after-care services

19.126 Responsibility disputes

Other mental health cases

19.128 *Re F (a child)* (1999) 2 CCLR 445, CA
Guardianship could not be imposed on a person with severe mental impairment unless that was associated with abnormally aggressive or seriously irresponsible conduct which, on the facts, was not made out by F's desire to continue to live with neglectful parents

19.129 *R (X) v Secretary of State for the Home Department* (2001) 4 CCLR 92, CA
The Secretary of State for the Home Department is entitled to remove mental patients from the UK using immigration powers and by-passing the MHA 1983

19.130 *Seal v Chief Constable of South Wales* [2007] UKHL 31, (2007) 10 CCLR 695
Proceedings issued without leave, where required under section 139 of the MHA 1983, were a nullity

19.131 *North Dorset NHS Primary Care Trust v Coombs* [2013] EWCA Civ 471, (2013) 16 CCLR 376
Psychiatric patients may pay for private care and, accordingly, recover the cost of such provision from a tortfeasor

19.132 *R (C) v Secretary of State for Justice* [2016] UKSC 2, (2016) 19 CCLR 5
There was no presumption of anonymity for mental patients challenging aspects of their treatment and care in the High Court but anonymity will be granted where that is necessary in the interests of the patient

19.1 Clinical commissioning groups (CCG) and local authorities provide health and social care to mentally disordered persons in the community, under the National Health Service Act 2006 (see chapter 18) and the Care Act 2014 (see chapters 7–12), often under the *Care Programme Approach* (see 'After-care services', at para 19.110 below).

19.2 In addition, specific provision is made by and under the Mental Health Act (MHA) 1983 for the reception, care and treatment in hospital, of mentally disordered patients, that is:

- persons affected by 'any disorder or disability of the mind', excluding dependence on alcohol or drugs; and
- for certain purposes only, persons with a 'learning disability' if that is 'associated with abnormally aggressive or seriously irresponsible conduct' (section 1 of the MHA 1983).

19.3 The main provisions of the Act are as follows:

- Part 2 of the MHA 1983 governs compulsory admission for the purposes of, inter alia, assessment (section 2) and treatment (section 3). It also makes provision for guardianship (sections 7–10) and community treatment orders (sections 17A–19A);
- Part 3 governs the detention and treatment of criminal offenders who are mentally disordered patients;
- Part 4 deals with compulsory treatment and part 4A deals with the treatment of community patients not recalled to hospital;
- Part 5 sets out the functions of the Mental Health Review Tribunal for Wales and the First-tier Tribunal (Health, Education and Social Care Chamber) in England.

19.4 A number of key terms are defined in section 145 of the MHA 1983, as follows:

Interpretation

145(1) In this Act, unless the context otherwise requires–

...

'hospital' means–

(a) any health service hospital within the meaning of the National Health Service Act 2006 or the National Health Service (Wales) Act 2006; and

(b) any accommodation provided by a local authority and used as a hospital by or on behalf of the Secretary of State under that Act; and

(c) any hospital as defined by section 206 of the National Health Service (Wales) Act 2006 which is vested in a Local Health Board; ...

'medical treatment' includes nursing, psychological intervention and specialist mental health habilitation, rehabilitation and care (but see also subsection (4) below);

'patient'... means a person suffering or appearing to be suffering from mental disorder; ...

(4) Any reference in this Act to medical treatment, in relation to mental disorder, shall be construed as a reference *to* medical treatment the purpose of which is to alleviate, or prevent a worsening of, the disorder or one or more of its symptoms or manifestations.

19.5 There is important statutory guidance, issued under section 118 of the Mental Health Act 1983, the *Mental Health Act 1983: Code of Practice.*[1]

19.6 What follows is a brief overview of the main statutory provisions and cases, with a focus on those issues most likely to crop up in the professional life of the social care practitioner.

19.7 For further information, reference should be made to a specialist practitioners' textbook, such as the *Mental Health Act Manual.*[2] It should also be noted that mentalhealthlaw.co.uk contains access to legislation, codes, articles and other useful material and has case-law updates and a case-law database.

Detention and treatment

Introduction

19.8 Section 2 makes provision for detention for the purposes of assessment. The central statutory provision is section 3 of the MHA 1983, which makes provision for detention for hospital treatment as follows:

> **Admission for treatment**
>
> **3**(1) A patient may be admitted to a hospital and detained there for the period allowed by the following provisions of this Act in pursuance of an application (in this Act referred to as '*an application for admission for treatment*') made in accordance with this section.
>
> (2) An application for admission for treatment may be made in respect of a patient on the grounds that–
>
> (a) he is suffering from mental disorder of a nature or degree which makes it appropriate for him to receive medical treatment in a hospital; and
>
> (b) [...]
>
> (c) it is necessary for the health or safety of the patient or for the protection of other persons that he should receive such treatment and it cannot be provided unless he is detained under this section ; and
>
> (d) appropriate medical treatment is available for him.
>
> (3) An application for admission for treatment shall be founded on the written recommendations in the prescribed form of two registered medical practitioners, including in each case a statement that in the opinion of the practitioner the conditions set out in subsection (2) above are complied with; and each such recommendation shall include–
>
> (a) such particulars as may be prescribed of the grounds for that opinion so far as it relates to the conditions set out in paragraphs (a) and (d) of that subsection; and
>
> (b) a statement of the reasons for that opinion so far as it relates to the conditions set out in paragraph (c) of that subsection, specifying whether other methods of dealing with the patient are available and, if so, why they are not appropriate.
>
> (4) In this Act, references to appropriate medical treatment, in relation to a person suffering from mental disorder, are references to medical treatment which is appropriate in his case, taking into account the nature

1 www.gov.uk/government/uploads/system/uploads/attachment_data/file/435512/MHA_Code_of_Practice.PDF.

2 Richard Jones. Published annually by Sweet & Maxwell.

and degree of the mental disorder and all other circumstances of his case.

19.9 Under section 3:

- the expression 'nature or degree' is disjunctive but it can be difficult to disentangle the two concepts;[3]
- 'nature' generally refers to the category of mental disorder which the patient suffers, whilst 'degree' generally refers to the current intensity of the symptoms;[4]
- thus, where a patient is taking medication and is asymptomatic, their mental disorder will not be of a *'degree'* that warrants hospital treatment, but it could be of a *'nature'* that requires hospital treatment and detention for that purpose if, without hospital treatment and detention the patient is likely to cease taking medication, deteriorate and become a risk to himself or others;[5]
- the word *'necessary'* is, however, a strong one;[6]
- all the other relevant circumstances need to be considered, such as the patient's age and gender, where they live, where their family and social contacts are, their cultural background, the medical and other services available to them in the community and any offending history;
- the need must be for treatment *'in a hospital'*, which requires that there is a need for at least some initial *'in-patient'* treatment before a leave of absence is granted under section 17 of the Mental Health Act 1983, for example, on the basis of ongoing treatment 'at' hospital on an out-patient basis[7];
- section 3(2)(d) requires only that *'appropriate'* medical treatment is available ie the treatment need not be such as to be likely to alleviate or prevent a deterioration in the patient's condition;
- it is hard to imagine a case where *'appropriate'* medical treatment is not available, including for patients with a personality disorder: as noted above, '*'medical treatment'* includes nursing, psychological intervention and specialist mental health habilitation, rehabilitation and care' and 'Any reference in this Act to medical treatment, in relation to mental disorder, shall be construed as a reference *to* medical treatment the purpose of which is to alleviate, or prevent a worsening of, the disorder or one or more of its symptoms or manifestations' (section 145).[8]

3 *R v Mental Health Review Tribunal for the Thames Region ex p Smith* (1999) 47 BMLR 104.

4 *R v Mental Health Review Tribunal for the Thames Region ex p Smith* (1999) 47 BMLR 104.

5 *R v Mental Health Review Tribunal for the Thames Region ex p Smith* (1999) 47 BMLR 104; *R (H) v Mental Health Review Tribunal, North and East London Region* [2001] EWCA Civ 415, [2001] MHLR 48.

6 *R v Mental Health Review Tribunal for the Thames Region ex p Smith* (1999) 47 BMLR 104; *Reid v Secretary of State for Scotland* [1999] 2 AC 512.

7 *R v Barking, Havering and Brentwood Community Health NHS Trust ex p* B [1999] 1 FLR 106, (1999) 2 CCLR 5; *R (DR) v Mersey Care NHS Trust* [2002] EWHC 1810 (Admin), [2002] MHLR 386.

8 *DL-H v Devon Partnerships NHS Trust* [2010] UKHT 102 (AAC), [2010] MHLR 162.

19.10 Applications for admission for treatment (as well as for assessment or for a guardianship application) must be made in accordance with the provisions of sections 11–14 of the MHA 1983:

- applications are made to the managers of the hospital where admission is sought and a place is available (section 11(2)) and the managers scrutinise whether the application is lawful;
- applications may be made by a 'nearest relative' (see para 19.25 below) or an approved mental health professional ('AMHP'), providing that the applicant has personally seen the patient within the 14 days before the date of the application (section 11(1) and (5));
- before or within a reasonable time after applying for the admission of a patient for assessment the AMHP must take such steps as are practical to inform the person, if any, appearing to be the nearest relative of the application and of the nearest relative's power to order the patient's discharge (section 11(3));
- an AMHP must not apply for the admission of a patient for treatment if the nearest relative objects or (unless it is not reasonably practicable or would involve unreasonable delay) the AMHP has not undertaken proper consultation (ideally directly) with the person, if any, appearing to be the nearest relative of the patient (section 11(4));
- the consultation can and should involve the AMHP disclosing confidential medical information to the nearest relative, sufficient to enable the nearest relative properly to consider the exercise of their powers;[9]
- there are medical recommendations signed by two registered medical practitioners, or a joint recommendation signed by two registered medical practitioners (section 12);
- providing that the registered medical practitioners have personally examined with the patient, either at the same time or within five days of each other (section 12 (1)); and
- providing that at least one of the registered medical practitioners has been approved for the purposes of section 12 of the MHA 1983 by the Secretary of State and, if that practitioner does not have previous experience of the patient, the other recommendation is made, if practicable, by a practitioner who has (section 12(2)); and
- providing neither the AMHP or the registered medical practitioners have a '*conflict of interest*', as defined in section 12A and The Mental Health (Conflicts of Interest)(England) Regulations 2008, or the Welsh equivalent (section 12(3)): and
- prescribed forms are used, as required by the Mental Health (Hospital, Guardianship and Treatment (England) Regulations 2008[10] and regulation 33 of the Mental Health (Hospital, Guardianship, Community Treatment and Consent to Treatment) (Wales) Regulations 2008.[11]

9 *R (S) v Plymouth CC* [2002] EWCA Civ 388, (2002) 5 CCLR 251; *GD v Edgware Community Hospital and Barnet LBC* [2008] EWHC 3572 (Admin), [2008] MHLR 282.

10 SI No 1184.

11 SI No 2439.

A period of detention will be unlawful if, inter alia:

- the AMHP or doctors have not personally seen the patient;[12]
- the AMHP has failed to take reasonably practicable steps properly to consult with the nearest relative;[13]
- the AMHP has made the application despite objection by the nearest relative.[14]

It is implicit in the statutory scheme that a further application may not be made after a tribunal has directed that the patient be discharged, unless the AMHP has formed the reasonable and bona fide opinion that he has information, not known by the tribunal, that puts a significantly different complexion on the case (there is no need for there to have been a change of circumstances).[15] If professionals consider that a tribunal decision to direct discharge is wrong, their remedy was to apply for a judicial review and a stay of the tribunal's decision but now would be to appeal to the Upper Tribunal and apply for a stay.[16]

Cases

19.11 *R (Barker) v Barking, Havering and Brentwood Community Healthcare NHS Trust* (1999) 2 CCLR 5, CA

A detained patient on hospital leave remained detained and liable to recall to hospital if in receipt of, and still needing, hospital treatment, which included monitoring and testing

Facts: Ms Barker had a history of personality disorder and repeated admissions to hospital in a psychotic state. She was detained under section 3 of the MHA 1983 and then, later, allowed section 17 leave under which Ms Barker spent five days a week living at home, subject to conditions attached to her leave. Her psychiatrist renewed Ms Barker's section 3 detention, under section 20 of the MHA 1983. Ms Barker submitted that section 20 was inapplicable because she was no longer 'detained' or in receipt of, or needing, 'medical treatment in a hospital'.

Judgment: the Court of Appeal (Lord Woolf MR, Hobhouse and Thorpe LJJ) held that a patient continues to be 'detained' in hospital, for the purposes of the MHA 1983, while on section 17 leave; and that while assessments on their own did not amount to 'hospital treatment', the requirement to return to hospital to be monitored, and a liability to be recalled and subjected to hospital treatment under supervision with urine and other tests, did amount to '*hospital treatment*':

> If Mr Gledhill's approach is right it creates considerable difficulties in treating the many patients like the appellant who should be treated partly as an

12 *R v Managers of South Western Hospital ex p M* [1994] 1 All ER 161; *R (M) v The Managers, Queen Mary's Hospital* [2008] EWCA Civ 1112, [2008] MHLR 306.

13 *GD v Edgware Community Hospital and Barnet LBC* [2008] EWHC 3572 (Admin), [2008] MHLR 282.

14 *TTM v Hackney LBC* [2011] EWCA Civ 4.

15 *R v East London and the City Mental Health Trust ex p von Brandenburg* [2003] UKHL 58, [2004] 2 AC 280.

16 *R (H) v Ashworth Hospital Authority* [2002] EWCA Civ 923, [2003] 1 WLR 127.

> inpatient and partly as an outpatient as described by Dr Taylor in the case of the appellant. In such cases the activities which take place as part of the inpatient treatment may all individually be capable of being performed without the treatment taking place in the hospital, yet for the treatment as a whole to be successful there will often need to be an inpatient element to the treatment which means it is in fact 'appropriate for him to receive medical treatment in a hospital' and 'that it cannot be provided unless he continues to be detained'. The requirement that the patient has to return to hospital and be monitored and is liable to be recalled and from time to time is subjected to the discipline of being treated in hospital as an inpatient under direct supervision with urine and other tests is an essential part of the treatments. They enable the patient to attempt the process of rehabilitation in the wider community which would be more precarious otherwise. This appears to be just the type of treatment contemplated by the second half of the definition of treatment contained in section 145 of the Act. As the Code of Practice states in paragraph 20.1, leave 'can be an important part of a patient's treatment plan.'
>
> ...
>
> Mrs Justice Hale in *Mental Health Law* suggests the change in language may be a draftsman's slip. On my reading of the 1959 Act 'liable to be detained' is used both to cover a person who is detained and a person who would be detained if he were not on leave. The opening words of section 20(3) require the responsible medical officer to examine those who are 'liable to be detained'. This literally applies to those on leave but it must also refer to those who are 'detained'. It is to the managers of the hospital where the 'patient is detained' that the report is to be furnished. However I do not find it inappropriate to describe the hospital of a patient who is on leave in this way. As Mr Grace submits the detention does not have to be continuous, as section 17 makes clear, but even when on leave the patient still has a hospital at which he is detained when not on leave. Equally he will for the purpose of section 20(4) continue to be detained whether when the report is furnished he is in hospital or liable to be required to return to hospital.
>
> No help is therefore available to Mr Gledhill from McCullough J's judgment. The same is true as to the distinction which he seeks to draw between assessment and treatment. The fact that assessment by itself cannot amount to treatment for section 3 does not mean that assessment cannot be a legitimate treatment under sections 3 and 20. Often assessment or monitoring of progress will be an important part of treatment. This will certainly be the case where as here there is an evolving programme of treatment.

The Court of Appeal also explained that, in detention cases, judicial review was the appropriate remedy, rather than habeas corpus, where '*what is in issue is the propriety of some prior administrative act*', rather than where '*what is in issue is whether some precedent fact going to jurisdiction is in issue*' (15D–H).

19.12 *R v Mental Health Review Tribunal for the Thames Region ex p Smith* (1999) 47 BMLR 104, [1999] COD 148, CA

The 'nature' of a patient's illness is not a static condition; it can be necessary to detain an asymptomatic patient who has ceased to take his medication and who has a history of relapse in such circumstances

Facts: Mr Smith sought a judicial review of the decision of the Mental Health Review Tribunal (MHRT) not to direct his conditional discharge.

Judgment: Popplewell J dismissed the application and held as follows:

> Mr Singh, on behalf of the Tribunal, submits that the words have a plain meaning compared with the use of the words 'severe degree' in section 5. They govern not merely the admission of patients but their continued detention and, although there is no authority in support of either contention, he submits that there are two pieces of evidence (if that is the right way to describe them) which assist the court. The first is that part of the report of a Committee of Inquiry presided over by Sir Lewis-Blom Cooper, than whom no one has greater experience in this field. I need not set out the facts giving rise to that inquiry. It is called 'The Falling Shadow'. Chapter 18 at page 161 says this:
>
> > 'We have indicated above our view that, even when asymptomatic, he could be said, both in a clinical and a legal sense, to be 'suffering from mental illness'. As to the 'nature or degree' of that illness, we see no inherent difficulty in applying this concept to a condition which is asymptomatic at the time of assessment, provided there is adequate material from past history to guide the clinician. Just because an illness is asymptomatic when assessed, does not mean that it cannot have gradations of severity, or in the statutory language gradations of 'nature or degree'. The issue concerns the features of the underlying condition, and in the example before us there was extensive history from which to assess the severity of that condition when unmodified by drugs. The wording of the phase is deliberately disjunctive. We are aware, however, that psychiatrists sometimes interpret the phrase conjunctively but it may be sufficient to consider the nature of the mental disorder without waiting for the development of 'degree' in its severity.'
>
> It is submitted in this case by Mr Rabinder Singh that the word 'then' in the section is of very great importance. The other material before me upon which he relies is in a book called 'Mental Health Review Tribunals, Law and Practice' by Mr Anselm Eldergill. He is a solicitor. He has been a Mental Health Act Commissioner and he is on the Mental Health Review Tribunal Panel of Solicitors. In his book, at page 213, he sets out his views about the matter. They are arguments which Mr Rabinder Singh adopts as part of his argument before me and I therefore set them out in full detail:
>
> > 'Where there is evidence of mental disorder, the use of compulsory powers requires that it is of a 'nature or degree' which either makes in-patient treatment appropriate or warrants the patient's detention for assessment or reception into guardianship ('the diagnostic question'). Practitioners and tribunals commonly confine their consideration of a patient's mental state to the degree of mental disorder present, seemingly interpreting the words 'nature' and 'degree' as essentially interchangeable. Accordingly, a patient is considered not to be detainable if his condition has responded to medication and is no longer acute. This approach takes no real account of the nature of the particular disorder and mistakenly quotes its 'degree' with its 'severity'. As such, there is

a failure to give due weight to the chronicity of the disorder and the prognosis.'

Then under 'Degree' he says this:

> 'The word 'degree' focuses attention on the extent to which the person's mental disorder is currently active. If a patient is acutely ill, his condition characterised by obvious and gross abnormalities in his mental state, the degree of mental disorder present will generally be of a level which satisfies the first ground of application. It is noteworthy that the emergency power to detain a patient for six hours under section 5(4) is exercised by a nurse only if it appears to him that the patient is suffering from mental disorder 'to such a degree that it is necessary for his health or safety or for the protection of others or for him to be immediately restrained from leaving the hospital.'The criteria do not refer to the nature of the patient's disorder. This reflects the fact that the purpose of the power is immediate restraint and reinforces the view that the word 'degree' is directed towards the present exacerbations and manifestations of a patient's disorder, rather its nature as revealed by its long-term consequences.
>
> '*Nature*'
>
> Many mental disorders wax and wane because they are cyclical in nature, because the patient enjoys periods of remission–for example, during periods of low stress–or because they are intermittently alleviated by a course of treatment. A particular patient may have a long history of readmissions indicative of a severe, chronic condition which is resistant to treatment or a record of poor compliance with informal treatment following previous discharges. Although the degree of disorder may be quite low at any given time, either in absolute terms or relative to his known optimum level of functioning, the serious nature of the disorder is revealed by its historical course. Likewise, with illnesses of recent onset, the prognosis associated with the diagnosis may point strongly towards the probability of a serious, further deterioration of the patient's condition in the near future. In both instances, it may be the nature of the disorder rather than its degree which brings the patient within the first of the grounds for making an application.'

Then he goes on in the next paragraph:

> '... it is not necessary as a matter of law to wait until the condition becomes acute before compelling the patient to receive the treatment which will prevent the otherwise inevitable further decline.
>
> *Mental Health Review Tribunals*
>
> Within the context of section 3 tribunal proceedings, a patient may have responded to treatment and be in remission by the time the hearing takes place. As such, and given the importance which attaches to a citizen's liberty in English law, the degree of mental disorder which remains may be insufficient to warrant a continuance of his liability to detention. The tribunal is not, however, obliged to discharge unless it is also satisfied that the nature of the patient's disorder, evidenced by his medical history or the outcome usually associated with such conditions, also makes liability to detention inappropriate. Similarily, where the degree of disorder apparently at the time of the hearing is quite low but the patient's recent mental state has been subject to marked fluctuations, the nature of disorder may mean that the tribunal cannot be satisfied that the first of the grounds for discharge is made out.'

I turn back then to the Tribunal's findings. The evidence about the Applicant's condition, at the time the Tribunal had to consider it, was static. He made excellent progress. He was in a stable condition and it is quite clear that the illness was not of a degree which of itself made it appropriate for him to be liable to be detained. The reason for that was because he has a chronic condition which was static. However, the nature of the condition was that it might cease to be static so that the interpretation that nature is in some way unchanging in one view may be right, but the effect of the condition is that because of its very nature it may not remain static. It seems to me that if the facts upon which the Tribunal rely have shown that it may not be static, that goes to the nature of the condition. The degree in the instant case, in relation to his condition, was not relevant because it was static and stable.

In my judgment there is a reason for the distinction, of which this case is perhaps a good example. If one had simply to look at the degree it would have been right for the discharge to take place, but the nature of the condition was such that it was clear that he should not be discharged. It may well be that in a great number of cases that nature and degree involve much the same questions–I hesitate to give examples–and it may be that Tribunals will be wise, if they have any doubts about it, to include them both.

However, that in my judgment in the instant case is not a ground for setting aside this Tribunal's decision which seems to me, on the material before it, to have properly applied the law. While at first sight Mr Bowen's argument has immense attraction, I think on analysis that it is, in the result, flawed and I pay tribute to the reasons set out by Mr Eldergill in his book which seems to me sufficiently to set out the various problems which can arise in the interpretation and the conclusion to which he has come.

19.13 *R (Wilkinson) v RMO Broadmoor Hospital* [2001] EWCA Civ 1546, (2002) 5 CCLR 121

The court would decide for itself whether the criteria for forcible medical treatment were met and could hear oral evidence subject to cross examination if necessary

Facts: Mr Wilkinson had been detained in Broadmoor for a number of years, as a result of a criminal conviction resulting in a hospital order with restriction. Mr Wilkinson strongly disagreed with his responsible medical officer's (RMO's) decision to treat him with anti-psychotic medication. In the circumstances that pertained, such treatment could be administered only with consent, or on the basis of a written certificate from another RMO that the patient was 'incapable of understanding the nature, purpose and likely effects of that treatment or has not consented to it but that, having regard to the likelihood of its alleviating or preventing a deterioration of his condition, the treatment should be given' (section 58 of the Mental Health Act 1983). Another RMO had certified that Mr Wilkinson was incapable of understanding the treatment and he was forcibly treated on a number of occasions before he brought an application for judicial review, supported by a report from an independent psychiatrist as to his capacity and the likely benefit of the treatment. Mr Wilkinson sought an order providing for oral evidence and cross-examination of both RMOs and his own psychiatrist.

Judgment: the Court of Appeal (Simon Brown, Brooke and Hale LJJ) held that had Mr Wilkinson brought an action for damages in the tort of assault, under section 7 of the Human Rights Act (HRA) 1998, or for declaratory relief in the Family Division, the court could and would have entertained oral evidence: the fact that he had proceeded by way of judicial review should not make any difference to the way the court approached the substantive issue. Conflicting views were expressed as to whether the hospital trust was vicariously liable for the RMO (if not, a claim under section 7 of the HRA 1998 would still require leave under section 139 of the MHA 1983).

19.14 *R (H) v Ashworth Hospital Authority* [2002] EWCA Civ 923, (2002) 5 CCLR 390

Tribunals are required to provide adequately reasoned decisions. If the authorities consider that the decision of a tribunal to discharge a patient is unlawful their remedy is to seek a judicial review and apply for a stay, which may be granted even though the patient has been discharged

Facts: the MHRT directed H's discharge from hospital, contrary to the opinion of the majority of the doctors and when no after-care arrangements were in place. The hospital authority then re-detained H pursuant to a further application under section 3 of the MHA 1983.

Judgment: the Court of Appeal (Simon Brown, Mummery and Dyson LJJ) held that the further application had been unlawful in that there had not been any materially changed circumstances since the decision of the MHRT but that the MHRT's decision had been irrational and inadequately reasoned and would be quashed; the authorities should have sought a judicial review of the MHRT's decision and applied for a stay of the discharge (which could have been granted even after H had left hospital). Dyson LJ said this:

> 66. The judge concluded that the tribunal's decision was unreasonable in the Wednesbury sense because no reasonable tribunal could have made an order that H should be discharged immediately into the community without at the very least being satisfied that suitable after-care arrangements were in place. The evidence before the tribunal could not have given it confidence that such arrangements had been or would be made. The judge referred to the evidence of Ms Ariola which I have mentioned at paragraph 15 above, and to the fact that the tribunal had little or no information from the section 117 authorities. The question of after-care was fundamental to the issues before the tribunal. In these circumstances, the tribunal should not simply have ordered immediate discharge. It should have either deferred discharge to a future date under section 72(3) or adjourned and called for information from the section 117 authorities. The course that it took was an unjustified 'step in the dark'.
>
> 67. In my view the judge was right. This was a case in which, if the criteria for discharge were to be met, it was obvious that suitable after-care should be available. H was a man who had been detained in Ashworth for about six years. He had a history of serious violence, and previous attempts to release him into the community had been unsuccessful. The tribunal accepted that H was still suffering from schizophrenia. The issue was whether it was of a 'nature or degree which makes it appropriate for him to be liable to

be detained in a hospital for medical treatment': section 72(1)(b)(i) of the Act. The tribunal was also required to have regard to 'the likelihood of the patient, if discharged, being able to care for himself, to obtain the care he needs or to guard against serious exploitation': section 72(2). The answer to the question whether H's mental illness was of a nature or degree which made it appropriate for him to be liable to be detained in a hospital for medical treatment was (to put it no higher) very likely to be heavily influenced by the after-care arrangements that were to be provided following his discharge. I refer to the observations of Lord Bridge of Harwich in *R v Oxford Regional Mental Health Review Tribunal ex p Secretary of State for the Home Department* [1988] AC 120, 127D, about the power under section 73(2) to order the conditional discharge of restricted patients. As Miss Morris points out, the tribunal cannot assume that any, still less any suitable, after-care services will be provided, since section 117 does not impose an absolute duty on the health and social services authorities to provide the services. The duty is no more than to use reasonable endeavours to provide after-care services: see *R (K) v Camden and Islington Health Authority* [2002] QB 198.

68. In agreement with the judge, I would therefore hold that H was a patient in respect of whom it was essential that the tribunal considered the availability of suitable after-care services when deciding whether to order his immediate discharge from hospital. If the tribunal had any doubt as to whether such services would be available, it should have adjourned to obtain any necessary information. I regard the alternative of a deferral under section 72(2) as less satisfactory. Section 72(3) authorises a tribunal to 'direct the discharge of a patient on a future date specified in the direction'. Under this subsection, therefore, the tribunal must specify a particular date for discharge. But if the tribunal is in doubt as to whether suitable after-care arrangements will be made available, it is difficult to see how it can specify a particular date for discharge. In cases of doubt, the safer course is to adjourn. On the facts of the present case, the tribunal could not reasonably have assumed that the services would be provided as soon as H was discharged into the community. For that reason alone, in my opinion the tribunal's decision was one which no reasonable tribunal could properly have made.

69. I would endorse the general observation of the judge:

> 'In general, in a case in which after-care is essential, and satisfaction of the discharge criteria depends on the availability of suitable after-care and accommodation, as in H's case, a tribunal should not direct immediate discharge at a time when no after-care arrangements are in place and there is no time for them to be put in place. The tribunal should consider whether to exercise its power under section 72(3A) to recommend that the RMO should make a supervision application. If it considers that to be inappropriate (and it should be borne in mind that the previous unwillingness of an RMO to make an application may not persist in the face of the tribunal's views) or unnecessary, and there is uncertainty as to the putting in place of the after-care arrangements on which satisfaction of the discharge criteria depends, the tribunal should adjourn pursuant to rule 16 to enable them to be put in place, indicating their views and giving appropriate directions: cf *Ex p Hall* [2000] 1 WLR 1323, per Kennedy LJ at 1352D '

...

75. Mr Walker submits that the judge was wrong to hold that the reasons of the tribunal were inadequate. He says that the judge adopted too strict

an approach. It is by no means unusual to find a tribunal decision containing reasons as brief as those in this case. The judge failed to take sufficient account of the fact that this decision was published to an informed audience who were aware of the issues and the details of the case. He also failed to pay sufficient regard to the practical realities of the workload imposed on tribunals and the limited resources that are available to them. The reality is that tribunal hearings are held at hospitals, members are part-time, and they do not have a wealth of administrative back-up to assist them. The judge found (correctly) that the tribunal gave adequate reasons for being satisfied that the discharge criteria were met, but he was wrong to hold that they were required to give any reasons for not deferring discharge until after-care arrangements were in place. This was a 'subsidiary' question, and not part of the decision 'by which the tribunal determines an application': see rule 23(2).

76. I cannot accept Mr Walker's submissions. I am in no doubt that the reasons given by the tribunal in this case were inadequate. But before I explain why, I want to make two preliminary general comments. The first concerns Mr Walker's reference to the problems of excessive workload and inadequate resources. If tribunals do not have the time and back-up resources that they need to discharge their statutory obligation to provide adequate reasons, then the time and resources must be found. I absolutely reject the submission that reasons which would be inadequate if sufficient resources were available may be treated as adequate simply because sufficient resources are not available. Either the reasons are adequate or they are not, and the sufficiency of resources is irrelevant to that question. The adequacy of reasons must be judged by reference to what is demanded by the issues which call for decision. What is at stake in these cases is the liberty of detained patients on the one hand, and their safety as well as that of other members of the public on the other hand. Both the detained persons and members of the public are entitled to adequate reasons.

77. I note in passing that the Rules require reasons to be given within seven days of a decision. That is not an unreasonable period within which to produce adequate reasons. I note further that the handbook issued to tribunal members in September 2000 contains the following advice about reasons:

> 'Tribunals must give detailed reasons, based on the evidence and the logical application of sound judicial principles, for their decisions (this has been given substance by decisions in the High Court). The reasons need not be elaborate but they must deal with the substantive points, which have been raised and must show the parties the basis on which the tribunal has acted. It is not sufficient merely to repeat the statutory grounds. It is not usually necessary to review the evidence at length. It is important to say which evidence has been accepted and often which has been rejected. It is not usually necessary to give lengthy reasons for acceptance or rejection of evidence. The reasons for the decision will be agreed by the tribunal members at the conclusion of the hearing, put in writing and signed by the president.'

78. This correctly states that reasons should be given dealing with the 'substantive' points. It does not expressly state, but it does imply, that reasons must be given for the acceptance or rejection of disputed evidence, although it is not usually necessary for these to be lengthy. In my opinion this advice is both useful and consistent with the law.

79. My second general preliminary comment concerns the significance of the so-called 'informed audience' point. This was not identified in *English* as being relevant to the adequacy of reasons given by a judge of a lower

court. And yet, in ordinary civil litigation, a judgment will usually be given to an audience that is at least as informed as the audience at a tribunal hearing. (I leave out of account those few cases where a judgment may be reported on the grounds that it is of public interest.) Although it is true that, in some cases, the interests of others who are not parties to civil litigation may be affected by a court decision, it is at least arguable that the 'informed audience' point has less force in relation to a mental health review tribunal decision than to a decision by a lower court in the civil justice system. First, the ASW considering whether to make an application for readmission pursuant to section 3 may well not have any prior knowledge of the case, let alone the reports on the patient and the oral evidence and argument that was deployed before the tribunal. In the light of *von Brandenburg* it is essential that an ASW who is contemplating making such an application should know the facts and circumstances which a tribunal took into account when deciding to discharge a patient, and the reasons for its decision. Secondly, it is highly questionable whether a patient will always be able to supplement exiguous tribunal reasons with an accurate recollection of the evidence and arguments before the tribunal when he later considers a decision. Accordingly, I do not accept that the 'informed audience' point can properly be relied on to justify as adequate a standard of reasoning in tribunals which would not be regarded as adequate in a judgment by a judge. It does not follow that tribunals are obliged to produce decisions which are as long as judgments by a judge often tend to be. Far from it. A brief judgment is no less likely to be adequately reasoned than a lengthy one.

80. Against the background of these two general comments, I shall now identify the two principal reasons why I consider that the tribunal's reasons were inadequate in this case. First, as often happens, the tribunal was required to resolve a difference of opinion between experts as to whether the patient should be discharged. In such cases, it is important that the tribunal should state which expert evidence (if any) it accepts and which it rejects, giving reasons. This is as important in a case where the tribunal rejects evidence in favour of discharge as it is in a case where the tribunal rejects evidence which advocates continued detention. It is not enough for the tribunal simply to state that it prefers the evidence of A and B to that of C and D. It must give reasons. As the handbook states, these may be brief, but in some cases something more elaborate is required. It must at least indicate the reasoning process by which it has decided to accept some and reject other evidence. What this court said in *Flannery v Halifax Estate Agencies Ltd (trading as Colleys Professional Services)* [2000] 1 WLR 377, 381–382 is as apt in relation to the decisions of tribunals as it is to lower courts generally. In giving the judgment of the court, Henry LJ said, at p 382, that the reach of what is required to fulfil the duty to give reasons depends on the subject matter:

> 'Where there is a straightforward factual dispute whose resolution depends simply on which witness is telling the truth about events which he claims to recall, it is likely to be enough for the judge (having, no doubt, summarised the evidence) to indicate simply that he believes X rather than Y; indeed there may be nothing else to say. But where the dispute involves something in the nature of an intellectual exchange, with reasons and analysis advanced on either side, the judge must enter into the issues canvassed before him and explain why he prefers one case over the other. This is likely to apply particularly in litigation where as here there is disputed expert evidence; but it is not necessarily limited to such cases.'

81. In my view this passage applies with even greater force where the tribunal decides to reject most of the expert evidence and adopt the minority view. The present case is a graphic illustration. Here, there were ranged against Dr Williams several other highly qualified doctors who had written apparently well-reasoned reports. All of these other doctors said that H should not be discharged, although they expressed differing views as to whether he should remain at Ashworth or be transferred to an MSU. Even Dr Williams advised in his report that H should be made subject to a supervision application under section 25A, saying that 'supervised discharge is the most appropriate step forward for his own health and safety and for the protection of others'. Such an application can only be made in respect of a patient who is liable to be detained in a hospital for treatment. It was only at the hearing, when he realised that the RMO would not make a supervision application, that he stated unequivocally that H should be discharged from liability to detention. There was, therefore, powerful, if not overwhelming, expert evidence against discharge. If the tribunal decided to reject all of that evidence it was obliged to give cogent reasons for doing so. It is to be supposed that, before deciding to reject the evidence of the experts who opposed discharge, it carefully considered each report as well as the oral evidence given by Dr Croy. In his first witness statement, Mr Simms says that the tribunal did not find Dr Croy to be an 'impressive witness'. As regards the reports of the other doctors, he says that it carefully considered the report of Dr Heads, but he makes no reference to its consideration of the reports of the other doctors, and, as has already been seen, there is no reference in the written reasons to any of the doctors (apart from Dr Williams). The reasons given for deciding to accept the evidence of Dr Williams in preference to that of the other experts were wholly inadequate. The other doctors were aware of the four points that seem to have impressed the tribunal (see paragraph 19 above), and yet advised as they did. In view of (a) the number of doctors who disagreed with Dr Williams, including the two independent doctors instructed on behalf of H, (b) the fact that previous attempts to discharge H into the community had failed, and (c) the fact that he had not experienced life in the community for a number of years, the tribunal was required to explain carefully why it felt able to reject the opinions of the other doctors.

82. My second reason is that I do not accept Mr Walker's submission that the tribunal was not required to give any reasons for not adjourning in order to see whether suitable after-care arrangements, or not making an order for discharge at a deferred date. As I explained at paragraph 67, the question of what after-care services will be available in the community is relevant to the issue of whether the statutory criteria are met. That was certainly the case here. Mr Walker does not suggest otherwise. In my view the judge was right to say that the tribunal took a step in the dark. And yet, it gave no reasons for doing so. Ms Ariola's report was sufficient to put it on notice that the local authority might be unable or unwilling to provide after-care services to H. In my view the judge was right to hold that the reasons given by the tribunal were inadequate.

Comment: the appropriate remedy would now be to appeal to the Upper Tribunal and apply for a stay.

19.15 ## *HL v United Kingdom* Application no 45508/99, (2004) 7 CCLR 498

A person is detained when the hospital exercises complete control over him and that detention is unlawful if it is not governed by clear rules with provision for review and effective court review

Facts: HL suffered from autism and lacked the capacity to consent to residence, care or medical treatment. After a period of hospital treatment (intensive behavioural therapy) lasting seven years he had been discharged to the care of paid carers. About three years later, HL became distressed at a day centre and was taken to hospital. The hospital deemed it necessary to keep HL in hospital and provide him with intensive behavioural therapy, excluding the carers from visiting him for a period of time.

Judgment: the European Court of Human Rights held that HL had been deprived of his liberty in that the hospital exercised complete and effective control over him and that his deprivation of liberty had not been lawful because in the UK, there were no fixed rules or provisions for review of the detention of persons lacking mental capacity and because habeas corpus and judicial review were not, in all the circumstances, effective remedies.

19.16 ## *R v East London and the City Mental Health NHS Trust ex p von Brandenburg* [2003] UKHL 58, (2004) 7 CCLR 121

A patient may be detained, notwithstanding a tribunal's decision to direct his discharge, where there are reasonable and bona fide grounds to believe that there is information, not known to the tribunal, which puts a significantly different complexion on the case

Facts: Mr von Brandenburg sought a judicial review of the authorities' application to re-admit him compulsorily to hospital under section 2 of the MHA 1983, on the basis that there had not been a material change of circumstances since a decision by the MHRT to direct his discharge.

Judgment: the House of Lords (Lords Bingham, Steyn, Hobhouse, Scott and Rodger) held that a further application can be made when the applicant has formed the reasonable and bona fide opinion that he has information not known to the tribunal which puts a significantly different complexion on the case. Lord Bingham said this:

> **Governing principles**
>
> 6. The differences between the parties to this appeal do not lack practical importance for those charged with the difficult and sensitive task of administering the mental health regime established by the 1983 Act. But the differences are relatively narrow, and it is convenient to begin by rehearsing certain familiar overriding principles, not in themselves controversial. First, the common law respects and protects the personal freedom of the individual, which may not be curtailed save for a reason and in circumstances sanctioned by the law of the land. This principle is reflected in, but does not depend on, Article 5(1) of the European Convention on Human Rights. It can be traced back to chapter 29 of Magna Carta 1297 and before that to chapter 39 of Magna Carta 1215. But, secondly, the law may properly provide for the compulsory detention in hospital of those who suffer from mental disorder if detention is judged to be necessary for the health or safety of the patient or the protection of others. The necessity for such detention

in appropriate cases is recognised by article 5(1)(e) of the Convention, and has long been given effect in domestic law. Under the legislation now current, it is a precondition of an emergency application under section 4 of the 1983 Act, and an application for admission for assessment under section 2, and an application for admission for treatment under section 3, that the subject should be judged to be suffering from a mental disorder of a kind which warrants his detention in a hospital or makes it appropriate for him to receive treatment in a hospital and that detention is necessary for the health or safety of the patient or the protection of others. Thus the personal freedom of the individual may be lawfully curtailed in such cases, provided the strict statutory conditions are observed.

7. The third relevant principle is of more recent vintage. It is that a person compulsorily detained on mental health grounds should have the right to take proceedings by which the lawfulness of his detention may be decided by a court and his release ordered if the detention is not lawful. This right is expressed in Article 5(4) of the Convention, but was not adequately protected in the case of patients subject to restriction by the Mental Health Act 1959, which gave a mental health review tribunal no more than an advisory role in such cases. In *X v United Kingdom* (1981) 4 EHRR 188, which concerned a restricted patient, a violation of Article 5(4) was found because the mental health review tribunal enjoyed a power to advise only and not the power which a court would have to direct the discharge of a detained person. This deficiency was remedied by the Mental Health (Amendment) Act 1982 and now by the 1983 Act. In the case of patients who are not restricted, the tribunal's powers (so far as relevant) were laid down in section 72(1) of the 1983 Act. Before amendment in 2001, the subsection read:

> '*Powers of tribunals*
>
> '72(1) Where application is made to a Mental Health Review Tribunal by or in respect of a patient who is liable to be detained under this Act, the tribunal may in any case direct that the patient be discharged, and–(a) the tribunal shall direct the discharge of a patient liable to be detained under section 2 above if they are satisfied–(i) that he is not then suffering from mental disorder or from mental disorder of a nature or degree which warrants his detention in a hospital for assessment (or for assessment followed by medical treatment) for at least a limited period; or (ii) that his detention as aforesaid is not justified in the interests of his own health or safety or with a view to the protection of other persons; (b) the tribunal shall direct the discharge of a patient liable to be detained otherwise than under section 2 above if they are satisfied–(i) that he is not then suffering from mental illness, psychopathic disorder, severe mental impairment or mental impairment or from any of those forms of disorder of a nature or degree which makes it appropriate for him to be liable to be detained in a hospital for medical treatment; or (ii) that it is not necessary for the health or safety of the patient or for the protection of other persons that he should receive such treatment; or (iii) in the case of an application by virtue of paragraph (g) of section 66(1) above, that the patient, if released, would not be likely to act in a manner dangerous to other persons or to himself.'

By subsection (3) the tribunal was empowered, as it did in this case, to direct the discharge of a patient on a future date specified in the direction.

8. Fourthly, the rule of law requires that effect should be loyally given to the decisions of legally-constituted tribunals in accordance with what is decided. It was clearly established by the House in *P v Liverpool Daily Post and Echo Newspapers plc* [1991] 2 AC 370 that a mental health review

tribunal is a court to which the law of contempt applies. It follows that no one may knowingly act in a way which has the object of nullifying or setting at nought the decision of such a tribunal. The regime prescribed by Part V of the 1983 Act would plainly be stultified if proper effect were not given to tribunal decisions for what they decide, so long as they remain in force, by those making application for the admission of a patient under the Act. It is not therefore open to the nearest relative of a patient or an ASW to apply for the admission of the patient, even with the support of the required medical recommendations, simply because he or she or they disagree with a tribunal's decision to discharge. That would make a mockery of the decision.

9. In applying these principles, account must be taken of certain important considerations.

(1) While doctors may be expected to exercise their best professional judgment in diagnosing the condition and assessing the cases of those suffering from mental disorder, and prescribing treatment, their conclusions will rarely be capable of scientific verification. There will often be room for a bona fide difference of professional opinion. In *Johnson v United Kingdom (*1997) 27 EHRR 296, para 61, the European Court of Human Rights said: 'It must also be observed that in the field of mental illness the assessment as to whether the disappearance of the symptoms of the illness is confirmation of complete recovery is not an exact science.'

(2) As the Master of the Rolls pointed out in para 30 of his judgment quoted above, the condition of many of those suffering from mental disorder will not be static. Episodes of acute illness may be followed by episodes of remission. Thus it does not follow that a tribunal decision, however sound when made, will remain so. Other things being equal, the longer the period since the decision was made the greater the chance that the patient's mental condition may have altered, whether for better or worse.

(3) It is plain from the language of sub-paragraphs (a)(i) and (b)(i) of section 72(1), quoted above, that the focus of the tribunal's inquiry into the mental health of the patient is on whether he is not 'then suffering' from mental disorder or mental illness. 'Then' refers to the time of the tribunal's review and the tribunal has no power to consider the validity of the admission which gave rise to the liability to be detained: see *Ex p Waldron* [1986] QB 824, 846. The tribunal will doubtless endeavour to assess a patient's condition in the round, and in considering issues of health, safety and public protection under sub-paragraphs (a)(ii) and (b)(ii) of section 72(1) it cannot ignore the foreseeable future consequences of discharge, but the temporal reference of 'then' is clear and the tribunal is not called upon to make an assessment which will remain accurate indefinitely or for any given period of time.

(4) If an unrestricted patient, compulsorily detained, seeks to be discharged, and the responsible doctors (including the current RMO) agree that the conditions for detaining him are no longer satisfied, he may be discharged and there will be no occasion for a tribunal hearing. Thus hearings will take place where (as here) a patient seeks to be discharged and the responsible doctors, or some of them, judge that he should not be discharged. Where an order for discharge is made by the tribunal, it will (unless the resisting doctors revise their opinion during the hearing) indicate that the tribunal has not accepted their judgment. A conscientious doctor whose opinion has not been accepted by the tribunal will doubtless ask himself whether the tribunal's view is to be preferred and whether his own opinion should be revised. But if, having done so, he adheres to his original opinion he cannot be obliged to suppress or alter it. His professional duty to his patient,

and his wider duty to the public, require him to form, and if called upon express, the best professional judgment he can, whether or not that coincides with the judgment of the tribunal.

(5) Account must be taken of section 13 of the 1983 Act, which so far as relevant provides:

> '(1) It shall be the duty of an approved social worker to make an application for admission to hospital or a guardianship application in respect of a patient within the area of the local social services authority by which that officer is appointed in any case where he is satisfied that such an application ought to be made and is of the opinion, having regard to any wishes expressed by relatives of the patient or any other relevant circumstances, that it is necessary or proper for the application to be made by him.
>
> '(2) Before making an application for the admission of a patient to hospital an approved social worker shall interview the patient in a suitable manner and satisfy himself that detention in a hospital is in all the circumstances of the case the most appropriate way of providing the care and medical treatment of which the patient stands in need.'

It is plainly of importance that the ASW is subject to a statutory duty to apply for the admission of a patient where he is satisfied that such an application ought to be made and is of the opinion specified.

Conclusion

10. The problem at the heart of this case is to accommodate the statutory duty imposed on ASWs (by whom, in practice, most applications for admission are made) within the principles referred to in paras 6, 7 and 8 above. The correct solution is in my opinion that proposed by the Master of the Rolls, although I would express it in slightly different terms. In doing so, I do not find it necessary to make detailed reference to the European Convention. Consistently with the principle identified in para 8 above, an ASW may not lawfully apply for the admission of a patient whose discharge has been ordered by the decision of a mental health review tribunal of which the ASW is aware unless the ASW has formed the reasonable and bona fide opinion that he has information not known to the tribunal which puts a significantly different complexion on the case as compared with that which was before the tribunal. It is impossible and undesirable to attempt to describe in advance the information which might justify such an opinion. I give three hypothetical examples by way of illustration only.

(1) The issue at the tribunal is whether the patient, if discharged, might cause harm to himself. The tribunal, on the evidence presented, discounts that possibility and directs the discharge of the patient. After the hearing, the ASW learns of a fact previously unknown to him, the doctors attending the patient and the tribunal: that the patient had at an earlier date made a determined attempt on his life. Having taken medical advice, the ASW judges that this information significantly alters the risk as assessed by the tribunal. (2) At the tribunal hearing the patient's mental condition is said to have been stabilised by the taking of appropriate medication. The continuing stability of the patient's mental condition is said to depend on his continuing to take that medication. The patient assures the tribunal of his willingness to continue to take medication and, on the basis of that assurance, the tribunal directs the discharge of the patient. Before or after discharge the patient refuses to take the medication or communicates his intention to refuse. Having taken medical advice, the ASW perceives a real risk to the patient or others if the medication is not taken. (3) After the

tribunal hearing, and whether before or after discharge, the patient's mental condition significantly deteriorates so as to present a degree of risk or require treatment or supervision not evident at the hearing. In cases such as these the ASW may properly apply for the admission of a patient, subject of course to obtaining the required medical support, notwithstanding a tribunal decision directing discharge. The position of the patient's nearest relative, in those cases where he or she makes the application with knowledge of the tribunal decision, does not differ in principle from that of the ASW, although the nearest relative could not in many cases be expected to be familiar with the evidence or appreciate the grounds on which the tribunal had based its decision.

19.17 *R (B) v Dr SS and others* [2006] EWCA Civ 28, (2006) 9 CCLR 280

Compulsory treatment of detained patients, where the criteria of the MHA 1983 were met, was compatible with the ECHR

Facts: B was detained in Broadmoor under sections 37 and 41 of the MHA 1983. He refused consent to certain treatment and sought a judicial review of the decision to treat him compulsorily.

Judgment: the Court of Appeal (Lord Phillips MR, Thorpe and Rix LJJ) held that B lacked capacity to consent and that section 58 of the MHA 1983 was ECHR-compliant: it permitted compulsory treatment where that was likely to alleviate or prevent a deterioration in the patient's condition but English law also required the SOAD (second opinion appointed doctor) to be satisfied that medical treatment was in the patient's best interests:

> 67. Where the challenge is not to the grounds for detention but to the treatment itself, careful consideration must be given to the procedure to ensure, in so far as is possible, that there are not protracted and expensive legal proceedings requiring oral evidence from medical witnesses where there is no prima facie case that anything untoward has occurred. Both Silber J and Charles J gave consideration to procedure at the end of their judgments. We heard no argument about this and will not comment on it, save to say that some of the observations might be thought to suggest that any mental patient ought to be able to challenge treatment proposed under section 58 by a full hearing with evidence from medical experts additional to those already involved. It is, of course, essential that the requirements of Article 6 of the Convention are satisfied but this does not mean that permission must be given for judicial review proceedings where the papers do not disclose any arguable grounds for this.
>
> 68. Section 58 imposes preconditions to compulsory treatment which ought to ensure that this is not imposed unless there is a convincing therapeutic case for it. They will only do so, however, if the SOAD satisfies himself or herself that the treatment in question should be imposed. This requires a truly independent assessment, not merely approval of the RMO's decision on the basis that it is not manifestly unsound. If section 58 is properly complied with issues requiring the cross-examination of medical witnesses should not often arise.

19.18 *R (K) v West London Mental Health NHS Trust* [2006] EWCA Civ 118, (2006) 9 CCLR 319

The NHS is not required to make the provision recommended by clinicians as it could take into account cost and other views

Facts: K was a restricted patient under a hospital order, at Broadmoor. His RMO wished to transfer him to an MSU (medium secure unit), but whereas a local private facility assessed K as suitable, the local NHS facility did not and the Trust refused to pay for the private cost.

Judgment: the Court of Appeal (Waller, Arden and Dyson LJJ) held that the Trust was not bound to make the provision recommended by the RMO: it was entitled to take into account other clinical views, the views of the NHS facility as to cost-effectiveness and resources considerations generally.

19.19 *R (TF) v Secretary of State for Justice* [2008] EWCA Civ 1457, (2009) 12 CCLR 245

Where a transfer order was flawed the detention was unlawful and the court could not make it lawful on the basis that the Secretary of State could have achieved detention lawfully

Facts: TF had served a custodial sentence for robbery but on the day of his release was served with a hospital transfer order purporting to be made under section 47 of the MHA 1983. TF sought a judicial review. At first instance, Cox J held that the transfer order had been unlawful, in that neither of the doctors' recommendations gave reasons in support of their view that hospital treatment would alleviate mental illness or prevent deterioration. However, in the light of subsequent medical evidence garnered by the Secretary of State, she declined in the exercise of her discretion to quash the transfer order, order TF's release and require the Secretary of State to pay damages. TF appealed.

Judgment: the Court of Appeal (Waller, Thomas and Aikens LJ), having reviewed the position and confirmed that the transfer order was unlawful, allowed TF's appeal: the Secretary of State had not had the power to make a transfer order, so the detention was unlawful, and the Court could not make it lawful by exercising a discretion.

19.20 *TTM (by his litigation friend TM) v Hackney LBC* [2011] EWCA Civ 4, (2011) 14 CCLR 154

While a hospital acts lawfully by detaining a patient on the basis of an application that appears valid, if the application is not valid, the detention is still unlawful and action lies against the AMHP

Facts: in good faith, but incorrectly, the AMHP applied for TTM's detention under section 3 of the MHA 1983, on the basis that the nearest relative did not object.

Judgment: the Court of Appeal (Toulson and Jackson LJJ) held that the hospital managers had acted lawfully, by virtue of section 6(3) of the Mental Health Act 1983, because the application for admission appeared valid on its face but that did not mean that the AMHP's unlawful application was cured. TTM was entitled at common law and under Article 5 ECHR to damages and if necessary section 139 of the MHA 1983 (requirement to obtain leave) would have to be read down to achieve that result.

19.21 **MS v United Kingdom Application no 24527/08, (2012) 15 CCLR 549**

In the particular circumstances, it had been incompatible with Article 3 ECHR to detain a severely mentally ill man in police custody for four days before transferring him to a MSU

Facts: MS had been held in a police cell for two days before being transferred to a medium secure hospital, despite obvious signs that he was mentally unwell and that his behaviour was deteriorating. His claim in negligence was dismissed.

Judgment: the European Court of Human Rights held that MS had been in dire need of psychiatric treatment and his condition had deteriorated very badly whilst in the police cell so that, although there had not been any intention to humiliate or debase him, his treatment had been incompatible with Article 3 ECHR.

19.22 **Bostridge v Oxleas NHS Foundation Trust [2015] EWCA Civ 79, (2015) 18 CCLR 144**

Although a period of detention was unlawful, only nominal damages were awarded because the illegality had been immaterial, in the sense that had the Trust appreciated its error it would have done things differently with exactly the same result as far as concerned the detention

Facts: Mr Bostridge was detained under section 3 of the MHA 1983, discharged by the First-tier Tribunal (FTT), made subject to a Community Treatment Order (CTO) and then recalled into hospital detention pursuant to the CTO. That period of detention was unlawful because the CTO was unlawful, in that a CTO can only be made in respect of a patient who is liable to hospital detention whereas, at the time, Mr Bostridge had just been discharged by the FTT. As soon as the mistake came to light, Mr Bostridge was discharged from his unlawful detention and immediately re-detained, lawfully, under section 3 of the 1983 Act. The Trust also adduced evidence that, had it been appreciated that the CTO was unlawful, Mr Bostridge would have been detained in any event under section 3 of the 1983 Act, rather than the CTO, and his treatment would have been exactly the same. On that basis, the first instance judge awarded only nominal damages in respect of the period of admitted false imprisonment, pursuant to the CTO. Mr Bostridge appealed.

Judgment: the Court of Appeal (Vos and Clarke LJJ, Sir Terence Etherton) dismissed the appeal, holding that normally only nominal damages would be awarded in a case where the individual would have been in exactly the same position, even if the tort of false imprisonment had not been committed and the position was no different under Article 5 ECHR.

Comment: the burden is on the public authority to assert and prove that the unlawful detention in fact made no difference.[17] However, this decision is likely to impact considerably on DOLS cases, under the Mental Capacity Act 2005, where quite often a deprivation of liberty is effected in breach of provisions of the admittedly rather complex DOLS machinery

17 *R (EO) v Secretary of State for the Home Department* [2013] EWHC 1236 (Admin) para 74.

but where, in many cases, the individual concerned would have been detained in any event, in exactly the same way. In other cases, of course, the evidence might lead the Court to conclude that, had lawful steps been taken, the person would not have been detained or, in any event, that a less restrict approach would have been taken, in which case substantial damages may be awarded. It makes an interesting comparison with the *TF* case, above para 19.19.

19.23 *Lee-Hirons v Secretary of State for Justice* [2016] UKSC 46, (2016) 19 CCLR 383

A conditionally discharged patient recalled to hospital was not entitled to written reasons at the time of his recall; he was entitled to an oral explanation at the time and written reasons within 72 hours but the failure to provide such reasons did not render his detention unlawful or found a claim for damages

Facts: Mr Lee-Hirons was conditionally discharged and then later recalled to hospital. At the time of his recall he was told orally that the reason for the recall was that his mental condition had deteriorated. He was then given fuller written reasons 15 days later, rather than three days later, as required by the Secretary of State's policy.

Judgment: the Supreme Court (Hale, Kerr, Wilson, Reed and Toulson JJSC) held that the brief explanation provided to Mr Lee-Hirons at the time of his recall satisfied all that the common law and the ECHR required and that neither the common law nor the ECHR required a recalled patient to be provided with contemporaneous written reasons. The failure to provide Mr Lee-Hirons with written reasons within three days was in breach of the Secretary of State's policy and therefore unlawful at common law; but it did not render the detention unlawful (because there was no direct link between the breach of duty and the detention) or found a claim for damages (because it involved no tort and the effects were insufficient grave to warrant an award under the Human Rights Act 1998).

19.24 *WD v Belgium* Application no 73548/13, 6 September 2016

The lengthy detention of a mentally disordered sex offender without suitable treatment was in breach of the ECHR

Facts: WD was a sex offender suffering from mental disorders who had been detained for nine years in a prison psychiatric wing and had not been provided with suitable treatment, which had had a negative impact on his psychological well-being.

Judgment: the European Court of Human Rights held that Belgium had treated WD incompatibly with Articles 3 and 5(1) ECHR; there had also been breaches of Articles 5(4) and 13 ECHR. The breach of Articles 3 and 5(1) ECHR arose out of a structural problem in Belgian law, such that treatment in prison was often inadequate whereas facilities outside prison were limited and the authorities could not require provision to be made. The court accordingly applied the pilot-judgment procedure and gave the Belgian government two years to remedy the situation. It also ordered Belgium to pay WD €16,000 in respect of non-pecuniary damage.

Nearest relatives

The importance of nearest relatives

19.25 The nearest relative provisions are at sections 24–30 of the MHA 1983 and are important because the nearest relative has many functions to play: not least, unless displaced, nearest relatives are entitled to object to the detention of mentally disordered patients who are not excluded criminal offenders. The role of nearest relatives was explained by Maurice Kay J in *R (M) v Secretary of State for Health*:[18]

> 4. The nearest relative plays an important part in the scheme of the Act. He may make an application for admission for assessment (section 2), an emergency application for admission for assessment (section 4) and an application for admission for treatment (section 3). No application for admission or treatment under section 3 may be made by an approved social worker without first consulting with the nearest relative unless the social worker considers that such consultation is not reasonably practicable or would involve unreasonable delay (section 11(4)). The manager of a psychiatric institution in which a patient is detained has to inform the nearest relative in writing about, amongst other things, the right to apply to a Mental Health Review Tribunal, the right to be discharged, the right to receive and send correspondence and the right to consent to or refuse treatment (section 132 (4)). A nearest relative may order the discharge of a patient who is detained under section 3 (section 23). Prior to exercising this important power the nearest relative can appoint a medical practitioner to examine the patient and the appointed practitioner can require the production of records relating to the detention or treatment of the patient (section 24). The right to order discharge under section 23 is limited when the responsible medical officer certifies that the patient would, if released, be likely to be a danger to himself or others (section 25). Where a patient is to be discharged other than by the order of the nearest relative, the detaining authority is required to notify the nearest relative of the forthcoming discharge unless the patient requests that no such information is supplied (section 133(2)).
>
> 5. In addition to the power to order a discharge under section 23 the nearest relative may apply to a Mental Health Review Tribunal for the discharge of the patient pursuant to section 66. Moreover if someone else makes an application to the Mental Health Review Tribunal, the nearest relative must receive notice of the proceedings pursuant to rule 7(d) of the Mental Health Review Tribunal Rules. The nearest relative then becomes a party to the proceedings in the Tribunal 'unless the context otherwise requires' (rule 2(1)). Once a party to the proceedings, the nearest relative is entitled to be informed as to their progress and may be represented in the proceedings, may appear at the hearing and take such part in the proceedings as the Tribunal thinks proper (rule 22(4)). As a party, he will also receive the decision of the Tribunal and the reasons for it (rules 24 and 23). Where the nearest relative is the applicant to the Tribunal he may appoint a registered medical practitioner to visit and examine the patient and that practitioner may require production of and inspect any records relating to the detention and treatment of the patient (section 76(1)). As the applicant, the nearest relative may attend the Tribunal hearing, be heard by the tribunal, call witnesses and cross examine the witnesses (rule 22(4)). Moreover, as an appli-

18 [2003] EWHC 1094 (Admin).

cant, he also receives a copy of every document received by the Tribunal (rule 12(1)). Some of these provisions may be modified by the Tribunal in the interests of the patient.

19.26 In addition to the functions noted by Maurice Kay J, the nearest relative:

- is entitled to require the social services authority to arrange for an AMHP to consider the patient's case with a view to making an application for admission to hospital (and, where the AMHP does not make such an application they must give written reasons): section 13(4) of the MHA 1983;
- is entitled to require the Independent Mental Health Advocacy Service to visit and seek to talk with the patient and offer their services (which the patient may decline): section 130B(5) of the MHA 1983.

19.27 A period of detention will be unlawful if, inter alia:

- the AMHP fails to take reasonably practicable steps properly to consult with the nearest relative;[19]
- the AMHP makes the application despite objection by the nearest relative.[20]

19.28 There is guidance about the functions of nearest relatives at Chapter 5 of the *Mental Health Act 1983: Code of Practice.*

Who are nearest relatives?

19.29 'Relatives' are defined in section 26(1) and (2):

Definition of 'relative' and 'nearest relative'

26(1) In this Part of this Act 'relative' means any of the following persons:
(a) husband or wife or civil partner;
(b) son or daughter;
(c) father or mother;
(d) brother or sister;
(e) grandparent;
(f) grandchild;
(g) uncle or aunt;
(h) nephew or niece.

(2) In deducing relationships for the purposes of this section, any relationship of the half-blood shall be treated as a relationship of the whole blood, and an illegitimate person shall be treated as the legitimate child of
(a) his mother, and
(b) if his father has parental responsibility for him within the meaning of section 3 of the Children Act 1989, his father.

19.30 The 'nearest relative' is essentially the relative that is highest up the above list, with the proviso that –

- where there is a tie:
  - relatives of the whole blood are preferred to relatives of half-blood; and

19 *GD v Edgware Community Hospital and Barnet LBC* [2008] EWHC 3572 (Admin), [2008] MHLR 282.

20 *TTM v Hackney LBC* [2011] EWCA Civ 4.

  - older relatives are preferred to younger; except that:
- the relative
  - with whom the patient ordinarily resides, or did ordinarily reside before becoming a hospital in-patient; or
  - is or was cared for by (whether or not they share or shared the same accommodation)
- will be treated as the nearest relative; and
- if there are two such, preference between them will be decided as above (in accordance with blood and age):

  section 26(3) and (4).

19.31 Section 26(5) excludes persons who otherwise would be nearest relatives on the grounds that (n short) they are not ordinarily resident in the UK (etc), are under 18 or are a permanently separated spouse or civil partner.

19.32 Section 26(6) a non-relative with whom the patient has ordinarily resided for at least five years, or did so reside before becoming a hospital in-patient, is to be treated as a relative at the bottom of the relative's list. That means that they will also become the nearest relative, by virtue of section 26(4); unless a relative higher up the list is living with or caring for the patient.

19.33 The nearest relative may delegate their functions to another person, in accordance with regulation 24 of the Mental Health (Hospital, Guardianship and Treatment) (England) Regulations 2008[21] and regulation 33 of the Mental Health (Hospital, Guardianship, Community Treatment and Consent to Treatment) (Wales) Regulations 2008.[22] The nearest relative is entitled to take back their powers, at any time.

Appointment or displacement

19.34 The county court may appoint a nearest relative (usually a social services authority):

- on the application of the patient, any relative of the patient, any other person with whom the patient lives or lived before hospital admission, or an AMHP;
- when a patient does not have a nearest relative, or it is not reasonably practicable to ascertain whether he or she has one or who it is (section 29(3)(a) and (b)).

19.35 The county court may displace a nearest relative (usually in favour of a social services authority):

- on the application of the patient, any relative of the patient, any other person with whom the patient lives or lived before hospital admission, or an AMHP;
- on the ground, essentially, of inability to act or unreasonableness:

> **29**(3) An application for an order under this section may be made upon any of the following grounds, that is to say–
>
> ...

21 SI No 1184.

22 SI No 2439.

(b) that the nearest relative of the patient is incapable of acting as such by reason of mental disorder or other illness;
(c) that the nearest relative of the patient unreasonably objects to the making of an application for admission for treatment or a guardianship application in respect of the patient;
(d) that the nearest relative of the patient has exercised without due regard to the welfare of the patient or the interests of the public his power to discharge the patient under this Part of this Act, or is likely to do so; or
(e) that the nearest relative of the patient is otherwise not a suitable person to act as such.

19.36 For a nearest relative to be displaced on the unreasonableness ground, the unreasonableness has to have existed both at the date of the application and at the date of the court hearing[23] and, in addition, the unreasonableness must be objectively established and outside the range of divergent approaches that reasonable persons may adopt.[24]

19.37 The scheme is flexible:

- an application for displacement can be made at the same time as, or later than, an application for detention under section 3 of the MHA 1983;[25]
- it is preferable to use other powers under the MHA 1983 to detain and extend detention, before displacing a nearest relative and detaining the patient under section 3;[26]
- an application can be made ex parte without notice, although that is not usually good practice;[27]
- displacement proceedings extend assessment detentions (under section 29(4)) but, in such cases, to avoid a breach of Article 5(4) ECHR, the Secretary of State should refer the case to the tribunal to ensure there is sufficient court review;[28]
- the displacement order will usually set a date for when the displacement ends; otherwise, it ends automatically when the patient is discharged (section 30);
- if that does not happen, the patient, the replacement nearest relative or the displaced nearest relative may apply to discharge or vary the order (under section 30).

19.38 A nearest relative should in general be provided with sufficient medical information so as to be able to exercise their powers appropriately and, in particular, to consider whether it would be reasonable to discharge a patient or object to their admission.[29]

23 *Lewis v Gibson* [2005] EWCA Civ 587, (2005) 8 CCLR 399.
24 *W v L* [1974] QB 711.
25 *R v Central London County Court ex p Ax London* [1999] QB 1260, (1999) 2 CCLR 256.
26 *R v Central London County Court ex p Ax London* [1999] QB 1260, (1999) 2 CCLR 256.
27 *R (Holloway) v Oxfordshire CC* [2007] EWHC 776 (Admin), [2007] MHLR 225.
28 *R (H) v Secretary of State for Health* [2005] UKHL 60, [2006] 1 AC 441.
29 *R (S) v Plymouth CC* [2002] EWCA Civ 388, (2002) 5 CCLR 251; *GD v Edgware Community Hospital and Barnet LBC* [2008] EWHC 3572 (Admin), [2008] MHLR 282.

19.39 Further, the displacement of a nearest relative does not take away their continued legitimate interest in the patient's treatment and care.[30]

19.40 The displacement provisions are at section 29:

Appointment by court of acting nearest relative

29(1) The county court may, upon application made in accordance with the provisions of this section in respect of a patient, by order direct that the functions of the nearest relative of the patient under this Part of this Act and sections 66 and 69 below shall, during the continuance in force of the order, be exercisable by the person specified in the order.

(1A) If the court decides to make an order on an application under subsection (1) above, the following rules have effect for the purposes of specifying a person in the order–

(a) if a person is nominated in the application to act as the patient's nearest relative and that person is, in the opinion of the court, a suitable person to act as such and is willing to do so, the court shall specify that person (or, if there are two or more such persons, such one of them as the court thinks fit);

(b) otherwise, the court shall specify such person as is, in its opinion, a suitable person to act as the patient's nearest relative and is willing to do so.

(2) An order under this section may be made on the application of–

(za) the patient;

(a) any relative of the patient;

(b) any other person with whom the patient is residing (or, if the patient is then an in-patient in a hospital, was last residing before he was admitted); or

(c) an approved mental health professional.

(3) An application for an order under this section may be made upon any of the following grounds, that is to say–

(a) that the patient has no nearest relative within the meaning of this Act, or that it is not reasonably practicable to ascertain whether he has such a relative, or who that relative is;

(b) that the nearest relative of the patient is incapable of acting as such by reason of mental disorder or other illness;

(c) that the nearest relative of the patient unreasonably objects to the making of an application for admission for treatment or a guardianship application in respect of the patient;

(d) that the nearest relative of the patient has exercised without due regard to the welfare of the patient or the interests of the public his power to discharge the patient ... under this Part of this Act, or is likely to do so; or

(e) that the nearest relative of the patient is otherwise not a suitable person to act as such.

(4) If, immediately before the expiration of the period for which a patient is liable to be detained by virtue of an application for admission for assessment, an application under this section, which is an application made on the ground specified in subsection (3)(c) or (d) above, is pending in respect of the patient, that period shall be extended–

(a) in any case, until the application under this section has been finally disposed of; and

(b) if an order is made in pursuance of the application under this section, for a further period of seven days; and for the purposes of this subsection an application under this section shall be deemed to

30 *Surrey County Council Social Services v McMurray*, 11 November 1994, CA.

have been finally disposed of at the expiration of the time allowed for appealing from the decision of the court or, if notice of appeal has been given within that time, when the appeal has been heard or withdrawn, and 'pending' shall be construed accordingly.

(5) An order made on the ground specified in subsection (3)(a), (b) or (e) above may specify a period for which it is to continue in force unless previously discharged under section 30 below.

(6) While an order made under this section is in force, the provisions of this Part of this Act (other than this section and section 30 below) and sections 66, 69, 132(4) and 133 below shall apply in relation to the patient as if for any reference to the nearest relative of the patient there were substituted a reference to the person having the functions of that relative and (without prejudice to section 30 below) shall so apply notwithstanding that the person who was the patient's nearest relative when the order was made is no longer his nearest relative; but this subsection shall not apply to section 66 below in the case mentioned in paragraph (h) of subsection (1) of that section.

Cases

19.41 *R v Central London CC ex p Ax London* (1999) 2 CCLR 256, CA

A nearest relative can be displaced on an interim basis but unless there are cogent reasons a final displacement decision should be made prior to detention under section 3 of the MHA 1983

Facts: the county court made an ex parte order under section 29(3) of the MHA 1983, displacing Mr London's nearest relative. Mr London claimed that the court did not have jurisdiction to make such an order on an interim basis that, consequently, his detention had been unlawful.

Judgment: the Court of Appeal (Henry, Robert Walker and Stuart-Smith LJJ) held that the court did have jurisdiction to make an interim order displacing a nearest relative, by virtue of section 38 of the County Courts Act 1984 and, in any event, a hospital is bound to treat county court orders as validly made, so that a decision made to detain, on their basis, is lawful even if it transpires later that the orders were invalid. However, in the absence of cogent reasons, a final displacement decision should be made prior to any application for compulsory admission under section 3: where a person was being detained under section 2 of the MHA 1983, for assessment, that detention could be extended under section 29(4), until such time as displacement proceedings concluded.

Comment: see the *Homerton* case below para 19.50, which modified the approach here by determining that cogent reasons were not required for acting under section 3 before applying to displace a nearest relative.

19.42 *Barnet LBC ex p Robin* (1999) 2 CCLR 454, CA

A nearest relative could be displaced not because of what she had done in the past but because what the evidence showed she was likely to do in the future; the appeal to the Court of Appeal was probably in relation to facts as well as law

Facts: Jacob Robin had suffered from a mental impairment since adolescence but, with one exception, his hospital treatment had been voluntary.

As a result of his deterioration, and increasing violence, it had been decided to detain him under section 3 of the MHA 1983 and to apply to displace his mother, as his nearest relative, under section 29: the reason for that application was that, in the past, Jacob's mother had consistently removed him prematurely from his voluntary placements.

Judgment: the Court of Appeal (Simon Brown, Mummery and Mantell LJJ) held that whilst Mrs Robin had not exercised her powers of discharge as nearest relative, in the past, since Jacob Robin had not been compulsorily detained, on the evidence, she was likely to use those powers unreasonably in the future. However, it appeared that an appeal to the Court of Appeal under section 29 of the MHA 1983 lay in relation to matters of fact as well as matters of law.

19.43 *Dewen v Barnet Healthcare Trust and Barnet LBC* (2001) 4 CCLR 239, CA

Approved mental health professionals are under a duty of honesty, not of reasonable enquiry

Facts: before detaining Mr Dewen, under section 3 of the MHA 1983, the approved social worker consulted his youngest daughter, as his nearest relative, under section 26: she did not object to the detention. Mr Dewen then sought a judicial review of the lawfulness of his detention, on the basis that his true nearest relative was his son, who was older than his daughter, and section 26 placed the elder before the younger.

Judgment: the Court of Appeal (Otton LJ and Hooper J) rejected Mr Dewen's case: the approved social worker had not been under a duty of reasonable enquiry, but of honesty, and consequently had discharged the duty to consult the person 'appearing to be the nearest relative'. In any event, carers displaced other relatives and the younger daughter fell within that description: it was only necessary to provide more than minimal care, for these purposes:

> The question which this court has to consider is not, in deciding whether the application for determination for treatment was validly made, whether Mr Millington, the approved social worker, consulted with the person who was legally correct as the 'nearest relative', but whether Lorraine Dewen appeared to him to be that relative. That, to my mind, is a correct analysis of section 11(4). This section and subsection has to be construed strictly. It involves the liberty or loss of liberty of a person, particularly a person under a mental disorder. It imposes no duty of reasonable inquiry on Mr Millington in relation to deciding who is the nearest relative. I accept Mr Foster's argument on behalf of the respondent that such an imposition would, in the circumstances in which most decisions have to be made, be an intolerable one. It is not surprising that Parliament did not impose it. In support of that contention, he referred to the decision of *Whitbread v Kingston and District NHS Trust* 1998 39 BMLR 94, and in particular a passage at pages 101–102. Accordingly, as I assess the situation, the court cannot and should not inquire into the reasonableness of Mr Millington's decision, only into the honesty of his assertion that it appeared that Lorraine Dewen was the nearest relative. His honesty has not been impugned.

19.44 ## *R (S) v Plymouth CC* [2002] EWCA Civ 388, (2002) 5 CCLR 251

Fairness required disclosure of the son's mental health records to his mother, in nearest relative displacement proceedings

Facts: C suffered from a mental disorder and mental impairment. His mother, who was his nearest relative, opposed his being made subject to a guardianship order but, despite requests by her, she had not been shown the material on which that proposed application would be based, on the ground that it was confidential and C lacked capacity to consent to its disclosure to his mother.

Judgment: the Court of Appeal (Kennedy (dissenting in part), Clarke and Hale LJJ) held that such material would have to be disclosed in any proceedings to displace the nearest relative and that such proceedings were likely if the mother continued to object. For that reason, and because of the importance under the ECHR of involving the mother, disclosure would be ordered – not just to the mother's lawyers and expert, but also (Kennedy LJ dissenting) to the mother personally. Hale LJ said this:

> 48. Hence both the common law and the Convention require that a balance be struck between the various interests involved. These are the confidentiality of the information sought; the proper administration of justice; the mother's right of access to legal advice to enable her to decide whether or not to exercise a right which is likely to lead to legal proceedings against her if she does so; the rights of both C and his mother to respect for their family life and adequate involvement in decision-making processes about it; C's right to respect for his private life; and the protection of C's health and welfare. In some cases there might also be an interest in the protection of other people, but that has not been seriously suggested here.
>
> 49. C's interest in protecting the confidentiality of personal information about himself must not be underestimated. It is all too easy for professionals and parents to regard children and incapacitated adults as having no independent interests of their own: as objects rather than subjects. But we are not concerned here with the publication of information to the whole wide world. There is a clear distinction between disclosure to the media with a view to publication to all and sundry and disclosure in confidence to those with a proper interest in having the information in question. We are concerned here only with the latter. The issue is only whether the circle should be widened from those professionals with whom this information has already been shared (possibly without much conscious thought being given to the balance of interests involved) to include the person who is probably closest to him in fact as well as in law and who has a statutory role in his future and to those professionally advising her. C also has an interest in having his own wishes and feelings respected. It would be different in this case if he had the capacity to give or withhold consent to the disclosure: any objection from him would have to be weighed in the balance against the other interests, although as *W v Egdell* [1990] Ch 359 shows, it would not be decisive. C also has an interest in being protected from a risk of harm to his health or welfare which would stem from disclosure; but it is important not to confuse a possible risk of harm to his health or welfare from being discharged from guardianship with a possible risk of harm from disclosing the information sought. As *In re D (Minors) (Adoption Reports: Confidentiality)* [1996] AC 593 shows, he also has an interest in decisions about his future being properly informed.

50. That balance would not lead in every case to the disclosure of all the information a relative might possibly want, still less to a fishing exercise amongst the local authority's files. But in most cases it would lead to the disclosure of the basic statutory guardianship documentation. In this case it must also lead to the particular disclosure sought. There is no suggestion that C has any objection to his mother and her advisers being properly informed about his health and welfare. There is no suggestion of any risk to his health and welfare arising from this. The mother and her advisers have sought access to the information which her own psychiatric and social work experts need in order properly to advise her. That limits both the context and the content of disclosure in a way which strikes a proper balance between the competing interests.

19.45 *Lewis v Gibson and MH* [2005] EWCA Civ 587, (2005) 8 CCLR 399

It was unnecessary to seek a best interests declaration but the court ought to joint the patient as a party in displacement applications

Facts: after the daughter was admitted to hospital under section 2 of the MHA 1983, the local authority obtained an order in the county court displacing the appellant as her daughter's nearest relative, enabling the local authority to assume guardianship for the daughter and make arrangements for her to live away from the appellant, in a supported living arrangement.

Judgment: the Court of Appeal (Thorpe, Smith and Wall LJJ) held that once the criteria in section 29 of the MHA 1983 were made out, the county court judge was entitled to displace a nearest relative and not required to refuse to do so, on the basis that the local authority should seek the alternative remedy of a best interests declaration. The court ought to join the patient as interested party in such applications.

19.46 *R (H) v Secretary of State for Health* [2005] UKHL 60, [2006] 1 AC 441

The machinery for detaining persons under section 2 of the MHA 1983 during displacement proceeds was ECHR compliant

Facts: H had been detained under section 2 of the MHA 1983 and an application was made to displace her mother, who objected to H being received into guardianship, as H's nearest relative. The displacement proceedings dragged on and as a result H was detained under section 2 well beyond the usual 28 days. The Court of Appeal held that sections 2 and 29(4) of the MHA 1983 were incompatible with Article 5(4) ECHR insofar as they made no provision for a patient's detention to be reviewed in circumstances where the patient was incapable of exercising the right of review and their detention was extended because of nearest relative displacement proceedings.

Judgment: the House of Lords (Lords Bingham Hope, Rodger, Lady Hale and Lord Brown) allowed the Secretary of State's appeal, on the basis that the scheme could be operated consistently with Article 5(4), in particular by the Secretary of State exercising his power to refer cases to the MHRT.

Comment: H's complaint to the European Court of Human Rights was upheld, in *MH v United Kingdom* (below at para 19.48).

19.47 *GD v Hospital Managers Edgware Community Hospital* [2008] EWHC 3572 (Admin), [2008] MHLR 282

GD's detention had been unlawful because there had not been more than a 'nod in the direction of consultation' which seriously inhibited the chances of the nearest relative having any effective input into the process or any proper opportunity to object: habeas corpus was granted

Facts: GD was detained under section 3 of the MHA 1983 and claimed that he was being detained unlawfully because of the social worker's failure to engage in proper consultation with his father and nearest relative (because of a concern that he would object).

Judgment: Burnett J held that the GD's detention had been unlawful because of inadequate steps to consult with GD's nearest relative:

> *Discussion*
>
> 34. This case is concerned with an application for admission for treatment made by an approved social worker, namely Mr Scheuring. The complaint, as I have said, is that he failed to comply with the mandatory requirements of section 11(4) of the Act. It is plain, on the authority of *In re S-C (Mental Patient: Habeas Corpus)* [1996] 1 QB 599, that a failure to comply with these provisions renders the subsequent detention for treatment unlawful. Section 11(4) contains two distinct parts. The first is that if the nearest relative objects to the application for admission for treatment, that application shall not be made. That is why the question of whether GD's father objected on this occasion is of importance and was explored at length in evidence.
>
> 35. It should be noted, however, that there are other provisions within the Act which enable objections to be overridden in certain circumstances, and also for those responsible for the treatment of somebody considered to be in urgent need of attention to use other mechanisms.
>
> 36. The second requirement is that no such application shall be made, except after consultation with the person appearing to be the nearest relative, unless:
>
>> '... it appears to that social worker that in the circumstances such consultation is not reasonably practicable or would involve unreasonable delay.'
>
> 37. There is no issue in this case but that GD's father was the nearest relative. That was known to Mr Scheuring. I am not therefore concerned with the statutory definition of 'nearest relative', nor with a dispute about whether the social worker had identified the correct nearest relative and the basis upon which he did so. It is to be noted, however, that section 11(4) requires consultation with the person 'appearing to be the nearest relative' and it also relieves the social worker of that obligation if 'it appears' that consultation is not reasonably practicable and so forth.
>
> 38. It is plain that the language of the subsection is directed towards the subjective knowledge of the social worker concerned. Indeed, for Parliament to have imposed an objective test in those circumstances would have been unduly oppressive and probably counterproductive.
>
> 39. In what circumstances can the view of the social worker on these matters be challenged? In *Re D (Mental Patient: Habeas Corpus)* [2000] 2 FLR 848, the Court of Appeal was concerned with the issue which arose because the social worker consulted someone who turned out not to be the nearest

relative, but who appeared to the social worker to be so. In paragraphs 15 and 16 of his judgment, Otton LJ dealt with the matter:

> '(15) The question which this court has to consider is not, in deciding whether the application for determination for treatment was validly made, whether Mr JM, the approved social worker, consulted with the person who was legally correct as the 'nearest relative', but whether L appeared to him to be that relative. That, to my mind, is a correct analysis of s 11(4). This section and subsection has to be construed strictly. It involves the liberty or loss of liberty of a person, particularly a person under a mental disorder. It imposes no duty of reasonable inquiry on Mr JM in relation to deciding who is the nearest relative. I accept Mr Foster's argument on behalf of the respondent that such an imposition would, in the circumstances in which most decisions have to be made, be an intolerable one. It is not surprising that Parliament did not impose it. In support of that contention, he referred to the decision of *Whitbread v Kingston and District NHS Trust* (1998) 39 BMLR 94, and in particular a passage at 101–102. Accordingly, as I assess the situation, the court cannot and should not inquire into the reasonableness of Mr JM's decision, only into the honesty of his assertion that it appeared that L was the nearest relative. His honesty has not been impugned.
>
> (16) We have to ask the following question: Was his decision, in concluding that L was the nearest relative, plainly wrong?'

He went on to conclude on the evidence that there was much which made it appear in that case that the person consulted by the social worker was the nearest relative. The complaint was thus not upheld.

40. In *R (WC) v South London & Maudsley NHS Trust* [2001] EWHC 1025 (Admin), [2001] 1 MHLR 187, Scott Baker J (as he then was) came to a similar conclusion, confirming that the test was a subjective one with which the court would not interfere unless, for example, the social worker had failed to apply the legal test in section 26, which explains who is to be regarded as the nearest relative, or acted in bad faith or in some way reached a conclusion which was plainly wrong.

41. What both these judgments demonstrate is no more than a well-recognised proposition that when a statute imposes a subjective test of the sort one sees in section 11(4) of the Act, this court will not interfere with the decision made save on well-recognised public law grounds.

42. Furthermore, in that review exercise, given the circumstances engaged in cases of this sort, the court will inevitably be sensitive to the difficulties faced be those who have to make difficult decisions, sometimes in fast-moving and tense circumstances. The question might be, for example, whether it was open to the decision-maker on the information available to him to reach the conclusion he did. In both *Re D* and the case of *WC* the court used the words 'plainly wrong' as shorthand for that concept.

43. Ms Street, who appeared, as I say, on behalf of the defendants, submitted that unless the assertion contained in Form 9, from which I have read, was dishonest, this court should not interfere. She focused on the word 'dishonest' because it had been found in paragraph 15 of the judgment of Otton LJ in *Re D*.

44. In my judgment, that is too austere an approach. The court should look at the question on a wider basis because it is concerned with the legality of the process. In doing so, the court will recognise that the decisions can only be questioned on a public law basis and, as I have already indicated, in an

environment where some sensitivity to the difficulties faced by those making the decisions is required.

45. Scott Baker J alluded to bad faith. Misuse of power, which is an aspect of the same thing, would be another label that might be attached. Both are classic grounds of review which, if made out, would result in the process under consideration being adjudged unlawful. His reference to misconstruing section 26 was also an example of his recognising that a decision might be flawed because a wrong legal approach had been taken.

46. The duty to consult is one which exists to enable there to be a dialogue about the action proposed in respect of a mentally ill individual. The person consulted is entitled to have his views taken into account and, importantly, the consultation possess should enable the nearest relative to object to the proposed course if he wishes. The consultation must be a real exercise and not a token one. If an objection is made, it does not have to be a reasonable one. It does not have to be one which judged objectively is sensible. But it has the effect of stopping the proposed course of action, whilst of course not shutting out alternatives available under the Act.

47. Ms Street submits that as events unfolded, it was not reasonably practicable to make contact with GD's father until the morning of the assessment. That being the case, it was not possible to engage in consultation before the application was made. To have delayed the application to enable consultation to take place would have resulted in unreasonable delay. So she submits that those matters were apparent to Mr Scheuring and his conclusion cannot be challenged.

48. Mr Simblet submitted that the evidence leads inexorably to the conclusion that there was no proper attempt to engage in consultation in this case at all. Mr Scheuring's conclusion was thus flawed for that reason, because the statutory procedure was in effect sidelined. He emphasised that the role of the nearest relation is an important one under the legislation and that it cannot matter that the social worker concerned, as a result of information provided to him by colleagues, has formed the view that GD's father was unlikely to be helpful. He submits that Mr Scheuring has candidly admitted that he delayed attempts to make contact with GD's father and essentially boxed himself into the corner in which he found himself on the morning of Saturday, 14th June. Whilst he would accept that ordinarily there is no need to search uphill and down dale for the nearest relation, in this instance there was a calculated decision not to do so whilst the whole process was in its early stages and being set up. Thus, he submits, it could not have appeared to Mr Scheuring for the purposes of section 11(4) that it was not reasonably practicable to consult.

49. Furthermore, Mr Simblet submits that the events on the morning of Saturday, 14th June, provide further support for the submission that I have just summarised and possibly an additional point. There was, submitted Mr Simblet, absolutely no reason why the assessment had to take place immediately at the family home. Mr Scheuring was in possession of a warrant which entitled him to convey GD to a place of safety for the purposes of an assessment to be carried out there. So, he asks rhetorically, why not attempt to make contact with GD's father, then convey GD to the unit, and only thereafter undertake the assessment and follow it by the application, if necessary.

50. It is quite clear, as was recognised by Mr Simblet on behalf of the applicant, that at all times Mr Scheuring and the other professionals were motivated only by what they perceived to be in the best interests of GD. His mother also shared that motivation and was desperately trying to confront

a serious deterioration in her son's health. But, submits Mr Simblet, that motivation cannot be used as a justification for what in effect was a circumventing of the statutory mechanisms found in section 11(4). Conflicts within families and between members of a patient's family and the professionals are not uncommon, but there are other mechanisms available under the legislation to ensure that the patient is appropriately protected and treated.

Conclusion

51. I accept that Mr Scheuring and those who were engaged with him in the days leading up to the assessment and admission to hospital were motivated only by the best interests of the patient, GD. However, I have come to the conclusion, on both the written and oral evidence, that in seeking to protect the best interests of GD they calculated that they should do no more than nod in the direction of consultation as contemplated by section 11(4). They set in motion a course of events which was designed to leave consultation with GD's father to the very last moment, and thus seriously inhibit the chances of his having any effective input into the process and the chances of his having an opportunity to make an objection. In those circumstances, what in my judgment they contemplated could not properly be considered consultation at all. In my judgment, this amounted to a misuse of power, albeit for the best of motives, that infected the application process from beginning to end.

19.48 *MH v United Kingdom* Application no 11577/06, (2014) 58 EHRR 35

MS's rights under Article 5 ECHR had been breached during a period of detention under section 2 of the MHA 1983 when she had been unable to apply to the tribunal to be discharged, because of her lack of the mental capacity to do so, and no one else was entitled or required to make the application on her behalf

Facts: H had been detained under section 2 of the MHA 1983 and an application was made to displace her mother, who objected to H being received into guardianship, as H's nearest relative. The displacement proceedings dragged on and as a result H was detained under section 2 well beyond the usual 28 days. The Court of Appeal held that sections 2 and 29(4) of the MHA 1983 were incompatible with Article 5(4) ECHR insofar as they made no provision for a patient's detention to be reviewed in circumstances where the patient was incapable of exercising the right of review and their detention was extended because of nearest relative displacement proceedings.

Judgment: the European Court of Human Rights held that H's detention had been unlawful during its initial period in that, although she had been entitled in principle to apply to the MHRT for discharge, she had lacked the capacity to do so and no special safeguards had been made available to ensure that this right was made practical and effective in such cases. However, after H's detention had been automatically extended, the Secretary of State had secured a MHRT tribunal within a month, which was not unreasonable: the exercise by the Secretary of State of the power of referring cases to the MHRT was capable of removing any potential incompatibility with the ECHR, in the legislation.

19.49 *R (Holloway) v Oxfordshire CC* [2007] EWHC 776 (Admin), (2007) 10 CCLR 264

An interim displacement order and the ensuing detention were both lawful despite failure to notify the nearest relative of the displacement hearing, but that had been very poor practice

Facts: H had a long history of paranoid schizophrenia and hospital admissions but his mother had indicated that she objected to a further planned compulsory admission. Oxford applied to court for an order under section 29(3) of the MHA 1983, displacing H's mother as his nearest relative. The judge granted an interim order, at a hearing that Oxford had not notified to the mother, although it could have done, therefore she had not been represented.

Judgment: Beatson J held that Oxford's failure to notify the mother was very poor practice, and that it would have been good practice for the court to undertake enquiries with a view to possibly adjourning until the mother had been notified, but that, nonetheless, the interim displacement order remained valid, so that H's detention on its basis had been valid.

19.50 *R (M) v Homerton University Hospital* [2008] EWCA Civ 197

It is desirable but not legally necessary for displacement proceedings to be concluded before the patient is detained under section 3 of the MHA 1983

Facts: M and her mother both had a history of mental disorder and M had a life-threatening form of anorexia. Her mother applied to discharge her from detention for assessment under section 2 of the MHA 1983. The hospital blocked the discharge under section 25 of the MHA 1983, applied to displace the mother under section 29, secured interim displacement orders and then detained M under section 3 of the MHA 1983 before the final hearing of the section 29 proceedings.

Judgment: the Court of Appeal (Hallet and Buxton LJJ, Sir Peter Gibson) held that whilst it might be desirable for section 29 proceedings to be concluded before an application is made under section 3 there was no legal requirement to that effect or anything implicit in the legislation that required there to be exceptional circumstances if that course was not taken, nor was the procedure adopted incompatible with the ECHR: M's detention had not been arbitrary but on proper grounds and subject to review.

19.51 *R (V) v South London and Maudsley NHS Foundation Trust* [2010] EWHC 742 (Admin), (2010) 13 CCLR 181

Habeas corpus was granted when the approved mental health professional knew full well that the patient had a nearest relative who could be contacted, but had not done so

Facts: the social worker completed an application for compulsory admission stating that the claimant's nearest relative was unknown, when the social worker knew that the claimants nearest relative was his mother, had sought to contact her (unsuccessfully) and there were still several hours left in which to make continued efforts to make contact before the claimant's existing detention expired.

Judgment: Wyn Williams J granted habeas corpus on the basis that the decision by the social worker had been *Wednesbury* unreasonable.

19.52 *TW v Enfield LBC* [2013] EWCA Civ 362, (2014) 17 CCLR 264

An AMHP need not consult a nearest relative when the patient objects, providing the AMHP balances the patient's right to privacy (against the nearest relative) under Article 8 ECHR, with the patient's right to liberty (which the nearest relative could support) under Article 5

Facts: the AMHP failed to consult TW's nearest relative, her father, before applying for her compulsory admission, because TW alleged that her father had abused her sexually and had insisted that her case details should not be disclosed to her family. However, TW then sought to bring proceedings against the AMHP/local authority for unlawful detention, because of the failure to consult her father. She was initially refused permission to proceed.

Judgment: the Court of Appeal (Arden, Aikens and Clarke LJJ) allowed TW's appeal, holding that the 'reasonably practicable' test in section 11(4) of the MHA 1983 required the AMHP to balance the patient's right to liberty under Article 5 ECHR against her right to privacy under Article 8 but that it was arguable that, in this case, the AMHP had treated Article 8 as decisive:

> 51. In a case where an ASW's statutory obligation to consult the 'nearest relative' under section 11(4) would constitute an interference with the patient's Article 8(1) rights to private life, the decision of the ASW on whether it is or is not 'reasonably practicable' to consult the 'nearest relative' will depend on whether that is justified and proportionate to do so in the particular circumstances of the case. In the English cases on section 11(4) I have cited above it has been held that the issue of whether or not to consult will depend upon the subjective knowledge and judgment of the social worker concerned and that the court will not interfere with a decision save on well-recognised public law grounds. However, those decisions did not fully take into account the need to ensure that section 11(4) is interpreted (as far as possible) in a way compatible with the patient's Convention rights. Normally, proportionality is not assessed by reference simply to the subjective conclusion of the person making the judgment. Nor, strictly speaking, is proportionality to be judged solely on 'public law grounds'. However, a court will accord a decision-maker a wide margin of judgment as to what is proportional in a particular case.
>
> 52. In some circumstances, of which the present case is an example, this balance will be a difficult exercise. But I think that my analysis demonstrates that one principle is clear: as a matter of construction of section 11(4), a patient's assertion, even if founded on fact and even if reasonable, that consultation would lead to an infringement of her Article 8(1) rights cannot, as a matter of law, lead automatically to the conclusion that it is 'not reasonably practicable' to consult the 'nearest relative'. Nor is an ASW's conclusion that such consultation would lead to an infringement of the patient's Article 8(1) rights enough, in law, to lead to the decision that there should be no such consultation under section 114). Equally, as a matter of construction of section 11(4), it must be wrong in law for the ASW

to conclude that because consultation with TW's 'nearest relative' would require disclosure of details of TW's case and that would therefore constitute an interference with TW's Article 8(1) rights, that must necessarily lead to the conclusion that it was 'not reasonably practicable' to consult the 'nearest relative'.

53. It must also follow, with respect to Bennett J, that his analysis on the construction of section 11(4) by reference to the patient's Article 8 rights was incomplete. In my view, in that regard *R (E) v Bristol CC* [2005] EWHC 74 (Admin), [2005] 1 MHLR 2873 should not be followed. But, as I have stated above, I would accept what I might call Bennett J's 'domestic law' analysis and construction of section 11(4) and the word 'practicable'. It is only the Convention rights aspect of construction in which he erred.

Discharges from detention

19.54 For present purposes, one can divide detained patients into three broad categories: unrestricted patients, patients who are subject to restriction orders, and patients who are subject to restriction or limitation directions.

Unrestricted patients

19.55 Within this category are Part II patients who are detained under sections 2 or 3, and unrestricted Part III patients (ie those who have been made subject to a hospital order under section 37, but not to a restriction order under section 41; or prisoners transferred by the Secretary of State for Justice to hospital under sections 47 or 48 but who have not also been made subject to a restriction direction under section 49). Transferred prisoners with determinate sentences who remain in hospital after expiry of their restrictions will become unrestricted patients, commonly referred to as 'notional' section 37 patients.

19.56 There are other compulsory powers in Part II which include: guardianship (sections 7 and 8); supervised community treatment (sections 17A ff); short-term holding powers (sections 4 and 5).

19.57 In all of these cases, the Secretary of State for Justice has no statutory role.

19.58 Under section 23, a Part II patient detained under section 2 or 3 may be discharged without the need for a tribunal hearing by their nearest relative, responsible clinician or the hospital managers. An unrestricted Part III patient may be discharged by the responsible clinician or the hospital managers, again under section 23, which is modified for this type of patient by paragraph 8 of Part 1 of Schedule 1 to the 1983 Act.

19.59 Similarly under section 23, patients subject to guardianship may be discharged by the responsible clinician, the local social services authority, or the nearest relative. Patients subject to supervised community treatment may be discharged by the responsible clinician, the hospital managers, or the nearest relative.

19.60 In the case of patients in this category, under section 72 of the MHA 1983, the First-tier Tribunal has a discretion to direct discharge, and a duty to direct discharge if certain criteria for lawful detention are not satisfied.

Patients subject to restriction orders

19.61 Within this category of patients are those who have who have been made subject to a hospital order under section 37 with a restriction order under section 41. In these cases, the Secretary of State for Justice has a statutory role. There is also a range of interim powers to send people involved in criminal proceedings to hospital, under sections 35, 36 and 38. However, the Secretary of State for Justice does not have a statutory role in respect of these patients.

19.62 Under section 23 as modified by paragraph 7 of Part II of Schedule 2 to the 1983 Act, the responsible clinician and the hospital managers may discharge these patients, but only with the consent of the Secretary of State. The Secretary of State has his/her own powers of discharge, including absolute or conditional discharge, and recall (from conditional discharge) under section 42. Under section 42(1), the Secretary of State also has the power to lift the restriction order if satisfied that it is no longer required to protect the public from serious harm.

19.63 The First-tier Tribunal has no general discretion to direct discharge in these cases, but under section 73 it must do so when certain criteria for lawful detention are not satisfied. The discharge may be absolute or conditional.

19.64 A patient who has already been conditionally discharged may be absolutely discharged by the First-tier Tribunal under section 75.

Patients subject to restriction and limitation directions

19.65 Within this category of patients are those who have been made subject to hospital and limitation directions under section 45A, and those who have been transferred from prison to hospital under sections 47 or 48 and have additionally made subject to restriction direction under section 49.

19.66 The Secretary of State has the same powers under section 42 as above. In addition, under section 50, the Secretary of State may direct that the patient be remitted to prison (or the institution in which the patient would have otherwise been detained – such as immigration detention) where he or she is notified by the responsible clinician that that there is no further need or purpose for detention in hospital.

19.67 However, as mentioned in paragraph 5 above, if a patient remains detained in hospital beyond the date of the expiry of their sentence, the restriction or limitation direction ceases to have effect, but they remain lawfully detained in hospital as if, on the sentence expiry date, they had been made the subject to a section 37 hospital order without restrictions. The statutory mechanism for this process is convoluted, but the result is that the patient becomes what is often called a 'notional section 37' patient, and would fall into the first category above. This does not apply to indeterminate sentence prisoners, because they do not have a sentence expiry date.

19.68 While the restriction or limitation direction applies, the First-tier Tribunal cannot direct discharge, but under section 74 it must decide whether it *would have* granted an absolute or conditional discharge, had section 73 applied, ie had the patient been subject to a hospital order under section 37 and a restriction order under section 41.

19.69 Where the tribunal decides the patient would have been entitled to conditional discharge, it may also recommend that if the patient is not discharged as a result (see below), they should remain in hospital rather than be remitted to prison. That is what happened in the appellant's case.

19.70 Additionally, if the tribunal decides that it would have directed discharge, the Secretary of State has a discretion under section 74(2)(b) to notify the tribunal that the patient can be so discharged. The Secretary of State considers such cases and decides whether there are exceptional circumstances that would indicate the exercise of the discretion is appropriate. More usually in the case of indeterminate sentence prisoners, the result of a tribunal notification of a patient's entitlement to discharge, along with a recommendation that they remain detained in hospital rather than be remitted, is that the patient's case is brought before the Parole Board to consider release from the sentence under section 28 of the Crime (Sentences) Act 1997.

Applications and references to the tribunal

Applications

19.71 Section 66 governs the right of unrestricted patients and in some cases their nearest relative to apply to the First-tier Tribunal. The right to apply, and the frequency with which applications may be made, is determined by reference to the particular compulsory power to which they are subject.

19.72 Section 70 governs the right of all restricted patients to apply to the First-tier Tribunal. That includes patients subject to restriction orders, restriction directions, and limitation directions, although section 69(2)(b) provides an additional initial right to apply to the tribunal for patients who are made subject to a restricted transfer direction.

References

19.73 The 1983 Act requires the case of every detained patient to be brought before the tribunal, even where a patient has never sought a tribunal hearing. This is achieved by requirements for patients' cases to be referred to the tribunal after certain intervals.

19.74 Under sections 67 and 71 the Secretary of State has a discretion to refer any patient's case to the First-tier Tribunal at any time.

19.75 If a patient does not apply to the tribunal within certain time periods, then their case must be referred to the tribunal. In the case of unrestricted patients, the reference must be made by the hospital managers under section 68; in the case of restricted patients, the reference must be made by the Secretary of State under section 71.

Tribunals' lack of power

19.76 The Tribunals have no power to determine:

- whether the initial admission was lawful; or
- whether the hospital is suitable in terms of its level of security, the treatment available, its proximity to family members and so forth;[31] although the tribunal can make recommendations about such matters, under section 72(3).

Mental Health Act 1983 s72

19.77 The main statutory power of discharge by the tribunal is at section 72 of the MHA 1983 (section 73 addresses the absolute or conditional discharge of restricted patients), the main provisions of which require the tribunal to focus on what the consequences of a discharge would be, and are as follows:

> **Powers of tribunals**
>
> 72(1) Where application is made to the appropriate tribunal by or in respect of a patient who is liable to be detained under this Act or is a community patient, the tribunal may in any case direct that the patient be discharged, and–
>
> (a) the tribunal shall direct the discharge of a patient liable to be detained under section 2 above if it is not satisfied–
>
> (i) that he is then suffering from mental disorder or from mental disorder of a nature or degree which warrants his detention in a hospital for assessment (or for assessment followed by medical treatment) for at least a limited period; or
>
> (ii) that his detention as aforesaid is justified in the interests of his own health or safety or with a view to the protection of other persons;
>
> (b) the tribunal shall direct the discharge of a patient liable to be detained otherwise than under section 2 above if it is not satisfied–
>
> (i) that he is then suffering from mental disorder or from mental disorder of a nature or degree which makes it appropriate for him to be liable to be detained in a hospital for medical treatment; or
>
> (ii) that it is necessary for the health of safety of the patient or for the protection of other persons that he should receive such treatment; or
>
> (iia) that appropriate medical treatment is available for him; or
>
> (iii) in the case of an application by virtue of paragraph (g) of section 66(1) above, that the patient, if released, would be likely to act in a manner dangerous to other persons or to himself ...
>
> (1A) In determining whether the criterion in subsection (1)(c)(iii) above is met, the tribunal shall, in particular, consider, having regard to the patient's history of mental disorder and any other relevant factors, what risk there would be of a deterioration of the patient's condition if he were to continue not to be detained in a hospital (as a result, for example, of his refusing or neglecting to receive the medical treatment he requires for his mental disorder).
>
> (2) ...

31 *Re S (Care Plan)* [2002] UKHL 10, [2002] 2 AC 291.

(3) A tribunal may under subsection (1) above direct the discharge of a patient on a future date specified in the direction; and where a tribunal does not direct the discharge of a patient under that subsection the tribunal may–
   (a) with a view to facilitating his discharge on a future date, recommend that he be granted leave of absence or transferred to another hospital or into guardianship; and
   (b) further consider his case in the event of any such recommendation not being complied with.

(3A) Subsection (1) above does not require a tribunal to direct the discharge of a patient just because it thinks it might be appropriate for the patient to be discharged (subject to the possibility of recall) under a community treatment order; and a tribunal–
   (a) may recommend that the responsible clinician consider whether to make a community treatment order; and
   (b) may (but need not) further consider the patient's case if the responsible clinician does not make an order.

19.78 As far as concerns the operation of section 72:

- the burden of proof is on the detaining authority;[32]
- the tribunal *must* direct discharge if they are not satisfied as to any of the criteria in section 72(1)(a) (in the case of section 2 patients) or section 72(1)(b) (in the case of section 3 patients);
- the burden of proof is the civil standard of balance of probabilities, flexibly applied, but no more than cogent evidence accepted as correct is needed to justify continued detention;[33]
- whilst the discharge criteria in section 72 mirror the admission criteria in section 3, the question is not simply whether the patient would be detained under section 3, as at the date of the tribunal hearing (since, as a patient, they will be receiving medication and care in hospital) but whether discharge into the community will result in a likelihood of the patient not complying with treatment or, for whatever reasons, deteriorating so that the criteria for discharge are not met;[34]
- it is usually essential that the tribunal has evidence of what after-care services will be in place and, otherwise, what the patient's circumstances will be, relevant to future risks. If there is uncertainty, the tribunal should adjourn with directions,[35] although that is not an absolute rule;[36]
- the power of deferral can be used when it is clear that satisfactory after-care will be provided, but time is needed to put them in place;[37]
- as noted above, at para 19.7, where a patient is taking medication and is a-symptomatic, their mental disorder will not be of a *'degree'* that warrants hospital treatment, but it could be of a *'nature'* that requires

32 *R (N) v Mental Health Review Tribunal (Northern Region)* [2005] EWCA Civ 1605, [2006] 4 All ER 194.

33 *R (H) v Mental Health Review Tribunal, North and East London Region* [2000] MHLR 242; *Re D* [2008] UKHL 33, [2008] 1 WLR 1499.

34 *R (N) v Mental Health Review Tribunal (Northern Region)* [2005] EWCA Civ 1605, [2006] 4 All ER 194; *Re D* [2008] UKHL 33, [2008] 1 WLR 1499.

35 *R (H) v Ashworth Hospital Authority* [2002] EWCA Civ 923, [2003] 1 WLR 127.

36 *M v West London Mental Health NHS Trust* [2013] EWCA Civ 1010.

37 *R (H) v Ashworth Hospital Authority* [2002] EWCA Civ 923, [2003] 1 WLR 127.

hospital treatment and detention for that purpose if, without hospital treatment and detention the patient is likely to cease taking medication, deteriorate and become a risk to himself or others;[38]

- the tribunal has to weigh the interests of the patient against those of the public and determine whether detention is proportionate to the risks involved to the public (and, in some cases, to the patient).[39]

Discharges in criminal cases

Introduction

19.79 Mental patients who are detained in hospital as a result of a criminal conviction may be:

- ordinary restricted patients (under section 79), who are subject to a restriction order (under section 41); or
- restricted patients (under section 79), who are more serious offenders and are subject to a limitation direction (under section 145(1)), a restriction direction (under section 49) or a transfer direction (under section 48).

19.80 In the latter case, of restricted patients who are subject to a limitation direction or restriction direction, or a transfer direction:

- these patients are liable to continue to serve sentences of imprisonment if they no longer require hospital treatment;
- accordingly, the function of the tribunals is to notify the Secretary of State, after the conclusion of the hearing, whether in their opinion the patient would be entitled to an absolute or conditional discharge, if the patient was an ordinary restricted patient: section 74(1) of the MHA 1983;
- if the conclusion is that the patient would be entitled to conditional discharge, the tribunal may recommend that, if the patient is not discharged, the patient should remain in hospital and not be transferred to prison: section 74(1);
- in the case of sentenced prisoners, subject to hospital and limitation directions, or a restricted transfer direction, the Secretary of State has a discretion whether to consent to the patient's discharge: section 74;
- if the patient has already served their minimum tariff, they are entitled to apply to the Parole Board for release in the same way as other prisoners and, if the Secretary of State refuses to consent to their discharge under section 74, he or she will automatically refer the case to the Parole Board.

38 *R (H) v Mental Health Review Tribunal, North and North East London Region* [2001] EWCA Civ 415, (2001) 4 CCLR 119; *R (Secretary of State for the Home Department) v Mental Health Review Tribunal* [2002] EWHC 1128 (Admin), [2002] MHLR 241.

39 *R (H) v Mental Health Review Tribunal, North and North East London Region* [2001] EWCA Civ 415, (2001) 4 CCLR 119; *R (Secretary of State for the Home Department) v Mental Health Review Tribunal* [2002] EWHC 1128 (Admin), [2002] MHLR 241; *Smirek v Williams* [2000] EWCA Civ 3025, [2000] MHLR 38.

Conditional discharges

19.81 The cases of ordinary restricted patients are dealt with by the tribunals under section 73 of the MHA 1983, under which patients may be 'absolutely discharged' or 'conditionally discharged'.

19.82 In the case of restricted patients, the tribunal has no general discretion to direct discharge, but must direct the absolute discharge of a patient where:

- the tribunal is not satisfied that:
  - the patient is then suffering from mental disorder or from mental disorder of a nature or degree which makes it appropriate for him or her to be liable to be detained in hospital for medical treatment; or that
  - it is necessary for the health or safety of the patient or for the protection of other persons that he or she should receive such treatment; or that
  - appropriate medical treatment is available for him or her;
- and the tribunal is satisfied that it is not appropriate for the patient to be liable to be recalled to hospital for further treatment:
  section 73(1).

19.83 The tribunal has no general discretion to direct the conditional discharge of a restricted patient, but must so direct where the tribunal is not satisfied that:

- the patient is then suffering from mental disorder or from mental disorder of a nature or degree which makes it appropriate for him or her to be liable to be detained in hospital for medical treatment; or that
- it is necessary for the health or safety of the patient or for the protection of other persons that he or she should receive such treatment; or that
- appropriate medical treatment is available for him or her;
- but are also not satisfied that it is not appropriate for the patient to be liable to be recalled to hospital for further treatment:
  section 73(1) and (2).

19.84 The tribunal 'may defer a direction for the conditional discharge of a patient until such arrangements as appear to the tribunal to be necessary for that purpose have been made to its satisfaction ...' (section 72(7)).

19.85 All of this creates a flexible regime enabling the tribunal to ensure that a patient is only discharged when conditions in the community will be suitable, and to maintain residual control over patients.[40]

19.86 Conditions usually require the restricted patient to reside in a particular place, to accept a certain level of supervision and to undergo a defined level of treatment. Having said that, there is no limit on the conditions that may be imposed, other than that:

- they must be relevant, rational, capable of being fulfilled and for a proper purpose that is consistent with the legislation;[41] and

40 *R v Merseyside Mental Health Review Tribunal ex p K* [1990] 1 All ER 694; *R (H) v Secretary of State for the Home Department* [2002] EWCA Civ 646, [2003] QB 320.

41 *R (SH) v Mental Health Review Tribunal* [2007] EWHC 884 (Admin), [2007] MHLR 234.

- they must not result in the patient continuing to be deprived of liberty in hospital, or elsewhere;[42]
- they must not be such as to, in effect, make the discharge conditional on the agreement of some other body, such as the Ministry of Justice.[43]

19.87 Conditionally discharged patients are not subject to the compulsory treatment provisions in Part 4 of the MHA 1983 so, if the patient does not comply with conditions relating to treatment, the only remedy is recall to hospital.[44]

19.88 The purpose of a conditional discharge is to make the restricted patient liable to be recalled to hospital detention, by the Secretary of State, if any of the conditions are broken: section 73(4). This seems primarily designed to protect the public, but the regime is also supportive of the patient and protective of the patient.[45]

19.89 The Secretary of State will monitor the conditionally discharged patient in the community and has power to vary the conditions, under section 73(5).

19.90 Where a restricted patient is no longer mentally disordered:[46]

- their conditional (but not absolute) discharge may be deferred for a reasonable, limited period; however,
- ultimately, they must be discharged, whether or not the authorities have been able to put in place arrangements relevant to the conditions that the tribunal wanted to attach to the discharge; although
- the discharge may be absolute, or conditional (so as to make the patient subject to the power of recall).

19.91 Where the restricted patient remains mentally disordered:[47]

- their discharge may be deferred for a reasonable period, and their detention will remain lawful, while the authorities make efforts to arrange community services;
- if, however, the tribunal's view is that such services are not an essential precondition of discharge, the patient must be discharged whether or not those services are put in place.

19.92 Where the patient remains mentally disordered but the tribunal determines that the criteria for conditional discharge are met, *providing that* the authorities arrange specified community services then:[48]

42 *Secretary of State for Justice v RB* [2011] EWCA Civ 1608, [2012] 1 WLR 2043.

43 *R (Secretary of State for the Home Department) v Mental Health Review Tribunal* [2007] EWHC 2224 (Admin), [2008] MHLR 212.

44 *R (SH) v Mental Health Review Tribunal* [2007] EWHC 884 (Admin), [2007] MHLR 234.

45 *R v Merseyside Mental Health Review Tribunal ex p K* [1990] 1 All ER 694; *R (H) v Secretary of State for the Home Department* [2002] EWCA Civ 646, [2003] QB 320.

46 *R (H) v Secretary of State for the Home Department* [2003] UKHL 59, [2004] 2 AC 253, (2004) 7 CCLR 147.

47 *R (H) v Secretary of State for the Home Department* [2003] UKHL 59, [2004] 2 AC 253, (2004) 7 CCLR 147.

48 *R (H) v Secretary of State for the Home Department* [2003] UKHL 59, [2004] 2 AC 253, (2004) 7 CCLR 147.

- the tribunal should defer directing a conditional discharge whilst the authorities responsible for after-care endeavour to make arrangements for the provision of the necessary services;
- the tribunal should keep the situation under review by means of adjournments and directions;
- the after-care authorities are under a duty of best endeavour and not an absolute duty to provide services that match the tribunal's conditions;
- if the after-care authorities do not use their best endeavours they will be susceptible to judicial review;
- if, however, they cannot provide the services that the tribunal considers to be a necessary precondition of discharge then, in principle, the patient will remain lawfully detained;
- for example (a recurrent theme), after-care authorities cannot compel psychiatrists to act contrary to their conscientious professional judgment so that, for example, where discharge is conditional on psychiatric supervision in the community, but no psychiatrist is willing to undertake such supervision because in their judgment the risks are too great, the after-care authorities cannot compel a psychiatrist to undertake supervision and that proposed condition will remain unfulfilled;
- if difficulties arise the tribunal may (i) continue to defer and impose directions or give advice; (ii) amend or vary its proposed conditions to seek to overcome any difficulties; (iii) order a conditional discharge without specific conditions, thereby making the patient simply subject to recall; or (iv) decide that the patient should remain detained in hospital for treatment;
- patients must not be left in limbo in case there is a breach of Article 5(4) ECHR (the right to a regular review of the lawfulness of detention): the tribunal must ensure that it keeps the situation under review in the light of any changes in the patient's condition and/or any difficulties implementing its conditions.

19.93 Applications concerning conditionally discharged restricted patients are made under section 75 of the MHA 1983, under which provision the tribunal can, among other things, vary conditions or absolutely discharge the patient.[49]

Cases

19.94 *R v Camden and Islington Health Authority ex p K* (2001) 4 CCLR 170, CA

A patient remains lawfully detained when she continues to suffer from a mental disorder that warrants hospital detention and treatment unless psychiatric supervision in the community can be provided and, despite the authorities using reasonable endeavours, psychiatric supervision in the community cannot be provided because no psychiatrist can be found willing to provide it

Facts: disagreeing with K's responsible medical officer, the MHRT ordered that K (a restricted patient) be discharged conditionally, to live at home

49 For the process and criteria, see *R (SC) v Mental Health Review Tribunal* [2005] EWHC 17 (Admin), (2005) MHLR 31.

under psychiatric supervision. No doctor could be found in K's home area, willing to supervise her. Wider enquiries proved fruitless. On the invitation of K's RMO, the Secretary of State referred her case back to the MHRT. K sought a judicial review, submitted that the health authority's failure to arrange psychiatric supervision was in breach of section 117 of the MHA 1983.

Judgment: the Court of Appeal (Lord Phillips MR, Buxton and Sedley LJJ) held that the health authority had not acted unlawfully. It had acted with reasonable diligence to make appropriate arrangements, but did not have the power to compel consultants to act in a manner that consultants were unable to reconcile with the exercise of their professional judgment:

> 20. The relevant provisions of section 117(2) are set out at paragraph 19 of Burton J's judgment. On their face they require the Health Authority to provide after care services for persons who cease to be detained and leave hospital. Decisions at first instance, to which I am about to refer, have held that the duty of a Health Authority extends to making arrangements for the care of a patient before that patient is discharged. Before Burton J, the respondent Authority reserved its position as to whether these decisions were correct. Before us it has made the following limited concessions:
>
> (a) A Health Authority has power to take preparatory steps before discharge of a patient;
>
> (b) It will normally be the case that, in the exercise of this discretionary power, an authority should give way to a tribunal decision, and should use reasonable endeavours to fulfill the conditions imposed by such a decision, insofar as they relate to medical care;
>
> (c) Failure to use such endeavours, in the absence of strong reasons, would be likely to be an unlawful exercise of discretion.
>
> ...
>
> 29. In my judgment section 117 imposes on Health Authorities a duty to provide after care facilities for the benefit of patients who are discharged from mental hospitals. The nature and extent of those facilities must, to a degree, fall within the discretion of the Health Authority which must have regard to other demands on its budget. In relation to the duty to satisfy conditions imposed by a tribunal, I would endorse the concession made by the respondent Authority as to the extent of its duty.

There was, moreover, no breach of Article 5 ECHR, given that K still suffered from a mental disorder for which treatment was necessary, in hospital if community services were not available.

19.95 *R (C) v Mental Health Review Tribunal London South and South West Region* (2001) 4 CCLR 284, CA

It was incompatible with Article 5(4) ECHR routinely to list discharge hearings under section 72 of the MHA 1983 eight weeks after the application

Facts: Mr C, who had been detained under section 3 of the MHA 1983, after his wife had been displaced as his nearest relative, complained of delay in securing a hearing before the Mental Health Review Tribunal for the hearing of his application to be discharged: it took eight weeks.

Judgment: the Court of Appeal (Lord Phillips MR, Lord Mustill, Jonathan Parker LJ) allowed Mr C's appeal and held that the tribunal had a practice of fixing hearing dates eight weeks after the date of the application and that this was a matter of administrative convenience rather than necessity, in that some cases the requisite evidence could be available, and the case heard, much sooner. That inevitably meant that some applications did not get the speedy hearing required by Article 5(4) ECHR, so the eight-week practice was unlawful.

19.96 *R (H) v Ashworth Hospital Authority* [2002] EWCA Civ 923, (2002) 5 CCLR 390

It had been irrational for the tribunal to direct discharge without ensuring that adequate after-care arrangements would be in place and it had been unlawful not to give reasons why some evidence was preferred to other evidence; however, the authorities should have applied for judicial review and a stay; their further application for H's detention was unlawful given that it was for the same reasons that the tribunal had rejected

Facts: the MHRT directed H's discharge, although no after-care arrangements were in place. A few days later H was re-detained. The hospital applied for a judicial review of the MHRT's decision. H applied for a judicial review of the hospital's and social worker's decision to re-detain him.

Judgment: the Court of Appeal (Simon Brown, Mummery and Dyson LJJ) held that the MHRT decision had indeed been *Wednesbury* irrational and, also, that it was unlawful because of the MHRT's failure to record adequate reasons for explaining why it preferred some rather than other evidence. However, it also been unlawful to re-detain H in circumstances where, on analysis, the reasons for that were the same as those considered and rejected by the MHRT. In such a case, the appropriate course was to apply for a judicial review of the MHRT's decision. In an appropriate (strong) case, the Administrative Court could grant a stay of an order discharging the patient, including (Simon Brown dissenting on this point) after the patient had left the hospital:

> 48. To summarise, I consider that there is jurisdiction to grant a stay even after the decision of the tribunal has been fully implemented. But the jurisdiction should be exercised sparingly, and where it is exercised, the court should decide the judicial review application, if at all possible, within days of the order of stay.
>
> ...
>
> 59. It seems to me that, when considering whether to resection a patient who has only very recently been discharged by a tribunal, the question that the professionals must ask themselves is whether the sole or principal ground on which they rely is one which in substance has been rejected by the Tribunal. If it is, then in my view, they should not resection. In deciding whether the grounds on which they rely are ones which have been very recently rejected by the tribunal, they should not be too zealous in seeking to find new circumstances. As in the present case, the tribunal will have made an assessment of the degree of the patient's insight into his mental problems, his willingness to comply with the treatment regime in the community, his willingness to engage with doctors, nurses, social workers and so on. If experience of what happens when he is released shows that the tribunal seriously misjudged the patient, then that might well be sufficient evidence of new circumstances: a straightforward application of the 'proof

of the pudding' principle. But if the professionals form the view that the tribunal's assessment was wrong not on the basis of what happens upon release, but simply on the basis of their assessment at interview before the patient has actually left the hospital, then it may well be difficult for them reasonably to justify a resection on the basis of circumstances of which the tribunal was unaware.

60. Nothing that I have said affects the ability of the professionals to resection a patient if he does or threatens to do something which imperils or might imperil his health or safety, or that of members of the public.

...

80. Against the background of these two general comments, I shall now identify the two principal reasons why I consider that the Tribunal's reasons were inadequate in this case. First, as often happens, the Tribunal was required to resolve a difference of opinion between experts as to whether the patient should be discharged. In such cases, it is important that the tribunal should state which expert evidence (if any) it accepts and which it rejects, giving reasons. This is as important in a case where the tribunal rejects evidence in favour of discharge as it is in a case where the tribunal rejects evidence which advocates continued detention. It is not enough for the tribunal simply to state that they prefer the evidence of A and B to that of C and D. They must give reasons. As the Handbook states, these may be brief, but in some cases something more elaborate is required. They must at least indicate the reasoning process by which they have decided to accept some and reject other evidence. What this court said in *Flannery v Halifax Estate Agencies Limited* [2000] 1 WLR 377, 381G–382D is as apt in relation to the decisions of tribunals as it is to lower courts generally. ...

82. My second reason is that I do not accept Mr Walker's submission that the Tribunal were not required to give any reasons for not adjourning in order to see whether suitable after-care arrangements, or not making an order for discharge at a deferred date. As I explained at paragraph 67, the question of what after-care services will be available in the community is relevant to the issue of whether the statutory criteria are met. That was certainly the case here. Mr Walker does not suggest otherwise. In my view, the judge was right to say that the Tribunal took a step in the dark. And yet, they gave no reasons for doing so. Ms Ariola's report was sufficient to put them on notice that the local authority might be unable or unwilling to provide after-care services to H. In my view, the judge was right to hold that the reasons given by the Tribunal were inadequate.

19.97 ### *R (KB and others) v Mental Health Review Tribunal and the Secretary of State for Health* [2002] EWHC 639 (Admin), (2002) 5 CCLR 458

Endemic delays in hearing applications to be discharged from detention, caused by a chronic shortage of administrative resources, were incompatible with Article 5(4) ECHR

Facts: the claimants were detained mental patients who had experienced delays in securing a hearing in the MHRT of their applications for discharge.

Judgment: Stanley Burnton J held that this was a long-standing problem, caused by inadequate administrative support and a shortage of resources; and there was no justification for the delays; accordingly, the claimants' right to a speedy hearing under Article 5(4) ECHR had been breached and damages would be awarded (at a further hearing):

> 45. Normally, the question whether the Government allocates sufficient resources to any particular area of state activity is not justiciable. A decision as to what resources are to be made available often involves questions of policy, and certainly involves questions of discretion. These are matters for policy makers rather than judges: for the executive rather than the judiciary: cf *X (Minors) v Bedfordshire County Council* [1995] 2 AC 633 and *R v Cambridge Health Authority ex p B* [1995] 1 WLR 898, 906D-F; see too the speech of Lord Slynn of Hadley in *R v Chief Constable of Sussex ex p International Trader's Ferry Ltd* [1999] 2 AC 418 at 439A-B, and the judgment of Moses J in *Hooper v Secretary of State for Work and Pensions* [2002] EWHC 191 (Admin) at paragraph 100. However, as has been seen, when issues are raised under Articles 5 and 6 as to the guarantee of a speedy hearing or of a hearing within a reasonable time, the Court may be required to assess the adequacy of resources, as well as the effectiveness of administration; and it is common ground that the Court must do so in the present cases.
>
> 46. It is at this point that I must mention an important qualification. In general a court is ill-equipped to determine general questions as to the efficiency of administration, the sufficiency of staff levels and the adequacy of resources. It is one thing to instruct a team of management consultants to go out into the field to study and to report on the efficiency and adequacy of the Tribunal system and its practices; it is another to expect a judge, in the confines of a two-day hearing, to reach sensible and reliable conclusions as to whether, for example, the practice of allocating hearing dates before it is known whether a panel will be available is an aid or a hindrance to speedy hearings. Not only is the time available to the court limited: so is the evidence; and such expertise as the judge may have is, notwithstanding the title to this Division of the High Court, legal, rather than administrative.
>
> 47. In my judgment, the correct approach in a case that raises issues of this kind is, first, to consider whether the delays in question are, on the face of it, inconsistent with the requirement of a speedy hearing. If they are, the onus is on the State to excuse the delay. It may do so by establishing, for example, that the delay has been caused by a sudden and unpredictable increase in the workload of the tribunal, and that it has taken effective and sufficient measures to remedy the problem. But if the State fails to satisfy that onus, the claimant will have established a breach of his right under Article 5(4).

19.98 *R (KB and others) v Mental Health Review Tribunal* [2003] EWHC 193 (Admin), (2003) 6 CCLR 96

Damages were awarded for delayed discharge hearings, in breach of Article 5(4) ECHR (i) where the patient would probably have been discharged at an earlier hearing and/or (ii) for distress caused by the delay

Facts: the claimants were detained mental patients. The court had earlier held that delays in determining their applications for discharge had been incompatible with Article 5 ECHR.[50] It now assessed their claims for damages.

50 *R (KB and others) v Mental Health Review Tribunal* [2002] EWHC 639 (Admin), (2002) 5 CCLR 458.

Judgment: Stanley Burnton J held that it would be contrary to the case-law of the ECtHR to award damages for the loss of a chance of a favourable decision: it was necessary for a claimant to prove that, on the balance of probabilities, they would have been discharged (notwithstanding the opposition of the hospitals and the generally low success rate in such cases). Nonetheless, damages could be awarded for distress caused by the delay:

> 73. Thus, even in the case of mentally ill claimants, not every feeling of frustration and distress will justify an award of damages. The frustration and distress must be significant: 'of such intensity that it would in itself justify an award of compensation for non-pecuniary damage'. In my judgment, an important touchstone of that intensity in cases such as the present will be that the hospital staff considered it to be sufficiently relevant to the mental state of the patient to warrant its mention in the clinical notes.

19.99 *R v East London and the City Mental Health NHS Trust ex p von Brandenburg* [2003] UKHL 58, (2004) 7 CCLR 121

It is unlawful to re-detain a patient simply because of a disagreement with the tribunal's direction to discharge the patient but it is lawful to do so where the AMHP forms the bona fide and rational opinion that there is new material that puts a different complexion on the case

Facts: on the 31 March the MHRT ordered that Mr von Brandenburg should be discharged on the 7 April (to allow time for after-care arrangements), but on the 6 April the approved social worker (ASW) applied for Mr von Brandenburg to be compulsorily admitted, relying on a report from the same RMO who had opposed discharge earlier, before the MHRT. Mr von Brandenburg sought a judicial review, submitting that his further admission was unlawful in that the circumstances had not changed.

Judgment: the House of Lords (Lords Bingham, Steyn, Hobhouse, Scott and Rodger) held that it would not be lawful to make a further application for re-admission simply because of a disagreement with the view of the MHRT, but it was lawful to do so where the ASW forms the bona fide and reasonable opinion that there is new material, not known to the MHRT, that puts a different complexion on the case. The ASW was not under a duty to inquire as to whether there had been an earlier MHRT although he was under a general duty of enquiry into the patient's background, which might reveal that information. The ASW was under a limited duty to explain why a further application was being made, in the face of the MHRT's decision to discharge.

19.100 *R (H) v Secretary of State for the Home Department* [2003] UKHL 59, (2004) 7 CCLR 147

Tribunals must keep deferred conditional discharges under review so as to comply with Article 5(4) ECHR but a patient remained lawfully detained where the patient suffered from a mental disorder that warranted compulsory treatment in hospital unless community services were available and it had not been possible to arrange for those services despite using reasonable endeavours

Facts: H had been made the subject of a hospital order in 1995 with restriction. In 1999, the MHRT concluded that he was not suffering from mental illness but should remain liable to be recalled to hospital. It adjourned the hearing for the hospital to draw up a care plan but that did not occur because the hospital could not locate a psychiatrist willing to supervise IH in the community. In February 2000 the MHRT re-convened and reached the same conclusion but still the hospital could not find a psychiatrist willing to supervise IH in the community. In March 2002 the MHRT re-convened and decided that IH had suffered from a mental illness throughout. H sought a judicial review and damages for unlawful detention between February 2000 and March 2002.

Judgment: the House of Lords (Lords Bingham, Steyn, Hobhouse, Scott and Rodger) held that H had been left in limbo for too long, so that his rights under Article 5(4) ECHR had been breached: tribunals must keep under view deferred conditional discharges. However, at no time had IH been unlawfully detained. At all times, IH had suffered from a mental disorder that required hospital treatment under detention, unless community supervision and treatment was available. As to that, the after-care authorities were not under an absolute duty to make provision but a duty to use reasonable endeavours, which they had discharged. Lord Bingham said this:

> *Conclusions*
>
> 25. This regrettably lengthy prologue enables me, I hope fairly, to review Mr Owen's main submissions summarised in para 7 above more briefly than would otherwise have been possible.
>
> 26. I do not accept that, because the tribunal lacked the power to secure compliance with its conditions, it lacked the coercive power which is one of the essential attributes of a court. What Article 5(1)(e) and (4) require is that a person of unsound mind compulsorily detained in hospital should have access to a court with power to decide whether the detention is lawful and, if not, to order his release. This power the tribunal had. Nothing in Article 5 suggests that discharge subject to conditions is impermissible in principle, and nothing in the Convention jurisprudence suggests that the power to discharge conditionally (whether there are specific conditions or a mere liability to recall), properly used, should be viewed with disfavour. Indeed, the conditional discharge regime, properly used, is of great benefit to patients and the public, and conducive to the Convention object of restricting the curtailment of personal liberty to the maximum, because it enables tribunals to ensure that restricted patients compulsorily detained in hospital represent the hard core of those who suffer from mental illness, are a risk to themselves or others and cannot be effectively treated and supervised otherwise than in hospital. If there is any possibility of treating and supervising a patient in the community, the imposition of conditions permits that possibility to be explored and, it may be, tried.
>
> 27. When, following the tribunal's order of 3 February 2000, it proved impossible to secure compliance with the conditions within a matter of a few months, a violation of the appellant's article 5(4) right did occur. It occurred because the tribunal, having made its order, was precluded by the authority of the Oxford case from reconsidering it. The result was to leave the appellant in limbo for a much longer period than was acceptable or compatible with the Convention. I would accordingly endorse the Court of Appeal's decision to set aside the Oxford ruling and I would adopt the ruling it gave in para 71 of its judgment quoted above. Evidence before

the House shows that that ruling is already yielding significant practical benefits. Mr Owen was, I think, right to submit that the tribunal could have achieved the same result, consistently with the Oxford case, by a judicious use of its power to adjourn and by proleptic indication of the conditions it had in mind to impose, but it is undesirable to restrict the procedural freedom of tribunals in a field as important and sensitive as this, where personal liberty and safety and public protection are all at stake: the outcome should not turn on procedural niceties.

28. There was no time between 3 February 2000 and 25 March 2002 when the appellant was, in my opinion, unlawfully detained, and there was thus no breach of Article 5(1)(e). There is a categorical difference, not a difference of degree, between this case and that of *Johnson*. Mr Johnson was a patient in whose case the Winterwerp criteria were found not to be satisfied from June 1989 onwards. While, therefore, it was reasonable to try and ease the patient's reintegration into the community by the imposition of conditions, the alternative, if those conditions proved impossible to meet, was not continued detention but discharge, either absolutely or subject only to a condition of liability to recall. His detention became unlawful shortly after June 1989 because there were, as all the doctors agreed, no grounds for continuing to detain him. The present case is quite different. There was never a medical consensus, nor did the tribunal find, that the Winterwerp criteria were not satisfied. The tribunal considered that the appellant could be satisfactorily treated and supervised in the community if its conditions were met, as it expected, but the alternative, if these conditions proved impossible to meet, was not discharge, either absolutely or subject only to a condition of recall, but continued detention. The appellant was never detained when there were no grounds for detaining him. To the extent that Buxton and Sedley LJJ differed from the Master of the Rolls on this point in K, the opinion of the latter is to be preferred.

29. The duty of the health authority, whether under section 117 of the 1983 Act or in response to the tribunal's order of 3 February 2000, was to use its best endeavours to procure compliance with the conditions laid down by the tribunal. This it did. It was not subject to an absolute obligation to procure compliance and was not at fault in failing to do so. It had no power to require any psychiatrist to act in a way which conflicted with the conscientious professional judgment of that psychiatrist. Thus the appellant can base no claim on the fact that the tribunal's conditions were not met. This conclusion makes it unnecessary, in my opinion, to address a question on which the House heard argument, but which was not considered below, whether in a context such as this psychiatrists were or could be a hybrid public authority. Determination of that question is best left to a case in which it is necessary to the decision. We are nonetheless grateful to the Royal College of Psychiatrists for its submissions on this point.

30. I do not consider that the violation of Article 5(4) which I have found calls for an award of compensation since (a) the violation has been publicly acknowledged and the appellant's right thereby vindicated, (b) the law has been amended in a way which should prevent similar violations in future, and (c) the appellant has not been the victim of unlawful detention, which Article 5 is intended to avoid.

19.101 *R (H) v Secretary of State for Health* [2005] UKHL 60, [2006] 1 AC 441

The machinery for detaining persons under section 2 of the MHA 1983 during displacement proceeds was ECHR compliant

Facts: H had been detained under section 2 of the MHA 1983 and an application was made to displace her mother, who objected to H being received into guardianship, as H's nearest relative. The displacement proceedings dragged on and as a result H was detained under section 2 well beyond the usual 28 days. The Court of Appeal held that sections 2 and 29(4) of the MHA 1983 were incompatible with Article 5(4) ECHR insofar as they made no provision for a patient's detention to be reviewed in circumstances where the patient was incapable of exercising the right of review and their detention was extended because of nearest relative displacement proceedings.

Judgment: the House of Lords (Lords Bingham Hope, Rodger, Lady Hale and Lord Brown) allowed the Secretary of State's appeal, on the basis that the scheme could be operated consistently with Article 5(4), in particular by the Secretary of State exercising his power to refer cases to the MHRT.

Comment: H's complaint to the European Court of Human Rights was upheld to a limited extent, in *MH v United Kingdom* (below para 19.102).

19.102 *MH v United Kingdom* Application no 11577/06, (2014) 58 EHRR 35

Special safeguards were required to ensure that patients who lacked capacity were able to apply for discharge from detention under section 2 of the MHA 1983 within the initial period of detention of 28 days; if detention under section 2 is then extended because of proceedings to displace a nearest relative, Article 5(4) ECHR may be satisfied by the Secretary of State referring the case to the tribunal

Facts: H had been detained under section 2 of the MHA 1983 and an application was made to displace her mother, who objected to H being received into guardianship, as H's nearest relative. The displacement proceedings dragged on and as a result H was detained under section 2 well beyond the usual 28 days. The Court of Appeal held that sections 2 and 29(4) of the MHA 1983 were incompatible with Article 5(4) ECHR insofar as they made no provision for a patient's detention to be reviewed in circumstances where the patient was incapable of exercising the right of review and their detention was extended because of nearest relative displacement proceedings.

Judgment: the European Court of Human Rights held that H's detention had been unlawful during its initial period in that, although had been entitled in principle to apply to the MHRT for discharge, she had lacked the capacity to do so and no special safeguards had been made available to ensure that this right was made practical and effective in such cases. However, after H's detention had been automatically extended, the Secretary of State had secured a MHRT hearing within a month, which was not unreasonable: the exercise by the Secretary of State of the power of referring cases to the MHRT was capable of removing any potential incompatibility with the ECHR, in the legislation.

Comment: The government has responded by amending MHA 1983 to introduce independent mental health advocates (at sections 130A–130L) and making further provision in the *Mental Health Act 1983: Code of Practice.*

19.103 *Kolanis v United Kingdom* Application no 517/02, (2006) 9 CCLR 297

It was lawful to continue to detain a patient who suffered from a mental disorder warranting treatment in hospital and detention even though the patient could be discharged if services were available in the community if such services were not available; however, there would be a breach of Article 5(4) ECHR unless there continued to be regular court review

Facts: K, a restricted patient, was directed to be discharged conditionally, inter alia, on psychiatric supervision in the community, but the tribunal deferred the discharge. K's RMO was unable to find a doctor in the community prepared to supervise her and K's judicial review of that failure was dismissed. K remained in detention though meanwhile her case was referred back to the MHRT.

Judgment: the European Court of Human Rights held that K's detention continued to be lawful under Article 5(1) ECHR (as the MHRT had adjudged her discharge to be appropriate only if appropriate provision could be made in the community), but that the delay of over a year in referring her case back to the MHRT had been incompatible with Article 5(4)(in that new issues relating to the lawfulness of K's detention had arisen on account of the failure to make community provision for her) and K was entitled to compensation, assessed at £6,000.00, for the loss of her opportunity to be released and frustration.

19.104 *R (SH) v Mental Health Review Tribunal* [2007] EWHC 884 (Admin), (2007) 10 CCLR 306

Discharge on condition that the patient took specified medication did not amount to compulsory treatment, merely a condition which, if broken, would justify recall

Facts: SH was detained under a hospital order, with a restriction. He was granted a conditional discharge, on condition that he comply with prescribed medication. SH sought judicial review of that condition.

Judgment: Holman J held that the condition was lawful. It was not irrational or unlawful. It did not remove SH's absolute right to refuse medical treatment on each occasion he attended for his fortnightly medication. (If he did refuse, then the Secretary of State would consider his power of recall). Holman J said this:

> 17. The general effect of section 73 is, accordingly, that the tribunal must direct the absolute discharge of a patient if they (a) are not satisfied, in paraphrase, that he is still ill and his detention for assessment or treatment is warranted or justified; and (b) are satisfied that it is not appropriate for him to remain liable to be recalled. But, if only the first but not the second limb

applies, then the tribunal must direct conditional discharge. The critical difference between absolute and conditional discharge is that if the patient is only conditionally discharged, he may be recalled by the Secretary of State. The tribunal themselves do not necessarily have to impose any actual condition (see words '(if any)' in subsection(4)b)) but may do so. The Secretary of State has a wide power himself to impose conditions at any subsequent time, and from time to time vary any condition whether imposed by the tribunal or by himself.

18. The references to conditions are entirely general and open ended and there are no express words in sections 73, 75 or elsewhere limiting the scope or effect of any condition which may be attached. Clearly, however, the law imports or requires some limitations. A condition could not lawfully be capricious and must be relevant and for a proper purpose within the scope of the statute. It is not suggested that condition 1 is not relevant and for a proper purpose.

19. Mr Hugh Southey, on behalf of the claimant, submits that section 73(4)(b) is subject also to the principle of legality as described by Lord Hoffmann in *R v Secretary of State for the Home Department ex p Simms* [2004] 2 AC 115 at 131E to G, where he said:

> '... the principle of legality means that Parliament must squarely confront what it is doing and accept the political cost. Fundamental rights cannot be overridden by general or ambiguous words. This is because there is too great a risk that the full implications of their unqualified meaning may have passed unnoticed in the democratic process. In the absence of express language or necessary implication to the contrary, the courts therefore presume that even the most general words were intended to be subject to the basic rights of the individual. In this way the courts of the United Kingdom, though acknowledging the sovereignty of Parliament, apply principles of constitutionality little different from those which exist in countries where the power of the legislature is expressly limited by a constitutional document.'

20. I fully accept that that principle applies to this case and operates as a limitation to the scope of a condition which may lawfully be imposed. The question in issue, however, is whether condition 1, properly understood and applied, does override any fundamental right of SH.

19.105 *Rayner and Marsh v Secretary of State for the Home Department* [2007] EWHC 1028 (Admin), (2007) 10 CCLR 464

Recalled conditionally discharged patients were entitled to an immediate referral of their case to the tribunal

Facts: the claimants were conditionally discharged patients recalled to hospital by the Secretary of State and they complained about delays in having their cases reviewed by the MHRT.

Judgment: Holman J held that the system was compatible with Article 5 ECHR in that section 75 of the MHA 1983 required an immediate referral (unless the circumstances positively required otherwise). In cases where there had been unjustified delay, that would be unlawful and damages could be awarded.

19.106 *R (TF) v Secretary of State for Justice* [2008] EWCA Civ 1457, (2009) 12 CCLR 245

The absence of adequate reasons in medical recommendations meant that the detention had been unlawful and the fact that, later, other doctors were found who did provide adequate reasons justifying detention did not make the earlier detention lawful

Facts: TF had served a custodial sentence for robbery but on the day of his release was served with a hospital transfer order purporting to be made under section 47 of the MHA 1983. TF sought a judicial review. At first instance, Cox J held that the transfer order had been unlawful, in that neither of the doctors' recommendations gave reasons in support of their view that hospital treatment would alleviate mental illness or prevent deterioration. However, in the light of subsequent medical evidence garnered by the Secretary of State, she declined in the exercise of her discretion to quash the transfer order, order TF's release and require the Secretary of State to pay damages. TF appealed.

Judgment: the Court of Appeal (Waller, Thomas and Aikens LJJ), having reviewed the position and confirmed that the transfer order was unlawful, allowed TF's appeal: the Secretary of State had not had the power to make a transfer order, so the detention was unlawful, and the Court could not make it lawful by exercising a discretion.

19.107 *Secretary of State for Justice v RB* [2011] EWCA Civ 1608, [2012] 1 WLR 2043, [2012] MHLR 131

It is not lawful to discharge a patient to a facility which is not a hospital and where he or she will be detained otherwise than for the purposes of treatment

Facts: the Upper Tribunal directed RB's discharge on condition that he lived in a care home in circumstances that amounted to a deprivation of liberty.

Judgment: the Court of Appeal (Maurice Kay, Moses and Arden LJJ) held that neither the MHA 1983 not the ECHR permitted conditional discharge to an institution other than a hospital, where the patient would be detained otherwise for the purposes of treatment and without appropriate medical treatment being available for the patient. Maurice Kay LJ said:

> *The 'prescribed by law' issue*
>
> 52. This is the most difficult issue. No person could fail to have sympathy with the decision of the Upper Tribunal in the circumstances of this case. The proposed conditional discharge would no doubt be more beneficial to RB than his continued detention in hospital. There is also the point made by Bean J in *IT v Secretary of State for the Home Department* [2008] MHLR 290 about this being a 'curious area of human rights jurisprudence': see para 33 above. The Secretary of State is in the unusual position of seeking to argue against a conditional discharge on the terms sought on the basis of human rights jurisprudence when (a) those terms would produce a more humane result and (b) RB is content with those terms.
>
> 53. At the end of the day, however, I accept the submission of Mr Chamberlain that the original order made against RB authorised, and authorised only, detention in a hospital: see section 37 and section 41(3)(a) of the 1983 Act

set out above. That conclusion seems to me to be the starting point. The consequence of that conclusion is that Mr Burrows is driven to rely for the authority to deprive RB of his liberty on the wording of section 73(2), which is wholly silent on that important point. The right to liberty of the person is a fundamental right. It has been so regarded since at least the time of the well-known provisions of clause 39 of Magna Carta, which in due course found its reflection in article 9 of the Universal Declaration of Human Rights and article 5 of the Convention. A person cannot have his right to liberty taken away unless that is the clear effect of a statute: see per Lord Hoffmann in *R v Secretary of State for the Home Department ex p Simms* [2000] 2 AC 115, 131:

> 'Fundamental rights cannot be overridden by general or ambiguous words. This is because there is too great a risk that the full implications of their unqualified meaning may have passed unnoticed in the democratic process. In the absence of express language or necessary implication to the contrary, the courts therefore presume that even the most general words were intended to be subject to the basic rights of the individual. In this way the courts of the United Kingdom, though acknowledging the sovereignty of Parliament, apply principles of constitutionality little different from those which exist in countries where the power of the legislature is expressly limited by a constitutional document.'

54. It is not enough that the patient is given a right to apply to the court under section 73 if he does not know the legal basis on which he could lawfully be subjected to an order for conditional discharge to an institution other than a hospital on terms that he continued to be deprived of his liberty: see *HL v United Kingdom* 40 EHRR 761 quoted in para 11 above. In this case, section 73(2) would not assist him because the only operative provision would be paragraph (b) of that subsection. The effect of this provision would be, for instance, that a patient who did not need to be detained in hospital for the purposes of any treatment, could be conditionally discharged on terms that involved a deprivation of liberty simply on the basis that the tribunal was not satisfied that it was not appropriate that he should not be liable to be recalled to hospital for further treatment. That provision simply does not address the reasons why in any particular case there is a need for him also to be deprived of his liberty.

55. The aim of the Strasbourg jurisprudence is, of course, to protect the individual against arbitrary action by the state. But that statement demonstrates important limitations on the jurisprudence. There is no Convention right to a particular type of treatment or care in detention. I would, therefore, dispute the conclusion of Bean J on that basis. If his comment (see para 33 above) were carried to its logical conclusion, Strasbourg jurisprudence would require the United Kingdom to provide a particular form of care for a person in RB's decision. The thrust of that jurisprudence is, however, the provision of certain procedural guarantees as a bulwark against arbitrary detention by the state.

56. As I have already pointed out, in fact the relevant jurisprudence of the Strasbourg court on this point is moulded by the doctrine of subsidiarity. It has been left to the United Kingdom Parliament to decide what is the right place for a person in the position of RB to be detained. That means that, if there is dissatisfaction with the statutory scheme, that is a matter to be taken up in Parliament unless RB can succeed under the next issue. Although a conclusion adverse to that of the Upper Tribunal is less liberal towards the individual, that result (again, unless RB succeeds under the

next issue) is in law simply a function of human rights protection based on a international human rights instrument which adopts a principle of subsidiarity.

57. The points made by Mr Chamberlain underline this point because they show that Parliament could not have intended to create, as he puts it, a new species of detention that is potentially more detrimental to personal liberty than detention under the 1983 Act. This is because the 1983 Act does not specify the circumstances in which a tribunal can order a conditional discharge on terms that there is a deprivation of liberty. Moreover, section 73 appears, on its face, to be wide enough, on the Upper Tribunal's interpretation, to authorise detention for the purposes of containment rather than treatment, which is contrary to the policy of the 1983 Act: see para 24 above.

19.108 *DC v Nottinghamshire Healthcare NHS Trust* [2012] UKUT 92 (AAC), (2012) 15 CCLR 537

The tribunal was entitled to adjourn proceedings for evidence to be adduced as to what conditions might be appropriate to attach to a conditional discharge

Facts: DC was a restricted patient, who appealed the decision of the First-tier Tribunal not to order his deferred conditional discharge, but to adjourn for further evidence to decide the appropriate conditions.

Judgment: Upper Tribunal Judge Jacobs held that before a deferred conditional discharge was made, conditions for the discharge had to be identified and included in the direction; the purpose of deferral was to allow time for the specified arrangements to be made. Accordingly the First-tier Tribunal had acted appropriately.

19.109 *R (South Staffordshire & Shropshire Healthcare NHS Foundation Trust) v St George's Hospital Managers* [2016] EWHC 1196 (Admin), (2016) 19 CCLR 253

The decision of an independent panel exercising the function of hospital discharge was amenable to judicial review but such panels are not required to take into account decisions about discharge by the First-tier Tribunal

Facts: X was in his 60s and had long-standing mental health problems. He had been detained under section 3 of the MHA 1983. The First-tier Tribunal decided not to discharge him. Then, the independent panel appointed by the NHS Foundation Trust to exercise its powers under section 23 of the MHA 1983 decided to discharge him. The NHS Foundation Trust sought a judicial review of that decision.

Judgment: Cranston J held that the independent panel was sufficiently separate from the NHS Foundation Trust to be amenable to judicial review at the suit of the Trust but that its decision had been lawful – the First-tier Tribunal's decision had simply not been, under the relevant statutory machinery, a relevant consideration that the independent panel had been required to consider, let alone follow, and its decision had been rational on the evidence before it.

After-care services

Introduction

19.110 Persons who cease to be detained under certain provisions of the MHA 1983 (sections 3, 37, 45A, 47 and 48) are entitled to after-care services from the relevant CCG (or, in Wales, Local Health Board) and local authority, until both organisations are satisfied that the person is no longer in need of such services.

After-care services comprise any service within reason necessary to meet a need arising from a person's continued mental disorder including (most commonly) medication, counselling and accommodation plus care and social support.[51] The statutory definition is as follows:

117(6) In this section, 'after-care services', in relation to a person, means services which have both of the following purposes–
(a) meeting a need arising from or related to the person's mental disorder; and
(b) reducing the risk of a deterioration of the person's mental condition (and, accordingly, reducing the risk of the person requiring admission to a hospital again for treatment for mental disorder).

19.111 In addition:

- the duty to provide services arises on the actual discharge of the patient but, while there is no duty to monitor the patient's progress, the authorities have a power to take preparatory steps before discharge and are under a duty to use reasonable endeavours to fulfil the conditions imposed by a conditional discharge or similar;[52]
- the duty to provide after-care services applies to patients with leave of absence from hospital;
- there is a duty to provide social care but a duty only to use reasonable endeavours to provide professional medical services because medical professionals remain entitled to decline to provide a service they consider to be clinically inappropriate;[53]
- no charge can be made for services under section 117(3),[54] although the preferred accommodation and top up provisions now apply to accommodation provided under section 117(3) (see 'Preferred accomodation', paras 9.45–9.52 above);
- under section 117(3) of the MHA 1983, the clinical commissioning group/local authority responsible for providing after-care services is the one for the area where the patient was ordinarily resident before his or her detention or, if the patient had no settled residence, where

51 *R (Mwanza) v Greenwich LBC* [2010] EWHC 1462 (Admin), (2010) 13 CCLR 454 at paras 61–67; *R (Afework) v Camden LBC* [2013] EWHC 1637 (Admin) at para 19.

52 *R v Camden and Islington Health Authority ex p K* [2001] EWCA Civ 240, [2002] QB 198, (2001) 4 CCLR 170; *W v Doncaster MBC* [2004] EWCA Civ 378, [2004] MHLR 201; *R (B) v Camden LBC* [2005] EWHC 1366 (Admin), (2005) 8 CCLR 422.

53 *R (H) v Secretary of State for the Home Department* [2003] UKHL 59, [2004] 2 AC 253, (2004) 7 CCLR 147.

54 *R v Manchester CC ex p Stennett* [2002] UKHL 34, [2002] 2 AC 1127, (2002) 5 CCLR 500.

the patient was present before his or her detention, or (if that cannot be established) the area where he or she is sent on discharge;

- after-care services will usually be delivered under the Care Programme Approach, which requires joint, multi-disciplinary working between social and health care professionals. See the following:
  - *Refocusing the Care Programme Approach: Policy and Positive Practice Guidance* (DoH, March 2008);[55]
  - in Wales, *Delivering the Care Programme Approach in Wales: Interim Policy Implementation Guidance* (July 2010);[56]
  - the national strategy and standards documents, *No health without mental health: a cross-government mental health outcomes strategy for people of all ages* (2 February 2011);[57]
  - *No health without mental health: implementation framework* (24 July 2012);[58] and
  - in Wales, *Together for Mental Health: a strategy for mental health and wellbeing in Wales.*[59]

19.112 Section 117, as amended by the Care Act 2014, now reads as follows:

After-care

117(1) This section applies to persons who are detained under section 3 above, or admitted to a hospital in pursuance of a hospital order made under section 37 above, or transferred to a hospital in pursuance of a hospital direction made under section 45A above or a transfer direction made under section 47 or 48 above, and then cease to be detained and (whether or not immediately after so ceasing) leave hospital.

(2) It shall be the duty of the clinical commissioning group or Local Health Board and of the local social services authority to provide or arrange for the provision of, in co-operation with relevant voluntary agencies, after-care services for any person to whom this section applies until such time as the clinical commissioning group or Local Health Board and the local social services authority are satisfied that the person concerned is no longer in need of such services ; but they shall not be so satisfied in the case of a community patient while he remains such a patient.

(2A) [...]

(2B) Section 32 above shall apply for the purposes of this section as it applies for the purposes of Part II of this Act.

(2C) References in this Act to after-care services provided for a patient under this section include references to services provided for the patient–

(a) in respect of which direct payments are made under

(i) sections 31 to 33 of the Care Act 2014 (as applied by Schedule 4 to that Act),

(ii) ...

55 http://webarchive.nationalarchives.gov.uk/20130107105354/http:/www.dh.gov.uk/prod_consum_dh/groups/dh_digitalassets/@dh/@en/documents/digitalasset/dh_083649.pdf.

56 http://gov.wales/topics/health/publications/health/guidance/cpa/?lang=en.

57 www.mhpf.org.uk/sites/default/files/documents/publications/dh_124058.pdf.

58 www.gov.uk/government/uploads/system/uploads/attachment_data/file/216870/No-Health-Without-Mental-Health-Implementation-Framework-Report-accessible-version.pdf.

59 http://gov.wales/topics/health/nhswales/mental-health-services/strategy/?lang=en.

(iii) regulations under section 12A(4) of the National Health Service Act 2006,

(b) which would be provided under this section apart from those sections (as so applied) or the regulations.

(2D) Subsection (2), in its application to the clinical commissioning group, has effect as if the words 'provide or' were omitted.

(2E) The Secretary of State may by regulations provide that the duty imposed on the clinical commissioning group by subsection (2) is, in the circumstances or to the extent prescribed by the regulations, to be imposed instead on another clinical commissioning group or the National Health Service Commissioning Board.

(2F) Where regulations under subsection (2E) provide that the duty imposed by subsection (2) is to be imposed on the National Health Service Commissioning Board, subsection (2D) has effect as if the reference to the clinical commissioning group were a reference to the National Health Service Commissioning Board.

(2G) Section 272(7) and (8) of the National Health Service Act 2006 applies to the power to make regulations under subsection (2E) as it applies to a power to make regulations under that Act.

(3) In this section 'the clinical commissioning group or Local Health Board' means the clinical commissioning group or Local Health Board, and 'the local social services authority' means the local social services authority

(a) if, immediately before being detained, the person concerned was ordinarily resident in England, for the area in England in which he was ordinarily resident;

(b) if, immediately before being detained, the person concerned was ordinarily resident in Wales, for the area in Wales in which he was ordinarily resident; or

(c) in any other case for the area in which the person concerned is resident or to which he is sent on discharge by the hospital in which he was detained.

(4) Where there is a dispute about where a person was ordinarily resident for the purposes of subsection (3) above–

(a) if the dispute is between local social services authorities in England, section 40 of the Care Act 2014 applies to the dispute as it applies to a dispute about where a person was ordinarily resident for the purposes of Part 1 of that Act;

(b) if the dispute is between local social services authorities in Wales, the dispute is to be determined by the Welsh Ministers;

(c) if the dispute is between a local social services authority in England and a local social services authority in Wales, it is to be determined by the Secretary of State or the Welsh Ministers.

(5) The Secretary of State and the Welsh Ministers shall make and publish arrangements for determining which of them is to determine a dispute under subsection (4)(c); and the arrangements may, in particular, provide for the dispute to be determined by whichever of them they agree is to do so.

(6) In this section, 'after-care services', in relation to a person, means services which have both of the following purposes–

(a) meeting a need arising from or related to the person's mental disorder; and

(b) reducing the risk of a deterioration of the person's mental condition (and, accordingly, reducing the risk of the person requiring admission to a hospital again for treatment for mental disorder).

19.113 Section 117 is supplemented by Regulations:

- the Care and Support and After-care (Choice of Accommodation) Regulations 2014;[60]
- the Mental Health (After-care under Supervision) Regulations 1996.[61]

19.114 Guidance is found in the English Code of Practice to the MHA 1983 and the Welsh Code of Practice to the MHA 1983.

19.115 In addition, MIND has published a guide: *After-care under section 117 of the Mental Health Act,*[62] as has Rethink.[63]

Cases

19.116 *Clunis v Camden and Islington Health Authority* (1997–8) 1 CCLR 214, CA

Health and social services authorities do not owe a duty of care to patients, to discharge their duty to provide after-care services in a reasonably careful manner and, in any event, a patient who, in consequence, killed a man knowing that was wrong, would not be permitted to sue because of the ex turpi causa principle

Facts: Mr Clunis relapsed and killed a man not long after being discharged from psychiatric detention and was convicted of manslaughter on the grounds of diminished responsibility. Mr Clunis sued for damages, on the basis that the health authority had negligently failed to provide him with adequate after-care services under the MHA 1983, in particular so as monitor his mental state. His claim was struck out and his appeal dismissed.

Judgment: the Court of Appeal (Beldam and Potter LJJ, Bracewell J) held that:

(1) the maxim *ex turpi causa non oritur action* applied, given that Mr Clunis had known that his actions were wrong, so as to attract criminal responsibility:

> 'In the present case we consider the defendant has made out its plea that the plaintiff's claim is essentially based on his illegal act of manslaughter; he must be taken to have known what he was doing and that it was wrong, notwithstanding that the degree of his culpability was reduced by reason of mental disorder. The court ought not to allow itself to be made an instrument to enforce obligations alleged to arise out of the plaintiff's own criminal act and we would therefore allow the appeal on this ground.'

(2) section 117(2) MHA 1983 did not give rise to a common law duty of care in negligence:

60 SI No 2670.

61 SI No 294.

62 www.mind.org.uk/information-support/legal-rights/aftercare-under-section–117-of-the-mental-health-act/.

63 Avaiable at www.rethink.org/living-with-mental-illness/mental-health-laws/section–117-aftercare.

'After care services are not defined in the Act. They would normally include social work, support in helping the ex-patient with problems of employment, accommodation or family relationships, the provision of domiciliary services and the use of day centre and residential facilities. No doubt an assessment of the patient's needs would in the first instance be made by the hospital which discharged him. It was for that purpose in this case that the defendant authority sought to arrange appointments with the plaintiff. In that respect, its actions through Dr Sergeant were essentially in the sphere of administrative activities in pursuance of a scheme of social welfare in the community. Bearing in mind the ambit of the obligations under section 117 of the Act and that they affect a wide spectrum of health and social services, including voluntary services, we do not think that Parliament intended so widespread a liability as that asserted by Mr Irwin. The question of whether a common law duty exists in parallel with the authority's statutory obligations is profoundly influenced by the surrounding statutory framework. See per Lord Browne-Wilkinson *in X v Bedfordshire CC* at page 739C, and per Lord Hoffmann in *Stovin v Wise* [1996] AC 923 at 952F–953A. So, too, in this case, the statutory framework must be a major consideration in deciding whether it is fair and reasonable for the local health authority to be held responsible for errors and omissions of the kind alleged. The duties of care are, it seems to us, different in nature from those owed by a doctor to a patient whom he is treating and for whose lack of care in the course of such treatment the local health authority may be liable.

Nor do we think that Dr Sergeant should be held liable for a failure to arrange for a mental health assessment more speedily. The suggestion that because local police had reported that the plaintiff was waving screwdrivers and knives about and talking about devils illustrates to our mind the difficulty of holding her responsible in this case. Under sec. 136 of the Mental Health Act a constable finding a person in a public place who appears to be suffering from a mental disorder and to be in immediate need of care or control may:

> '... if he thinks it necessary to do so in the interests of that person or for the protection of other persons, remove that person to a place of safety ...'

We doubt if even this language, though specifically requiring the constable to act in the interests of a mentally disordered person, creates a duty to take care which gives rise to a claim for damages at the suit of the disordered person. Moreover as Lord Browne-Wilkinson pointed out in *X v Bedfordshire CC* (supra), the question whether a doctor owes a duty of care to a patient in certifying that a patient is fit to be detained under the Mental Health Acts was left undecided in *Everett v Griffiths* [1920] 3 KB 163; [1921] 1 AC 361 and still remains open for decision in an appropriate case. We have no doubt that it would not be right to hold Dr Sergeant or the defendant health authority liable to the plaintiff in damages for failure to arrange the plaintiff's assessment for the purposes of section 117 more speedily than she did.

For these reasons we do not think the plaintiff can establish a cause of action arising from a failure by the defendant health authority or Dr Sergeant to carry out their functions under sec. 117 of the Mental Health Act. Nor do we think that it would be fair or reasonable to hold the defendant responsible for the consequences of the plaintiff's criminal act.

In our view the defendant's application should have succeeded on both grounds and we would allow the appeal.

Comment: Section 117(1) and (2) remain materially the same; consequently the Court of Appeal's description of the nature of after-care services and the absence of any common law duty of care still apply.

19.117 *R v Camden and Islington Health Authority ex p K* (2001) 4 CCLR 170, CA

A patient remains lawfully detained where she continues to suffer from a mental disorder that warrants hospital detention and treatment unless psychiatric supervision in the community can be provided and, despite the authorities using reasonable endeavours, psychiatric supervision in the community cannot be provided because no psychiatrist can be found willing to provide it

Facts: disagreeing with K's responsible medical officer, the MHRT ordered that K (a restricted patient) be discharged conditionally, to live at home under psychiatric supervision. No doctor could be found in K's home area, willing to supervise her. Wider enquiries proved fruitless. On the invitation of K's RMO, the Secretary of State referred her case back to the MHRT. K sought a judicial review, submitted that the health authority's failure to arrange psychiatric supervision was in breach of section 117 of the MHA 1983.

Judgment: the Court of Appeal (Lord Phillips MR, Buxton and Sedley LJJ) held that the health authority had not acted unlawfully. It had acted with reasonable diligence to make appropriate arrangements, but did not have the power to compel consultants to act in a manner that consultants were unable to reconcile with the exercise of their professional judgment:

> 20. The relevant provisions of section 117(2) are set out at paragraph 19 of Burton J's judgment. On their face they require the Health Authority to provide after care services for persons who cease to be detained and leave hospital. Decisions at first instance, to which I am about to refer, have held that the duty of a Health Authority extends to making arrangements for the care of a patient before that patient is discharged. Before Burton J, the respondent Authority reserved its position as to whether these decisions were correct. Before us it has made the following limited concessions:
>
> (a) A Health Authority has power to take preparatory steps before discharge of a patient;
>
> (b) It will normally be the case that, in the exercise of this discretionary power, an authority should give way to a tribunal decision, and should use reasonable endeavours to fulfill the conditions imposed by such a decision, insofar as they relate to medical care;
>
> (c) Failure to use such endeavours, in the absence of strong reasons, would be likely to be an unlawful exercise of discretion.
>
> ...
>
> 29. In my judgment section 117 imposes on Health Authorities a duty to provide after care facilities for the benefit of patients who are discharged from mental hospitals. The nature and extent of those facilities must, to a degree, fall within the discretion of the Health Authority which must have regard to other demands on its budget. In relation to the duty to satisfy conditions imposed by a tribunal, I would endorse the concession made by the respondent Authority as to the extent of its duty.

There was, moreover, no breach of Article 5 ECHR, given that K still suffered from a mental disorder for which treatment was necessary, in hospital if community services were not available.

19.118 *R v Manchester CC ex p Stennett* [2002] UKHL 34, (2002) 5 CCLR 500

It was not lawful to charge for after-care services

Facts: the claimants sought a judicial review of charges imposed on them for after-care services under section 117 of the MHA 1983, in particular for the provision of residential accommodation.

Judgment: the House of Lords (Lords Slynn, Mackay, Steyn, Hutton and Millet) held that after-care services, including residential accommodation, were provided under section 117 of the MHA 1983 and not under the community care statutes. Since section 117 contained no charging provision, consequently it was unlawful to charge for after-care services.

Comment: this remains the position, except that it is now possible for a person entitled to accommodation as after-care under section 117 of the MHA 1983 to choose their '*preferred accommodation*' under section 30 of the Care Act 2014 and '*top up*' the cost, that is, pay the difference between the sum the local authority would usually expect to pay for accommodation and the actual cost (in cases where the preferred accommodation is more expensive than reasonable quality accommodation that meets the patient's needs, available in the local market): see 'Preferred accommodation' at paras 9.45–9.52 above.

19.119 *R (W) v Doncaster MBC* [2004] EWCA Civ 378, [2004] MHLR 201

Local authorities were not under a duty to make arrangements for after-care services before the tribunal directed discharge and, when the tribunal ordered conditional discharge, were not under an absolute duty but a duty to make reasonable endeavours to make provision to satisfy the conditions: meanwhile, the patient's continued detention was lawful

Facts: the MHRT conditionally discharged W but the conditions proved impracticable to fulfil. After eight months, W re-applied to the MHRT, who conditionally discharged him again, on varied conditions. W claimed damages for false imprisonment and breach of his rights under Article 5 ECHR.

Judgment: the Court of Appeal (Judge, Mance and Scott Baker LJJ) dismissed the claim, holding that W had always been lawfully detained and that (i) the duty to provide after-care services only arises upon the patient ceasing to be detained leaving hospital; (ii) the authorities were under a duty to make reasonable endeavours to make arrangements required as the conditions of a conditional discharge or a deferred conditional discharge; (iii) in a non-contentious case, the authorities should seek to finalise an after-care plan for consideration by the tribunal; a breach of section 117 did not in itself give rise to a cause of action for damages or create a right to damages under Article 5 ECHR, against the after-care authority or the hospital; (iv) in this case, Doncaster had been faced with a number of issues leading to delay but it had used reasonable endeavours.

19.120 *R (H) v Secretary of State for the Home Department* [2003] UKHL 59, (2004) 7 CCLR 147

Tribunals must keep deferred conditional discharges under review so as to comply with Article 5(4) ECHR but a patient remained lawfully detained where the patient suffered from a mental disorder that warranted compulsory treatment in hospital unless community services were available and it had not been possible to arrange for those services despite using reasonable endeavours

Facts: the claimant had been made the subject of a hospital order in 1995 with restriction. In 1999, the MHRT concluded that he was not suffering from mental illness but should remain liable to be recalled to hospital. It adjourned the hearing for the hospital to draw up a care plan but that did not occur because the hospital could not locate a psychiatrist willing to supervise IH in the community. In February 2000 the MHRT re-convened and reached the same conclusion but still the hospital could not find a psychiatrist willing to supervise IH in the community. In March 2002 the MHRT re-convened and decided that IH had suffered from a mental illness throughout. IH sought a judicial review and damages for unlawful detention between February 2000 and March 2002.

Judgment: the House of Lords (Lords Bingham, Steyn, Hobhouse, Scott and Rodger) held that IH had been left in limbo for too long, so that his rights under Article 5(4) ECHR had been breached: tribunals must keep under view deferred conditional discharges. However, at no time had IH been unlawfully detained. At all times, IH had suffered from a mental disorder that required hospital treatment under detention, unless community supervision and treatment was available. As to that, the after-care authorities were not under an absolute duty to make provision but a duty to use reasonable endeavours, which they had discharged. Lord Bingham said this:

> *Conclusions*
>
> 25. This regrettably lengthy prologue enables me, I hope fairly, to review Mr Owen's main submissions summarised in para 7 above more briefly than would otherwise have been possible.
>
> 26. I do not accept that, because the tribunal lacked the power to secure compliance with its conditions, it lacked the coercive power which is one of the essential attributes of a court. What Article 5(1)(e) and (4) require is that a person of unsound mind compulsorily detained in hospital should have access to a court with power to decide whether the detention is lawful and, if not, to order his release. This power the tribunal had. Nothing in article 5 suggests that discharge subject to conditions is impermissible in principle, and nothing in the Convention jurisprudence suggests that the power to discharge conditionally (whether there are specific conditions or a mere liability to recall), properly used, should be viewed with disfavour. Indeed, the conditional discharge regime, properly used, is of great benefit to patients and the public, and conducive to the Convention object of restricting the curtailment of personal liberty to the maximum, because it enables tribunals to ensure that restricted patients compulsorily detained in hospital represent the hard core of those who suffer from mental illness, are a risk to themselves or others and cannot be effectively treated and supervised otherwise than in hospital. If there is any possibility of treating

and supervising a patient in the community, the imposition of conditions permits that possibility to be explored and, it may be, tried.

27. When, following the tribunal's order of 3 February 2000, it proved impossible to secure compliance with the conditions within a matter of a few months, a violation of the appellant's Article 5(4) right did occur. It occurred because the tribunal, having made its order, was precluded by the authority of the Oxford case from reconsidering it. The result was to leave the appellant in limbo for a much longer period than was acceptable or compatible with the Convention. I would accordingly endorse the Court of Appeal's decision to set aside the Oxford ruling and I would adopt the ruling it gave in para 71 of its judgment quoted above. Evidence before the House shows that that ruling is already yielding significant practical benefits. Mr Owen was, I think, right to submit that the tribunal could have achieved the same result, consistently with the Oxford case, by a judicious use of its power to adjourn and by proleptic indication of the conditions it had in mind to impose, but it is undesirable to restrict the procedural freedom of tribunals in a field as important and sensitive as this, where personal liberty and safety and public protection are all at stake: the outcome should not turn on procedural niceties.

28. There was no time between 3 February 2000 and 25 March 2002 when the appellant was, in my opinion, unlawfully detained, and there was thus no breach of Article 5(1)(e). There is a categorical difference, not a difference of degree, between this case and that of *Johnson*. Mr Johnson was a patient in whose case the Winterwerp criteria were found not to be satisfied from June 1989 onwards. While, therefore, it was reasonable to try and ease the patient's reintegration into the community by the imposition of conditions, the alternative, if those conditions proved impossible to meet, was not continued detention but discharge, either absolutely or subject only to a condition of liability to recall. His detention became unlawful shortly after June 1989 because there were, as all the doctors agreed, no grounds for continuing to detain him. The present case is quite different. There was never a medical consensus, nor did the tribunal find, that the Winterwerp criteria were not satisfied. The tribunal considered that the appellant could be satisfactorily treated and supervised in the community if its conditions were met, as it expected, but the alternative, if these conditions proved impossible to meet, was not discharge, either absolutely or subject only to a condition of recall, but continued detention. The appellant was never detained when there were no grounds for detaining him. To the extent that Buxton and Sedley LJJ differed from the Master of the Rolls on this point in K, the opinion of the latter is to be preferred.

29. The duty of the health authority, whether under section 117 of the 1983 Act or in response to the tribunal's order of 3 February 2000, was to use its best endeavours to procure compliance with the conditions laid down by the tribunal. This it did. It was not subject to an absolute obligation to procure compliance and was not at fault in failing to do so. It had no power to require any psychiatrist to act in a way which conflicted with the conscientious professional judgment of that psychiatrist. Thus the appellant can base no claim on the fact that the tribunal's conditions were not met. This conclusion makes it unnecessary, in my opinion, to address a question on which the House heard argument, but which was not considered below, whether in a context such as this psychiatrists were or could be a hybrid public authority. Determination of that question is best left to a case in which it is necessary to the decision. We are nonethe-

less grateful to the Royal College of Psychiatrists for its submissions on this point.

30. I do not consider that the violation of article 5(4) which I have found calls for an award of compensation since (a) the violation has been publicly acknowledged and the appellant's right thereby vindicated, (b) the law has been amended in a way which should prevent similar violations in future, and (c) the appellant has not been the victim of unlawful detention, which Article 5 is intended to avoid.

19.121 *R (B) v Camden LBC* [2005] EWHC 1366 (Admin), (2005) 8 CCLR 422

Local authorities were entitled to carry out preparatory steps but were not under a duty to monitor patients to consider the exercise of this discretion. They came under a duty to exercise reasonable endeavours to make arrangements for after-care services when a tribunal has provisionally determined that a conditional discharge is appropriate. They are entitled to explore funding issue. In this case, the authority's ineffective action had not been causative of B's continued detention but, even if it had done, B would not have been entitled to damages under Article 5 ECHR

Facts: the MHRT directed B's conditional discharge on the 11 September 2003. Camden had not been involved in that hearing and it took it until around June 2004 to make the necessary arrangements. B sued for damages for delayed provision under section 117 of the MHA 1983, contending that the delay had violated his rights under Articles 5 and 8 ECHR.

Judgment: Stanley Burnton J held that although Camden had a power to undertake preparatory steps, section 117 of the MHA 1983 did not impose a duty on Camden to monitor B, prior to the MHRT hearing, to see whether it ought to undertake preparatory steps; Camden could expect to be notified, where appropriate. Camden did come under a duty to make reasonable endeavours to put after-care arrangements in place, once the tribunal had decided that, in principle, a conditional discharge was appropriate. However, it had been entitled to defer making provision whilst it explored the availability of funding from elsewhere for some of the provision. B could not show that any delay caused by ineffectual action by Camden had resulted in additional detention as other conditions of his discharge, also, had not been met. In any event, damages under Article 5 ECHR did not flow from any failure to make arrangements under section 117, even where that caused prolonged detention because the hospital detaining B could not have acted differently in national law, other than by continuing to detain B:

91. In *W*, the Court of Appeal considered the question whether a social services authority which is in breach of its duty under section 117 prolonged the detention of a patient in hospital was liable to the patient for having caused a breach of his rights under Article 5. At [68] and [69], Scott Baker LJ said:

'68. Mr Jay submits that even if there was a breach of Article 5 on the facts Mr Gordon is shooting at the wrong target in seeking to recover damages from the Respondent. He submits that the hospital detaining W could not have acted differently under domestic law. It is not logical,

> he argues to be unable to proceed against the detaining authority and yet recover damages against a third party. The true remedy against a section 117 body is judicial review and not damages. He further submits that the *Martin v Watson* does not extend to false imprisonment: see *Davidson v Chief Constable of Wales and another* [1994] 2 All ER 597. Just as the claimant in that case was imprisoned without a remedy, so it would be with W.
>
> 69. I can see the force of these arguments. I do not think that W is able to identify the respondent as a public authority liable for his detention under Article 5. But I do not think the case ever gets as far as this because in my view the respondent did nothing to cause the unlawful detention of W. It neither knowingly tried to nullify the decision of the tribunal nor failed to use its best endeavours to implement the conditions it had directed.'

Neither of the other members of the Court of Appeal specifically referred to this issue, but they both agreed with the judgment of Scott Baker LJ. The statement of the Scott Baker LJ was self-evidently *obiter*, and Mr Bowen submitted that I should not follow it. I consider that I should do so, not only because it was the considered opinion of the Court of Appeal but also because of the earlier consistent decision of Crane J in *R (A) v Secretary of State for the Home Department* [2003] 1 WLR 330, and the dictum of Buxton LJ *K* at [49].

92. Furthermore, in the present case, B was never detained in circumstances in which the *Winterwerp* requirements (helpfully summarised in *H* in the Court of Appeal at [29]) were not satisfied. The judgments of Simon Brown LJ and Laws LJ in *Cawser v Home Secretary* [2003] EWCA Civ 1522, [2004] 1 PLR 166 are inconsistent with the proposition that Camden's breach of its duties under section 117 involves liability for an infringement of Article 5.

93. It follows that, even if Camden had been in breach of its duties to B under section 117 or section 47, and that breach had prolonged his detention under the Mental Health Act 1983, Camden would not have been liable to damages under sections 6 and 8 of the Human Rights Act 1998.

19.122 *R (B) v Lambeth LBC* [2006] EWHC 2363 (Admin), (2007) 10 CCLR 84

A local authority is under a duty to secure alternative accommodation under section 117 straightaway when it has assessed the need as existing

Facts: B faced housing possession proceedings brought by her landlord, Lambeth, on account of her nuisance to neighbours. However, Lambeth owed her the after-care duty under section 117 of the MHA 1983. It undertook an assessment, that the problem with the neighbours was insoluble and B required alternative accommodation. It did not, however, intend to offer her alternative accommodation until shortly before the hearing of the possession proceedings.

Judgment: Deputy High Court Judge Gilbart held that Lambeth was plainly in breach of section 117 of the MHA 1983 and that in the light of its own assessment it was untenable for it to suggest that B's accommodation would remain suitable until a possession order was made.

19.123 *R (Mwanza) v Greenwich LBC* [2010] EWHC 1462 (Admin), (2010) 13 CCLR 454

After-care services must address needs arising from a patient's mental disorder and may not address other needs that patient might have

Facts: Mr Mwanza and his family were unlawfully present in the UK. Mr Mwanza had received various support services under section 117 of the MHA 1983 but the PCT and local authority ultimately decided to cease their duty under that section. Afterwards, facing destitution on account of his and his family's immigration status, Mr Mwanza sought accommodation and support, either under section 117 or under section 21 of the National Assistance Act 1948.

Judgment: Hickinbottom J held that the duty to provide after-care services is a duty to provide services that are necessary to meet needs arising from a person's mental disorder. That can involve a duty to meet needs such as the need to work and have a roof over one's head where that is necessary to meet needs arising from a person's mental disorder. No duty arises, however, to meet such needs, where a mental patient simply needs such provision because they do not have it, and cannot secure it, as in this case, where Mr Mwanza's need for accommodation was caused by his immigration status, which prevented him from working, and not from his mental condition:

> 61. Section 117 requires the relevant authorities to provide a patient on discharge from section 3 with 'after-care services'. 'After-care services' are not defined in the statute. Mr Armstrong submitted that the term was wide in scope: the authorities were bound to provide any service that prevented possible deterioration in the former patient's mental condition, and reduced the chance of relapse and readmission. Ms Richards for Greenwich Council submitted that the services required to be provided under section 117 were restricted to those that addressed a need deriving from or related to the patient's mental disorder and, consequently, the provision of 'ordinary accommodation' (ie housing without any care element) and the provision of financial support to cover basic living costs (eg food) was incapable of falling within its scope.
>
> 62. I do not accept Mr Armstrong's submission that section 117 requires the relevant authorities to provide a former section 3 patient with any and all services simply because those services do or may prevent deterioration or relapse of a mental condition, or require readmission, for the following reasons.
>
> 63. In relation to the scope of section 117 services, the respected commentary on the 1983 Act by Richard Jones says (Mental Health Act Manual, 12th Edition, at paragraph 1–1053)
>
> > 'It is suggested that an after-care service is a service which is (1) provided in order to meet an assessed need that arises from a person's mental disorder; and (2) aimed at reducing that person's chance of being readmitted to hospital for treatment for that disorder.'
>
> 64. Mr Armstrong sought to persuade me that the relevant service was defined in terms of Mr Jones' second limb only – but I do not agree. The duty derives from a provision in mental health legislation; and it is described as a duty to provide 'after-care services'. As Ms Richards submitted, section 117 is not concerned with the provision of support and accommodation

at large, but rather with the provision, to the specified category of patients who have been detained on account of their mental disorder, of services tailored to meet needs arising from that disorder. An after-care service must, in my judgment, be a service that is necessary to meet a need arising from a person's mental disorder.

65. It may be that, if a former patient were unemployed or homeless, that would increase the chance of deterioration in his mental condition – but, in my judgment, that would not require an authority under section 171 to provide employment or housing, as Mr Armstrong's submission suggested. The need for work or the need for a roof over one's head *simpliciter* are common needs, and do not arise from mental disorder. Section 171 does not impose a general responsibility on the relevant authorities to house or provide an income to a former patient. Of course, a patient's mental disorder may make it more difficult for him to look for housing or employment on discharge from section 3 – and it may therefore give rise to a need for assistance in doing so. But that is a different need and a different issue.

66. That, it seems to me, is the principle. In practice, the assessment of needs that do arise from a mental disorder may of course give rise to difficult issues. It is for the relevant authorities – the local authority and the health authority – to reach their own view as to what need the person has, and, in making an assessment under section 47 of the 1990 Act, they enjoy a discretion as to what if any services are required to meet such needs. As Lord Phillips MR said in *R (K) v Camden and Islington Health Authority* [2001] EWCA Civ 240 at [29]:

> 'The nature and extent of those [after-care] facilities must, to a degree, fall within the discretion of the [authorities] which must have regard to other demands in [their] budget.'
>
> The reference to 'nature', as well as 'extent', of the services in my view emphasises both the potential broad scope of section 117 and the wide discretion of the authorities within that scope. They are The recognition of this discretion, given to the authorities by Parliament, appears to me to be vital.

67. Therefore, I agree with Mr Jones' suggested criteria for after-care services quoted above. However, I do not agree when later in the same paragraph he says:

> 'The provision of accommodation meets a basic human need that relates to all individuals, irrespective of their mental health. Ordinary accommodation cannot therefore be said to constitute a service that is provided to meet a need that arises from a person's mental disorder'

insofar as that suggests that, as a matter of law, ordinary accommodation can never fall within the scope of section 117, a submission also made by Ms Richards before me. As a proposition, that goes too far – although I accept that it is difficult readily to envisage in practice circumstances in which a mere roof over the head would, on the facts of a particular case, be necessary to meet a need arising from a person's mental disorder. That difficulty, it seems to me, explains why, in the legal authorities to which I was referred, where there is discussion of the scope section 117 services, bare accommodation is not mentioned. In my view, that reflects a dearth of practical examples, rather than a principle of law.

19.124 *R (Afework) v Camden LBC* [2013] EWHC 1637 (Admin)

Accommodation need only be provided as an after-care service when the patient is required to occupy specialised accommodation to meet needs arising out of the condition that led to his or her detention

Facts: an issue arose as to whether Mr Afework was entitled to accommodation under section 117(2) of the MHA 1983 (for which no charge could be made) and, later on, whether he was entitled to accommodation under section 117(2) or section 21 of the National Assistance Act 1948.

Judgment: Mostyn J held that Mr Afework has never been entitled to accommodation under section 117(2) of the MHA 1983 because initially he had been able to function independently in his own accommodation, albeit with social work support and then subsequently, when he required specialist accommodation, that was not because a supervening brain injury, not for the reasons that had led to his earlier detention under the Mental Health Act 1983. Mostyn J reviewed the authorities and concluded as follows:

> 19. I therefore hold that as a matter of law section 117(2) is only engaged vis-à-vis accommodation if:
>
> i) The need for accommodation is a direct result of the reason that the ex-patient was detained in the first place ('the original condition');
>
> ii) The requirement is for enhanced specialised accommodation to meet needs directly arising from the original condition; and
>
> iii) The ex-patient is being placed in the accommodation on an involuntary (in the sense of being incapacitated) basis arising as a result of the original condition.

Comment: this seems very restrictive.

19.125 *Richards v Worcestershire CC* [2016] EWHC 1954 (Ch)

A patient could be entitled to bring private law proceedings in restitution, to reclaim money spent by him on after-care services

Facts: Worcestershire had provided the claimant with residential accommodation and other services for years after his discharge from detention under section 3 of the MHA 1983. He brought a claim for restitution of the charges he had paid, on the basis that he had been entitled to such provision free of charge, as an after-care service. Worcestershire applied to strike out his claim on the basis that (i) it was not possible to bring such a restitutionary claim; and (ii) in any event, any claim had to be brought by way of judicial review.

Judgment: Newey J held that (i) in principle, a person who had paid for care services that were shown to have been the responsibility of a local authority under section 117 of the MHA 1983, but which in error the local authority failed to provide without charge, was entitled to bring a claim for restitution; and (ii) such a claim could be properly brought as a private law action, at least in a case such as the present where there was no allegation that the local authority had failed properly to assess and meet needs.

Responsibility disputes

19.126 The Care Act 2014 has amended section 117 of the MHA 1983 to make it considerably clearer which authority bears responsibility for the provision of after-care services. The authority responsible will be:

- the authority where the patient was ordinarily resident immediately before being detained, if that was in England or Wales; otherwise,
- the authority for the area in which the person concerned was resident; otherwise,
- if the patient has no residence, that can be ascertained, the local authority for the area to which the patient is sent on discharge:[64]

> **117**(3) In this section 'the clinical commissioning group or Local Health Board' means the clinical commissioning group or Local Health Board, and 'the local social services authority' means the local social services authority
> (a) if, immediately before being detained, the person concerned was ordinarily resident in England, for the area in England in which he was ordinarily resident;
> (b) if, immediately before being detained, the person concerned was ordinarily resident in Wales, for the area in Wales in which he was ordinarily resident; or
> (c) in any other case for the area in which the person concerned is resident or to which he is sent on discharge by the hospital in which he was detained.
>
> (4) Where there is a dispute about where a person was ordinarily resident for the purposes of subsection (3) above–
> (a) if the dispute is between local social services authorities in England, section 40 of the Care Act 2014 applies to the dispute as it applies to a dispute about where a person was ordinarily resident for the purposes of Part 1 of that Act;
> (b) if the dispute is between local social services authorities in Wales, the dispute is to be determined by the Welsh Ministers;
> (c) if the dispute is between a local social services authority in England and a local social services authority in Wales, it is to be determined by the Secretary of State or the Welsh Ministers.
>
> (5) The Secretary of State and the Welsh Ministers shall make and publish arrangements for determining which of them is to determine a dispute under subsection (4)(c); and the arrangements may, in particular, provide for the dispute to be determined by whichever of them they agree is to do so.

19.127 There is guidance at Chapters 19–21 and Annex H of the *Care and Support Statutory Guidance*, specifically at paragraphs 19.42–19.48 in relation

64 *R v Mental Health Tribunal ex p Hall* [2000] 1 WLR 1323; *R v Sunderland CC v South Tyneside Council* [2012] EWCA Civ 1232, (2012) 15 CCLR 701, at para 46 ('the case of no residence is a last resort, an ultimate default position, which should not be held to apply except in extreme and clear circumstances, which it is not necessary to define or even illustrate for the purposes of this appeal').

to after-care (see 'Ordinary residence', chapter 12 above). There is also NHS guidance: *Who Pays: Determining responsibility for payments to providers* (August 2013).[65]

The case-law in this area is to be found above in chapter 12 at paras 12.53–12.56.

Other mental health cases

19.128 *Re F (a child)* (1999) 2 CCLR 445, CA

Guardianship could not be imposed on a person with severe mental impairment unless that was associated with abnormally aggressive or seriously irresponsible conduct which, on the facts, was not made out by F's desire to continue to live with neglectful parents

Facts: F's brother and sisters had been taken into local authority care because of parental neglect and the risk of sexual abuse on the part of adults with whom the parents had associated; but F was over 16 and so could not be made subject to a care order. Nonetheless, her mental age had been assessed as between the 5- to 8-year-old range and she was highly vulnerable. The local authority therefore applied for a guardianship order, under section 7 of the MHA 1983 (which would give the authority the power to prevent F returning home) and for an order displacing F's father as her 'nearest relative'.

Judgment: the Court of Appeal (Evans, Thorpe and Mummery LJJ) held that section 7(2) of the MHA 1983 permitted a guardianship application to be made on the ground of 'severe mental impairment' but, as defined in section 2, that also required there to be abnormally aggressive or seriously irresponsible conduct. F's determination to return home could not be construed as 'seriously irresponsible' as she had given cogent reasons for wishing to return home, which is what the great majority of children taken into care did, as soon as they were able. It would have been preferable if the local authority had invoked the wardship jurisdiction, as F had remained under 18 years of age; that jurisdiction was child-centred and considerably more flexible.

19.129 *R (X) v Secretary of State for the Home Department* (2001) 4 CCLR 92, CA

The Secretary of State for the Home Department is entitled to remove mental patients from the UK using immigration powers and by-passing the MHA 1983

Facts: the claimant was a foreign national, unlawfully present in the UK, detained in hospital pursuant to section 48 of the MHA 1983. He challenged the Secretary of State for the Home Department's decision to remove him from the UK.

Judgment: the Court of Appeal (Schiemann and Tuckey LJJ, Sir Swinton Thomas) held that while the Secretary of State for the Home Department

65 www.england.nhs.uk/wp-content/uploads/2014/05/who-pays.pdf.

did not have power under the MHA 1983 to remove X from hospital without permission from the MHRT, under section 86, he did have power to bypass the MHA 1983 and remove X under the Immigration Act 1971 and his decision to do so was, on the facts, rational and compliant with the ECHR.

19.130 *Seal v Chief Constable of South Wales* [2007] UKHL 31, (2007) 10 CCLR 695

Proceedings issued without leave, where required under section 139 of the MHA 1983, were a nullity

Facts: S brought proceedings against the South Wales police, in relation to action taken by them under section 136 of the MHA 1983. The police responded that the proceedings were a nullity, in that Mr Seal had not obtained leave under section 139 of the MHA 1983 (section 139 provides that, inter alia, no one shall be liable for anything purportedly done under MHA 1983 unless the act was in in bad faith or without reasonable care and that no patient may bring civil proceedings in respect of any such act without the leave of the High Court).

Judgment: the House of Lords (Lords Bingham, Browne-Wilkinson and Carswell; Lord Woolf and Baroness Hale dissenting) held that section 139 of the MHA 1983 had not been intended to be merely procedural, but to confer a substantial protection such as to invalidate proceedings brought without leave. The purpose of section 139 was to provide reassurance and protection to mental health professionals and it was compatible with Article 6 ECHR.

Comment: Mr Seal's complaint was rejected by the European Court of Human rights.[66]

19.131 *North Dorset NHS Primary Care Trust v Coombs* [2013] EWCA Civ 471, (2013) 16 CCLR 376

Psychiatric patients may pay for private care and, accordingly, recover the cost of such provision from a tortfeasor

Facts: Mr Coombs had a lengthy psychiatric history, but then sustained significant head injuries as a result of the negligence of the PCT, which worsened his psychiatric condition. Mr Coombs claimed and was awarded damages for private psychiatric treatment and the PCT appealed that.

Judgment: the Court of Appeal (Rix, Aikens and Black LJJ) held that there was nothing in the statutory scheme or public policy that prevented a psychiatric patient, or others, from paying for care privately, as other private patients in hospitals do; so the damages award in that respect was lawful.

19.132 *R (C) v Secretary of State for Justice* [2016] UKSC 2, (2016) 19 CCLR 5

There was no presumption of anonymity for mental patients challenging aspects of their treatment and care in the High Court but anonymity will be granted where that is necessary in the interests of the patient

66 *Seal v United Kingdom* (2012) 54 EHRR 6, [2011] MHLR 1.

Facts: C had been convicted of murder, then transferred to hospital as a mental patient. After many years in detention, the First-tier Tribunal recommended that he was suitable for conditional discharge but the Secretary of State for Justice refused to allow C trial periods of unescorted leave in the community. C sought a judicial review of that decision. His application was refused and the High Court revoked C's anonymity order. The Court of Appeal upheld that revocation.

Judgment: the Supreme Court (Hale, Clarke, Wilson, Carnwath and Hughes JJSC) held that there was no presumption of anonymity in the High Court and above, in relation to mental patients challenging aspects of their care and treatment under the MHA 1983, but that an anonymity order should be made in this case otherwise the patient's integration into the community would be jeapordised.

Comment: although this is a judgment on particular facts the analysis of the Supreme Court, allowing the appeal from decisions by the High Court and Court of Appeal, suggests that there will be very few cases indeed, if any, where anonymity may be refused in this type of case – perhaps where there is no real prospect of the mental patient being discharged into the community, at all, or in the foreseeable future.

CHAPTER 20

Housing and community care

continued

20.39 *R (Morris) v Westminster CC* [2005] EWCA Civ 1184, [2006] 1 WLR 505
The exclusion of a British parent from homelessness assistance, because her child was subject to immigration control, was incompatible with Articles 8 and 14 ECHR

20.40 *R (Limbuela) v Secretary of State for the Home Department* [2005] UKHL 66, (2006) 9 CCLR 30
It was necessary to provide accommodation and support to asylum-seekers who were destitute or faced imminent destitution, to avoid a breach of Article 3 ECHR

20.41 *R (Mooney) v Southwark LBC* [2006] EWHC 1912 (Admin), (2006) 9 CCLR 670
Care assessments had not identified a care need requiring the provision of accommodation: this was a housing case only

20.42 *Barber v Croydon LBC* [2010] EWCA Civ 51, [2010] HLR 26
It was unlawful to seek to evict a vulnerable person incompatibly with the local authority's own policy on dealing with anti-social behaviour committed by vulnerable persons and irrational

20.43 *Manchester City Council v Pinnock* [2010] UKSC 45, [2011] 2 AC 104
It can be disproportionate, in breach of Article 8 ECHR, to order a person to give up possession of their home, but the rights of the public landowner will almost always prevail

20.44 *Bah v United Kingdom* Application no 56328/07, (2012) 54 EHRR 21
States were entitled to treat persons differently, for the purposes of housing assistance, on the basis of their or their dependants' immigration status and States enjoyed a wide margin of appreciation in that respect

20.45 *R (SL) v Westminster CC* [2013] UKSC 27, (2013) 16 CCLR 161
A need for 'care and attention' was a need for more than accommodation and monitoring

20.46 *Hotak, Kanu and Johnson v Southwark LBC and Solihull MBC* [2015] UKSC 30, [2015] 2 WLR 1341
A homeless person is in priority need if he or she is vulnerable compared with the average person not the average homeless person

20.47 *Nzolameso v City of Westminster* [2015] UKSC 22, (2015) 18 CCLR 201
Housing authorities had to consider their duty to safeguard and promote the welfare of children when assessing what accommodation would be suitable for a homeless family

20.48 *Akerman-Livingstone v Aster Communities Ltd* [2015] UKSC 15, [2015] AC 1399
The court should not ordinarily determine summarily a possession claim defendant on disability discrimination grounds that appeared to be substantial because, unlike defences under the ECHR, it was not the case that a tenant's rights under the Equality Act 2010 would almost always be outweighed by the landlord's property rights

20.49 *R (SG) v Haringey LBC* [2015] EWHC 2579 (Admin), (2015) 18 CCLR 444
A local authority need only provide accommodation under the Care Act 2014 in response to an accommodation-related need

20.50 *R (H) v Ealing LBC* [2016] EWHC 841 Admin, [2016] HLR 20
A Housing Allocation Scheme must not be discriminatory or breach the PSED

Introduction

20.1 The relationship between housing and adult social care ought to be seamless but is often, in practice, difficult:

- the possibility of securing accommodation under adult social care provisions can be of vital importance to homeless, vulnerable adults who are not entitled to mainstream provision (whether because of their immigration status,[1] or earlier conduct[2]);
- that incoming pressure on social care resources is exacerbated by the fact that it is relatively easy to exclude persons, or discharge duties towards persons, under the Housing Acts[3] and because, in many areas, housing officers are considerably tougher in their approach than their social services counterparts;
- on the other hand, the courts have increasingly emphasised the need for adults seeking accommodation under social care provisions to demonstrate that their need truly is a social care need,[4] whilst adult and children's social care budgets have come under such pressure that both managers and practitioners simply have to be tougher, within the law, than before;
- at the other end of the process, the courts have tried to balance legitimate grounds for seeking possession, such as rent arrears and neighbour nuisance, against the special difficulties that tenants with needs for care and support may face.[5]

20.2 The major legal and practical difficulty arises out of the fact that there are large numbers of vulnerable individuals and families who fall between legal stools because:

- they may qualify for assistance under the Housing Act 1996 or the Care Act 2014, but need a different type of provision that is generally made under the enactment under which they qualify;
- they are excluded from assistance under the Housing Act 1996 for immigration reasons or because of having become intentionally homeless, or having refused an offer of 'suitable accommodation';
- their needs are insufficient to qualify them under the Care Act 2014 but they have also fallen foul of a decision that they do not have sufficient vulnerability so as to achieve 'priority need' under the Housing Act 1996, when nonetheless they are vulnerable and so still need special help.

1 *R (Clue) v Birmingham CC* [2010] EWCA Civ 460, (2010) 13 CCLR 276.
2 *R v Bristol CC ex p Penfold* (1997–8) 1 CCLR 315, QBD.
3 *R v Kensington and Chelsea RLBC ex p Kujtim* [1999] 4 All ER 161, (1999) 2 CCLR 340.
4 *R (Mwanza) v Greenwich LBC* [2010] EWHC 1462 (Admin), (2010) 13 CCLR 454; *R (M) v Slough BC* [2008] UKHL 52, (2008) 11 CCLR 733; *R (SL) v Westminster CC* [2013] UKSC 27, (2013) 16 CCLR 161.
5 *Akerman-Livingstone v Aster Communities Ltd* [2015] UKSC 15, [2015] AC 1399.

Housing provision under the Care Act 2014

20.3 Section 8 of the Care Act 2014 allows local authorities to, on the face of it, provide any type of accommodation:

> **How to meet needs**
> 8(1) The following are examples of what may be provided to meet needs under sections 18 to 20–
> (a) accommodation in a care home or in premises of some other type;
> (b) care and support at home or in the community;
> (c) counselling and other types of social work;
> (d) goods and facilities; (e) information, advice and advocacy.
> (2) The following are examples of the ways in which a local authority may meet needs under sections 18 to 20–
> (a) by arranging for a person other than it to provide a service;
> (b) by itself providing a service;
> (c) by making direct payments.
> (3) 'Care home' has the meaning given by section 3 of the Care Standards Act 2000.

20.4 Section 8(1)(a) of the Care Act 2014 plainly encompasses the provision of what might be termed 'ordinary accommodation'.

20.5 On the other hand section 23 of the Care Act 2014 prevents a local authority meeting needs under sections 2 and 18–20 of the Care Act 2014 by doing anything which it or another local authority 'is required to do under – (a) the Housing Act 1996':

> **Exception for provision of housing etc**
> **23**(1) A local authority may not meet needs under sections 18 to 20 by doing anything which it or another local authority is required to do under–
> (a) the Housing Act 1996, or
> (b) any other enactment specified in regulations.
> (2) 'Another local authority' includes a district council for an area in England for which there is also a county council.
> (3) For the purposes of its application in relation to the duty in section 2(1) (preventing needs for care and support), this section is to be read as if, in subsection (1), for 'meet needs under sections 18 to 20' there were substituted 'perform the duty under section 2(1)'.

20.6 Read out of context, section 23 could mean almost anything:

- at one extreme, it could prevent local authorities ever providing 'ordinary accommodation' under the Care Act 2014, since that is a form of provision that local authorities can be required to make under the Housing Act 1996;
- at the other extreme, it could allow local authorities to provide 'ordinary accommodation' under the Care Act 2014 whenever they are not under a duty, owed to a person individually, to provide that person with accommodation under the Housing Act 1996.

20.7 The simplest solution is that a local authority may provide ordinary accommodation, and any other service within reason, to an adult whom it assesses as needing care and support within the meaning of sections 18 and 19 of the Care Act 2014; and that the exercise or non-exercise of that power is a question for the judgment of the local authority, subject only to the usual public law constraints.

20.8 That approach seems to be fit the new statutory scheme whilst remaining connected with long-standing social services practice, endorsed by the courts, to provide 'ordinary accommodation', in appropriate cases, to persons who met the statutory criteria for residential accommodation under section 21 of the National Assistance Act 1948, whether or not they happened also to meet the statutory criteria for assistance under the Housing Acts – for example, in the case of young adults with a mental disorder or learning disability, who simply need a certain amount of support and a safety net, in order to occupy ordinary accommodation in the community.[6] It seems very unlikely that section 23 of the Care Act 2014 was intended to end that beneficial overlap, which seems consistent with the *Care and Support Statutory Guidance* which emphasises, at Chapter 10, the importance of the individual's wishes as to how their care should be delivered and, probably at least as important in this context, the need for local authorities to signpost and broker services, and liaise with the housing department/ housing authority (see paragraphs 10.10–10.26).

20.9 The potentially tricky issue is to define what an 'appropriate case' would be, under the current legislation.

20.10 In *R (SL) v Westminster CC*,[7] the Supreme Court held that a person only became entitled to residential accommodation under section 21 of the National Assistance Act 1948 (which imposed a duty to provide residential accommodation 'for persons aged eighteen or over who by reason of age, illness, disability or any other circumstances are in need of care and attention which is not otherwise available to them') where the person in question had a need for the sort of care that was normally provided in a home (whether ordinary or specialised) or that would be effectively useless if the applicant had no home.

20.11 The initial judicial indication is that the same approach applies under the Care Act 2014, in the sense that a local authority may not provide 'accommodation' under section 8 of the Care Act 2014 unless the applicant needs the sort of care that is normally provided in a home (whether ordinary or specialised) or that would be effectively useless if he or she had no home: *R (SG) v Haringey LBC*.[8] That may be right, but one could not expect a different answer, from a High Court Judge seeking to make sense of rather disparate materials in a way that gives proper effect to a recent decision of the Supreme Court, albeit in a somewhat different statutory context.

20.12 It could be that an appellate court might take a somewhat broader view, of the kind outlined above at para 20.8. On the other hand, the view might be taken that, nowadays, there are many different ways in which ordinary accommodation can be provided to vulnerable persons (see below at paras 20.17–20.18) and that, as a matter of policy, accommodation under the Care Act 2014 should be reserved for relatively limited classes of case.

20.13 Otherwise, because of the provisions of Part 6 of the Housing Act 1996, a local authority plainly may not meet needs under the Care Act 2014 by 'allocating' a person social housing (that is, selecting a person to be a secure

6 *R (Wahid) v Tower Hamlets LBC* [2002] EWCA Civ 287, (2002) 5 CCLR 239.

7 [2013] UKSC 27, (2013) 16 CCLR 161.

8 [2015] EWHC 2579 (Admin), (2015) 18 CCLR 444.

or introductory tenant of housing accommodation held by them, or some other person, or nominating a person to be an assured tenant of housing accommodation held by a private registered provider of social housing or registered social landlord: section 159 of the Housing Act 1996).

20.14 That is because Part 6 of the Housing Act 1996 provides that allocations of social housing are to be made pursuant to each housing authority's published Housing Allocation Scheme (HAS), drawn by it to reflect local priorities, subject to broad statutory parameters in the Housing Act 1996 and associated regulations.

20.15 Otherwise, whilst local authorities may not 'allocate' social housing to persons with care needs, otherwise than through their Housing Allocation Scheme, neither section 23 of the Care Act 2014 nor Part 6 of the Housing Act 1996 prevent local authorities discharging their duty under sections 18 to 20 of the Care Act 2014 by providing 'ordinary accommodation' by:

- making an allocation to a person who is already a secure or introductory tenant, or an assured tenant of a private registered provider of social housing or a registered social landlord, where the allocation does not involve a 'transfer' within section 159(4B), because such allocations are excluded from Part 6 of the Housing Act 1996, by virtue of section 159(4A);
- granting or arranging for non-secure tenancies or licenses of social housing;
- making arrangements with private sector providers for the provision of housing accommodation;
- revising their Housing Allocation Scheme to provide for additional allocations to be made to persons referred by social services for reasons connected with the Care Act 2014.

Housing provision under the Housing Acts

20.16 There is nothing to prevent housing authorities from, in appropriate cases:

- providing temporary accommodation to persons with care and support needs under Part 7 of the Housing Act 1996, providing it is 'suitable accommodation' for them; or from
- allocating 'suitable' social housing to persons with care and support needs under Part 6 of the Housing Act 1996, although the combination of Part 6 of the Housing Act 1996 and section 23 of the Care Act 2014 means that the only lawful method of so doing is to include criteria in the local Housing Allocation Scheme which will have that effect.

In practice, housing authorities do provide accommodation to persons with care and support needs through both these routes, usually in liaison with their social services department/local social services authority. Providing the situation is not exploited so as to finesse or curtail duties owed under the Care Act 2014, this practice seems entirely beneficial.

Housing allocations under the Housing Act 1996

20.17 It is very common for local authority Housing Allocation Schemes to include provision for sheltered housing to be provided for certain elderly residents and for supported housing to be provided for certain vulnerable groups, eg persons with mental disorders, or substance abuse problems, women fleeing domestic violence, offenders, adults with a history of rough sleeping and so forth.[9]

20.18 That is consistent with the duty, at section 166A of the Housing Act 1996, to accord preferential treatment within the Housing Allocation Scheme, to members of certain vulnerable groups:

166A(3) As regards priorities, the scheme shall, subject to subsection (4), be framed so as to secure that reasonable preference is given to–
(a) people who are homeless (within the meaning of Part 7);
(b) people who are owed a duty by any local housing authority under section 190(2), 193(2) or 195(2) (or under section 65(2) or 68(2) of the Housing Act 1985) or who are occupying accommodation secured by any such authority under section 192(3);
(c) people occupying insanitary or overcrowded housing or otherwise living in unsatisfactory housing conditions;
(d) people who need to move on medical or welfare grounds (including any grounds relating to a disability); and
(e) people who need to move to a particular locality in the district of the authority, where failure to meet that need would cause hardship (to themselves or to others).

The scheme may also be framed so as to give additional preference to particular descriptions of people within one or more of paragraphs (a) to (e) (being descriptions of people with urgent housing needs).

The scheme must be framed so as to give additional preference to a person with urgent housing needs who falls within one or more of paragraphs (a) to (e) and who–
(i) is serving in the regular forces and is suffering from a serious injury, illness or disability which is attributable (wholly or partly) to the person's service,
(ii) formerly served in the regular forces,
(iii) has recently ceased, or will cease to be entitled, to reside in accommodation provided by the Ministry of Defence following the death of that person's spouse or civil partner who has served in the regular forces and whose death was attributable (wholly or partly) to that service, or
(iv) is serving or has served in the reserve forces and is suffering from a serious injury, illness or disability which is attributable (wholly or partly) to the person's service.

For this purpose 'the regular forces' and 'the reserve forces' have the meanings given by section 374 of the Armed Forces Act 2006.

(4) People are to be disregarded for the purposes of subsection (3) if they would not have fallen within paragraph (a) or (b) of that subsection without the local housing authority having had regard to a restricted person (within the meaning of Part 7).

(5) The scheme may contain provision for determining priorities in allocating housing accommodation to people within subsection (3); and the factors which the scheme may allow to be taken into account include–
(a) the financial resources available to a person to meet his housing costs;

9 See, just as an example, Islington LBC's current HAS, at http://www.islington.gov.uk/publicrecords/library/Housing/Business-planning/Policies/2015-2016/(2015-07-14)-Housing-allocation-scheme-2015.pdf.

(b) any behaviour of a person (or of a member of his household) which affects his suitability to be a tenant;
(c) any local connection (within the meaning of section 199) which exists between a person and the authority's district.

(6) Subject to subsection (3), the scheme may contain provision about the allocation of particular housing accommodation–
(a) to a person who makes a specific application for that accommodation;
(b) to persons of a particular description (whether or not they are within subsection (3)).

20.19 In addition, there is scope within the statutory scheme for housing authorities to allocate social housing to achieve a range of locally desirable objectives:

Including local priorities alongside the statutory reasonable preference categories

4.19 As the House of Lords made clear in the case of *R (Ahmad) v Newham LBC*, s166A(3) only requires that the people encompassed within that section are given 'reasonable preference'. It 'does not require that they should be given absolute priority over everyone else'. This means that an allocation scheme may provide for other factors than those set out in s166A(3) to be taken into account in determining which applicants are to be given preference under a scheme, provided that:

- they do not dominate the scheme, and
- overall, the scheme operates to give reasonable preference to those in the statutory reasonable preference categories over those who are not.

The Secretary of State would encourage authorities to consider the scope to take advantage of this flexibility to meet local needs and local priorities.

4.20 The House of Lords also made clear that, where an allocation scheme complies with the reasonable preference requirements and any other statutory requirements, the courts should be very slow to interfere on the ground of alleged irrationality.

Local lettings policies

4.21 Section 166A(6)(b) of the 1996 Act enables housing authorities to allocate particular accommodation to people of a particular description, whether or not they fall within the reasonable preference categories, provided that overall the authority is able to demonstrate compliance with the requirements of s166A(3). This is the statutory basis for so-called 'local lettings policies' which may be used to achieve a wide variety of housing management and policy objectives.[10]

20.20 In addition, Housing Allocation Schemes must not be discriminatory or drawn up in breach of the public sector equality duty (PSED) (see chapter 5).[11]

20.21 Social housing allocations are governed by Part 6 of the Housing Act 1996, supplemented by delegated legislation and statutory guidance:

- Allocation of Housing (Procedure) Regulations 1997;
- Allocation of Housing and Homelessness (Eligibility) (England) Regulations 2006;

10 *Allocation of accommodation: guidance for local housing authorities in England* (2012), at https://www.gov.uk/government/uploads/system/uploads/attachment_data/file/5918/2171391.pdf.

11 *R (H) v Ealing LBC* [2016] EWHC 841 Admin, [2016] HLR 20.

- Allocation of Housing and Homelessness (Miscellaneous Provisions) (England) Regulations 2006;
- Allocation of Housing (Reasonable and Additional Preference) Regulations 1997;
- Allocation of Housing and Homelessness (Review Procedures) Regulations 1999;
- Allocation of Housing (Qualification Criteria for Armed Forced) (England) Regulations 2012;
- Homelessness (Suitability of Accommodation) (England) Order 2012;
- Allocation of Housing (Qualification Criteria for Right to Move) (England) Regulations 2015;
- *Supplementary Guidance on the homelessness changes in the Localism Act 2011 and on the Homelessness (Suitability of Accommodation) (England) Order 2012* (November 2012);[12]
- *Allocation of accommodation: guidance for local housing authorities in England* (2012, updated 2013);[13]
- *Providing social housing for local people: Statutory guidance on social housing allocations for local authorities in England* (December 2013);[14] and
- *Right to Move: Statutory guidance on social housing allocations for local housing authorities in England* (March 2015).[15]

20.22 In 2009, the House of Lords signalled a more restrained approach, on the part of the courts, to challenges to the content of local authority HAS.[16]

Assistance for homeless persons under the Housing Act 1996

20.23 Assistance for homeless persons is provided under Part 7 of the Housing Act 1996, under which various duties may be owed, in particular the rehousing duty, which is owed to persons who are:

- '*homeless*' (defined at sections 175–178);
- '*eligible*' (in immigration terms, defined at sections 185 and 186);
- in '*priority need*' (section 189);
- and not '*intentionally homeless*' (section 190).

20.24 The critical provision, the gateway for many homeless persons in need of care and support, is the 'priority need' definition, at section 189 of Housing Act 1996:

> **Priority need for accommodation.**
> **189**(1) The following have a priority need for accommodation–
> (a) a pregnant woman or a person with whom she resides or might reasonably be expected to reside;

12 https://www.gov.uk/government/uploads/system/uploads/attachment_data/file/270376/130108_Supplementary_Guidance_on_the_Homelessness_changes_in_the_Localism_Act_2011_and_on_the_Homelessness_Order_2012.pdf.

13 https://www.gov.uk/government/uploads/system/uploads/attachment_data/file/5918/2171391.pdf.

14 https://www.gov.uk/government/uploads/system/uploads/attachment_data/file/269035/131219_circular_for_pdf.pdf.

15 https://www.gov.uk/government/uploads/system/uploads/attachment_data/file/418437/Right_to_move_-_statutory_guidance.pdf.

16 *R (Ahmad) v Newham LBC* [2009] UKHL 14, [2009] HLR 31.

(b) a person with whom dependent children reside or might reasonably be expected to reside;
(c) a person who is vulnerable as a result of old age, mental illness or handicap or physical disability or other special reason, or with whom such a person resides or might reasonably be expected to reside;
(d) a person who is homeless or threatened with homelessness as a result of an emergency such as flood, fire or other disaster.

(2) The Secretary of State may by order–
(a) specify further descriptions of persons as having a priority need for accommodation, and
(b) amend or repeal any part of subsection (1).

(3) Before making such an order the Secretary of State shall consult such associations representing relevant authorities, and such other persons, as he considers appropriate.

(4) No such order shall be made unless a draft of it has been approved by resolution of each House of Parliament.

20.25 Recently the Supreme Court has signalled a more liberal approach to assessing who falls within section 189(1)(c) of the Housing Act 1996.[17]

20.26 Part 7 of the Housing Act 1996 is supplemented by delegated legislation and statutory guidance as follows:

- Allocation of Housing and Homelessness (Eligibility) (England) Regulations 2006;
- Allocation of Housing and Homelessness (Eligibility) (Wales) Regulations 2014;
- Allocation of Housing and Homelessness (Miscellaneous Provisions) (England) Regulations 2006;
- Allocation of Housing and Homelessness (Review Procedures) Regulations 1997;
- Homeless Persons (Priority Need)(Wales) Order 2001;
- Homelessness (Decisions on Referrals) Order 1998;
- Homelessness (England) Regulations 2000;
- Homelessness (Wales) Regulations 2000;
- Homeless Persons (Priority Need)(England) Order 2001;
- Homelessness (Suitability of Accommodation(England) Order 2012;
- Homelessness (Suitability of Accommodation(Wales) Order 2006;
- *Homelessness Code of Guidance for Local Authorities* (July 2006);
- *Supplementary Guidance on the homelessness changes in the Localism Act 2011 and on the Homelessness (Suitability of Accommodation)(England) Order 2012* (November 2012).

17 *Hotak v Southwark LBC* [2015] UKSC 30, [2015] 2 WLR 1341.

Accommodation through the Local Government Act 2000 and/or the Localism Act 2011 and/or special purpose vehicles

20.27 The Supporting People scheme is a shadow of its former self,[18] nonetheless although grant funding is reduced and is no longer ring-fenced such provision still has a valuable role to play. The statutory basis is section 93 of the Local Government Act 2000, which provides inter alia:

> **Grants for welfare services**
>
> **93** (1) The Secretary of State may, with the consent of the Treasury, pay grants to local authorities in England towards expenditure incurred by them [...]
>
> (a) in providing, or contributing to the provision of, such welfare services as may be determined by the Secretary of State, or
>
> (b) in connection with any such welfare services.
>
> (2) The National Assembly for Wales may pay grants to local authorities in Wales towards expenditure incurred by them [...]
>
> (a) in providing, or contributing to the provision of, such welfare services as may be determined by the Assembly, or
>
> (b) in connection with any such welfare services.
>
> (3) The amount of any grants under this section and the manner of their payment are to be such as may be determined by the Secretary of State or the Assembly (as the case may be).

20.28 In addition, as noted above at Chapter 13, Welsh local authorities have a GWP (general well-being power) under sections 1–4 of the Local Government Act 2000 whilst English local authorities have a GPC (general power of competence) under sections 1–8 of the Localism Act 2011, which is wide enough to allow them to provide housing to any individuals or types of individuals who are not statutorily excluded from such provision.

20.29 In addition, some local authorities utilise 'special purpose rental vehicles' – trading companies set up under section 95 of the Local Government Act 2003 and/or section 1 of the Localism Act 2011 to provide tenancies at affordable rents, but for commercial purposes, outside of their housing revenue account and/or to provide tenancies to members of vulnerable groups, for non-commercial purposes.

Eviction

20.30 At the other end of the process, the courts have grappled with ways of factoring into the housing possession process, usually under the Housing Act 1985 (secure tenancies, etc) or the Housing Act 1988 (assured tenancies, etc), the fact that some tenants/occupiers have care and support needs, are especially vulnerable and may be less able to comply with tenancy terms, for disability-related reasons.

18 Its rise and fall is charted in this Parliamentary Briefing Paper, at http://researchbriefings.parliament.uk/ResearchBriefing/Summary/RP12-40 , and the archived material that constituted the scheme when in full flow and constituted by earmarked grants can still be found at http://webarchive.nationalarchives.gov.uk/20100210162740/http:/www.spkweb.org.uk/.

20.31 That can be done:

- through the requirement, where it exists, that possession should only be ordered when it is *'reasonable'* to do so;[19]
- through allowing an Article 8 ECHR defence;[20]
- through allowing a public law defence; [21]
- through allowing a defence based on discrimination in breach of the Equality Act 2010.[22]

Cases

20.32 For additional cases relevant to housing possession claims against adults with care and support needs, see above chapter 6 on Discrimination and chapter 5 on the PSED.

20.33 *R v Bristol CC ex p Penfold* (1997–8) 1 CCLR 315, QBD

A mentally unwell single parent who had become intentionally homeless might need accommodation in order to meet her need for care

Facts: Ms Penfold was a homeless single parent who suffered from anxiety and depression. She was no longer entitled to assistance under the Housing Acts. Bristol declined to assess Ms Penfold's needs under the National Health Service and Community Care Act 1990, on the ground that she did not appear to be a person who 'may' need services and, in any event, there was no realistic prospect of the local authority providing her with accommodation under any of the community care legislation, given its straightened resources and the applicant's accommodation history.

Judgment: Scott Baker J held, at 322E, as follows:

> It seems to me that Parliament has expressed section 47(1) in very clear terms. The opening words of the subsection, the first step in the three stage process, provide a very low threshold test. The reference is to community care services the authority *may* provide or arrange for. And the services are those of which the person *may* be in need. If that test is passed it is mandatory to carry out the assessment. The word *shall* emphasises that this is so ... As a matter of logic, it is difficult to see how the existence or otherwise of resources to meet a need can determine whether or not that need exists ... Even if there is no hope from the resources point of view of meeting any needs identified in the assessment, the assessment may serve a useful purpose in identifying for the local authority unmet needs which will help it to plan for the future ... Resource implications in my view play no part in the decision whether to carry out an assessment.

19 *Croydon LBC v Moody* (1999) 2 CCLR 92, CA.

20 *Manchester CC v Pinnock* [2010] UKSC 45, [2011] 2 AC 104 ('64. Sixthly, the suggestions put forward on behalf of the Equality and Human Rights Commission, that proportionality is more likely to be a relevant issue "in respect of occupants who are vulnerable as a result of mental illness, physical or learning disability, poor health or frailty", and that "the issue may also require the local authority to explain why they are not securing alternative accommodation in such cases" seem to us well made.').

21 *Shane Barber v Croydon LBC* [2010] EWCA Civ 51, [2010] HLR 26; *Kay v Lambeth LBC* [2006] UKHL 10, [2006] 2 AC 465.

22 *Akerman-Livingstone v Aster Communities Ltd* [2015] UKSC 15, [2015] 2 WLR 721.

20.34 ## *R v Wigan MBC ex p Tammadge* (1997–8) 1 CCLR 581, QBD

A local authority was under a duty to meet a family's need for larger, adapted accommodation under care legislation, having assessed a need as existing for such provision under that legislation

Facts: the social services complaints review panel concluded that the applicant and her family were in urgent need of re-housing for health and care reasons. Wigan accepted that and ascertained that the most cost-effective solution was to knock together two adjacent houses in its area. However, Wigan then decided not to undertake that course because 'the potential benefits ... do not justify the significant costs'.

Judgment: Forbes J held that while resources were relevant to a limited extent when determining whether and if so what needs existed for residential accommodation under section 21 of the National Assistance Act 1948, once a need has been assessed as existing, the authority is under a duty to make provision for that need. That applied in this case and Wigan was ordered to undertake the work that it had itself determined as being the most cost-effective solution:

> I have come to the firm conclusion that Mr Gordon's submissions are correct. In my view, the social services complaints review panel's (SSCRP's) finding as to Mrs Tammadge's need for larger accommodation is perfectly clear from the wording in which that particular conclusion is expressed. Moreover, that conclusion is entirely in keeping with views of Wigan's own professionally qualified staff and advisers, as expressed both before and after the hearing before the SSCRP. I am therefore satisfied that, by a date no later than 22 October 1996 (when it was acknowledged that Wigan had accepted the SSCRP finding: see above), Mrs Tammadge's need for larger accommodation was established. I reject Miss Patterson's submissions to the contrary. As a result, from that date Wigan have been obliged to make provision of such accommodation to Mrs Tammadge and her family: see *ex p M* at pages 1009–1010. Once the duty had arisen in this way, it was not lawful of Wigan to refuse to perform that duty because of a shortage of or limits upon its financial resources or for any of the other reasons expressed in Mr Walker's letters of 30 July and 28 August 1997: see *ex p Sefton* at page 58 and also at page 67I–J, where Lord Woolf said this:
>
>> 'However, in this case it is clear from the evidence that Sefton accepted that Mrs Blanchard met its own threshold as a person in need of care and attention. What it was seeking to do was to say that because of its lack of resources notwithstanding this it was not prepared to meet the duty which was placed upon it by the section. This it was not entitled to do.'
>
> Accordingly, for those reasons, I have come to the firm conclusion that Wigan's decision not to provide Mrs Tammadge with larger accommodation is unlawful and must be quashed. Having regard to my conclusion on the central issue in this case and to the present length of this judgment, I do not propose to say anything further about Mrs Gordon's submissions on his core propositions four and five, except to acknowledge the compelling nature of his submissions with regard to core proposition four, which submissions are fully set out in his helpful written skeleton argument.

Comment: the principle should still apply under section 18 of the Care Act 2014 and, in relation to carers, under section 20.

20.35 *Marzari v Italy* Application no 36448/97, (2000) 30 EHRR CD 218

A positive duty could arise under the ECHR to provide housing assistance to a seriously disabled person, if the consequences were sufficiently severe

Facts: Mr Marzari claimed that a number of housing-related difficulties experienced by him, connected with his serious disability, resulted from violations of his rights under Article 8 ECHR.

Judgment: the European Court of Human Rights declared the application inadmissible on its facts, but did accept that a positive obligation could arise under Article 8 ECHR, to provide housing assistance to a disabled person:

> The court considers that, although Article 8 does not guarantee the right to have one's housing problem solved by the authorities, a refusal of the authorities to provide assistance in his respect to an individual suffering from a severe disease might in certain circumstances raise an issue under Article 8 of the Convention because of the impact of such refusal on the private life of the individual. The court recalls in his respect that, while the essential object of Article 8 is to protect the individual against arbitrary interference by public authorities, this provision does not merely compel the State to abstain from such interference: in addition to this negative undertaking, there may be positive obligations inherent in effective respect for private life. A State has obligations of his type where there is a direct and immediate link between the measures sought by an applicant and the latter's private life (*Botta v Italy* (1998) 26 EHRR 241, paras 33–34).

20.36 *R (Patrick) v Newham LBC* (2001) 4 CCLR 48, QBD

Referring a homeless woman with care needs to a housing charity did not amount to a discharge of the duty to assess or meet her needs

Facts: Ms Patrick, a single woman who suffered from physical and mental ill health, was evicted on the ground of neighbour nuisance and found intentionally homeless. Newham had purported to discharge its duty towards her under section 21 of the National Assistance Act 1948, by offering her accommodation provided by a charity, which she had refused. Ms Patrick then slept rough.

Judgment: Henriques J held that Newham had failed in breach of statutory duty to assess Ms Patrick's needs and had not discharged its duty under section 21:

> 27. Her solicitor in her witness statement says that she did not take up the accommodation provided by HOST because she believed she was being sent to Sunderland and not to Southwark. In any event, Southwark was a distance away from her sister and from her medical support network.
>
> 28. Since the offer of accommodation was on 28 April and the certificate of mental incapacity to handle her affairs was granted on 9 May, it requires no mental gymnastics to conclude that her decision to reject the offer of accommodation at Southwark was neither considered nor likely to have been well informed.
>
> 29. It is of particular significance that the respondent knew that solicitors were acting for the applicant as they had written on her behalf on 5 April.

30. Further, they had informed the respondent that they could obtain no clear instructions from the applicant due to her mental health and enclosed a note from her general practitioner.

31. If the respondent sought to put an end to its section 21 duties to provide accommodation, they ought in my judgment at the very least to have ensured that the applicant was legally represented when the offer was made to her to ensure not only that she understood what the offer was, both in terms of location and services offered, but also that she understood the legal consequences or potential legal consequences of refusing the offer.

32. Since she may well not have understood what was being offered and its location, I am not prepared to find that her refusal of it was unreasonable.

33. In the exercise of its duty to provide accommodation a local authority must have a concurrent duty to explain fully and to the point of comprehension any offer it may make. I am not persuaded that the local authority has discharged its duty. In my judgment the duty to provide Part III accommodation continues pursuant to section 21 of the 1948 Act.

20.37 *R (Wahid) v Tower Hamlets LBC* [2002] EWCA Civ 287, (2002) 5 CCLR 239

Local authorities are only required to provide accommodation under social care legislation when the qualifying criteria under such legislation are met

Facts: Mr Wahid was mentally unwell and lived with his family in suitable accommodation. Tower Hamlets concluded that Mr Wahid had a medical and social need for better accommodation (to be met under the Housing Acts) but did not need 'care and attention', so as to trigger the duty to provide residential accommodation under section 21 of the National Assistance Act 1948.

Judgment: the Court of Appeal (Pill, Mummery and Hale LJJ) upheld Tower Hamlets' decision: whilst residential accommodation could be ordinary accommodation, it was a precondition of such a duty arising that the applicant had been assessed as needing 'care and attention', which means more than just housing:

30. I agree that this appeal should be dismissed for the reasons given by Pill LJ. Some basic points may deserve emphasis given the recent expansion of litigation in this field. Under section 21(1)(a) of the National Assistance Act 1948, local social services authorities have a duty to make arrangements for providing residential accommodation for people over 18 (who are ordinarily resident in their area or in urgent need) where three inter-related conditions are fulfilled:

(1) the person is in need of care and attention;

(2) that need arises by reason of age, illness, disability or any other circumstances; and

(3) that care and attention is not available to him otherwise than by the provision of residential accommodation under this particular power.

Three further points are also relevant:

(1) it is for the local social services authority to assess whether or not these conditions are fulfilled and, if so, how the need is to be met, subject to the scrutiny of the court on the ordinary principles of judicial review;

(2) section 21 does not permit the local social services authority to make provision which may or must be made by them or any other authority under an enactment other than Part III of the 1948 Act (see s21(8)); but

(3) having identified a need to be met by the provision of residential accommodation under section 21, the authority have a positive duty to meet it which can be enforced in judicial review proceedings (see *R v Sefton MBC ex p Help the Aged and Others* [1997] 4 All ER 532, (1997) 1 CCLR 57, CA; *R v Kensington and Chelsea RLBC ex p Kujtim* [1999] 4 All ER 161, (1999) 2 CCLR 340, CA).

31. Mr Goudie's argument, skilfully and attractively though it was put, was ultimately circular. It is common ground that the 'residential accommodation' which may be provided under section 21 includes ordinary housing (see, on this point, *R v Newham LBC ex p Medical Foundation for the Care of Victims of Torture* (1997–98) 1 CCLR 227; *R v Bristol CC ex p Penfold* (1997–98) 1 CCLR 315; *R (Batantu) v Islington LBC* (2001) 4 CCLR 445). I agree with Stanley Burnton J, at first instance in this case (see (2001) 4 CCLR 455, at para 27), that there are several indications in the Act that the kind of accommodation originally envisaged was in a residential home or hostel. This is the power under which local authorities provided elderly and aged people's homes or arranged accommodation in such homes run by others. However, it can no longer be assumed that a need for care and attention can only be properly met in an institutional setting. There are people who are undoubtedly in need of care and attention for whom local social services authorities wish to provide residential accommodation in ordinary housing. The most obvious examples are small groups of people with learning disabilities who are able to live in ordinary houses with intensive social services support; or single people with severe mental illnesses who will not receive the regular medication and community psychiatric nursing they need unless they have somewhere to live. Whatever the words 'residential accommodation' may have meant in 1948, therefore, they are a good example of language which is 'always speaking' and can be change its meaning in the light of changing social conditions (see the observations of this court in *R v Westminster CC ex p M, P, A and X* (1997–98) 1 CCLR 85 at 90). Hence, Mr Knafler, in common with others who have appeared for local social services authorities, has conceded that 'residential accommodation' can mean ordinary housing without the provision of any ancillary services.

32. But it does not follow that because residential accommodation can mean ordinary housing and the claimant is in need of ordinary housing, a duty arises to provide him with that housing under section 21(1)(a). That duty is premised on an unmet need for 'care and attention' (a 'condition precedent', as this court put it in the *Westminster* case, at p93E). These words must be given their full weight. Their natural and ordinary meaning in this context is 'looking after': this can obviously include feeding the starving, as with the destitute asylum-seekers in the *Westminster* case. Ordinary housing is not in itself 'care and attention'. It is simply the means whereby the necessary care and attention can be made available if otherwise it will not (I do not understand this court to have rejected that part of the local authority's argument in the *Westminster* case, at p93B–D).

20.38 *R (Bernard) v Enfield LBC* [2002] EWHC 2282 (Admin), (2002) 5 CCLR 577

A serious failure to provide the services required under section 21 of the National Assistance Act 1948, which had severe repercussions on Ms Bernard's family and private law, breached Article 8 ECHR

Facts: Mrs Bernard and her family had become intentionally homeless but meanwhile occupied temporary accommodation provided under the Housing Act 1996. Being unable to secure suitable, alternative accommodation, because of Mrs Bernard's disability, they sought a community care assessment from Enfield. Enfield assessed Mrs Bernard as being wholly wheelchair dependent, but as being unable to use her wheelchair in her home, confining her to the living room, where she had no privacy and was in discomfort, as being wholly dependent on her husband and as being unable to gain access to the bathroom without great difficulty, although she was doubly incontinent: it concluded that the family needed assistance to move to suitable adapted accommodation. Enfield failed to secure the family's rehousing and meanwhile Mrs Bernard's circumstances remained dire: not only did she lack privacy, and any ability to mobilise within the home, she was incontinent in the living room several times a day, so that her husband had to clean her and her clothes/bedding and the carpets.

Judgment: Sullivan J noted that Enfield accepted that, in substance, it had assessed Mrs Bernard as requiring to be moved to suitable, adapted accommodation so as to trigger the duty to provide residential accommodation in section 21 of the National Assistance Act 1948. He held that Enfield's failure to discharge that duty, for about 20 months, did not quite reach the threshold of inhuman or degrading treatment in breach of Article 3 ECHR, but that it was an unjustified breach of Mrs Bernard's rights under Article 8, for which damages would be awarded of £10,000 (£8,000 for Mrs Bernard and £2,000 for her husband):

> 32. I accept the defendant's submission that not every breach of duty under section 21 of the 1948 Act will result in a breach of Article 8. Respect for private and family life does not require the state to provide every one of its citizens with a house: see the decision of Jackson J in *Morris v Newham LBC* [2002] EWHC 1262 (Admin) paragraphs 59 to 62. However, those entitled to care under section 21 are a particularly vulnerable group. Positive measures have to be taken (by way of community care facilities) to enable them to enjoy, so far as possible, a normal private and family life. In *Morris* Jackson J was concerned with an unlawful failure to provide accommodation under Part VII of the Housing Act 1996, but the same approach is equally applicable to the duty to provide suitably adapted accommodation under the 1948 Act. Whether the breach of statutory duty has also resulted in an infringement of the claimants' Article 8 rights will depend upon all the circumstances of the case. Just what was the effect of the breach in practical terms on the claimants' family and private life?
>
> 33. Following the assessments in September 2000 the defendant was under an obligation not merely to refrain from unwarranted interference in the claimants' family life, but also to take positive steps, including the provision of suitably adapted accommodation, to enable the claimants and their children to lead as normal a family life as possible, bearing in mind the

second claimant's severe disabilities. Suitably adapted accommodation would not merely have facilitated the normal incidents of family life, for example the second claimant would have been able to move around her home to some extent and would have been able to play some part, together with the first claimant, in looking after their children. It would also have secured her 'physical and psychological integrity'. She would no longer have been housebound, confined to a shower chair for most of the day, lacking privacy in the most undignified of circumstances, but would have been able to operate again as part of her family and as a person in her own right, rather than being a burden, wholly dependent upon the rest of her family. In short, it would have restored her dignity as a human being.

34. The Council's failure to act on the September 2000 assessments showed a singular lack of respect for the claimants' private and family life. It condemned the claimants to living conditions which made it virtually impossible for them to have any meaningful private or family life for the purposes of Article 8. Accordingly, I have no doubt that the defendant was not merely in breach of its statutory duty under the 1948 Act. Its failure to act on the September 2000 assessments over a period of 20 months was also incompatible with the claimants' rights under Article 8 of the Convention.

Section 8(3) of the Act

It does not follow that the claimants are entitled to an award of damages. Under section 8(1) the court 'may grant such relief or remedy or make such order within its powers as it considers just and appropriate'. Section 8(3) provides:

'No award of damages is to be made unless, taking account of all the circumstances of the case, including–

(a) any other relief or remedy granted, or order made, in relation to the act in question (by that or any other court), and

(b) the consequences of any decision (of that or any other court) in respect of that act,

the court is satisfied that the award is necessary to afford just satisfaction to the person in whose favour it is made.

(4) In determining–

(a) Whether to award damages, or

(b) The amount of an award,

the court must take into account the principles applied by the European Court of Human Rights in relation to the award of compensation under Article 41 of the Convention.'

20.39 *R (Morris) v Westminster CC* [2005] EWCA Civ 1184, [2006] 1 WLR 505

The exclusion of a British parent from homelessness assistance, because her child was subject to immigration control, was incompatible with Articles 8 and 14 ECHR

Facts: Ms Morris was a British citizen but, because her daughter was not, they were excluded from housing assistance when homeless, under the provisions of Part 7 of the Housing Act 1996.

Judgment: the Court of Appeal (Auld, Sedley and Jonathan Parker LJJ, Jonathan Parker LJ dissenting) held that the exclusion was a violation of rights under Articles 8 and 14 ECHR. Pending the government amending that legislation, alternative provision could be used, potentially.

Comment: the European Court of Human Rights took a different view, in *Bah v United Kingdom* (see para 20.44 below).

20.40 *R (Limbuela) v Secretary of State for the Home Department* [2005] UKHL 66, (2006) 9 CCLR 30

It was necessary to provide accommodation and support to asylum-seekers who were destitute or faced imminent destitution, to avoid a breach of Article 3 ECHR

Facts: four healthy, able-bodied asylum-seekers faced destitution because they claimed asylum late, by virtue of section 55 of the Nationality, Immigration and Asylum Act 2002.

Judgment: the House of Lords (Lords Bingham, Hope, Scott, Lady Hale and Lord Brown) held that a decision to exclude certain asylum-seekers from asylum support was an intentionally inflicted act for which the Secretary of State was responsible and it amounted to 'treatment' for the purposes of Article 3 ECHR. That treatment would be 'inhuman or degrading' when a person was obliged to sleep in the street or go seriously hungry or became unable to satisfy the most basic requirements of hygiene. The duty to avoid inhuman or degrading treatment required the Secretary of State to provide support to avert imminent destitution.

20.41 *R (Mooney) v Southwark LBC* [2006] EWHC 1912 (Admin), (2006) 9 CCLR 670

Care assessments had not identified a care need requiring the provision of accommodation: this was a housing case only

Facts: Mrs Mooney was herself physically disabled and was the single parent of three boys, two of whom had severe disabilities. She had waited for suitable accommodation for a long time and ultimately brought proceedings to secure it, via section 21 of the National Assistance Act (NAA) 1948 or section 17 of the Children Act (CA) 1989.

Judgment: Jackson J held that the community care assessments undertaken by Southwark had not identified that Mrs Mooney had a need for 'care and attention' falling within NAA 1948 s21 and CA 1989 s17 did not impose a duty to rehouse the entire family – this was a housing case:

> 54. (iv) Nowhere in the various assessments is there any suggestion that the claimant has a need for care and attention by reason of her disability and that such care and attention is not available to her otherwise than by the provision of accommodation under section 21.
>
> 55. (v) On the contrary, the assessments arrive at a different conclusion. The assessments conclude that the proper course is for the social services department to provide additional support for the family, and also to make a priority housing nomination under the Council's housing allocation policy. Such a nomination would enable the claimant to access suitable accommodation under Pt VI of the Housing Act 1996. In taking this course, the social services department was acting in a manner envisaged by section 47(3) of the 1990 Act (although in this instance both the social services department and the housing department were part of the same Council).

56. (vi) The fact that the provision of suitable accommodation can be achieved under the Housing Act 1996 brings into play section 21(8) of the 1948 Act. That subsection prevents section 21(1) from imposing an obligation upon the Council in the circumstances of this case.

...

65. The first limb of this alternative case is based upon section 21 of the 1948 Act and therefore cannot succeed. The second limb of the alternative case is based upon section 17 of the Children Act 1989. That provision cannot be relied upon as imposing a positive duty on the Council to re-house the whole family: see the reasoning of the House of Lords in *R (G) v Barnet LBC* [2004] 2 AC 208. It is no doubt for this reason that Mr Kolinsky, very sensibly, did not press the claimant's alternative case in oral argument.

20.42 *Barber v Croydon LBC* [2010] EWCA Civ 51, [2010] HLR 26

It was unlawful to seek to evict a vulnerable person incompatibly with the local authority's own policy on dealing with anti-social behaviour committed by vulnerable persons and irrational

Facts: Mr Barber, who had learning difficulties and a personality disorder, and who suffered from severe depression, assaulted the caretaker of his block. Croydon brought possession proceedings.

Judgment: the Court of Appeal (Rix, Richards and Patten LJJ) held that whilst the assault had been serious, Croydon's pursuit of possession proceedings was unlawful in public law: Croydon had mis-construed and failed to comply with its policy on dealing with anti-social behaviour committed by vulnerable persons, which required them to explore options other than eviction and, in all the circumstances, its approach had been irrational. On behalf of the Court of Appeal, Patten LJ said this:

15. The legality of this decision falls to be considered in private law proceedings by the Council for possession of its property. The ability of a defendant in such proceedings to raise by way of defence in the action a public law challenge to the decision to bring the claim rather than proceeding separately by way of judicial review was recognised in *Wandsworth LBC v Winder (No 1)* [1985] AC 461. More recently, the House of Lords has given extensive consideration to the grounds of any such challenge in possession proceedings particularly in relation to an Article 8 defence.

16. In *Kay v Lambeth LBC* [2006] 2 AC 465 the majority view was that judges in the county court trying such cases should proceed on the assumption that domestic law strikes a fair balance and is compatible with the occupier's convention rights. This led Lord Hope to limit possible challenges to a local authority's otherwise established right to possession to two types of case: (a) those in which exceptionally it was arguable that the law giving the right to possession was incompatible with Article 8; and (b) cases where the decision to exercise the legal right to obtain possession was one which no reasonable person would consider justifiable: see [110] at 517D.

17. These gateways were considered further by Lord Hope in the subsequent decision in *Doherty v Birmingham City Council* [2008] UKHL 57 but the guidance set out in *Kay* remained intact and any further analysis is unnecessary for the purposes of this appeal. Gateway (b) is essentially a conventional public law test, although one which is broader than a strict formulation of the *Wednesbury* principle: see *Doherty* at [55].

...

44. Judged by any ordinary standards, the assault on Mr Baah was serious and obviously unacceptable. But the Council's policy on vulnerable people is to explore alternative solutions which may lead to the prevention of anti-social behaviour (ASB) in the future. Although there may be cases where the risk of future ASB by such a tenant is unlikely to be countered by anything less than their removal, the requirement to consult the specialist agencies is likely to ensure that the recovery of possession is confined as a remedy to cases where it is actually necessary in order to prevent a repetition of such behaviour. Given the absence of any misbehaviour by Mr Barber prior to May 22 or subsequently, and having regard to Dr Owen's assessment of him, it was, I think, incumbent upon Mr Hunt to consult the other agencies and to take advice as to whether some alternative remedy such as an ABC would solve the problem. As I read it, the Council's policy is not (and certainly ought not to be) that incidents of ASB involving persons with mental disabilities should be handled without regard to the existence of those disabilities and their responsibility for the conduct in question.

45. What Mr Hunt appears to have done is to treat this as an ordinary category 3 case to which the Council's policies on vulnerable people have no application. I think that approach was wrong in principle and led to a decision by him which no housing authority faced with the facts of this case could reasonably have taken.

46 The judge's endorsement of Mr Hunt's decision is objectionable in my view for the same reasons. He makes no mention of the relevance of an alternative remedy and considers the interaction between the Council and the health authorities only in relation to providing an explanation as to why Mr Barber's condition was not recognised earlier when the decision to serve the notice to quit was made. He seems to attach some weight to Mr Hunt's evidence that the case would be kept under review but that is something which should have been carried out before the making of an outright order for possession; not afterwards. Once that stage is reached the court ceases to have any control of the process. If, as I believe, steps should have been taken to explore other solutions, that should have occurred prior to the trial of the action. Absent such steps, the challenge to Mr Hunt's decision was, in my view, entitled to succeed.

Conclusions

47. For these reasons, I would allow the appeal and set aside the possession order. The consequence of Mr Barber having established a gateway (b) defence is that the action fails and should be dismissed. It was suggested by Mr Beglan that this might have the consequence that the Council would either be issue-estopped or prevented on *Henderson v Henderson* principles from seeking a possession order in a second action were it to carry out the consultation process I have identified but nevertheless ultimately conclude that the recovery of possession was, in all the circumstances, the appropriate remedy. I do not accept that. If *Wednesbury*-type public law defences are to be permitted to be run in private law proceedings for possession then an exception to the private law rules against re-litigating previously decided issues has to be recognised. In such cases, the court will not treat the second action as an abuse of process when it has been necessitated by the Council having to take further administrative steps (including reconsideration) in order to satisfy its public law obligations. In such cases, the second action will fall to be considered on its merits alone.

20.43 *Manchester City Council v Pinnock* [2010] UKSC 45, [2011] 2 AC 104

It can be disproportionate, in breach of Article 8 ECHR, to order a person to give up possession of their home, but the rights of the public landowner will almost always prevail

Facts: a local housing authority brought possession proceedings.

Judgment: the Supreme Court (Phillips, Hope, Rodger, Walker, Hale, Brown, Mance, Neuberger and Collins JJSC) held that when a public authority brought possession proceedings the court had power to assess the proportionality of making the order and, in making that assessment, to resolve any relevant dispute of fact:

> 61. First, it is only where a person's 'home' is under threat that Article 8 comes into play, and there may be cases where it is open to argument whether the premises involved are the defendant's home (eg where very short-term accommodation has been provided). Secondly, as a general rule, Article 8 need only be considered by the court if it is raised in the proceedings by or on behalf of the residential occupier. Thirdly, if an Article 8 point is raised, the court should initially consider it summarily, and if, as will no doubt often be the case, the court is satisfied that, even if the facts relied on are made out, the point would not succeed, it should be dismissed. Only if the court is satisfied that it could affect the order that the court might make should the point be further entertained.
>
> 62. Fourthly, if domestic law justifies an outright order for possession, the effect of Article 8 may, albeit in exceptional cases, justify (in ascending order of effect) granting an extended period for possession, suspending the order for possession on the happening of an event, or even refusing an order altogether.
>
> 63. Fifthly, the conclusion that the court must have the ability to assess the Article 8 proportionality of making a possession order in respect of a person's home may require certain statutory and procedural provisions to be revisited. For example, section 89 of the Housing Act 1980 limits the period for which a possession order can be postponed to 14 days, or, in cases of 'exceptional hardship', 42 days. And some of the provisions of CPR Pt 55, which appear to mandate a summary procedure in some types of possession claim, may present difficulties in relation to cases where Article 8 claims are raised. Again, we say no more on the point, since these aspects were not canvassed on the present appeal to any significant extent, save in relation to the legislation on demoted tenancies which we are about to discuss under the third issue.
>
> 64. Sixthly, the suggestions put forward on behalf of the Equality and Human Rights Commission, that proportionality is more likely to be a relevant issue 'in respect of occupants who are vulnerable as a result of mental illness, physical or learning disability, poor health or frailty', and that 'the issue may also require the local authority to explain why they are not securing alternative accommodation in such cases' seem to us well made.

20.44 *Bah v United Kingdom* Application no 56328/07, (2012) 54 EHRR 21

States were entitled to treat persons differently, for the purposes of housing assistance, on the basis of their or their dependants' immigration status and States enjoyed a wide margin of appreciation in that respect

Facts: Ms Bah had indefinite leave to remain in the United Kingdom whereas her son only had limited leave to remain, without recourse to public funds, on the basis of which she was excluded from entitlement to statutory housing assistance under Parts 6 and 7 of the Housing Act 1996, although she was helped to secure private sector accommodation, although that was more expensive.

Judgment: the European Court of Human Rights held that Ms Bah's differential treatment was on the basis of her son's immigration status and was justified for socio-economic purposes:

> 46. The Court finds therefore, in line with its previous conclusions, that the fact that immigration status is a status conferred by law, rather than one which is inherent to the individual, does not preclude it from amounting to an '*other status*' for the purposes of Article 14. In the present case, and in many other possible factual scenarios, a wide range of legal and other effects flow from a person's immigration status.
>
> 47. The Court recalls that the nature of the status upon which differential treatment is based weighs heavily in determining the scope of the margin of appreciation to be accorded to Contracting States. As observed above at [45], immigration status is not an inherent or immutable personal characteristic such as sex or race, but is subject to an element of choice. In the applicant's case, while she entered the United Kingdom as an asylum seeker, she was not granted refugee status. She cannot therefore be described as a person who was present in a contracting state because, as a refugee, she could not return to her country of origin. Furthermore, she subsequently chose to have her son join her in the United Kingdom. Given the element of choice involved in immigration status, therefore, while differential treatment based on this ground must still be objectively and reasonably justifiable, the justification required will not be as weighty as in the case of a distinction based, for example, on nationality. Furthermore, given that the subject matter of this case – the provision of housing to those in need – is predominantly socio-economic in nature, the margin of appreciation accorded to the Government will be relatively wide.
>
> 48. The court notes that while the Government argued before the Court of Appeal in the *R (Morris) v Westminster City Council* case that the differential treatment under the Housing Act 1996, as it was prior to amendment, was justified by the need to maintain immigration control and to prevent 'benefits tourism', the justification as presented to this Court was framed in terms of the need for the fair allocation of a scarce resource. The Government maintained that it was reasonable, in the allocation of social housing, to prioritise those who had a fixed and permanent right to be in the United Kingdom, or who had a priority need for housing due to dependants who had such a right.
>
> 49. The court finds that it is legitimate to put in place criteria according to which a benefit such as social housing can be allocated, when there is insufficient supply available to satisfy demand, so long as such criteria are not arbitrary or discriminatory. As the court has previously held, any welfare system, to be workable, may have to use broad categorisations to distinguish between different groups in need. The court also recalls its finding in the case of *Ponomaryov*, that states may be justified in distinguishing between different categories of aliens resident on its territory and in limiting the access of certain categories of aliens to '*resource-hungry public services*'. The court takes the view that social housing is such a public service.

20.45 *R (SL) v Westminster CC* [2013] UKSC 27, (2013) 16 CCLR 161

A need for 'care and attention' was a need for more than accommodation and monitoring

Facts: SL was a failed asylum-seeker with fresh representations who suffered from PTSD and depression. He was independent in self-care skills and had no cognitive difficulties but required practical assistance in arranging activities during the day and regular monitoring of his mental state (with general advice and encouragement), not normally at his home. Westminster concluded that SL did not require 'care and attention' for the purposes of section 21 of the National Assistance Act 1948.

Judgment: the Supreme Court (Neuberger, Hale, Mance, Kerr and Carnwath JJSC) agreed with Westminster, holding that SL had not needed anything beyond *'monitoring'* of his mental state, whereas a need for *'care and attention'* denoted a need that went beyond that and had to be the sort of care that was normally provided in a home (whether ordinary or specialised) or that would be effectively useless if the applicant had no home. In this case, even if what SL needed had amounted to *'care and attention'* it was in no way related to the provision of accommodation and, for that reason also, did not trigger the duty to provide residential accommodation.

20.46 *Hotak, Kanu and Johnson v Southwark LBC and Solihull MBC* [2015] UKSC 30, [2015] 2 WLR 1341

A homeless person is in priority need if he or she is vulnerable compared with the average person not the average homeless person

Facts: Mr Hotak had learning and mental health difficulties and Southwark decided that he was not in priority need because he had his brother's support. Mr Kanu had mental and physical health problems and Southwark decided that he was not in priority need because of support from his wife and son. Mr Johnson suffered from heroin addiction and a range of relatively low level physical and mental health problems and Solihull decided that he was not in priority need because he was not more vulnerable than the average homeless person.

Judgment: the Supreme Court (Neuberger, Hale, Clarke, Wilson and Hughes JJSC) held that the true question is whether the applicant was vulnerable compared with the average person, if made homeless, not compared with the average homeless person and that local authorities could take into account third party support, but only where it was available on a consistent and predictable basis.

20.47 *Nzolameso v City of Westminster* [2015] UKSC 22, (2015) 18 CCLR 201

Housing authorities had to consider their duty to safeguard and promote the welfare of children when assessing what accommodation would be suitable for a homeless family

Facts: Ms Nzolameso, a Westminster residents who had five young children, became unintentionally homeless. Westminster offered her accommodation in Milton Keynes then discharged its duty towards her, when she refused to accept it.

Judgment: the Supreme Court (Hale, Clarke, Reed, Hughes and Toulson JJSC) held that Westminster had acted unlawfully insofar as it had failed properly to assess and have regard to the need to safeguard and promote the welfare of the children, in breach of section 11 of the Children Act 2004, and insofar as it had failed properly to consider what accommodation closer to Westminster it might offer, if accommodation in Westminster was not available. As far as concerned the future:

> 39. Ideally, each local authority should have, and keep up to date, a policy for procuring sufficient units of temporary accommodation to meet the anticipated demand during the coming year. That policy should, of course, reflect the authority's statutory obligations under both the 1996 Act and the Children Act 2004. It should be approved by the democratically accountable members of the council and, ideally, it should be made publicly available. Secondly, each local authority should have, and keep up to date, a policy for allocating those units to individual homeless households. Where there was an anticipated shortfall of 'in borough' units, that policy would explain the factors which would be taken into account in offering households those units, the factors which would be taken into account in offering units close to home, and if there was a shortage of such units, the factors which would make it suitable to accommodate a household further away. That policy too should be made publicly available.

20.48 *Akerman-Livingstone v Aster Communities Ltd* [2015] UKSC 15, [2015] AC 1399

The court should not ordinarily determine summarily a possession claim defendant on disability discrimination grounds that appeared to be substantial because, unlike defences under the ECHR, it was not the case that a tenant's rights under the Equality Act 2010 would almost always be outweighed by the landlord's property rights

Facts: Mr A-L had a severe distress disorder and defended possession proceedings on the basis that they involved discrimination against him on the ground of his disability, contrary to section 15 of the Equality Act 2010. The county court judge made a possession order on the basis that such a defence fell to be considered in the same way as a defence under Article 8 ECHR, ie with the effect that a possession order would almost always be a proportionate means of achieving the twin aims of vindicating the local authority's property rights and enabling the authority to comply with its statutory duties in the allocation and management of its housing stock. He concluded that the defendant did not have a seriously arguable case and that there was no need for a full trial, so he made the possession order. The High Court and the Court of Appeal dismissed the defendant's appeals.

Judgment: the Supreme Court (Neuberger, Hale, Clarke, Wilson and Hughes JJSC) held that because of various recent developments, a trial judge would be bound to conclude that a possession order would be proportionate. However, the substantive right to equal treatment protected by section 35(1)(b) of the Equality Act 2010 was different from and stronger than the rights protected by Article 8 ECHR; once the possibility of disability discrimination was made out, the burden was on the landlord to show that there was no unfavourable treatment because of something arising in consequence of the tenant's disability contrary to section 15(1)(a), or that an order for possession was a proportionate means of achieving a legitimate aim under section 15(1)(b); that it could not be taken for granted that the aim of vindicating the landlord's property rights would almost always prevail over a tenant's right to have due allowances made for the consequences of his disability; that where social housing was involved the aim of enabling the local authority to comply with its statutory housing duties might have to give way to the equality rights of a particular disabled person; that, therefore, although such a claim could be dealt with summarily under CPR r55.8(1), that would not normally be an appropriate course if the claim were genuinely disputed on grounds which appeared to be substantial, where disclosure or expert evidence might be required; and that, accordingly, the judge in the county court had misdirected himself in his approach to the claim for possession.

20.49 *R (SG) v Haringey LBC* [2015] EWHC 2579 (Admin), (2015) 18 CCLR 444

A local authority need only provide accommodation under the Care Act 2014 in response to an accommodation-related need

Facts: SG was an asylum-seeker provided with asylum support. She suffered from severe mental health problems and needed help with self-care, preparing and eating food, simple tasks and medication. Haringey declined to provide residential accommodation to SG under section 21 of the National Assistance Act 1948 and then, later, under the Care Act 2014.

Judgment: Deputy High Court Judge Bowers held that the assessment under the Care Act 2014 was unlawful because (i) Haringey failed to ensure that SG was offered an independent advocate, under section 67(2) of the Care Act 2014; and (ii) Haringey failed to ask itself the correct question:

> 56. I first reiterate that the authorities already considered stand for these propositions, which I think continue to apply under the Care Act:
>
> (a) the services provided by the council must be accommodation-related for accommodation to be potentially a duty;
>
> (b) in most cases the matter is best left to the good judgment and common sense of the local authority;
>
> (c) 'accommodation-related care and attention' means care and attention of a sort which is normally provided in the home or will be 'effectively useless' if the claimant has no home.
>
> 57. Mr Burton submits there is a duty here to provide accommodation because it would be irrational not to do so in order to meet the adult's care and support needs. He has the lesser case, however, that the Council did not ask itself the correct questions. I agree with Mr Burton in the latter argument that the only suggestion that the question of whether or not the defendant was under a duty to provide accommodation was even considered by the defendant is contained in the pre-action letter. I also accept that there is no evidence that the defendant asked itself whether, even if services could have been provided in a non-home environment, they would

> have been rendered effectively useless if the claimant were homeless and sleeping on the street. This is so despite the fact that it was acknowledged that it was 'agreed that [the claimant] would benefit from some structured activities to minimise her PTSD symptoms but before that she needs help with the very basic practical support before she can be referred for more structured activities.' I thus think that the care plan has to be redone.

20.50 *R (H) v Ealing LBC* [2016] EWHC 841 (Admin), [2016] HLR 20

A Housing Allocation Scheme must not be discriminatory or breach the PSED

Facts: Ealing revised their Housing Allocation Scheme so that 20 per cent of their allocations would be made to existing tenants seeking to transfer, who had not been in breach of their tenancy agreements for specified periods of time, and to 'working households', defined as households which included a person who had been employed for at least 24 hours a week during 12 of the previous 18 months.

Judgment: HHJ Waksman QC, sitting as a Deputy High Court Judge, held that the quota for working households discriminated indirectly against people with disabilities, elderly people and women in breach of section 19 of the Equality Act 2010 in that although it pursued a legitimate objective the difference in treatment was not justified because it was not the least intrusive means of achieving that aim, in that Ealing had failed to include a discretion allowing them to override the quota for those who were unable to work because of disability, age or caring responsibilities. In addition, the quota was incompatible with Articles 8 and 14 ECHR and the process was in breach of the PSED at section 149 of the Equality Act 2010 in that Ealing's Equalities Analysis had failed to give proper consideration to how the quota might affect those with protected characteristics.

CHAPTER 21

Asylum-seekers and other overseas nationals

continued

21.23 *R (SG) v Haringey LBC* [2015] EWHC 2579 (Admin), (2015) 18 CCLR 444

A need that qualified for accommodation under the Care Act 2014 had to be accommodation-related

21.24 *R (GS) v Camden LBC [2016] EWHC 1762 (Admin), (2016) 19 CCLR 398*

Section 1 of the Localism Act 2011 could be used to provide accommodation to a person not entitled to accommodation under the Care Act 2014 and had to be so used insofar as necessary to avoid the breach of a person's ECHR rights

21.25 The statutory bar and local authority provision

Cases

21.29 *R (K) v Lambeth LBC* [2003] EWCA Civ 1150, (2003) 6 CCLR 484

It was not a breach of Article 8 ECHR to offer only travel assistance to leave the UK to a family who could reasonably be expected to leave the UK

21.30 *R (M) v Islington LBC* [2004] EWCA Civ 235, (2004) 7 CCLR 230

It was a breach of Article 8 ECHR to refuse to support this family under section 17 of the Children Act 1989

21.31 *R (Conde) v Lambeth LBC* [2005] EWHC 62 (Admin), (2005) 8 CCLR 486

It was not incompatible with EU law to refuse to accommodate a work-seeking family

21.32 *R (Limbuela) v Secretary of State for the Home Department* [2005] UKHL 66, (2006) 9 CCLR 30

It was incompatible with Article 3 ECHR to refuse to accommodate and support destitute asylum-seekers

21.33 *R (AW) v Croydon LBC* [2005] EWHC 2950 (Admin), (2006) 9 CCLR 252

It would be incompatible with the ECHR not to accommodate failed asylum-seekers with fresh claims that were not manifestly hopeless or abusive

21.34 *Blackburn-Smith v Lambeth LBC* [2007] EWHC 767 (Admin), (2007) 10 CCLR 352

On the facts, it had been lawful to offer travel assistance rather than accommodation

21.35 *R (Mwanza) v Greenwich LBC* [2010] EWHC 1462 (Admin), (2010) 13 CCLR 454

Accommodation could be provided under section 117 of the Mental Health Act 1983 only in order to address a need arising out of mental disorder

21.36 *R (Clue) v Birmingham CC* [2010] EWCA Civ 460, (2010) 13 CCLR 276

It was incompatible with Article 8 ECHR not to offer accommodation and support under section 17 of the Children Act 1989 to a mother and her children who had made an outstanding application for LTR under Article 8 ECHR, which was not manifestly abusive or hopeless

21.37 *R (Birara) v Hounslow LBC* [2010] EWHC 2113 (Admin), (2010) 13 CCLR 685

A failed asylum-seeker who had applied at port was lawfully present in the UK

21.38 *R (de Almeida) v Kensington & Chelsea RLBC* [2012] EWHC 1082 (Admin), (2012) 15 CCLR 318

A person who reasonably required assistance with domestic chores required 'care and attention'

21.39 *Pryce v Southwark LBC* [2012] EWCA Civ 1572, (2012) 15 CCLR 731
The sole carer of British children had a right of residence in the UK that qualified her for homelessness assistance

21.40 *R (KA) v Essex CC* [2013] EWHC 43 (Admin), (2013) 16 CCLR 63
It was incompatible with the ECHR to refuse accommodation to a destitute family whose claim for LTR under Article 8 ECHR had been refused, who were awaiting an appealable immigration decision and whose appeal would not be manifestly hopeless or abusive

21.41 *R (MK) v Barking and Dagenham LBC* [2013] EWHC 3486 (Admin)
Section 1 of the Localism Act 2011 could not be used to provide accommodation and support to a destitute individual, without children or care needs

21.42 *Sanneh and others v Secretary of State for Work and Pensions and others* [2015] EWCA Civ 49, (2015) 18 CCLR 5
Sole carers of British children had a right of residence under EU law and, also, a right to work and to a reasonable basic minimum for subsistence; but not to social security benefits

21.43 *R (Tigere) v Secretary of State for Business, Innovation and Skills* [2015] UKSC 57, [2015] 1 WLR 3820
It was incompatible with Article 2 of the 1st Protocol to the ECHR and Article 14 ECHR to exclude from student loans prospective students who had not clocked up three years of lawful, ordinary residence but who had lived in the UK for most of their lives, had been educated here, could not be removed save for grave misconduct and were treated throughout as members of UK society

21.44 *R (F) v Barking and Dagenham LBC* [2015] EWHC 2838 (Admin), (2015) 18 CCLR 754
It was desirable for the court to case manage jointly family law and support proceedings

21.45 *R (Kosi) v Secretary of State for the Home Department* (unreported)
Interim relief was granted, restraining the removal of a parent involved in contact proceedings

21.46 *Mirga v Secretary of State for Work and Pensions; Samin v Westminster City Council* [2016] UKSC 1
EU nationals who were not exercising rights of residence in the UK under EU law were not entitled to social assistance except perhaps in extreme circumstances and it was unnecessary for the authorities to undertake a 'proportionality exercise' in every case

21.47 United Kingdom Visas and Immigration support and local authority support

21.47 Machinery and introduction

Cases

21.59 *R (Mani and others) v Lambeth LBC and another* [2002] EWHC 735 (Admin), (2002) 5 CCLR 486
Adults who needed help with household chores needed 'care and attention'

21.60 *R (Westminster CC) v National Asylum Support Service* [2002] UKHL 38, (2002) 5 CCLR 511
Asylum support was residual and could not be provided for persons entitled to residential accommodation

continued

21.61 *R (Ouji) v Secretary of State for the Home Department* [2002] EWHC 1839 (Admin)
The local authority, not NASS, was responsible for the special needs of disabled children whose family was in receipt of asylum support

21.62 *R (Q) v Secretary of State for the Home Department* [2003] EWCA Civ 364, (2003) 6 CCLR 136
It was incompatible with Article 3 ECHR to refuse support to destitute asylum-seekers

21.63 *R (Mani) v Lambeth LBC* [2003] EWCA Civ 836, (2003) 6 CCLR 376
A person who needed help with domestic chores needed 'care and attention'

21.64 *R (A) v NASS and Waltham Forest LBC* [2003] EWCA Civ 1473, (2003) 6 CCLR 538
NASS was under a duty to accommodate a family with disabled children, not the local authority: but the accommodation had to be suitable for those children

21.65 *R (O) v Haringey LBC* [2004] EWCA Civ 535, (2004) 7 CCLR 310
The local authority was responsible for providing residential accommodation to a mother but the Secretary of State for the Home Department was responsible for funding the children's accommodation and support costs

21.66 *R (Limbuela) v Secretary of State for the Home Department* [2005] UKHL 66, (2006) 9 CCLR 30
It was incompatible with Article 3 ECHR to refuse support to destitute asylum-seekers

21.67 *R (AW) v Croydon LBC* [2005] EWHC 2950 (Admin), (2006) 9 CCLR 252
It was incompatible with the ECHR to refuse support to failed asylum-seekers who had outstanding further representations that were not manifestly hopeless or abusive

21.68 *R (AW) v Croydon LBC* [2007] EWCA Civ 266, (2007) 10 CCLR 225
Local authorities, not the Secretary of State for the Home Department, were responsible for accommodating failed asylum-seekers with a need for 'care and attention'

21.69 *R (M) v Slough BC* [2008] UKHL 52, (2008) 11 CCLR 733
A need for storage of medicine and a need for accommodation and basic living needs did not amount of a need for 'care and attention'

21.70 *R (YA) v Secretary of State for Health* [2009] EWCA Civ 225, (2009) 12 CCLR 213
A failed asylum-seeker who could not return to his country of origin was entitled to NHS care that was either immediately necessary or could not wait for his return to his country of origin

21.71 *R (Zarzour) v Hillingdon LBC* [2009] EWCA Civ 1529, (2010) 13 CCLR 157
A blind man who needed help when in new accommodation needed 'care and attention'

21.72 *R (VC) v Newcastle CC* [2011] EWHC 2673 (Admin), (2012) 15 CCLR 194
It had not lawful to decline to provide support to a destitute child, and the child's family, under section 17 of the Children Act 1989, on the basis that support might be available under section 4 of the Immigration and Asylum Act 1999

21.73 *R (SL) v Westminster CC* [2013] UKSC 27, (2013) 16 CCLR 161
A need for 'care and attention' had to be accommodation-related

21.74 *R (EAT) v Newham LBC* [2013] EWHC 344 (Admin), (2013) 16 CCLR 259
When in substance a person had applied for LTR under Article 8 ECHR, not Article 3 ECHR, only the local authority could provide support – the asylum support regime was inapplicable

21.75 *R (Refugee Action) v Secretary of State for the Home Department* [2014] EWHC 1033 (Admin), [2014] PTSR D18
The level of asylum support was in breach of the Reception Conditions Directive

Introduction

21.1 Parliament has legislated so as to limit local authority duties and powers in relation to asylum-seekers and other overseas nationals, hereafter referred to as persons subject to immigration control ('PSIC').

21.2 The easiest way of addressing such cases is as follows:

- first, assess whether the PSIC is entitled to, or may be provided with, a local authority service:
  - under the terms of the legislation governing that particular service;
  - taking into account anything in that legislation that imposes a special hurdle in relation to PSIC;

if the PSIC does not qualify, that is generally the end of the matter;

- second, if the PSIC qualifies thus far, consider whether:
  - the service falls within the list of barred services in paragraph 1 of Schedule 3 to the Nationality, Immigration and Asylum Act 2002; and if so whether
  - the PSIC falls within the list of excluded persons in paragraphs 2 and 4 to 7A of Schedule 3 to the Nationality, Immigration and Asylum Act 2002;

if the service is barred and the PSIC is excluded that could be the end of the matter, however, one must then consider whether:

- third, it is necessary for some provision to be made of a barred service, to an excluded person, in order to avoid the breach of a person's rights under EU law or the ECHR, in which case there is a duty to make that necessary level of provision available; or whether
- fourth, the PSIC is entitled to 'packing up' accommodation/assistance under the Withholding and Withdrawal of Support (Travel Assistance and Temporary Accommodation) Regulations 2002.

Limitations on local authority powers under the Care Act 2014

Adults

21.3 The starting point (for adults) is section 21 of the Care Act 2014, which prevents a local authority from providing 'care and support' to an 'adult' PSIC, or preventative services under section 2 of the Care Act 2014, in cases where the needs or future needs 'have arisen solely– (a) because the adult is destitute, or (b) because of the physical effects, or anticipated physical effects, of being destitute' as further defined.

21.4 PSIC is defined very widely, at section 115(9) of the Immigration and Asylum Act 1999, as follows:

> **115**(9) 'A person subject to immigration control' means a person who is not a national of an EEA State and who–
> (a) requires leave to enter or remain in the United Kingdom but does not have it;
> (b) has leave to enter or remain in the United Kingdom which is subject to a condition that he does not have recourse to public funds;

(c) has leave to enter or remain in the United Kingdom given as a result of a maintenance undertaking; or

(d) has leave to enter or remain in the United Kingdom only as a result of paragraph 17 of Schedule 4.

21.5 The first point to note is that section 21 of the Care Act 2014 does not prevent a local authority coming under a duty, or exercising a power, to provide 'support' to a 'carer' under section 20 of the Care Act 2014.

21.6 The second point is that, in any event, a duty could not arise by virtue of section 18 of the Care Act 2014 unless the applicant satisfied the universally applicable restriction in regulation 2 of the Care and Support (Eligibility Criteria) Regulations 2015[1] which, in short, provide that needs will only meet the eligibility criteria if they 'arise from or are related to a physical or mental impairment or illness' and 'as a consequence there is, or is likely to be, a significant impact on the adult's well-being' (reg 2(1)). It is hard to see how an eligible need ever could arise as a result of destitution. If so, the main purpose of section 21 of the Care Act 2014 must be to prevent a power arising under section 19, or a duty to take preventative steps, under section 2.

21.7 The third point is that, in any event, the Supreme Court acted under the previous regime to limit the responsibility of local authorities to provide accommodation as an adult social care service. In *R (SL) v Westminster CC*,[2] the Supreme Court held that a person only became entitled to residential accommodation under section 21 of the National Assistance Act 1948 (which imposed a duty to provide residential accommodation 'for persons aged eighteen or over who by reason of age, illness, disability or any other circumstances are in need of care and attention which is not otherwise available to them') where the person in question had a need for the sort of care that was normally provided in a home (whether ordinary or specialised) or that would be effectively useless if the applicant had no home. The initial judicial indication is that the same approach applies under the Care Act 2014, in the sense that a local authority may not provide 'accommodation' under section 8 of the Care Act 2014 unless the applicant needs the sort of care that is normally provided in a home (whether ordinary or specialised) or that would be effectively useless if he or she had no home: *R (SG) v Haringey LBC*:[3] see further above, at chapter 20 on housing provision under the Care Act 2014 at paras 20.3 and 20.12.

21.8 The fourth point is that a function of section 21 of the Care Act 2014 is to provide a sorting mechanism for distinguishing between PSIC who might (potentially) be accommodated and supported by the Secretary of State for the Home Department under section 4 or Part 6 of the Immigration and Asylum Act 1999 (eg because they are asylum-seekers or failed asylum-seekers) and PSIC who might (potentially be accommodated and supported by local authorities under the Care Act 2014. However, section 21 of the Care Act 2014 provides only one part of the sorting mechanism, the whole of which works as follows:

1 SI No 313.

2 [2013] UKSC 27, (2013) 16 CCLR 161.

3 [2015] EWHC 2579 (Admin), (2015) 18 CCLR 444.

- on its proper construction, the statutory scheme makes support from the Secretary of State for the Home Department largely residual, such that where a local authority has power to provide support to an adult, then the Secretary of State for the Home Department may not do so;[4]
- a local authority has power to provide accommodation plus support to persons who meet the criteria for such in the Care Act 2014 and who are:
  - asylum-seekers and other persons *not excluded* by Schedule 3 to the Nationality, Immigration and Asylum Act 2002;[5]
  - failed asylum-seekers who are in the UK in breach of the immigration laws, and other persons who *are excluded* by Schedule 3 to the Nationality, Immigration and Asylum Act 2002, insofar as it may be necessary to provide support to avoid a breach of a person's rights under the ECHR or EU law;[6] *providing that*
  - such persons need the sort of care that is normally provided in a home (whether ordinary or specialised) or that would be effectively useless if the applicant had no home;[7] and *unless those needs*
  - 'have arisen solely– (a) because the adult is destitute, or (b) because of the physical effects, or anticipated physical effects, of being destitute'.[8]

21.9 These 'sorting provisions' apply where there is a potential overlap between the powers of a local authority to provide both accommodation and support and those of the Secretary of State for the Home Department, eg in the case of asylum-seekers and failed asylum-seekers. This type of case is considered further below, at 'United Kingdom Visas and Immigration support' at para 21.47.

21.10 In some types of case, of course, there is no potential overlap and an adult who is a PSIC and also destitute will need to try to secure accommodation and support from a local authority because the Secretary of State for the Home Department has no express statutory power to provide them with support, primarily:

- adults who have dependent children and who are waiting for a decision on an application for leave to remain (LTR) under Article 8 ECHR, who may be provided with accommodation and support under section 17 of the Children Act 1989;[9]
- adults without dependent children who are waiting for a decision on an application for LTR under Article 8 ECHR, who may be provided with accommodation and support under the Care Act 2014 or the Localism

4 *R (Westminster CC) v National Asylum Support Service* [2002] UKHL 38, (2002) 5 CCLR 511.

5 See below, 'the statutory bar', para 21.25.

6 See below, 'the statutory bar', para 21.25.

7 *R (SL) v Westminster CC* [2013] UKSC 27, (2013) 16 CCLR 161; applied in *R (SG) v Haringey LBC* [2015] EWHC 2579 (Admin), (2015) 18 CCLR 444: but see the discussion above, at paras 20.10–20.15 and 20.45.

8 Care Act 2014 s21.

9 *R (Clue) v Birmingham CC* [2010] EWCA Civ 460, (2010) 13 CCLR 276.

Act 2011, although such cases are not without some difficulty:[10] see further, 'the statutory bar', at para 21.25 below.

21.11 The No Recourse to Public Funds Network has published 'Practice Guidance for Local Authorities (England): Assessing and Supporting Adults who have No Recourse to Public Funds'.[11]

Children

21.12 Unaccompanied asylum-seeking children will almost certainly qualify for accommodation under section 20 of the Children Act 1989, which does not impose any special criteria on children from abroad.

21.13 After they turn 18, they will in general continue to qualify for local authority support under the 'children leaving care machinery', up to the age of 21[12] – longer, if they continue to supported by the local authority to pursue a course of education or training.

21.14 Children living with their families (seeking asylum or LTR under the ECHR) will have their general accommodation and welfare needs met by the Secretary of State for the Home Department, by virtue of section 122 of the Immigration and Asylum Act 1999 – but the local authority will meet any special needs that they may have, under section 17 of the Children Act 1989.[13]

Cases

21.15 *R v Hammersmith & Fulham LBC ex p M, P, A and X* (1997–8) 1 CCLR 85, CA

A destitute person might require 'care and attention'

Facts: the applicants were healthy and able-bodied single males who were destitute asylum-seekers, not permitted to work and excluded from social security benefits and housing assistance. They sought residential accommodation under section 21 of the National Assistance Act 1948.

Judgment: the Court of Appeal (Lord Woolf MR, Waite and Henry LJJ) held that destitution would inevitably result in a person needing 'care and attention' within the meaning of section 21 of the National Assistance Act 1948:

> Asylum-seekers are not entitled merely because they lack money and accommodation to claim they automatically qualify under section 21(1)(a). What they are entitled to claim (and this is the result of the 1996 Act) is that they can as a result of their predicament after they arrive in this country reach a state where they qualify under the subsection because of the effect upon them of the problems under which they are labouring. In addition to the lack of food and accommodation is to be added their inability to speak the language, their ignorance of this country and the fact they have been subject to the stress of coming to this country in circumstances which at

10 *R (MK) v Barking and Dagenham LBC* [2013] EWHC 3486 (Admin).
11 www.nrpfnetwork.org.uk/Documents/Practice-Guidance-Adults-England.pdf.
12 *R (SO) v Barking and Dagenham LBC* [2010] EWCA Civ 1101, (2010) 13 CCLR 591.
13 *R (Ouji) v Secretary of State for the Home Department* [2002] EWHC 1839 (Admin).

least involve their contending to be refugees. Inevitably the combined effect of these factors with the passage of time will produce one or more of the conditions specifically referred to in section 21(1)(a). It is for the authority to decide whether they qualify. In making their decision, they can bear in mind the wide terms of the Direction to which reference has already been made, as contrary to Mr Beloff's submission the direction is not *ultra vires* and gives a useful introduction to the application of the subsection. In particular the authorities can anticipate the deterioration which would otherwise take place in the asylum seekers condition by providing assistance under the section. They do not need to wait until the health of the asylum seeker has been damaged. The result is that section 21(1)(a) should enable assistance to be provided at least in the case of some asylum seekers. It also means that an added burden has been placed upon local authorities which but for the 1996 Act would have had to be met in part by central government. This consequence is not however one for which the court can give any relief. This court's task is limited to seeking to clarify the proper interpretation and scope of section 21(1)(a) which having been done means this appeal should be dismissed.

Comment: this decision has now been substantially modified by the decisions of the House of Lords and Supreme Court in *Slough* (para 21.69) and *SL* (para 21.22 below). Nonetheless, it and *Limbuela* (para 21.32) remain powerful indicators that the courts will do everything possible to ensure that asylum-seekers are not left destitute.

21.16 *R (Ali) v Birmingham CC* [2002] EWHC 1511 (Admin), (2002) 5 CCLR 355

It could be lawful to use section 17 of the Children Act 1989 to offer assistance enabling a destitute family to leave the UK, rather than to remain here

Facts: families from abroad with children, who were ineligible for mainstream benefits, were not asylum-seekers and their children's needs could be met in their country of origin. On claims being made for support under section 17 of the Children Act 1989, on the basis that the families were destitute, Birmingham offered assistance to return to the country of origin, or accommodation for the children on their own. The families sought a judicial review, to compel the provision of 'family support'.

Judgment: Moses J dismissed the applications: although the children had been assessed as being children in need, Birmingham had a wide power to decide how to meet such needs and its decision was far from irrational (irrespective of whether claims of domestic violence in the country of origin were true); neither was there any breach of the ECHR; nor did it matter that no assessments had been completed under section 21 of the National Assistance Act 1948 because the issues and result would have been the same:

61. The submission of the claimants is, in my view, wrong in that it fails to distinguish between assessment of need and the Council's wide power to decide as to how that need can properly be met. The choice of the mother to leave the Netherlands was, as it seems to me, relevant to the distinct question as to how assessed needs could properly be met. If, in the light of the accommodation and support available in the Netherlands, the children were better off in a country where they spoke the language and where they

had hitherto stronger ties, then the Council was entitled to meet the need by funding the return of the family. The fact that the mother had exercised a choice to leave the Netherlands and was not compelled to do so was relevant to the question as to whether the needs could be met in the Netherlands. If she had no choice but to leave the Netherlands then her needs obviously could not be met there. Thus the fact that she did have a choice, in the judgment of the Council, which had been exercised, was relevant to the distinct issue as to what action the Council should take to meet the assessed need. In short, choice was relevant to the question of what ought to be done to meet the need.

Comment: for the proper approach where a family member cannot be expected to leave the UK because to do so would be incompatible with Article 8 ECHR, see *Clue* below at para 21.21.

21.17 *R (Mani and others) v Lambeth LBC and another* [2002] EWHC 735 (Admin), (2002) 5 CCLR 486

A need for help with domestic chores amounted to a need for 'care and attention'

Facts: Mr Mani and Mr Tasci had limited mobility as a result of physical disability and Mr J was seriously ill as a result of advanced HIV+: All three needed help with domestic tasks and were destitute asylum-seekers.

Judgment: the claimants' needs did not arise solely as a result of destitution so that, because regulations 6 and 23 of the Asylum Support Regulations 2000 required the local authorities to disregard the availability of Home Office support, they were under a duty to provide the claimants with residential accommodation under section 21 of the National Assistance Act 1948.

21.18 *R (M) v Islington LBC* [2004] EWCA Civ 235, (2004) 7 CCLR 230

It can be incompatible with Article 8 ECHR to use section 17 of the Children Act 1989 to offer travel assistance, rather than assistance to remain in the UK

Facts: Mrs M was a national of Guyana, who had separated from her British citizen partner, and who looked after a young child, also British. Pending the determination of her application for LTR she was destitute, and applied to Islington for accommodation and support and section 17 of the Children Act 1989. Islington determined to offer her and her child only travel assistance back to Guyana.

Judgment: the Court of Appeal (Waller, Buxton and Maurice Kay LJJ) held that (by a majority), Islington had power to offer accommodation pending any removal by the Secretary of State for the Home Department, even if that removal was a long way distant in the future, under the Withholding and Withdrawal of Support (Travel Assistance and Temporary Accommodation) Regulations 2002, which it had failed to consider exercising.

The court held unanimously that, if Islington lacked such power, that would interfere with the Article 8 rights of mother and child:

> 46. In paras 49–59 of his judgment Wilson J gave cogent reasons why the Convention rights at least under Article 8 of all of the child, Mrs M and Mr M are in issue in this case. All of those rights would be likely to be seriously

> affected if all that Islington could do were to exercise its powers under the Regulations, with the effects summarised in para 40 above. First, Mrs M is adamant that she will not leave the UK. Absent removal directions, she cannot be forced to do so; and since, as we have seen, Islington cannot fund her travel arrangements under Schedule 3 it is difficult to see how a destitute woman could leave, let alone find her way back to Guyana, even if she wanted to do so. Islington made it clear in its letter of 21 March 2003 that that would raise 'a real prospect' of the child being taken into care. I for my part would find it difficult not to see an offer of tickets with an alternative of no accommodation (made not for social reasons but in an attempt to enforce immigration control other than by the issuing of removal directions) as an unjustifiable interference with the Article 8 rights both of Mrs M and of the child. Second, as the judge pointed out, whilst Mrs M and the child may be able to maintain family life in Guyana, if the object of removing them there succeeds, there has to be substantial certainty on that point before removal can confidently be said not to raise issues under Article 8. Third, it would be quite unreasonable to expect Mr M, settled in the United Kingdom and separated from Mrs M, to follow her to Guyana. Depending on the strength of the bond between Mr M and the child, the Article 8 rights of both of them would be threatened by the prospect of the child's removal to Guyana.
>
> 47. While this would be in the first instance a matter for Islington, it might have found it difficult not to conclude that, on any view of Mrs M's possible reaction, the limitation of its powers to those under the Regulations will involve interference with the parties' Convention rights. I should also make plain that, in assessing any future decision that Islington might have made, the criterion would not simply be that of *Wednesbury* unreasonableness. The test of necessity under para 3 of Schedule 3 imposes a condition precedent to the exercise of a statutory function, under the (restored) Children Act powers. That test must be applied according to objective criteria, which the court retains the power to review.

Buxton and Waller LJJ agreed about the proper approach to assessment under the Children Act 1989, in these circumstances:

> 49. Islington would have to bear three considerations in mind before it could lawfully discharge its Children Act duty by an offer of tickets rather than by providing support, including accommodation, in the United Kingdom. First, it would have to be confident that the child will cease to be 'in need' if removed to Guyana. Wilson J, who has unrivalled experience in these matters, pointed to the detailed and circumstantial enquiry needed in this case, none of which appears to have taken place. Second, the various parties' Convention rights must be respected in any action taken under the Children Act, just as they are relevant to putative action under the Regulations. The considerations set out in para 46 above remain directly in point. Here again, because what is in issue is the state's positive obligation under Article 8 of the Convention to protect family life (see for instance *Marckx v Belgium* Case 6833/74 at para 31), Islington would have to act in the light of that obligation, and not simply reach a decision that is not *Wednesbury* unreasonable. Third, Islington would have to bear in mind the implications of seeking to remove a British citizen from the United Kingdom, as indicated in para 30 above.

21.19 *R (PB) v Haringey LBC* [2006] EWHC 2255 (Admin), (2007) 10 CCLR 99

It could be incompatible with Article 8 ECHR to refuse to provide support to a woman engaged in care proceedings involving her children

Facts: Ms PB was an unlawful overstayer, with an outstanding application for LTR under a child concession policy: she had five children and although one lived with the father and four were in foster care and subject to care proceedings, she had regular contact with them all. Ms PB was destitute and Haringey was refusing to provide her with accommodation under section 21 of the National Assistance Act 1948, in part on the ground that the sole cause of her need to 'care and attention' was destitution and/or its physical effects.

Judgment: Deputy High Court Judge Nicol held that Haringey had erred in law by failing to consider whether Ms PB's needs were also caused by her moderate depression and by failing to scrutinise with appropriate care her submission that if she had to return to Jamaica because of destitution, that would breach her rights under Article 8 ECHR: even if she applied for entry clearance from Jamaica to participate in the care proceedings, she would miss a crucial social work assessment of her relationship with the children.

21.20 *R (Mwanza) v Greenwich LBC* [2010] EWHC 1462 (Admin), (2010) 13 CCLR 454

Ordinary accommodation could only be provided under section 117 of the Mental Health Act 1983 when it answered a need arising out of mental disorder

Facts: Mr Mwanza and his family were unlawfully present in the UK. Mr Mwanza had received various support services under section 117 of the Mental Health Act 1983 but the PCT and local authority ultimately decided to cease their duty under that section. Afterwards, facing destitution on account of his and his family's immigration status, Mr Mwanza sought accommodation and support, either under section 117 or under section 21 of the National Assistance Act 1948.

Judgment: Hickinbottom J held that:

1) The duty to provide after-care services under section 117 of the Mental Health Act 1983 is a duty to provide services that are necessary to meet a need arising from a person's mental disorder. The need to work and the need for a roof over one's head are common needs and do not arise from mental disorder. This does not mean that a need for assistance in finding employment or housing on discharge cannot be provided and neither is it the case that provision of ordinary accommodation can never fall within section 117.

2) In this case, the need for accommodation came from the legal inability of the claimant and his wife to work due to their immigration status and could not be said to be due to the claimant's mental condition or any change in that condition.

3) In any event, there had been a proper decision in 2001 to discharge the claimant from further section 117 services, on the basis that it had been concluded by the claimant's absence and the lack of further problems that the claimant no longer needed them. Also, the challenge in this case had to be viewed as a challenge to the decision to treat section 117 responsibilities as discharged and gave rise to overwhelming arguments of delay in challenging the decision by way of judicial review.

4) The claim against Bromley council under section 21 of the National Assistance Act 1948 would be dismissed, since the claimant did not need any care and attention that could not be provided by his family looking after him and that assessment had not been challenged, nor could it be. It also appeared that the family's immigration status and the absence of any reliable evidence that there were any outstanding immigration appeals meant that the council was precluded from providing services under section 21.

21.21 *R (Clue) v Birmingham CC* [2010] EWCA Civ 460, (2010) 13 CCLR 276

It was incompatible with Article 8 ECHR not to offer accommodation and support under section 17 of the Children Act 1989 to a mother and her children who had made an outstanding application for LTR under Article 8 ECHR, which was not manifestly abusive or hopeless

Facts: Ms Clue was a Jamaican national who had unlawfully overstayed her leave to enter the UK, but who had an outstanding application for LTR with the Secretary of State for the Home Department, based on the long residence of her children. Having become destitute, she applied to Birmingham for support under section 17 of the Children Act 1989. Birmingham declined to provide any support, except such as would enable the family to return to Jamaica.

Judgment: the Court of Appeal (Dyson and Etherton LJJ, Sir Scott Baker) allowed Ms Clue's application for judicial review:

1) When enacting Schedule 3 to the 2002 Act, Parliament cannot reasonably have intended to confer a general power on local authorities to pre-empt the determination by the Secretary of State of applications for leave to remain. Save in hopeless or abusive cases, the duty imposed on local authorities to act so as to avoid a breach of an applicant's Convention rights does not require or entitle them to decide how the Secretary of State will determine an application for leave to remain or, in effect, determine such an application themselves by making it impossible for an applicant to pursue it.

2) There was no material before the court to suggest that the Secretary of State routinely exercises his discretion to determine an application for leave to remain notwithstanding that the applicant has left the UK. Accordingly, local authorities should approach their task on the footing that if, by withholding assistance, they require a person to return to his country of origin, that person's application for leave to remain will be treated by the Secretary of State as withdrawn.

3) Therefore when applying Schedule 3, a local authority should not consider the merits of an outstanding application for leave to remain. It is required to be satisfied that the application is not 'obviously hopeless or abusive'.

4) In circumstances where a person has made an application to the Secretary of State for leave to remain that raises Convention grounds and has made an application for assistance to the local authority that falls to be considered under Schedule 3 to the 2002 Act, the financial situation of the local authority is irrelevant when applying Article 8(2). The disposal of applications for leave should not depend on the vagaries of the budgetary considerations of local authorities.

5) Even if it had been legitimate for Birmingham to disregard the application for leave to remain and it had been entitled to decide for itself whether the withholding of assistance would breach the Convention rights of the claimant and her family, its assessment was nevertheless unlawful. The whole emphasis of the assessment was on the issue of respect for family life. There was no recognition that a return to Jamaica would interfere with the family's right to private life (their relationships and social, cultural and family ties in the UK) or that they understood that the private life rights of children who were born in the UK or came here at an early age were of particular weight.

6) The facts of the case exposed the problem created for local authorities by delays on the part of UKBA in dealing with applications for leave to remain by persons in the position of the claimant and her family. The Secretary of State had agreed to take steps to mitigate these problems, namely to prioritise consideration of cases involving applicants supported by local authorities in the same way as those of applicants supported by the Secretary of State and to review decision-making processes having regard to the need to safeguard and promote the welfare of children.

21.22 *R (SL) v Westminster* CC [2013] UKSC 27, (2013) 16 CCLR 161

A need for 'care and attention' had to be accommodation-related

Facts: SL was a failed asylum-seeker with fresh representations who suffered from PTSD and depression. He was independent in self-care skills and had no cognitive difficulties but required practical assistance in arranging activities during the day and regular monitoring of his mental state (with general advice and encouragement), not normally at his home. Westminster concluded that SL did not require 'care and attention' for the purposes of section 21 of the National Assistance Act 1948.

Judgment: the Supreme Court (Neuberger, Hale, Mance, Kerr and Carnwath JJSC) agreed with Westminster:

1) The meaning of 'care and attention' has been subject to authoritative guidance by Baroness Hale, with helpful elaboration by Lord Neuberger, in *R (M) v Slough Borough Council*[14] and the ordinary meaning of the statutory words does not support a more restrictive approach of limiting

14 [2008] UKHL 52, (2008) 11 CCLR 733.

it to personal care or services of a 'close and intimate nature'. What is involved in 'care and attention' must take its colour from its association with the duty to provide residential accommodation. It cannot be confined to that species of care and attention that can only be delivered in residential accommodation of a specialised kind but something well beyond mere monitoring of an individual's condition is required.

2) (*Obiter*) Assuming that L's needs did amount to a need for 'care and attention', the care and attention was available otherwise than by the provision of accommodation under National Assistance Act 1948 s21. The services provided by the Council were in no sense accommodation-related. They were entirely independent of his actual accommodation, however provided, or his need for it. The Court of Appeal was wrong in concluding that 'available 'means not merely available in fact but as implying also a requirement for care and attention to be 'reasonably practicable and efficacious'. Moreover, the need for accommodation cannot in itself constitute a need for care and attention. The care and attention has to be accommodation-related which means that it has at least to be care and attention of a sort which is normally provide in the home (whether ordinary or specialised) or will be effectively useless if the claimant has no home. On this part of section 21, the Court of Appeal in *R (Mani) v Lambeth LBC*[15]and *R (O) v Barking and Dagenham LBC*[16] erred in concluding that if an applicant's need for care and attention is to any extent made more acute by circumstances other than the lack of accommodation and funds, he qualifies for assistance under section 21(1)(a).

21.23 *R (SG) v Haringey LBC* [2015] EWHC 2579 (Admin), (2015) 18 CCLR 444

A need that qualified for accommodation under the Care Act 2014 had to be accommodation-related

Facts: SG was an asylum-seeker provided with asylum support. She suffered from severe mental health problems and needed help with self-care, preparing and eating food, simple tasks and medication. Haringey declined to provide residential accommodation to SG under section 21 of the National Assistance Act 1948 and then, later, under the Care Act 2014.

Judgment: Deputy High Court Judge Bowers held that the assessment under the Care Act 2014 was unlawful because (i) Haringey failed to ensure that SG was offered an independent advocate, under section 67(2) of the Care Act 2014; and (ii) Haringey failed to ask itself the correct question:

> 56. I first reiterate that the authorities already considered stand for these propositions, which I think continue to apply under the Care Act:
>
> (a) the services provided by the council must be accommodation-related for accommodation to be potentially a duty;
>
> (b) in most cases the matter is best left to the good judgment and common sense of the local authority;

15 [2003] EWCA Civ 836, (2003) 6 CCLR 376.

16 [2010] EWCA Civ 1101, (2010) 13 CCLR 591.

(c) 'accommodation-related care and attention' means care and attention of a sort which is normally provided in the home or will be 'effectively useless' if the claimant has no home.

57. Mr Burton submits there is a duty here to provide accommodation because it would be irrational not to do so in order to meet the adult's care and support needs. He has the lesser case, however, that the Council did not ask itself the correct questions. I agree with Mr Burton in the latter argument that the only suggestion that the question of whether or not the defendant was under a duty to provide accommodation was even considered by the defendant is contained in the pre-action letter. I also accept that there is no evidence that the defendant asked itself whether, even if services could have been provided in a non-home environment, they would have been rendered effectively useless if the claimant were homeless and sleeping on the street. This is so despite the fact that it was acknowledged that it was 'agreed that [the claimant] would benefit from some structured activities to minimise her PTSD symptoms but before that she needs help with the very basic practical support before she can be referred for more structured activities.' I thus think that the care plan has to be redone.

Comment: see the discussion of this case above at paras 20.3–20.12.

21.24 *R (GS) v Camden LBC* [2016] EWHC 1762 (Admin), (2016) 19 CCLR 398

Section 1 of the Localism Act 2011 could be used to provide accommodation to a person not entitled to accommodation under the Care Act 2014 and had to be so used insofar as necessary to avoid the breach of a person's ECHR rights

Facts: GS was a Swiss national of Afghan origin who suffered from a number of fairly severe physical and mental health problems and had become homeless and without the means to support herself but unable to bring herself to return to Switzerland. She was excluded from all forms of mainstream benefits apart from Personal Independence Payments, which she received.

Judgment: Mr Peter Marquand sitting as a Deputy High Court Judge held that, on the particular facts, it had been lawful for Camden to conclude that GS had not required 'care and support' for the purposes of the Care Act 2014 and that a need simply for accommodation did not amount to a need for 'care and support' (applying *R (SG) v Haringey LBC* [2015] EWHC 2579 (Admin), (2015) 18 CCLR 444). However, the Judge went on to hold that section 1 of the Localism Act 2011 empowered Camden to provide GS with accommodation and that it was, on the facts, required to do so to avoid a breach of her rights under the ECHR resulting from her homelessness and lack of sufficient means to support herself. In particular, the Judge distinguished *R (MK) v Barking and Dagenham LBC* [2003] EWHC 3486 (Admin), on the basis that because the Care Act 2014 post-dated the Localism Act 2011, the very broad power in section 1 of the Localism Act 2011 was not excluded because the Care Act 2014 did not include a 'post commencement limitation', as defined in section 2(2) and (4) of the Localism Act 2011, that is, 'a prohibition, restriction or other limitation expressly imposed by a statutory provision' that is 'expressed to apply – (i) to the general power, (ii) to all of the authority's powers, or (iii) to all of the authority's powers but with exceptions that do not include the general power'.

The statutory bar and local authority provision

21.25 The list of excluded services is set out in paragraph 1 of Schedule 3 to the Nationality, Immigration and Asylum Act 2002, the provisions relating to England being as follows:

1(1) A person to whom this paragraph applies shall not be eligible for support or assistance under–

(a) section 21 or 29 of the National Assistance Act 1948 (local authority: accommodation and welfare),

(b) section 45 of the Health Services and Public Health Act 1968 (local authority: welfare of elderly),

(c) section 12 or 13A of the Social Work (Scotland) Act 1968 (social welfare services),

(d) Article 7 or 15 of the Health and Personal Social Services (Northern Ireland) Order 1972 (SI No 1265 (NI 14)) (prevention of illness, social welfare, etc),

(e) ... section 192 of, and Schedule 15 to, the National Health Service (Wales) Act 2006 (social services),

(f) section 29(1)(b) of the Housing (Scotland) Act 1987 (interim duty to accommodate in case of apparent priority need where review of a local authority decision has been requested),

(g) section 17, 23C, 23CA, 24A or 24B of the Children Act 1989 (welfare and other powers which can be exercised in relation to adults),

(h) Article 18, 35 or 36 of the Children (Northern Ireland) Order 1995 (SI No 755 (NI 2)) (welfare and other powers which can be exercised in relation to adults),

(i) sections 22, 29 and 30 of the Children (Scotland) Act 1995 (provisions analogous to those mentioned in paragraph (g)),

(j) section 188(3) or 204(4) of the Housing Act 1996 (accommodation pending review or appeal),

(k) section 2 of the Local Government Act 2000 (promotion of well-being),

(ka) section 1 of the Localism Act 2011 (local authority's general power of competence),

(l) a provision of the Immigration and Asylum Act 1999,

(m) a provision of this Act, or Part 1 of the Care Act 2014 (care and support provided by local authority).

(2) A power or duty under a provision referred to in sub-paragraph (1) may not be exercised or performed in respect of a person to whom this paragraph applies (whether or not the person has previously been in receipt of support or assistance under the provision).

(3) An approval or directions given under or in relation to a provision referred to in sub-paragraph (1) shall be taken to be subject to sub-paragraph (2).

The classes of persons subject to the exclusion are:

- persons/dependants with refugee status abroad (paragraph 4 of Schedule 3);
- EEA nationals/dependants (paragraph 5);
- failed asylum-seekers (lawfully present) who have failed to co-operate with removal directions (paragraph 6);
- persons in the UK in breach of the immigration laws within the meaning of section 50A of the British Nationality Act 1981, unless they are

asylum-seekers (defined for these purposes at paragraph 17 of Schedule 3) (paragraph 7);
- failed asylum-seekers with dependent children who have been certified by the Secretary of State as failing without reasonable excuse to take reasonable steps to leave the UK (paragraph 7A).

21.26 Even if PSICs satisfy the eligibility criteria for accommodation and support and/or even if they surmount the hurdle at section 21 of the Care Act 2014 they must also not fall foul of Schedule 3 to the Nationality, Asylum and Immigration Act 2002, which prohibits local authorities from providing a range of services to some classes of PSIC, including but by no means limited to services under the Care Act 2014, except insofar as may be necessary to avoid a breach of a person's rights under the ECHR or EU law.

21.27 The exclusionary effect of Schedule 3 does not extend:
- to children, for whom local authorities may always provide services, irrespective of their immigration status;
- to the extent permitted by delegated legislation: the Withholding and Withdrawal of Support (Travel Assistance and Temporary Accommodation) Regulations 2002[17] permit and sometimes require local authorities to provide temporary accommodation pending the making of travel arrangements (for the PSIC to leave the UK) in certain circumstances;
- to the provision of any service insofar as it may be necessary to avoid a breach of EU or ECHR rights (paragraph 3 of Schedule 3 to the Nationality, Immigration and Asylum Act 2002):

> 3. Paragraph 1 does not prevent the exercise of a power or the performance of a duty if, and to the extent that, its exercise or performance is necessary for the purpose of avoiding a breach of–
> (a) a person's Convention rights, or
> (b) a person's rights under the EU Treaties.

21.28 The approach of the courts to paragraph 3 of Schedule 3 has been to treat it as being necessary to provide basic support in a case where, otherwise:
- the applicant would be pushed away from the UK as a result of not having their basic needs met (including accommodation and essential needs);
- *providing* that would be incompatible with their rights under the ECHR;
- *which will be the case,* where the applicant has an outstanding application for LTR on refugee or ECHR grounds that is not '*manifestly hopeless or abusive*'.[18]

17 SI No 3078.

18 *R (Clue) v Birmingham CC* [2010] EWCA Civ 460, (2010) 13 CCLR 276.

Cases

21.29 *R (K) v Lambeth LBC* [2003] EWCA Civ 1150, (2003) 6 CCLR 484

It was not a breach of Article 8 ECHR to offer only travel assistance to leave the UK to a family who could reasonably be expected to leave the UK

Facts: Ms K was a Kenyan citizen whose marriage to an Irish national had been determined by the Secretary of State for the Home Department to be a marriage of convenience. Ms K's appeal against that decision was pending but she was precluded meanwhile from mainstream benefits and sought assistance from Lambeth under section 17 of the Children Act 1989, for herself and her young child. Lambeth took the view that Ms K was excluded from eligibility by Schedule 3 to the Nationality, Immigration and Asylum Act 2002 and that it was unnecessary to provide her with support, to avoid a breach of ECHR rights.

Judgment: the Court of Appeal (Lord Phillips MR, Judge and Kay LJJ) held that it was unnecessary, for the purpose of respecting the family or private life of Ms K and her child, for them to remain in the UK pending her appeal: Ms K and her husband had already separated (and the child was not his) whereas Ms K could pursue her appeal from Kenya without real difficulty:

> 49. No authority has been placed before us which bears directly on the issue we have to resolve. We must decide it as a matter of principle. We do not consider that either Article 3 or Article 8 imposes a duty on the State to provide the appellant with support. She has not been granted leave to enter or remain in this country. She has been permitted to remain here to pursue an appeal in which she advances, inter alia, an Article 8 claim, which we consider to be clearly specious. Even if it were not, no infringement of Article 8 would result from requiring her to return to her own country pending the determination of her appeal. There is no impediment to her returning to her own country. A State owes no duty under the Convention to provide support to foreign nationals who are permitted to enter their territory but who are in a position freely to return home. Most people who fall into this category are given leave to enter on condition that they do not have recourse to public funds.

21.30 *R (M) v Islington LBC* [2004] EWCA Civ 235, (2004) 7 CCLR 230

It was a breach of Article 8 ECHR to refuse to support this family under section 17 of the Children Act 1989

Facts: Mrs M was a national of Guyana, who had separated from her British citizen partner, and who looked after a young child, also British. Pending the determination of her application for LTR she was destitute, and applied to Islington for accommodation and support under section 17 of the Children Act 1989. Islington determined to offer her and her child only travel assistance back to Guyana.

Judgment: the Court of Appeal (Waller, Buxton and Maurice Kay LJJ) held that (by a majority), Islington had power to offer accommodation pending any removal by the Secretary of State for the Home Department, even if that was some time distant in the future, under the Withholding and

Withdrawal of Support (Travel Assistance and Temporary Accommodation) Regulations 2002, which it had failed to consider exercising.

The court held unanimously that, if Islington lacked such power, that would interfere with the Article 8 rights of mother and child:

> 46. In paras 49–59 of his judgment Wilson J gave cogent reasons why the Convention rights at least under article 8 of all of the child, Mrs M and Mr M are in issue in this case. All of those rights would be likely to be seriously affected if all that Islington could do were to exercise its powers under the Regulations, with the effects summarised in para 40 above. First, Mrs M is adamant that she will not leave the UK. Absent removal directions, she cannot be forced to do so; and since, as we have seen, Islington cannot fund her travel arrangements under Schedule 3 it is difficult to see how a destitute woman could leave, let alone find her way back to Guyana, even if she wanted to do so. Islington made it clear in its letter of 21 March 2003 that that would raise 'a real prospect' of the child being taken into care. I for my part would find it difficult not to see an offer of tickets with an alternative of no accommodation (made not for social reasons but in an attempt to enforce immigration control other than by the issuing of removal directions) as an unjustifiable interference with the Article 8 rights both of Mrs M and of the child. Second, as the judge pointed out, whilst Mrs M and the child may be able to maintain family life in Guyana, if the object of removing them there succeeds, there has to be substantial certainty on that point before removal can confidently be said not to raise issues under Article 8. Third, it would be quite unreasonable to expect Mr M, settled in the United Kingdom and separated from Mrs M, to follow her to Guyana. Depending on the strength of the bond between Mr M and the child, the Article 8 rights of both of them would be threatened by the prospect of the child's removal to Guyana.
>
> 47. While this would be in the first instance a matter for Islington, it might have found it difficult not to conclude that, on any view of Mrs M's possible reaction, the limitation of its powers to those under the Regulations will involve interference with the parties' Convention rights. I should also make plain that, in assessing any future decision that Islington might have made, the criterion would not simply be that of *Wednesbury* unreasonableness. The test of necessity under para 3 of Schedule 3 imposes a condition precedent to the exercise of a statutory function, under the (restored) Children Act powers. That test must be applied according to objective criteria, which the court retains the power to review.

Buxton and Waller LJJ agreed about the proper approach to assessment under the Children Act 1989, in these circumstances:

> 49. Islington would have to bear three considerations in mind before it could lawfully discharge its Children Act duty by an offer of tickets rather than by providing support, including accommodation, in the United Kingdom. First, it would have to be confident that the child will cease to be 'in need' if removed to Guyana. Wilson J, who has unrivalled experience in these matters, pointed to the detailed and circumstantial enquiry needed in this case, none of which appears to have taken place. Second, the various parties' Convention rights must be respected in any action taken under the Children Act, just as they are relevant to putative action under the Regulations. The considerations set out in para 46 above remain directly in point. Here again, because what is in issue is the state's positive obligation under Article 8 of the Convention to protect family life (see for instance *Marckx v Belgium* Case 6833/74 at para 31), Islington would have

to act in the light of that obligation, and not simply reach a decision that is not *Wednesbury* unreasonable. Third, Islington would have to bear in mind the implications of seeking to remove a British citizen from the United Kingdom, as indicated in para 30 above.

21.31 *R (Conde) v Lambeth LBC* [2005] EWHC 62 (Admin), (2005) 8 CCLR 486

It was not incompatible with EU law to refuse to accommodate a work-seeking family

Facts: Mrs Conde was the mother of two young children and a Spanish national. Lambeth declined to provide her with accommodation and support under section 17 of the Children Act 1989, on the basis that she was ineligible by virtue of Schedule 3 to the Nationality, Immigration and Asylum Act 2002. Mrs Conde claimed that the exception in paragraph 3 of Schedule 3 applied, in that it was necessary to provide her with support to avoid a breach of her rights under EU law, in that she was a work-seeker, who required accommodation in order to secure employment and that it was discriminatory to refuse to provide it.

Judgment: Collins J held that accommodation was not sufficiently linked with facilitating access to employment to fall within the scope of EU rights afforded to work-seekers and that, in any event, there had not been any discrimination, because Mrs Conde had not been treated differently to a work-seeker who had arrived in Lambeth from a different part of the UK.

21.32 *R (Limbuela) v Secretary of State for the Home Department* [2005] UKHL 66, (2006) 9 CCLR 30

It was incompatible with Article 3 ECHR to refuse to accommodate and support destitute asylum-seekers

Facts: four healthy, able-bodied asylum-seekers faced destitution because they claimed asylum late, by virtue of section 55 of the Nationality, Immigration and Asylum Act 2002.

Judgment: the House of Lords (Lords Bingham, Hope, Scott, Lady Hale and Lord Brown) held that:

1) Article 3 imposes an absolute prohibition on torture or inhuman or degrading treatment or punishment. While the prohibition requires the state or public authority to refrain from treatment of the kind it describes, it may also require the state or public authority to do something to prevent its deliberate acts which would otherwise be lawful from amounting to the prohibited ill-treatment. There is no sound basis for the distinction drawn by the Court of Appeal between state violence and acts or omissions which arise in the administration or execution of government policy. Where inhuman or degrading treatment results from acts of omissions for which the state is directly responsible, the state is under an absolute obligation to refrain from it.

2) The regime imposed on those who do not make an asylum claim as soon as reasonably practicable after their arrival in the UK constitutes 'treatment' within the meaning of Article 3. The Secretary of State is

directly responsible for all the consequences that flow from the decision to withdraw support bearing in mind the prohibition on asylum-seekers from earning money in order to fend for themselves.

3) Whether treatment attains the minimum level of severity required in order to be 'inhuman or degrading' depends on all the circumstances of the case including the nature and context of the treatment. The test is not more exacting where the treatment is the result of legitimate government policy. Treatment will be inhuman or degrading if, to a seriously detrimental extent, it denies the most basic needs of any human being. Destitution for the purposes of section 95 of the 1999 Act is not sufficient to give rise to a breach of Article 3. The question is whether the treatment to which the asylum-seeker is being subjected by the entire package of restrictions and deprivations that surround him is so severe that it can properly be described as inhuman or degrading treatment. A variety of factors are relevant to that assessment including age, gender, health, availability of alternative support and the length of time that the person has spent or is likely to spend without support. The threshold will be crossed where a person has no means and no alternative sources of support, is unable to support himself and is denied shelter, food or the most basic necessities of life.

4) The purpose of section 55(5)(a) is to prevent a breach from taking place before it occurs. The Secretary of State is therefore under a duty to provide support as soon as the asylum-seeker makes it clear that there is an imminent prospect that a breach of Article 3 will occur because the conditions which he or she is having to endure are on the verge of reaching the necessary degree of severity.

5) In the claimants' cases, there was sufficient evidence to justify the conclusion that there was an imminent prospect that the way they were being treated by the Secretary of State would lead to a condition that was inhuman or degrading.

21.33 *R (AW) v Croydon LBC* [2005] EWHC 2950 (Admin), (2006) 9 CCLR 252

It would be incompatible with the ECHR not to accommodate failed asylum-seekers with fresh claims that were not manifestly hopeless or abusive

Facts: the claimants were failed asylum-seekers who were unlawfully present in the UK but had made fresh representations and may have been eligible for residential accommodation under section 21 of the National Assistance Act 1948.

Judgment: Lloyd Jones J held that:

1) A failed asylum-seeker who was in the UK in breach of immigration laws within the meaning of section 11 of the 2002 Act was, by virtue of para 7 of Schedule 3, ineligible for the support or assistance identified in para 1 of Schedule 3, subject to the exceptions in paras 2 and 3 of Schedule 3. There was nothing in the scheme or language of Schedule 3 to support the view that para 6 was intended to make exclusive provision for failed asylum-seekers to the exclusion of other categories of ineligibility. It was

the intention of Parliament, as a matter of policy, to distinguish between failed asylum-seekers who were in the UK in breach of immigration laws within para 7 of Schedule 3 and those who were not and to make more generous provision for the latter category.

2) If in the case of a failed asylum-seeker who satisfied the criteria for section 21(1) and (1A) of the National Assistance Act 1948 the provision of support were necessary for the purpose of avoiding a breach of Convention rights within the meaning of para 3 of Schedule 3 to the 2002 Act, that provision was to be made by a local authority pursuant to section 21 of the 1948 Act rather than by the Secretary of State pursuant to section 4 of the Immigration and Asylum Act 1999 ('hard cases support').

3) If the Article 3 ECHR threshold were otherwise met, the making of a purported fresh claim on UN Convention on Refugees/Article 3 ECHR grounds by a failed asylum-seeker did not always make it necessary for support to be provided in order to avoid a breach of Convention rights, under Schedule 3 para 3 to the 2002 Act, pending a decision by the Secretary of State on the representations. It would be necessary for the relevant public body to have regard to all the circumstances including, where appropriate, the matters which were alleged to constitute a fresh claim. It was necessary to proceed on a case-by-case basis. However, it was only in the clearest cases that it would be appropriate for the public body concerned to refuse relief on the basis of the manifest inadequacy of the purported fresh grounds. Where appropriate the individual would have recourse to judicial review to challenge such a decision.

Comment: see the Court of Appeal decision below, affirming the Judge's conclusion as to the division of responsibility between Croydon and the Secretary of State for the Home Department.

21.34 *Blackburn-Smith v Lambeth LBC* [2007] EWHC 767 (Admin), (2007) 10 CCLR 352

On the facts, it had been lawful to offer travel assistance rather than accommodation

Facts: Ms B-S was a Jamaican citizen, who was unlawfully present in the UK, with an adult daughter who was also a Jamaican citizen, and two much younger children who were British citizens but who no longer had contact with their father. Lambeth refused to provide any support or assistance beyond assistance to travel back to Jamaica, or accommodation for the children on their own, even though Ms B-S had an outstanding application for LTR on human rights grounds.

Judgment: Dobbs J held that Lambeth's stance had been lawful: there was no reason to suppose that the children's needs would not be adequately met in Jamaica and, even then, it may well not violate Article 8 ECHR to accommodate the children only.

21.35 *R (Mwanza) v Greenwich LBC* [2010] EWHC 1462 (Admin), (2010) 13 CCLR 454

Accommodation could be provided under section 117 of the Mental Health Act 1983 only in order to address a need arising out of mental disorder

Facts: Mr Mwanza and his family were unlawfully present in the UK. Mr Mwanza had received various support services under section 117 of the Mental Health Act 1983 but the PCT and local authority ultimately decided to cease their duty under that section. Afterwards, facing destitution on account of his and his family's immigration status, Mr Mwanza sought accommodation and support, either under section 117 or under section 21 of the National Assistance Act 1948.

Judgment: Hickinbottom J held that:

1) The duty to provide after-care services under section 117 of the Mental Health Act 1983 is a duty to provide services that are necessary to meet a need arising from a person's mental disorder. The need to work and the need for a roof over one's head are common needs and do not arise from mental disorder. This does not mean that a need for assistance in finding employment or housing on discharge cannot be provided and neither is it the case that provision of ordinary accommodation can never fall within section 117.

2) In this case, the need for accommodation came from the legal inability of the claimant and his wife to work due to their immigration status and could not be said to be due to the claimant's mental condition or any change in that condition.

3) In any event, there had been a proper decision in 2001 to discharge the claimant from further section 117 services, on the basis that it had been concluded by the claimant's absence and the lack of further problems that the claimant no longer needed them. Also, the challenge in this case had to be viewed as a challenge to the decision to treat section 117 responsibilities as discharged and gave rise to overwhelming arguments of delay in challenging the decision by way of judicial review.

4) The claim against Bromley council under section 21 of the National Assistance Act 1948 would be dismissed, since the claimant did not need any care and attention that could not be provided by his family looking after him and that assessment had not been challenged, nor could it be. It also appeared that the family's immigration status and the absence of any reliable evidence that there were any outstanding immigration appeals meant that the council was precluded from providing services under section 21.

21.36 *R (Clue) v Birmingham CC* [2010] EWCA Civ 460, (2010) 13 CCLR 276

It was incompatible with Article 8 ECHR not to offer accommodation and support under section 17 of the Children Act 1989 to a mother and her children who had made an outstanding application for LTR under Article 8 ECHR, which was not manifestly abusive or hopeless

Facts: Ms Clue was a Jamaican national who had unlawfully overstayed her leave to enter the UK, but who had an outstanding application for LTR with the Secretary of State for the Home Department, based on the long residence of her children. Having become destitute, she applied to Birmingham for support under section 17 of the Children Act 1989. Birmingham declined to provide any support, except such as would enable the family to return to Jamaica.

Judgment: the Court of Appeal (Dyson and Etherton LJJ, Sir Scott Baker) allowed Ms Clue's application for judicial review:

1) When enacting Schedule 3 to the 2002 Act, Parliament cannot reasonably have intended to confer a general power on local authorities to pre-empt the determination by the Secretary of State of applications for leave to remain. Save in hopeless or abusive cases, the duty imposed on local authorities to act so as to avoid a breach of an applicant's Convention rights does not require or entitle them to decide how the Secretary of State will determine an application for leave to remain or, in effect, determine such an application themselves by making it impossible for an applicant to pursue it.

2) There was no material before the court to suggest that the Secretary of State routinely exercises his discretion to determine an application for leave to remain notwithstanding that the applicant has left the UK. Accordingly, local authorities should approach their task on the footing that if, by withholding assistance, they require a person to return to his country of origin, that person's application for leave to remain will be treated by the Secretary of State as withdrawn.

3) Therefore when applying Schedule 3, a local authority should not consider the merits of an outstanding application for leave to remain. It is required to be satisfied that the application is not 'obviously hopeless or abusive'.

4) In circumstances where a person has made an application to the Secretary of State for leave to remain that raises Convention grounds and has made an application for assistance to the local authority that falls to be considered under Schedule 3 to the 2002 Act, the financial situation of the local authority is irrelevant when applying Article 8(2). The disposal of applications for leave should not depend on the vagaries of the budgetary considerations of local authorities.

5) Even if it had been legitimate for Birmingham to disregard the application for leave to remain and it had been entitled to decide for itself whether the withholding of assistance would breach the Convention rights of the claimant and her family, its assessment was nevertheless unlawful. The whole emphasis of the assessment was on the issue of respect for family life. There was no recognition that a return to Jamaica would interfere with the family's right to private life (their relationships and social, cultural and family ties in the UK) or that they understood that the private life rights of children who were born in the UK or came here at an early age were of particular weight.

6) The facts of the case exposed the problem created for local authorities by delays on the part of UKBA in dealing with applications for leave to remain by persons in the position of the claimant and her family. The Secretary of State had agreed to take steps to mitigate these problems, namely to prioritise consideration of cases involving applicants supported by local authorities in the same way as those of applicants supported by the Secretary of State and to review decision-making processes having regard to the need to safeguard and promote the welfare of children.

21.37 *R (Birara) v Hounslow LBC* [2010] EWHC 2113 (Admin), (2010) 13 CCLR 685

A failed asylum-seeker who had applied at port was lawfully present in the UK

Facts: Hounslow declined to provide further support to Ms Birara (a failed asylum-seeker with fresh representations pending) under the children leaving care provisions, to enable her to continue to pursue a nursing course because, in its view, Ms Birara was unlawfully present in the UK (so that Schedule 3 to the Nationality, Immigration and Asylum Act 2002 applied) and because, in any event, its policy was only to provide support after the age of 21 where it had resolved to do so before the applicant reached that age.

Judgment: Mrs Justice Dobbs held that because Ms Birara had applied for asylum at port she was lawfully present and that there were a number of deficiencies in the pathway plans, which meant that Hounslow had not properly considered whether it ought to continue to support Ms Birara after she turned 18; it followed that Hounslow had not properly considered its policy and whether to make an exception to it.

Comment: as noted above, paragraph 7 of Schedule 3 now applies when a person is in the UK in breach of the immigration laws within section 50A of the British Nationality Act 1981.

21.38 *R (de Almeida) v Kensington & Chelsea RLBC* [2012] EWHC 1082 (Admin), (2012) 15 CCLR 318

A person who reasonably required assistance with domestic chores required 'care and attention'

Facts: Mr de Almeida was terminally ill with AIDS and there was no real support available for him in Portugal; however, Kensington and Chelsea refused to provide him with accommodation and support under section 21 of the National Assistance Act 1948.

Judgment: Lang J held that Kensington and Chelsea had acted unlawfully: it had applied too strict a test, by asking whether Mr de Almeida was incapable of undertaking domestic tasks, when the correct approach was to ask whether he reasonably required support with such matters, which he plainly did, during periods of fluctuating ill health and, in the circumstances (the court not limiting itself to a review on traditional judicial review grounds), it would be incompatible with Articles 3 and 8 ECHR to require Mr de Almeida to spent his last short period of life in Portugal.

21.39 *Pryce v Southwark LBC* [2012] EWCA Civ 1572, (2012) 15 CCLR 731

The sole carer of British children had a right of residence in the UK that qualified her for homelessness assistance

Facts: Ms Pryce was unlawfully present in the UK, but was the sole carer of her three young British children. The issue was whether Ms Pryce had a right of residence in the UK under the *Zambrano* principle, so as to qualify for homelessness assistance under Part 7 of the Housing Act 1996.

Judgment: The county court judge had held not and Ms Pryce appealed. Shortly before the hearing in the Court of Appeal Southwark indicated a desire to concede the appeal and the Court of Appeal (Pill and Rimer LJJ, Burton J) approved the consent order and the agreed statement of reasons, on the basis that they appeared to be appropriate.

The agreed statement of the appellant and the local authority read as follows:

> 1. Article 20 ... contains treaty rights which are directly applicable in the UK national legal order by virtue of section 2(1) of the European Communities Act 1972 without the need for transposition into national law.
>
> 2. A person in respect of whom a refusal of a right of residence would be inconsistent with Article 20 ... in accordance with the principles established by the EU in *Ruiz Zambrano v ONEm* C–34/09 is not a person subject to immigration control for the purposes of s185 Housing Act 1996 or s7 Immigration Act 1988.
>
> 3. For the purposes of the Appellant's application for housing assistance, the Respondent (whose responsibility it is to make such a determination) has determined that the Appellant meets the requirements of the *Zambrano* principles.
>
> 4. The Appellant is such a person who derives a right of residence from the EU law and there being no issue as to habitual residence is eligible for assistance as homeless under s185(3) of the 1996 Act and the Homeless Regulations, regulation 6, as in force at all material times on 15 June 2011 onwards when she applied for assistance as homeless, including 30 September 2011 being the date of the review decision under appeal in these proceedings.
>
> 5. In the circumstances, the appeal ought to be allowed; the Order of HHJ Faber of 2 May 2012 ought to be set aside; and [the local authority's] review decision of 30 September 2011 ought to be varied pursuant to s204(3) of the 1996 Act to a decision that the Appellant is eligible for assistance under Section 185 of the 1996 Act.

Albeit that the court had not heard contrary submissions as to the effect of *Zambrano*, the local authority's concessions of fact and law appeared to be appropriate, though.

21.40 *R (KA) v Essex CC* [2013] EWHC 43 (Admin), (2013) 16 CCLR 63

It was incompatible with the ECHR to refuse accommodation to a destitute family whose claim for LTR under Article 8 ECHR had been refused, who were awaiting an appealable immigration decision and whose appeal would not be manifestly hopeless or abusive

Facts: KA and her husband, and their three children, were Nigerian citizens without a right to reside in the UK. The Secretary of State for the Home Department had refused various applications made by them for LTR, on a basis that did not carry a right of appeal, although the family would have a right of appeal on ECHR grounds if and when the Secretary of State for the Home Department made a removal decision. Essex declined to provide the family with accommodation and support under section 17 of the Children Act 1989 on the basis that it would not be a breach of Article 8 ECHR if the family had to return to Nigeria.

Judgment: Deputy High Court Judge Robin Purchas held that, since the family would in due course have a right of appeal that was neither manifestly hopeless or abusive, it would be a breach of the procedural protection afforded by Article 8 ECHR for Essex to refuse support, when that would drive the family to leave the UK.

21.41 *R (MK) v Barking and Dagenham LBC* [2013] EWHC 3486 (Admin)

Section 1 of the Localism Act 2011 could not be used to provide accommodation and support to a destitute individual, without children or care needs

Facts: Ms MK was an unlawful overstayer, who had become homeless. She sought accommodation and support under section 17 of the Children Act 1989, or under section 1 of the Localism Act 2011. However, she was not a child, or a former relevant child, nor did she care for a child. Barking and Dagenham refused to provide her with support.

Judgment: Deputy High Court Judge Bidder dismissed Ms MK's application for judicial review, on the basis that she did not fall within section 17 and on the basis that section 1 of the Localism Act 2011 did not enable Barking and Dagenham to provide support because there was a pre-commencement restriction or limitation on its powers, found in section 17 of the CA 1989 (in that support under that provision had to be for the purpose of safeguarding and promoting the welfare of children), and also in section 21 of the National Assistance Act 1948 and section 185 of the Housing Act 1985. He also held that neither *Limbuela* nor *Clue* imposed a free-standing duty to provide support.

Comment: it seems questionable whether this decision would have survived an appeal to the Court of Appeal. See now paras 20.3–20.12 and *R (GS) v London Borough of Camden* [2016] EWHC 1762 (Admin), (2016) 19 CCLR 398 at para 21.24 above.

21.42 *Sanneh and others v Secretary of State for Work and Pensions and others* [2015] EWCA Civ 49, (2015) 18 CCLR 5

Sole carers of British children had a right of residence under EU law and, also, a right to work and to a reasonable basic minimum for subsistence; but not to social security benefits

Facts: a number of cases were heard together, so that the Court of Appeal could determine when any right to reside in the UK arose under the *Zambrano* principle and, when such right arose, whether it carried with it the right not just to work but, also, to mainstream benefits.

Judgment: the Court of Appeal (Arden, Elias and Burnett LJJ) held that:

1) EU law conferred on a *Zambrano* carer a right to reside from the time when the carer ceased to be liable to be removed from the UK, eg on the birth of a child, upon becoming the primary carer of an EU national who would be forced to leave the EU but for the carer's presence.

2) In order for the child's citizenship right under Article 20 TFEU to be effective, member states had to make social assistance available to *Zambrano* carers, when it was essential to do so, to enable them to support themselves in order to be the carer. The right to such basic support was, however, a derivative right only and was exclusively governed by national law; and accordingly the EU principle of proportionality did not apply.

3) It was not necessary to show, in addition to destitution, that the *Zambrano* carer would be forced out of the EU for want of resources; if necessary, an assumption about being forced out would be made; the law looked to the substance, not the form, and practical reality, requiring that the *Zambrano* carer and the EU child must not be left without the resources essential for them to remain. It was not open to the court on the material before it to determine whether section 17 of the Children Act 1989 operated satisfactorily on the ground; but if section 17 assistance was available it would have the effect of ensuring that the basic needs of the child and the *Zambrano* carer were both properly looked after.

4)) A *Zambrano* carer could not claim to be entitled to social benefits under the EU principle of non-discrimination under Article 18 TFEU: the discrimination between *Zambrano* carers and other benefit claimants, resulting from the amending Regulations, was not direct discrimination on the grounds of nationality but indirect discrimination on other grounds which could be justified; further, a *Zambrano* carer was not a potential beneficiary of social assistance under the EU legislative scheme for cross-border social benefits so as to enable a claim to be brought under Article 18 TFEU; and EU law did not prohibit reverse discrimination, *ie* unfavourable treatment by a member state of some of its own nationals. Accordingly, the only protection from discrimination available to *Zambrano* carers or their children was that derived from Article 14 ECHR, but in order to show a violation of the Convention right it would have to be shown that the legislative policy was manifestly without foundation. This could not be done because: the difference in treatment did not leave the *Zambrano* carer and EU child destitute as they could have recourse to assistance under section 17 of the Children Act 1989; the carer could apply for long-term leave to remain with an abbreviated period for a condition restricting recourse to public funds; and there were deliberate policy reasons for treating *Zambrano* carers and their children differently from other TCNs or other EU children, including deterrence whose value was a matter for political judgment.

5) The Secretary of State had complied with the general public sector equality duty under section 149 of the Equality Act 2010: the amending Regulations had been made to uphold the position that had existed previously; in such circumstances, the impact of the Regulations and the equality duty was limited.

6) It was not appropriate to make a reference to the ECJ for a preliminary ruling.

21.43 *R (Tigere) v Secretary of State for Business, Innovation and Skills* [2015] UKSC 57, [2015] 1 WLR 3820

It was incompatible with Article 2 of the 1st Protocol to the ECHR and Article 14 ECHR to exclude from student loans prospective students who had not clocked up three years of lawful, ordinary residence but who had lived in the UK for most of their lives, had been educated here, could not be removed save for grave misconduct and were treated throughout as members of UK society

Facts: Ms Tigere was excluded from a student loan because she had not clocked up three years' lawful, ordinary residence in the UK, despite the fact that she had lived in the UK for many years and been educated in England throughout her school career, had been granted LTR with recourse to public funds, would qualify for ILR in a few years and had obtained a university place.

Judgment: the Supreme Court (Hale, Kerr and Hughes JJSC, Sumption and Reed JJSC dissenting), held, in passing that '45 ...There are indeed strong public policy reasons for insisting that any period of ordinary residence required before a person becomes entitled to public services be lawful ordinary residence'. A similar approach was taken in *R (YA) v Secretary of State for Health,*[19] but a different approach was taken in the context of last-ditch support for the destitute in *R v Wandsworth LBC ex p O.*[20]

21.44 *R (F) v Barking and Dagenham LBC* [2015] EWHC 2838 (Admin), (2015) 18 CCLR 754

It was desirable for the court to case manage jointly family law and support proceedings

Facts: F was unlawfully present in the UK and did not have any outstanding application for LTR. She had a 14-year-old son, but the father (from whom F was separated) had a residence order in relation to the son. There were family court proceedings in which F was seeking a residence order. The family court was unable to grant F shared residence unless she had accommodation and Barking and Dagenham declined to provide F with accommodation on the basis that her son did not live with her. F claimed that this was incompatible with her right to respect for her family life, under Article 8 ECHR.

Judgment: Deputy High Court Judge Cheema QC held that the family court was best placed to resolve this conundrum: 'I direct that this claim is transferred to a High Court Judge who is also nominated to sit in the Family Division so that a Case Management Hearing can take place as soon as possible, and certainly well before the November 2015 date presently fixed for the five-day hearing in the Family Court. The High Court Judge will be in the best position to look at the interests of J in the round and make the appropriate order in this claim and the family proceedings. Joinder of the

19 [2009] EWCA Civ 225, (2009) 12 CCLR 213.

20 [2000] 1 WLR 2539, (2000) 3 CCLR 237.

two sets of proceedings will also overcome a specific difficulty identified by the defendant, namely the absence of J's father from this case'.

21.45 *R (Kosi) v Secretary of State for the Home Department* (unreported)[21]

Interim relief was granted, restraining the removal of a parent involved in contact proceedings

Facts: Mr Kosi was an unlawful overstayer, in immigration detention and facing imminent removal from the UK on account of his unlawful presence and offending history.

Judgment: Laing J awarded Mr Kosi an injunction restraining his removal as it appeared that the Secretary of State for the Home Department had not properly taken into account a direction by the family court that regular contact would be Mr Kosi's child's best interests.

21.46 *Mirga v Secretary of State for Work and Pensions; Samin v Westminster City Council* [2016] UKSC 1

EU nationals who were not exercising rights of residence in the UK under EU law were not entitled to social assistance except perhaps in extreme circumstances and it was unnecessary for the authorities to undertake a 'proportionality exercise' in every case

Facts: Ms Mirga was a Polish national who had spent much of her life in England and had worked at various times but was now pregnant and had been refused Income Support. Mr Samin was an Austrian national who had come to the UK in 2005, was in poor health and had been refused housing assistance as a homeless person.

Judgment: the Supreme Court (Neuberger, Hale, Kerr, Clarke and Reed JJSC) held that the right to reside freely within the EU, and the right not to be discriminated against, under Articles 21 and 18 of the Treaty on the Functioning of the European Union, were conditional on EU citizens exercising a right of residence under EU law. Ms Mirga and Mr Samin were not economically and were not, for any other reason, residing in the UK in the exercise of rights under EU law and, accordingly, were not entitled to social security or housing assistance in order to give effect to Articles 21 and 18 of the TFEU. In addition, whilst in extreme circumstances it might be disproportionate, in breach Articles 21 and/or 18 to withhold such assistance from an EU whose presence was not pursuant to the exercise of rights under EU law, that did not require the authorities to undertake a proportionality assessment in every case.

21 Short summary is available only on Westlaw.

United Kingdom Visas and Immigration support and local authority support

Machinery and introduction

21.47 Often still referred to as 'NASS support' ('NASS' being the acronym of the long-since-disbanded National Asylum Support Service) asylum support is now provided by the Home Office directorate UKVI.

21.48 UKVI provides asylum support for asylum-seekers and their dependants under Part 6 of the Immigration and Asylum Act 1999 and for 'accommodation' for failed asylum-seekers and some other groups, and their dependants, under section 4.

21.49 The main issues that arise in relation to asylum support and section 4 accommodation relate to:

- eligibility;
- the level of support, especially where children are involved;
- the boundary between UKVI and local authority responsibility.

21.50 'Asylum support' comprises accommodation plus provision for essential living needs and limited additional expenses (section 96 of the Immigration and Asylum Act 1999). It is provided to asylum-seekers/their dependents who are 'destitute' in the sense that they are unable to secure adequate accommodation or other essential living needs (section 95). It is provided until final determination of the asylum claim/so long as the asylum-seeker's household contains a dependent child under 18 (section 94).

21.51 The primary legislation is fleshed out by the Asylum Support Regulations 2000, which regulate levels of provision in respect of essential living needs and which provide important machinery in regulations 9 and 23, the effect of which is that, in assessing whether an asylum-seeker/dependent is 'destitute', UKVI must take into account any support available to the applicant (including from a local authority) but local authorities must disregard the availability of asylum support: thus, making asylum support residual, provided only when local authority support is unavailable.

21.52 UKVI practice is informed by *Asylum Support: Policy Bulletins Instructions*.[22]

21.53 Under section 4 of the Immigration and Asylum Act 1999, the Secretary of State has power to provide or arrange for the provision of facilities for the accommodation of:

- failed asylum-seekers/dependants; and
- persons/dependants:
  - temporarily admitted to the UK;
  - released from immigration detention pending investigation of their claims; or
  - released on bail from any form of immigration detention.

21.54 Such provision is limited by the Immigration and Asylum (Provision of Accommodation to Failed Asylum-seekers) Regulations 2005. Not only

22 Collected at www.gov.uk/government/uploads/system/uploads/attachment_data/file/422990/Asylum_Support_Policy_Bulletin_Instructions_Public_v6.pdf.

must the applicant appear to be 'destitute' but the conditions in regulation 3(2) must apply:

> **3**(2) Those conditions are that–
> (a) he is taking all reasonable steps to leave the United Kingdom or place himself in a position in which he is able to leave the United Kingdom, which may include complying with attempts to obtain a travel document to facilitate his departure;
> (b) he is unable to leave the United Kingdom by reason of a physical impediment to travel or for some other medical reason;
> (c) he is unable to leave the United Kingdom because in the opinion of the Secretary of State there is currently no viable route of return available;
> (d) he has made an application for judicial review of a decision in relation to his asylum claim– (i) in England and Wales, and has been granted permission to proceed pursuant to Part 54 of the Civil Procedure Rules 1998, (ii) in Scotland, pursuant to Chapter 58 of the Rules of the Court of Session 1994 or (iii) in Northern Ireland, and has been granted leave pursuant to Order 53 of the Rules of Supreme Court (Northern Ireland) 1980; or
> (e) the provision of accommodation is necessary for the purpose of avoiding a breach of a person's Convention rights, within the meaning of the Human Rights Act 1998.[23]

21.55 In addition to regulation 3(2)(e) (which of course is but one alternative), the whole power of the UKVI to offer section 4 accommodation is subject to the statutory bar in Schedule 3 to the Nationality, Immigration and Asylum Act 2002. Accordingly it cannot be provided to a failed asylum-seeker, or any other category of section 4 applicant, who falls foul of Schedule 3 (for example, as a result of being in the UK in breach of the immigration laws within the meaning of section 50A of the British Nationality Act 1981) except insofar as it is necessary to make provision to avoid a breach of EU or ECHR rights. Regulation 3 appears to set out the circumstances where the Secretary of State accepts that it is necessary to make provision to avoid a breach of ECHR rights.

21.56 The approach of the courts to paragraph 3 of Schedule 3, has been to treat it as being necessary to provide basic support in a case where, otherwise:

- the applicant would be pushed away from the UK as a result of not having their basic needs met (including accommodation and essential needs);
- *providing* that would be incompatible with their rights under the ECHR;
- *which will be the case,* where the applicant has an outstanding application for LTR on refugee or ECHR grounds that is not '*manifestly hopeless or abusive*'.[24]

21.57 Finally, a refusal to provide asylum support or section 4 accommodation, or the provision of inadequate support, will be unlawful if it is incompatible with EU law, in the shape of Council Directive 2003/9/EC of

23 For example, because the applicant has an outstanding application for LTR on refugee or ECHR grounds which is not manifestly hopeless or abusive.

24 *R (Clue) v Birmingham CC* [2010] EWCA Civ 460, (2010) 13 CCLR 276.

27 January 2003 laying down minimum standards for the reception of asylum-seekers.[25]

21.58 As noted above, unaccompanied asylum-seeking children are accommodated under section 20 of the Children Act 1989. Children living with their families (seeking asylum or LTR under the ECHR) will have their general accommodation and welfare needs met by the Secretary of State for the Home Department, by virtue of section 122 of the Immigration and Asylum Act 1999 – but the local authority will meet any special needs that they may have, under section 17 of the Children Act 1989.[26]

Cases

21.59 *R (Mani and others) v Lambeth LBC and another* [2002] EWHC 735 (Admin), (2002) 5 CCLR 486

Adults who needed help with household chores needed 'care and attention'

Facts: Mr Mani and Mr Tasci had limited mobility as a result of physical disability and Mr J was seriously ill as a result of advanced HIV+: All three needed help with domestic tasks and were destitute asylum-seekers.

Judgment: Wilson J held that the claimants' needs did not arise solely as a result of destitution so that, because regulations 6 and 23 of the Asylum Support Regulations 2000 required the local authorities to disregard the availability of Home Office support, they were under a duty to provide the claimants with residential accommodation under section 21 of the National Assistance Act 1948.

21.60 *R (Westminster CC) v National Asylum Support Service* [2002] UKHL 38, (2002) 5 CCLR 511

Asylum support was residual and could not be provided for persons entitled to residential accommodation

Facts: Mrs Y-Ahmed, a destitute Kurdish asylum-seeker, suffered from spinal cancer and required care and attention. The issue was, whether Westminster was required to provide her with residential accommodation plus essential living needs, care and attention, or whether NASS was required to provide her with accommodation and essential living needs, with Westminster providing care.

Judgment: the House of Lords (Lord Steyn, Slynn, Hoffman, Millett and Rodger) held that:

1) Mrs Y-Ahmed fell prima facie within NAA 1948 s21(1) because her need for care and attention entailed a need to be provided with accommodation. The reasoning in *R v Hammersmith and Fulham LBC ex p M*[27] applied: unless she was given accommodation she would have nowhere to receive care and attention.

25 *R (Refugee Action) v Secretary of State for the Home* Department [2014] EWHC 1033 (Admin), [2014] PTSR D18.

26 *R (Ouji) v Secretary of State for the Home Department* [2002] EWHC 1839 (Admin).

27 (1997) 30 HLR 10.

2) Mrs Y-Ahmed was not excluded from NAA 1948 s21(1) by section 21(1A) of the Act as her need for care and attention had not arisen solely because she was destitute but also (and largely) because she was ill.

3) The existence of the duty under NAA 1948 s21(1) excluded Mrs Y-Ahmed from consideration for asylum support. Regulation 6(4) of the Asylum Support Regulations 2000 required that when the Secretary of State determined for the purposes of Immigration and Asylum Act 1999 s95(1) whether a person was destitute, he must take into account 'any other support' available to that person. As an infirm and destitute asylum seeker, support was available to Mrs Y-Ahmed under section 21(1) of the NAA 1948. 'Support' in regulation 6(4) was not limited to support from private sources.

Comment: see the later decisions of *Slough* and *SL* (paras 21.69 and 21.73 below), where it was in dispute whether the applicant had a need for care and attention.

21.61 *R (Ouji) v Secretary of State for the Home Department* [2002] EWHC 1839 (Admin)

The local authority, not NASS, was responsible for the special needs of disabled children whose family was in receipt of asylum support

Facts: Mr Ouji was an asylum-seeker who, with his family, was in receipt of asylum support under Part 6 of the Immigration and Asylum Act 1999. He sought additional levels of support in order to meet the needs of his disabled daughter.

Judgment: Mr Justice Collins held that Part 6 of the 1999 Act required the Secretary of State for the Home Department to meet 'essential living needs' only. Those were the kinds of needs that people in general had in order to have a reasonable minimum standard of existence by UK standards. They were the needs of an ordinary child or adult with no special peculiarities or disabilities. Any such special features were the responsibility of the local social services authority.

21.62 *R (Q) v Secretary of State for the Home Department* [2003] EWCA Civ 364, (2003) 6 CCLR 136

It was incompatible with Article 3 ECHR to refuse support to destitute asylum-seekers

Facts: the claimants were asylum-seekers excluded from asylum support by statute, subject to the ECHR if, as was the case, the Secretary of State for the Home Department concluded that they had failed to claim asylum as soon as reasonably practicable. Each had failed to claim asylum on arrival in the UK, but had done so a day or so later.

Judgment: the Court of Appeal (Lord Phillips MR, Clarke and Sedley LJJ) held that the test of 'as soon as reasonably practicable' was not limited to focussing on physical obstacles but required consideration of all the claimant's circumstances including what instructions or advice he had been given by an agent:

> 37. In the light of the considerations discussed above, we would define the test of whether an asylum seeker has claimed asylum 'as soon as reasonably practicable' as follows: 'On the premise that the purpose of coming to this country was to claim asylum and having regard both to the practical opportunity for claiming asylum and to the asylum seeker's personal circumstances, could the asylum seeker reasonably have been expected to claim asylum earlier than he or she did?'

The Court of Appeal went on to hold that the regime imposed on late-claiming asylum-seekers amounted to '*treatment*' for the purposes of Article 3 ECHR:

> 56. In our judgment the regime that is imposed on asylum seekers who are denied support by reason of section 55(1) constitutes 'treatment' within the meaning of Article 3. Our reasoning is as follows. Treatment, as the Attorney-General has pointed out, implies something more than passivity on the part of the State; but here, it seems to us, there is more than passivity. Asylum seekers who are here without a right or leave to enter cannot lawfully be removed until their claims have been determined because, in accordance with the United Kingdom's obligations under Article 33 of the Refugee Convention, Parliament has expressly forbidden their removal by what is now section 15 of the 1999 Act. But while they remain here, as they must do if they are to press their claims, asylum seekers cannot work (Asylum and Immigration Act 1996, section 8) unless the Home Secretary gives them special permission to do so (Immigration (Restrictions on Employment) Order 1996).

21.63 *R (Mani) v Lambeth LBC* [2003] EWCA Civ 836, (2003) 6 CCLR 376

A person who needed help with domestic chores needed 'care and attention'

Facts: Mr Mani had limited mobility as a result of physical disability. He needed help with domestic tasks and was a destitute asylum-seeker.

Judgment: the Court of Appeal (Simon Brown and Judge LJJ, Nelson J) held that the claimant's needs did not arise solely as a result of destitution so that, because regulations 6 and 23 of the Asylum Support Regulations 2000 required the local authorities to disregard the availability of Home Office support, they were under a duty to provide the claimants with residential accommodation under section 21 of the National Assistance Act 1948.

Comment: it seems likely that the same result will follow under the Care Act 2014 (the Asylum Support Regulations 2000 remain unchanged).

21.64 *R (A) v NASS and Waltham Forest LBC* [2003] EWCA Civ 1473, (2003) 6 CCLR 538

NASS was under a duty to accommodate a family with disabled children, not the local authority: but the accommodation had to be suitable for those children

Facts: Ms A was an asylum-seeker with two disabled children, with special accommodation, educational and care needs.

Judgment: the Court of Appeal (Brooke, Waller and Clarke LJJ) held that because of section 122 of the Immigration and Asylum Act 1999, the National Asylum Support Service (rather than Waltham Forest) was under a duty to provide the family with accommodation but that accommodation had to be adequate, taking into account the children's needs.

21.65 *R (O) v Haringey LBC* [2004] EWCA Civ 535, (2004) 7 CCLR 310

The local authority was responsible for providing residential accommodation to a mother but the Secretary of State for the Home Department was responsible for funding the children's accommodation and support costs

Facts: Ms O was an HIV+ Ugandan citizen with two dependent children, who had come to the UK to join her husband, but had then fled domestic violence from him. Pending the Secretary of State for the Home Department's determination of her application for LTR, she applied for support from Haringey.

Judgment: the Court of Appeal (the LCJ, Rix and Carnwath LJJ) held that Haringey was responsible for accommodating the mother, under section 21 of the National Assistance Act 1948, whereas the Secretary of State for the Home Department was responsible for accommodating the children, under section 122 of the Immigration and Asylum Act 1999: in practice, the whole family would have to be accommodated by Haringey, with the Secretary of State for the Home Department paying for the cost of accommodating the children.

21.66 *R (Limbuela) v Secretary of State for the Home Department* [2005] UKHL 66, (2006) 9 CCLR 30

It was incompatible with Article 3 ECHR to refuse support to destitute asylum-seekers

Facts: 4 healthy, able-bodied asylum-seekers faced destitution because they claimed asylum late, by virtue of section 55 of the Nationality, Immigration and Asylum Act 2002.

Judgment: the House of Lords (Lords Bingham, Hope, Scott, Lady Hale and Lord Brown) held that:

1) Article 3 imposes an absolute prohibition on torture or inhuman or degrading treatment or punishment. While the prohibition requires the state or public authority to refrain from treatment of the kind it describes, it may also require the state or public authority to do something to prevent its deliberate acts which would otherwise be lawful from amounting to the prohibited ill-treatment. There is no sound basis for the distinction drawn by the Court of Appeal between state violence and acts or omissions which arise in the administration or execution of government policy. Where inhuman or degrading treatment results from acts of omissions for which the state is directly responsible, the state is under an absolute obligation to refrain from it.

2) The regime imposed on those who do not make an asylum claim as soon as reasonably practicable after their arrival in the UK constitutes 'treatment' within the meaning of Article 3. The Secretary of State is directly responsible for all the consequences that flow from the decision to withdraw support bearing in mind the prohibition on asylum-seekers from earning money in order to fend for themselves.

3) Whether treatment attains the minimum level of severity required in order to be 'inhuman or degrading' depends on all the circumstances of the case including the nature and context of the treatment. The test is not more exacting where the treatment is the result of legitimate government policy. Treatment will be inhuman or degrading if, to a seriously detrimental extent, it denies the most basic needs of any human being. Destitution for the purposes of section 95 of the 1999 Act is not sufficient to give rise to a breach of Article 3. The question is whether the treatment to which the asylum-seeker is being subjected by the entire package of restrictions and deprivations that surround him or her is so severe that it can properly be described as inhuman or degrading treatment. A variety of factors are relevant to that assessment including age, gender, health, availability of alternative support and the length of time that the person has spent or is likely to spend without support. The threshold will be crossed where a person has no means and no alternative sources of support, is unable to support him or herself and is denied shelter, food or the most basic necessities of life.

4) The purpose of section 55(5)(a) is to prevent a breach from taking place before it occurs. The Secretary of State is therefore under a duty to provide support as soon as the asylum-seeker makes it clear that there is an imminent prospect that a breach of Article 3 will occur because the conditions which he or she is having to endure are on the verge of reaching the necessary degree of severity.

5) In the claimants' cases, there was sufficient evidence to justify the conclusion that there was an imminent prospect that the way they were being treated by the Secretary of State would lead to a condition that was inhuman or degrading.

21.67 *R (AW) v Croydon LBC* [2005] EWHC 2950 (Admin), (2006) 9 CCLR 252

It was incompatible with the ECHR to refuse support to failed asylum-seekers who had outstanding further representations that were not manifestly hopeless or abusive

Facts: the claimants were failed asylum-seekers who were unlawfully present in the UK but had made fresh representations and may have been eligible for residential accommodation under section 21 of the National Assistance Act 1948.

Judgment: Lloyd Jones J held that:

1) A failed asylum-seeker who was in the UK in breach of immigration laws within the meaning of section 11 of the 2002 Act was, by virtue of para 7 of Schedule 3, ineligible for the support or assistance identified in para 1 of Schedule 3, subject to the exceptions in paras 2 and 3 of Schedule 3. There was nothing in the scheme or language of Schedule 3 to support the view that para 6 was intended to make exclusive provision for failed asylum-seekers to the exclusion of other categories of ineligibility. It was the intention of Parliament, as a matter of policy, to distinguish between failed asylum-seekers who were in the UK in breach of immigration laws

within para 7 to Schedule 3 and those who were not and to make more generous provision for the latter category.

2) If in the case of a failed asylum-seeker who satisfied the criteria for section 21(1) and (1A) of the National Assistance Act 1948 the provision of support were necessary for the purpose of avoiding a breach of Convention rights within the meaning of para 3 of Schedule 3 to the 2002 Act, that provision was to be made by a local authority pursuant to section 21 of the 1948 Act rather than by the Secretary of State pursuant to section 4 of the Immigration and Asylum Act 1999 ('hard cases support').

3) If the Article 3 ECHR threshold were otherwise met, the making of a purported fresh claim on UN Convention on Refugees/Article 3 ECHR grounds by a failed asylum-seeker did not always make it necessary for support to be provided in order to avoid a breach of Convention rights, under Schedule 3 para 3 to the 2002 Act, pending a decision by the Secretary of State on the representations. It would be necessary for the relevant public body to have regard to all the circumstances including, where appropriate, the matters which were alleged to constitute a fresh claim. It was necessary to proceed on a case-by-case basis. However, it was only in the clearest cases that it would be appropriate for the public body concerned to refuse relief on the basis of the manifest inadequacy of the purported fresh grounds. Where appropriate the individual would have recourse to judicial review to challenge such a decision.

Comment: see the Court of Appeal decision below, affirming the Judge's conclusion as to the division of responsibility between Croydon and the Secretary of State for the Home Department.

21.68 *R (AW) v Croydon LBC* [2007] EWCA Civ 266, (2007) 10 CCLR 225

Local authorities, not the Secretary of State for the Home Department, were responsible for accommodating failed asylum-seekers with a need for 'care and attention'

Facts: the claimants were failed asylum-seekers who were unlawfully present in the UK but had made fresh representations and may have been eligible for residential accommodation under section 21 of the National Assistance Act 1948.

Judgment: the Court of Appeal (Sir Igor Judge, President, Laws and Scott Baker LJJ) held:

> A failed asylum-seeker who satisfies the criteria for section 21(1) and (1A) of the National Assistance Act 1948 is not destitute within the meaning of regulation 3 of the Immigration and Asylum (Provision of Accommodation to Failed Asylum-Seekers) Regulations 2005 and therefore is not entitled to support from the Secretary of State under section 4 of the 1999 Act. Where the provision of support to a person in that position is necessary for the purpose of avoiding a breach of Convention rights, that provision is to be made by a local authority pursuant to section 21 of the 1948 Act. Therefore the appeals are dismissed.

21.69 *R (M) v Slough BC* [2008] UKHL 52, (2008) 11 CCLR 733

A need for storage of medicine and a need for accommodation and basic living needs did not amount of a need for 'care and attention'

Facts: M, a citizen of Zimbabwe, claimed that removal to Zimbabwe would breach his rights under Article 3 ECHR. Meanwhile, since he was destitute, he applied to his local authority, Slough, for residential accommodation. Slough declined to make provision on the ground that, although M was destitute, he did not require '*care and attention*' within the meaning of section 21 of the National Assistance Act 1948, in that his only need was for accommodation, basic living needs, health care and refrigeration for his medication.

Judgment: the House of Lords (Lords Bingham, Scott, Lady Hale, Lords Brown and Neuberger) held that M did not require '*care and attention*':

1) The 'care and attention' that is needed under section 21(1)(a) is a wider concept than 'nursing or personal care'. Section 21 accommodation may be provided for the purpose of preventing illnesses as well as caring for those who are ill. But 'care and attention' must mean something more than 'accommodation'. The natural and ordinary meaning of 'care and attention' in this context is 'looking after', which means doing something for the person being cared for that he cannot or should not be expected to do for himself. It includes household tasks, protection from risks or personal care. This list is not exhaustive. The provision of medical care is expressly excluded.

2) Section 21(1)(a) requires a present need for care and attention but, if there is a present need, then the authority is empowered to intervene before it becomes worse.

3) M's needs did not amount to a 'need for care and attention'. His medical needs were being met by the National Health Service so, even if they did amount to a 'need for care and attention', he would not qualify.

4) As he did not fall within section 21(1)(a) it was not necessary to ask whether he would be excluded by section 21(1A).

5) (Per Lord Neuberger) The words 'which is not otherwise available to them' refer back to 'care and attention', not 'accommodation'.

21.70 *R (YA) v Secretary of State for Health* [2009] EWCA Civ 225, (2009) 12 CCLR 213

A failed asylum-seeker who could not return to his country of origin was entitled to NHS care that was either immediately necessary or could not wait for his return to his country of origin

Facts: YA was a failed Palestinian asylum-seeker who, however, was unable to return to Palestine because it was impossible to obtain a travel document that permitted it. He was seriously ill with liver disease, received NHS treatment and was then billed for about £9,000.00. The hospital then agreed to withdraw then bill and provide further treatment without charge. YA then substituted the Secretary of State for Health as defendant and challenged the lawfulness of the Secretary of State's guidance to health authorities.

Judgment: the Court of Appeal (Ward, Lloyd and Rimer LJJ) held that where a person's residence was unlawful (as in this case, albeit that YA had *'temporary admission'* to the UK) they cannot be ordinarily resident, or lawfully resident, so the Secretary of State was correct that the charging provisions under section 75 of the National Health Service Act 2006 and the National Health Service (Charges to Overseas Visitors) Regulations 1989 applied. However, trusts had a discretion to treat those who cannot or will not pay and the Secretary of State's guidance was unlawful, in that it failed to identify how that discretion was to be exercised in relation to different categories of treatment, in particular in the case of failed asylum-seekers unable to leave the UK:

> 74. The Guidance divides treatment into three categories. The first is 'immediately necessary treatment', referred to at paragraph 3.1 but further defined in paragraph 9 which makes it clear:
>
>> 'Trusts need to treat patients in need of immediately necessary care regardless of their ability to pay. This may be because their condition is life-threatening, or because if treatment is not given immediately it will become life-threatening, or because permanent serious damage will be caused by any delay ... Where immediately necessary treatment takes place and the Trust knows that payment is unlikely, treatment should be limited to that which is clinically necessary to enable the patient to return to their own country. This should not normally include routine treatment unless it is necessary to prevent a life-threatening situation. Any charge for such treatment will stand, but if it proves to be irrecoverable, then it should be written off.'
>
> This is clear enough in so far as it advises that certain treatment should be given irrespective of the ability to pay for it but it leaves unclear what, if any, investigation should be made as to when the patient is likely to return to his own country so as to be able to decide what limits should be placed on the treatment.
>
> 75. The second category is 'urgent treatment' which is treatment which is not immediately necessary but cannot wait until the patient returns home. The advice that is given by the Guidance is that when the patient is chargeable the Trust should 'wherever possible' seek deposits equivalent to the estimated full cost of the treatment in advance of providing any treatment. The problem here is that the Guidance is silent on what should happen when it is not possible to provide that deposit. No help is given in the case of those who cannot return home before the treatment does become necessary. What is to happen to the patient who cannot wait? In those respects the guidance is not clear and unambiguous and in so far as it purports to be dealing with a category of patients like those before us, the failed asylum-seekers who cannot be returned, it is seriously misleading.
>
> 76. As for non-urgent treatment, namely 'routine elective treatment which could in fact wait until the patient returned home', the advice given is that where the patient is chargeable, the Trust should not initiate treatment processes (even by putting the patient on a waiting list) until a full deposit has been obtained. The assumption has to be that the patient can return home before that routine elective treatment becomes necessary. Again, it is not clear what should be done for those who have no prospect of returning within a medically acceptable time. There is no suggestion that it may be

necessary to treat in those circumstances or even that it may be necessary to investigate the likelihood and length of any undue delay. Once again the Guidance is not clear enough.

21.71 *R (Zarzour) v Hillingdon LBC* [2009] EWCA Civ 1529, (2010) 13 CCLR 157

A blind man who needed help when in new accommodation needed 'care and attention'

Facts: Mr Zarzour was a blind, destitute asylum-seeker. He was living with two friends in a studio flat but that could not continue. Hillingdon assessed him as being able to undertake all activities of daily living once he had memorised his surroundings and, on that basis, concluded that he did not require 'care and attention' for the purposes of section 21 of the NAA 1948: if accommodated by the Secretary of State for the Home Department, Hillingdon would provide 'settling in' assistance under section 29 of the NAA 1948, until Mr Zarzour had memorised his surroundings.

Judgment: the Court of Appeal (Laws and Etherton LJJ, Lewison J) held that:

1) The authority's own findings in the assessment compelled a conclusion that the claimant was in need of care and attention because the claimant needed others to do what he could not do for himself, and a reasonable authority was bound to find that he fell within s21(1)(a).

2. The decision in *R (M) v Slough BC* had made only a very modest change to the law as explained in *R (Westminster CC) v NASS* and did not mean, in unqualified terms, that it was open to local authorities to look to see whether a person's needs might be met through section 29 of the 1948 Act and section 2 of the CSDPA 1970 with accommodation, if necessary, provided by the National Asylum Support Service: NASS support was intended to be residual and a local authority could consider the provision of services under section 29 and section 2 combined with NASS accommodation only if they had first concluded that the asylum-seeker was outwith section 21(1)(a).

21.72 *R (VC) v Newcastle CC* [2011] EWHC 2673 (Admin), (2012) 15 CCLR 194

It had not lawful to decline to provide support to a destitute child, and the child's family, under section 17 of the Children Act 1989, on the basis that support might be available under section 4 of the Immigration and Asylum Act 1999

Facts: Newcastle terminated provision of support for a destitute family from abroad, under section 17 of the Children Act 1989, on the basis that support was available under section 4 of the Immigration and Asylum Act 1999.

Judgment: the Divisional Court (Munby LJ and Langstaff J) held that Newcastle had acted unlawfully in that, once a child has been assessed as being in need by reason of destitution, for the purposes of section 17 of the Children Act 1989, a local authority will only be justified in declining to provide support, if the Secretary of State is willing or required to provide support under section 4 of the Immigration and Asylum Act 1999 and if such support would meet the child's needs, which is unlikely to be case, given that section 4 is aimed at meeting basic subsistence needs whereas section 17 is aimed at safeguarding and promoting the child's welfare:

> 86. There are, in my judgment, a number of what Ms Rhee calls key legislative indicators which together point to the conclusion to which I have come, that, in contrast to section 17, section 4 is a residuary power and that the mere fact that support is or may be available under section 4 does not of itself exonerate a local authority from what would otherwise be its powers and duties under section 17.
>
> 87. First, there is the contrast not merely between the level of support available under section 17 and section 4 but also between the very different purposes of the two statutory schemes. Ms Rhee accurately describes section 4 as providing 'an austere regime, effectively of last resort, which is made available to failed asylum-seekers to provide a minimum level of humanitarian support'. Section 17 in contrast is capable of providing a significantly more advantageous source of support, its purpose being to promote the welfare and best interests of children in need. As she says, section 4 support is intended to provide the minimum support necessary to avoid breach of a person's Convention rights; section 17 support is to be provided by reference to the assessed needs of the child. In short, as she puts it, section 4 and section 17 establish two discrete regimes established for different purposes.
>
> 88. Second, there is the striking fact that, in contrast to the position under section 95, Parliament has not excluded families who are or may be eligible for support under section 4 from local authority support under section 17.
>
> 89. Third, there is the careful exclusion of children from the ambit of the provisions in Schedule 3 to the 2002 Act removing various asylum-seekers or failed asylum-seekers from eligibility for support under section 17. As Ms Rhee says, this is of central importance, being a clear legislative indication that even children of failed asylum-seekers should be entitled to access section 17 support. Accordingly, as she points out, any exclusion from section 17 support for the dependent children of failed asylum-seekers must, if it exists, be found elsewhere. Yet, as we have seen, in contrast to the position of dependent children of asylum-seekers, there is no such exclusion in place in respect of dependent children of failed asylum-seekers. If a child is being provided with support under section 95, the legislative scheme gives priority to the provision of section 95 support over section 17 support: section 122(3) and (5). Not so in relation to support under section 4. So, it is to be inferred that the legislative intent is that where section 4 and section 17 are both theoretically engaged, the more advantageous support regime under section 17 is to apply.

21.73 *R (SL) v Westminster CC* [2013] UKSC 27, (2013) 16 CCLR 161

A need for 'care and attention' had to be accommodation-related

Facts: SL was a failed asylum-seeker with fresh representations who suffered from PTSD and depression. He was independent in self-care skills and had no cognitive difficulties but required practical assistance in arranging activities during the day and regular monitoring of his mental state (with general advice and encouragement), not normally at his home. Westminster concluded that SL did not require 'care and attention' for the purposes of section 21 of the National Assistance Act 1948.

Judgment: the Supreme Court (Neuberger, Hale, Mance, Kerr and Carnwath JJSC) agreed with Westminster:

1) The meaning of 'care and attention' has been subject to authoritative guidance by Baroness Hale, with helpful elaboration by Lord Neuberger, in *R (M) v Slough Borough Council*[28] and the ordinary meaning of the statutory words does not support a more restrictive approach of limiting it to personal care or services of a 'close and intimate nature'. What is involved in 'care and attention' must take its colour from its association with the duty to provide residential accommodation. It cannot be confined to that species of care and attention that can only be delivered in residential accommodation of a specialised kind but something well beyond mere monitoring of an individual's condition is required.

2) *(obiter)* Assuming that L's needs did amount to a need for 'care and attention', the care and attention was available otherwise than by the provision of accommodation under National Assistance Act 1948 s21. The services provided by the Council were in no sense accommodation-related. They were entirely independent of his actual accommodation, however provided, or his need for it. The Court of Appeal was wrong in concluding that 'available ' means not merely available in fact but as implying also a requirement for care and attention to be 'reasonably practicable and efficacious'. Moreover, the need for accommodation cannot in itself constitute a need for care and attention. The care and attention has to be accommodation-related which means that it has at least to be care and attention of a sort which is normally provide in the home (whether ordinary or specialised) or will be effectively useless if the claimant has no home. On this part of section 21, the Court of Appeal in *R (Mani) v Lambeth LBC*[29] and *R (O) v Barking and Dagenham LBC*[30] erred in concluding that if an applicant's need for care and attention is to any extent made more acute by circumstances other than the lack of accommodation and funds, he qualifies for assistance under section 21(1)(a).

21.74 *R (EAT) v Newham LBC* [2013] EWHC 344 (Admin), (2013) 16 CCLR 259

When in substance a person had applied for LTR under Article 8 ECHR, not Article 3 ECHR, only the local authority could provide support – the asylum support regime was inapplicable

Facts: Ms N and her child, EAT, had applied for LTR under Article 8 ECHR. The Secretary of State for the Home Department had refused that application, referring to Article 3 as well as Article 8 ECHR. Ms N and EAT had appealed. Newham refused to provide support for them, under section 17 of the Children Act 1989, on the basis that section 122 of the Immigration and Asylum Act 1999 applied, because Newham had reasonable grounds to believe that they had made a 'claim for asylum' (which includes a claim under Article 3 ECHR).

28 [2008] UKHL 52, (2008) 11 CCLR 733.
29 [2003] EWCA Civ 836, (2003) 6 CCLR 376.
30 [2010] EWCA Civ 1101, (2010) 13 CCLR 591.

Judgment: Deputy High Court Judge Powell QC held that it was necessary to consider the terms in which the application was expressed. In this case, only Article 8 was referred to. The Secretary of State for the Home Department decision referred to Article 3 ECHR in a 'belt and braces' way. Accordingly, Newham had not had reasonable grounds to believe that Ms N and EAT had applied for asylum.

21.75 *R (Refugee Action) v Secretary of State for the Home Department* [2014] EWHC 1033 (Admin), [2014] PTSR D18

The level of asylum support was in breach of the Reception Conditions Directive

Facts: Refugee Action sought a judicial review of the levels of asylum support paid under the Asylum Support Regulations 2000.

Judgment: Popplewell J held that the levels of support were, in a number of respects, below the minimum required by Council Directive 2003/9/EC of 27 January 2003 laying down minimum standards for the reception of asylum-seekers, insofar as the Secretary of State for the Home Department had:

- disregarded the following essential needs: (i) essential household goods such as washing powder, cleaning materials and disinfectant; (ii) nappies, formula milk and other special requirements of new mothers, babies and very young children; (iii) non-prescription medication; (iv) the opportunity to maintain interpersonal relationships and a minimum level of participation in social, cultural and religious life;
- failed to consider whether the following matters were essential needs: (i) travel by public transport to attend appointments with legal advisers, where it was not covered by legal aid; (ii) telephone calls to maintain contact with families and legal representatives, and for necessary communication to progress their asylum claims, such as with legal representatives, witnesses and others who may be able to assist with obtaining evidence in relation to the claim; and (iii) writing materials, where necessary for communication and for the education of children.

CHAPTER 22

Learning disability and autism

22.1 Introduction and statutory machinery

Cases

22.11 *R v Avon CC ex p M* (1999) 2 CCLR 185, [1994] 2 FCR 259
Needs can include an entrenched psychological need for a particular service

22.12 *R (Alloway) v Bromley LBC* [2004] EWHC 2108 (Admin), (2005) 8 CCLR 61
A local authority fetters its discretion if it rules out one service from the start on costs grounds and does not fairly compare the rival options

22.13 *Autism-Europe v France (complaint 13/2002)* (2004) 38 EHRR CD 265
The European Committee of Social Rights declared admissible a complaint that France was in breach of the revised European Social Charter by failing to ensure that children and adults were entitled to education in mainstream schools in sufficient numbers

22.14 *R (Bishop) v Bromley LBC* [2006] EWHC 2148 (Admin), (2006) 9 CCLR 635
Prior assessments were only required in service closure cases where there were exceptional circumstances

22.15 *R (JL) v Islington LBC* [2009] EWHC 458 (Admin), (2009) 12 CCLR 322
It is unlawful simply to apply a new eligibility policy without genuinely assessing needs; further, the local authority had not discharged the disability equality duty because there was no audit trail or other documentation demonstrating a proper approach

22.16 *R (B) v Worcestershire CC* [2009] EWHC 2915 (Admin), (2010) 13 CCLR 13
The closure decision was based on irrational premises

22.17 *AH v Hertfordshire Partnership NHS Foundation Trust* [2011] EWHC 276 (COP), (2011) 14 CCLR 301
It was not in the best interests of a severely learning disabled man to be moved from an NHS facility where he had lived for many years to a flat in London

22.18 *R (RO) v East Riding of Yorkshire Council* [2011] EWCA Civ 196, (2011) 14 CCLR 256
A placement at a specialist residential school may be under section 20 of the Children Act 1989 rather than under the Education Act 1996

continued

22.19 *The Commissioner of Police for the Metropolis v ZH* [2013] EWCA Civ 69, (2013) 16 CCLR 109

There had been a serious assault and breach of ECHR when the police restrained a young autistic adult with taking special care

22.20 *R (MM) v Hounslow LBC* [2015] EWHC 3731 (Admin), (2016) 19 CCLR 141

The assessment of a teenager with autism had been lawful and the local authority had been entitled to await the outcome of the judicial review before preparing a care plan

Introduction and statutory machinery

22.1 Adults with a learning disability and/or autism may well have needs for care and support within section 9 of the Care Act 2014, and their carers may have well have needs for support within section 10 of the Care Act 2014, in which case those needs fall to be assessed and met on a similar basis as other adults' and carers' needs. Having said that, over the last 15 years or so, there has been a specific focus on adults with a learning disability and autism.

22.2 The Autism Act 2009 came into force on the 12 January 2010:

- section 1 requires the Secretary of State to publish and keep under review an 'autism strategy',
- section 2 requires the Secretary of State to publish and keep under review guidance for the purpose of securing the implementation of the autism strategy; section 3 requires local authorities and NHS bodies to 'act under' this guidance.

22.3 The current autism strategy is:

- *Fulfilling and rewarding lives*[1] (March 2010) and *Think Autism – Fulfilling and rewarding lives, the strategy for adults with autism in England: an update* (April 2014);[2]
- for Wales, *ASD Strategic Action Plan for Wales;*[3]
- for Northern Ireland, Department of Health Social Services and Public Safety *Autism strategy (2013–2020) and action plan (2013–2016);*[4] and
- for Scotland, *The Scottish Strategy for Autism* (2011).[5]

22.4 The current statutory guidance is *Statutory guidance for Local Authorities and NHS organisations to support implementation of the Adult Autism Strategy* (March 2015) (England).[6]

22.5 As discussed above in at para 8.9, local authorities must ensure that every person undertaking assessments 'has the skills, knowledge and competence to carry out the assessment in question', 'is appropriately trained' and, where appropriate, seeks an expert view (regulation 5 of the Care and Support (Assessment) Regulations 2014. These provisions, together with the *Care and Support Statutory Guidance* in effect require persons who assess adults with autism to have specialist training:

> 6.85 When assessing particularly complex or multiple needs, an assessor may require the support of an expert to carry out the assessment, to ensure that the person's needs are fully captured. Local authorities should consider whether additional relevant expertise is required on a case-by-case basis, taking into account the nature of the needs of the individual, and the skills

1 http://webarchive.nationalarchives.gov.uk/20130107105354/http://www.dh.gov.uk/prod_consum_dh/groups/dh_digitalassets/@dh/@en/@ps/documents/digitalasset/dh_113405.pdf.

2 www.gov.uk/government/uploads/system/uploads/attachment_data/file/299866/Autism_Strategy.pdf.

3 www.asdinfowales.co.uk/home.php?page_id=5983.

4 www.dhsspsni.gov.uk/publications/autism-strategy-and-action-plan.

5 www.gov.scot/Resource/Doc/361926/0122373.pdf.

6 www.gov.uk/government/uploads/system/uploads/attachment_data/file/422338/autism-guidance.pdf.

of those carrying out the assessment. The local authority must ensure that the person is able to be involved as far as possible, for example by providing an interpreter where a person has a particular condition affecting communication – such as autism, blindness, or deafness.[7] See the Equality Act 2010 for necessary provisions around reasonable adjustments.

6.86 Where the assessor does not have the necessary knowledge of a particular condition or circumstance, they must consult someone who has relevant expertise. This is to ensure that the assessor can ask the right questions relating to the condition and interpret these appropriately to identify underlying needs. A person with relevant expertise can be considered as somebody who, either through training or experience, has acquired knowledge or skill of the particular condition or circumstance. Such a person may be a doctor or health professional, or an expert from the voluntary sector, but there is no obligation for the local authority to source an expert from an outside body if the expertise is available in house.

6.87 The Department has published guidance for certain groups of adults that refer to their assessment for care and support. Two specific areas are for people who are deafblind and people with autism and these pieces of guidance should be read with this guidance. *Think Autism 2014*, the April 2014 update to Fulfilling and Rewarding Lives, the strategy for adults with autism in England (2010), sets out that local authorities should:

- make basic autism training available for all staff working in health and social care;
- develop or provide specialist training for those in roles that have a direct impact on access to services for adults with autism; and
- include quality autism awareness training within general equality and diversity training programmes across public services.

6.88 The Care Act strengthens this guidance in relation to assessors having specialised training to assess an adult with autism. The Act places a legal requirement on local authorities that all assessors must have the skills, knowledge and competence to carry out the assessment in question. Where an assessor does not have experience in a particular condition (such as autism, learning disabilities, mental health needs or other conditions), they must consult someone with relevant experience. This is so that the person being assessed is involved throughout the process and their needs, outcomes and the impact of needs on their wellbeing are all accurately identified.

22.6 Learning disability strategy, emphasising the importance of ensuring that people with a learning disability have as much choice and control as possible over their lives, has been published in:

- *Valuing People: a new strategy for learning disability for the 21st Century* (March 2001);[8]
- *Improving the life chances of disabled people: final report* (January 2005);[9]

7 See also the Equality Act for necessary provisions around reasonable adjustments at www. legislation.gov.uk/ukpga/2010/15/contents.

8 www.gov.uk/government/uploads/system/uploads/attachment_data/file/250877/5086.pdf.

9 http://webarchive.nationalarchives.gov.uk/+/http:/www.cabinetoffice.gov.uk/media/cabinetoffice/strategy/assets/disability.pdf.

- *Good Learning Disability Partnership Boards: 'Making it happen for everyone'* (October 2009);[10]
- *Valuing People Now: a new three-year strategy for people with learning disabilities* (January 2009).[11]

22.7 One of the main initiatives of *Valuing People*, has been the setting up of local Learning Disability Partnership Boards, to implement aspects of the *Valuing People* programme.

22.8 In Wales, there is the *Statement on policy and practice for adults with a learning disability* (2007).[12]

22.9 A key recommendation of *Valuing People* was that local authorities close day centres and provide flexible, individual community support instead:

> 7.21 For decades, services for people with learning disabilities have been heavily reliant on large, often institutional, day centres. These have provided much needed respite for families, but they have made a limited contribution to promoting social inclusion or independence for people with learning disabilities. People with learning disabilities attending them have not had opportunities to develop individual interests or the skills and experience they need in order to move into employment.
>
> 7.22 Local councils currently spend over £300 million a year on day services of which more than 80% goes on over 60,000 day centre places that often focus on large, group activities. The most severely disabled people often receive the poorest service and the particular cultural needs of people from minority ethnic communities are too often not addressed.
>
> 7.23 Some local councils have done much to modernise their day services, but overall progress has been too slow. The barriers standing in the way of change include:
>
> - Difficulties in releasing resources tied up in buildings and staff;
> - Slow development of links with other services (including supported employment) and support in the wider community;
> - Tension between providing respite for families and fulfilling opportunities for the person;
> - Slow progress in introducing person-centred approaches to planning.
>
> 7.24 The Government wishes to see a greater emphasis on individualised and flexible services which will:
>
> - Support people in developing their capacity to do what they want;
> - Help people develop social skills and the capacity to form friendships and relationships with a wider range of people;
> - Enable people to develop skills and enhance their employability;
> - Help communities welcome people with learning disabilities.
>
> 7.25 These problems will be addressed through a five year programme to support local councils in modernising their day services. Our aim will be to ensure that the resources currently committed to day centres are focused on providing people with learning disabilities with new opportunities to lead full and purposeful lives. Securing the active involvement of people with learning disabilities and their families in redesigning services will be essential to the success of the programme. The Government recognises

10 http://webarchive.nationalarchives.gov.uk/20130107105354/http://www.dh.gov.uk/prod_consum_dh/groups/dh_digitalassets/documents/digitalasset/dh_107384.pdf.

11 http://webarchive.nationalarchives.gov.uk/20130107105354/http://www.dh.gov.uk/prod_consum_dh/groups/dh_digitalassets/documents/digitalasset/dh_093375.pdf.

12 This, with associated documents, can be found at http://gov.wales/docs/dhss/publications/100126policyen.pdf.

that, for many families, day centres have provided essential respite from the day to day demands of caring. The services that replace them must result in improvements for both users and their families. The needs of people with profound or complex disabilities will be carefully considered as part of the modernisation programme.

22.10 Although drafted with the best of intentions, this policy has coincided with a period of acute budgetary pressures on local authorities, with the result that those affected by this process have often been gravely concerned that local authorities will replace day centres with community provision that is (a) limited for persons with eligible needs only; and (b) in any event, inadequate. A number of judicial reviews have resulted (see chapter 16 on Care home and other service closures) and continue to result.

There are useful resources published by, among others:

- The National Autistic Society;[13]
- The Foundation for People with Learning Disabilities;[14]
- Learning Disability;[15]
- BILD;[16]
- the Learning Disability Coalition;[17] and
- Mencap.[18]

Cases

22.11 *R v Avon CC ex p M* (1999) 2 CCLR 185, [1994] 2 FCR 259

Needs can include an entrenched psychological need for a particular service

Facts: a social services complaints review panel concluded that, as a result of his Down's Syndrome, M had developed the entrenched view that it was necessary for him to live in residential accommodation at a place called Milton Heights, such that to place him elsewhere would cause serious damage to his health; thus, he had a strong psychological need to live there. The panel recommended a placement at Milton Heights for three years, to allow for M to develop his living skills and be prepared to move elsewhere. In response, Avon concluded that whilst M had a strong personal preference to live at Milton Heights, his needs could be met at Berwick Lodge, which was substantial cheaper.

Judgment: Henry J held that Avon was under a duty to meet needs, including psychological needs of the kind that the panel held existed in this case and that Avon had not had *Wednesbury* rational reasons for disagreeing with the panel's assessment:

> Examining their reasons in detail, the following comments can be made:
>
> - The panel correctly found that in law the assessment must be based on current needs.

13 www.autism.org.uk/.
14 www.learningdisabilities.org.uk/.
15 www.learningdisability.co.uk/.
16 www.bild.org.uk/.
17 www.learningdisabilitycoalition.org.uk/.
18 www.mencap.org.uk/learning-disability-explained/.

- The panel correctly found that in law need is clearly capable of including psychological need. In particular, that must be so when (as it was on the evidence before them) that psychological need was contributed to by the congenital Down's Syndrome condition itself. I have recited the evidence that the panel had had as to that. That evidence was all one way once Mr Passfield had agreed that he was not an expert on Down's Syndrome.
- Next, the panel had found that M's entrenched position was part of his psychological need. This is the crucial finding of fact. It is arrived at against the background, recited in these reasons, that M would not be forced to live anywhere against his will; that the only place he would presently consider would be Milton Heights, that that entrenched position was contributed to by the Down's Syndrome, and that his present needs included a need for a period of stability.

...

But the making of the final decision did not lie with the review panel. It lay with the social services committee. I would be reluctant to hold (and do not) that in no circumstances whatsoever could the social services committee have overruled the review panel's recommendation in the exercise of their legal right and duty to consider it. Caution normally requires the court not to say 'never' in any obiter dictum pronouncement. But I have no hesitation in finding that they could not overrule that decision without a substantial reason and without having given that recommendation the weight it required. It was a decision taken by a body entrusted with the basic fact-finding exercise under the complaints procedure. It was arrived at after a convincing examination of the evidence, particularly the expert evidence. The evidence before them had, as to the practicalities, been largely one way. The panel had directed themselves properly in law, and had arrived at a decision in line with the strength of the evidence before them. They had given clear reasons and they had raised the crucial factual question with the parties before arriving at their conclusion.

The strength, coherence, and apparent persuasiveness of that decision had to be addressed head on if it were to be set aside and not followed. These difficulties were not faced either by the respondents' officers in their paper to the social services committee, or by the social services committee themselves. Not to face them was either unintentional perversity on their part, or showed a wrong appreciation of the legal standing of that decision. It seems to me that you do not properly reconsider a decision when, on the evidence, it does not seem that that decision was given the weight it deserved. That is, in my judgment, what the social services committee failed to do here. To neglect to do that is not a question which merely, as is suggested in one of the papers, impugns the credibility of the review panel, but instead ignores the weight to which it is prima facie entitled because of its place in the statutory procedure, and further, pays no attention to the scope of its hearing and clear reasons that it had given.

It seems to me that anybody required, at law, to give their reasons for reconsidering and changing such a decision must have good reasons for doing so, and must show that they gave that decision sufficient weight and, in my judgment, it is that that the social services committee have here failed to do. Their decision must be quashed. As is often the case in Wednesbury quashings, it can be put in a number of ways: either unintentional perversity, or failure to take the review panel's recommendation properly into account, or an implicit error of law in not giving it sufficient weight.

22.12 *R (Alloway) v Bromley LBC* [2004] EWHC 2108 (Admin), (2005) 8 CCLR 61

A local authority fetters its discretion if it rules out one service from the start on costs grounds and does not fairly compare the rival options

Facts: Mr Alloway was a 19-year-old man who was autistic and suffered from learning disabilities. Bromley's community care assessment concluded that he should be placed at Hesley Village and College. However, the Council then purported to place him at a cheaper option at Robinia Care. Bromley concluded that Hesley was unnecessarily expensive for Mr Alloway's needs but did not assert that its decision-making was affected by, or justified by, any lack of resources on its part.

Judgment: Crane J quashed this decision and said this:

> 71. In my judgment, the defendant's decision-making was flawed. The 2003 decision not to send Stephen to Hesley Village at that stage is not, as I have indicated, flawed. But, by at least February 2004, it is clear, in my view, that Hesley had been ruled out as too expensive and not justified, even before any viable alternatives had been identified. Moreover, it had been ruled out as too expensive on grounds that were clearly, at least in part, wrong. I refer to the apparent error, repeated by Mr Wright in his placement assessment, about the possibility of additions to that sum, and also the lack, apparently, of any exploration of assistance from the health care trust for assistance with funding.
>
> 72. It is very probable that Hesley, even on an accurate calculation, is the most expensive, perhaps significantly the most expensive, but the evidence is that it does at least cater for Stephen's level of problems. Whether it provides more than he needs is, of course, another matter.
>
> 73. In relation to Solent, on the assumption that that placement is still a possibility, there appears to be no plan, certainly no plan in the evidence, for Stephen's care there. There is, in the annex to the acknowledgment of service, a breakdown of the costs in relation to Solent, but although quite plainly they have assessed Stephen and they think that they can manage him, the court really has no basis for forming any view, and nor, on what is before the court, would the defendant have any ability to form a view of the suitability of Solent.
>
> 74. In relation to Robinia, they have plainly carried out an assessment. That is included in the annex to the acknowledgment of service. I emphasise that I am not reaching any conclusion that Robinia, or indeed Solent, should be ruled out of consideration, but there is no evidence before the court of an informed decision based on a fair comparison of Robinia (or indeed Solent) and Hesley, including an accurate comparison of costs.
>
> 75. In relation to Hesley, my view as to the early ruling out of Hesley, does make it correct to say that the council fettered their discretion.

22.13 *Autism-Europe v France (complaint 13/2002)* (2004) 38 EHRR CD 265

The European Committee of Social Rights declared admissible a complaint that France was in breach of the revised European Social Charter by failing to ensure that children and adults were entitled to education in mainstream schools in sufficient numbers

Facts: Autism-Europe brought proceedings against France in reliance on Articles 15, 17 and E of the revised European Social Charter, which provide as follows:

Article 15 – The right of persons with disabilities to independence, social integration and participation in the life of the community

With a view to ensuring to persons with disabilities, irrespective of age and the nature and origin of their disabilities, the effective exercise of the right to independence, social integration and participation in the life of the community, the Parties undertake, in particular:

1. to take the necessary measures to provide persons with disabilities with guidance, education and vocational training in the framework of general schemes wherever possible or, where this is not possible, through specialised bodies, public or private;

...

Article 17 – The right of children and young persons to social, legal and economic protection

With a view to ensuring the effective exercise of the right of children and young persons to grow up in an environment which encourages the full development of their personality and of their physical and mental capacities, the Parties undertake, either directly or in co-operation with public and private organisations, to take all appropriate and necessary measures designed:

1. a) to ensure that children and young persons, taking account of the rights and duties of their parents, have the care, the assistance, the education and the training they need, in particular by providing for the establishment or maintenance of institutions and services sufficient and adequate for this purpose;

...

Article E – Non-discrimination

The enjoyment of the rights set forth in this Charter shall be secured without discrimination on any ground such as race, colour, sex, language, religion, political or other opinion, national extraction or social origin, health, association with a national minority, birth or other status.

Judgment: the Committee held as follows:

48. As emphasised in the General Introduction to its Conclusions of 2003 (p10), the Committee views Article 15 of the Revised Charter as both reflecting and advancing a profound shift of values in all European countries over the past decade away from treating them as objects of pity and towards respecting them as equal citizens – an approach that the Council of Europe contributed to promote, with the adoption by the Committee of Ministers of Recommendation (92) 6 of 1992 on a coherent policy for people with disabilities. The underlying vision of Article 15 is one of equal citizenship for persons with disabilities and, fittingly, the primary rights are those of 'independence, social integration and participation in the life of the community'. Securing a right to education for children and others with disabilities plays an obviously important role in advancing these citizenship rights. This explains why education is now specifically mentioned in the revised Article 15 and why such an emphasis is placed on achieving that education 'in the framework of general schemes, wherever possible'. It should be noted that Article 15 applies to all persons with disabilities regardless of the nature and origin of their disability and irrespective of their age. It thus clearly covers both children and adults with autism.

49. Article 17 is predicated on the need to ensure that children and young persons grow up in an environment which encourages the 'full development of their personality and of their physical and mental capacities'. This approach is just as important for children with disabilities as it is for others and arguably more in circumstances where the effects of ineffective or untimely intervention are ever likely to be undone. The Committee views Article 17, which deals more generally, *inter alia*, with the right to education for all, as also embodying the modern approach of mainstreaming. Article 17(1), in particular, requires the establishment and maintenance of sufficient and adequate institutions and services for the purpose of education. Since Article 17(1) deals only with children and young persons it is important to read it in conjunction with Article 15(1) as far as adults are concerned.

...

51. The Committee considers that the insertion of Article E into a separate Article in the Revised Charter indicates the heightened importance the drafters paid to the principle of non-discrimination with respect to the achievement of the various substantive rights contained therein. It further considers that its function is to help secure the equal effective enjoyment of all the rights concerned regardless of difference. Therefore, it does not constitute an autonomous right which could in itself provide independent grounds for a complaint. It follows that the Committee understands the arguments of the complainant as implying that the situation as alleged violates Arts 15(1) and 17(1) when read in combination with Article E of the Revised Charter. Although disability is not explicitly listed as a prohibited ground of discrimination under Art E, the Committee considers that it is adequately covered by the reference to 'other status'. Such an interpretative approach, which is justified in its own rights, is fully consistent with both the letter and the spirit of the Political Declaration adopted by the 2nd European conference of ministers responsible for integration policies for people with disabilities (Malaga, April, 2003), which reaffirmed the anti-discriminatory and human rights framework as the appropriate one for development of European policy in this field.

52. The Committee observes further that the wording of Article E is almost identical to the wording of Article 14 of the European Convention on Human Rights. As the European Court of Human Rights has repeatedly stressed in interpreting Article 14 and most recently in the *Thlimmenos* case [*Thlimmenos v Greece* (2001) 31 EHRR 15, para [44]], the principle of equality that is reflected therein means treating equals equally and unequals unequally. In particular it is said in the above-mentioned case:

> 'The right not to be discriminated against in the enjoyment of the rights guaranteed under the Convention is also violated when States without an objective and reasonable justification fail to treat differently persons whose situations are significantly different'.

In other words, human difference in a democratic society should not only be viewed positively but should be responded to with discernment in order to ensure real and effective equality.

In this regard, the Committee considers that Article E not only prohibits direct discrimination but also all forms of indirect discrimination. Such indirect discrimination may arise by failing to take due and positive account of all relevant differences or by failing to take adequate steps to ensure that the rights and collective advantages that are open to all are genuinely accessible by and to all.

53. The Committee recalls, as stated in its decision relative to Complaint No 1/1998 (*International Commission of Jurist v Portugal*, para [32]), that the implementation of the Charter requires the State Parties to take not merely legal action but also practical action to give full effect to the rights recognised in the Charter. When the achievement of one of the rights in question is exceptionally complex and particularly expensive to resolve, a State Party must take measures that allows it to achieve the objectives of the Charter within a reasonable time, with measurable progress and to an extent consistent with the maximum use of available resources. States Parties must be particularly mindful of the impact that their choices will have for groups with heightened vulnerabilities as well as for others persons affected including, especially, their families on whom falls the heaviest burden in the event of institutional shortcomings.

54. In the light of the afore-mentioned, the Committee notes that in the case of autistic children and adults, notwithstanding a national debate going back more than 20 years about the number of persons concerned and the relevant strategies required, and even after the enactment of the Disabled Persons Policy Act of June 30, 1975, France has failed to achieve sufficient progress in advancing the provision of education for persons with autism. It specifically notes that most of the French official documents, in particular those submitted during the procedure, still use a more restrictive definition of autism than that adopted by the World Heath Organisation and that there are still insufficient official statistics with which to rationally measure progress through time. The Committee considers that the fact that the establishments specialising in the education and care of disabled children (particularly those with autism) are not in general financed from the same budget as normal schools, does not in itself amount to discrimination, since it is primarily for States themselves to decide on the modalities of funding.

Nevertheless, it considers, as the authorities themselves acknowledge, and whether a broad or narrow definition of autism is adopted, that the proportion of children with autism being educated in either general or specialist schools is much lower than in the case of other children, whether or not disabled. It is also established, and not contested by the authorities, that there is a chronic shortage of care and support facilities for autistic adults.

Conclusion

For these reasons, the Committee concludes by 11 votes to 2 that the situation constitutes a violation of Arts 15(1) and 17(1) whether alone or read in combination with Article E of the revised European Social Charter.

22.14 *R (Bishop) v Bromley LBC* [2006] EWHC 2148 (Admin), (2006) 9 CCLR 635

Prior assessments were only required in service closure cases where there were exceptional circumstances

Facts: Bromley decided to close a day care facility attached to a care home, subject to alternative day services being made available for current service users. The claimant, a daughter of one of the service users, contended that the decision was irrational and undertaken without first assessing her mother's needs.

Judgment: Deputy High Court Judge Parker refused permission to apply for judicial review, on the basis that Bromley had rational reasons for wanting to close this day care facility (cost and over-capacity) and this was not the exceptional type of case which require Bromley to fully assess all the service users' needs before reaching its decision (applying *R v North and East Devon Health Authority ex p Coughlan,*[19] see above at para 16.27; and applying *R v Merton, Sutton and Wandsworth Health Authority ex p Perry,*[20] see above at para 16.28, eg the type of case where there is cause to believe that prior assessment is essential in order to ascertain whether suitable alternative provision is in fact available). Further, the likely impact was not such as to meet the Article 8 ECHR threshold.

22.15 *R (JL) v Islington LBC* [2009] EWHC 458 (Admin), (2009) 12 CCLR 322

It is unlawful simply to apply a new eligibility policy without genuinely assessing needs; further, the local authority had not discharged the disability equality duty because there was no audit trail or other documentation demonstrating a proper approach

Facts: JL suffered from autism and received 1,248 hours of support each year. Islington then changed its eligibility criteria, as a result of which disabled children with 'high needs' (such as JL) received only 624 hours each year. Islington later added a small number of additional hours to enable some respite provision to be made. JL sought a judicial review.

Judgment: Black J held that Islington had not undertaken a genuine assessment of JL's needs but simply applied their new eligibility policy, that an eligibility policy could not be used to determine whether or not a local authority was under a duty to act under section 20 of the Children Act 1989 (which imposed an absolute duty) and that Islington's policy was flawed in a number of respects, in particular in that it had the effect of excluding needs that Islington would have decided it was necessary to meet (under section 2 of the Chronically Sick and Disabled Persons Act 1970). In addition, Islington had failed to discharge its duty under section 49A of the Disability Discrimination Act 1995 when drawing up its criteria.

22.16 *R (B) v Worcestershire CC* [2009] EWHC 2915 (Admin), (2010) 13 CCLR 13

The closure decision was based on irrational premises

Facts: Worcestershire decided to close a day centre for adults with severe physical and learning disabilities, on the basis that their needs could be met significantly more cheaply elsewhere.

Judgment: Stadlen J held that Worcestershire's decision was irrational because it was not based on a detailed analysis or evidence necessary to support a reasoned and rational decision that the claimants' needs could be met more cheaply elsewhere: the community care assessments did not sufficiently define the level of support needed, including what staff ratio was required.

19 [1999] 2 WLR 622, (1999) 2 CCLR 285.
20 (2000) 3 CCLR 378, QBD.

22.17 *AH v Hertfordshire Partnership NHS Foundation Trust* [2011] EWHC 276 (COP), (2011) 14 CCLR 301

It was not in the best interests of a severely learning disabled man to be moved from an NHS facility where he had lived for many years to a flat in London

Facts: AH was a learning disabled adult who had spent most of his life in a long-stay hospital and, when it closed, moved to a specialist facility within the grounds of a former hospital, in a rural location. Pursuant to central government policy, *Valuing People,* that persons with a learning disability should have increased choice and control over their lives, the NHS decided to move AH, contrary to the wishes of all those concerned about him, to a flat in London, to be cared for by an agency and the local authority there. AH himself lacked the relevant capacity to oppose this move.

Judgment: Peter Jackson J held that the proposed move did not entail a single benefit for AH but would cause him significant upset possibly amounting to serious harm:

> 77. Although the ambition to maximise Alan's opportunities is laudable, it has not been possible to identify a single dependable benefit arising from the proposed move. The thesis is that it would provide him with a greater experience of ordinary life in a local community, and that this would improve his quality of life. Each element of this proposition is incongruous with the realities of Alan's life. His experience is so far from being ordinary that it is not useful to use ordinariness as a yardstick. Ealing is not local for Alan and there is no community there which would be meaningful for him. I also accept the evidence of the clinicians, the experts, and not least of Alan's committed parents, that the prospect of him living a more expansive and fulfilled life following a move is a chimera. It is more likely that it would lead to a deterioration from which he might – or might not – recover. It is not enough to say that *'the benefits of community living may matter to Alan'* if one cannot show that they will. Facing up to these realities does not in any way diminish or demean Alan, but values and respects him for who he is.
>
> 78. I agree that the prospect of a home for life for Alan is attractive and accept that there is no guarantee that an alternative of the quality now offered would be available if he had to move at some point in the future. Nevertheless, only the closure of SRS could justify the turmoil of a move and as this is not expected in the foreseeable future, there is no reason to anticipate it.
>
> ...
>
> 80. This case illustrates the obvious point that guideline policies cannot be treated as universal solutions, nor should initiatives designed to personalise care and promote choice be applied to the opposite effect. The very existence of SRS, after most of the institutional population had been resettled in the community, is perhaps the exception that proves this rule. These residents are not an anomaly simply because they are among the few remaining recipients of this style of social care. They might better be seen as a good example of the kind of personal planning that lies at the heart of the philosophy of care in the community. Otherwise, an unintended consequence of national policy may be to sacrifice the interests of vulnerable and unusual people like Alan.

22.18 *R (RO) v East Riding of Yorkshire Council* [2011] EWCA Civ 196, (2011) 14 CCLR 256

A placement at a specialist residential school may be under section 20 of the Children Act 1989 rather than under the Education Act 1996

Facts: RO had severe autism and ADHD, as a result of which East Riding placed him at a specialist residential school, from where he returned home every weekend and during school holidays. East Riding and the parents were in dispute, however, as to whether East Riding continued to accommodate RO under section 20 of the Children Act 1989, so that he retained his 'looked after' child (LAC) status (and would ultimately qualify for 'children leaving care services'). East Riding contended that it was providing RO with accommodation in the exercise of its functions under the Education Act 1996, rather than in the exercise of its social services functions.

Judgment: the Court of Appeal (Rix, Smith and Richards LJJ) held that the placement was under section 20 of the Children Act 1989:

1) section 22(3A) of the Children Act 1989 suggested that 'a looked after child's' welfare embraced his or her education and that, even in the context of education, the Children Act was to be regarded as the primary statute. The question of education was to be specifically considered as part of the 'corporate parents' role which an authority had to undertake when a child entered into the LAC regime. The statutory guidance, *Promoting the educational achievement of looked after children*, reflected the primary role which the Children Act played where a 'looked after child' was concerned, to provide for the right educational help. That guidance, and the statutory guidance, *Framework for the Assessment of Children in Need and their Families*, reflecting statute, required social services and education departments to work together to address the needs and welfare of the child.

2) Given that both the social services and education departments were persuaded of the need for the specialist residential placement, it was impossible to regard the special educational needs placement in this case on these particular facts as being provided wholly or mainly to meet RO's educational needs as distinct from being provided to meet both those needs and the needs for which he had become and was a looked after child. It was plain that RO required full-time accommodation in his specialist placement in order to give him the care, as well as the educational assistance, which his needs, and his parents' inability to cope with and control him, demanded.

3) The council did not ask itself, let alone give anxious scrutiny to, the question whether the factors which had led to respite care, when they were carried over into the placement at Horton House, necessitated a continuation of RO's LAC status. They merely assumed that the status came to an end with the ending of the respite care which had brought that status into being. That was a legal error more fundamental than irrationality.

4) The council's recognition that RO's needs and the limits of his parents' coping abilities meant that RO needed a residential placement brought the case within section 20(1)(c) of the Children Act 1989, and meant that

it would be wrong to regard the council to have been exercising a mere power rather than their statutory duty.

22.19 *The Commissioner of Police for the Metropolis v ZH* [2013] EWCA Civ 69, (2013) 16 CCLR 109

There had been a serious assault and breach of ECHR when the police restrained a young autistic adult with taking special care

Facts: ZH, who suffered from severe autism, epilepsy and learning disabilities, became fixated by the water at a local swimming pool and would not move away from the poolside. His carers knew that if he was touched he might jump into the pool (he was fully clothed at the time). The swimming pool manager called the police who after a brief conversation with the carers, that established that ZH was autistic, went up to him and touched him. ZH then jumped into the pool. The police then pulled ZH out of the pool and restrained him before taking him, soaking wet and agitated, to the police station. ZH sued.

Judgment: the Court of Appeal (Lord Dyson MR, Richards and Black LJJ) held that the first instance judge had been entitled to conclude that the police had breached ZH's rights under Articles 3, 5 and 8 ECHR, and that they were guilty of assault and false imprisonment and a breach of section 21B of the Disability Discrimination Act 1995. The police defence under the Mental Capacity Act 2005 failed: whilst sections 4–6 of that Act permitted certain acts to be done in connection with the care and treatment of persons lacking capacity if it is in their best interests, those statutory defences were pervaded by concepts of reasonableness, practicability and appropriateness, which were lacking in this case: the police could and should have consulted with ZH's carers about how best to handle him and could not have had a reasonable belief that their actions were in his best interests.

22.20 *R (MM) v Hounslow LBC* [2015] EWHC 3731 (Admin), (2016) 19 CCLR 141

The assessment of a teenager with autism had been lawful and the local authority had been entitled to await the outcome of the judicial review before preparing a care plan

Facts: MM was a 15-year-old boy who had autism and who lived with his mother in a two-bedroom maisonette on the upper floor of a block of flats. He sought a judicial review of Hounslow's assessment that he and his mother continued to require 12.5 hours of support a week.

Judgment: Deputy High Court Judge Sir Brian Keith held that (1) the assessment was rational in all the circumstances, including that the social worker had agreed with SENDIST that MM should attend a special school during the day, had reasonable grounds for concluding that MM's mother had somewhat exaggerated his behavioural difficulties, had arranged some provision of specialised short breaks and had made a referral to a challenging behaviour team; (2) it had also been rational not to assess MM as needing alternative accommodation, given that MM only used a wheelchair occasionally and that the flat had been made safe for his occupation and, in any event, it would not have been unlawful to decline to meet such an assessed need on the basis of *R (G) v Barnet LBC*;[21] (3) Hounslow's eligibility criteria were rational; (4) given that MM had mounted a challenge to the assessment, it had been reasonable for Hounslow to defer completion of a care plan until conclusion of the proceedings.

21 [2003] UKHL 57, (2003) 6 CCLR 500.

CHAPTER 23

Mental capacity

continued

23.29 *A Local Authority v DL, ML, GRL and JP* [2011] EWHC 1022 (Fam), (2011) 14 CCLR 441

The court retained an inherent jurisdiction to protect persons who, whilst not lacking mental capacity, were incapacitated from making a relevant decision by reason of constraint, coercion, undue influence or other vitiating factors

23.30 *Re MN (An Adult)* [2015] EWCA Civ 411, (2015) 18 CCLR 521

The Court of Protection has no power to require a public authority to provide different services, only to consider whether services on offer are in P's best interests, so any legal challenge to the sufficiency of services offered must be brought by way of judicial review

23.31 *RP v United Kingdom* Application no 38245/08, (2013) 16 CCLR 135, ECtHR

Providing there were adequate safeguards, it was compatible with Article 6 ECHR for the Official Solicitor to represent an incapacitated mother in care proceedings relating to her daughter

23.32 *P v Cheshire West and Chester Council, P and Q v Surrey County Council* [2014] UKSC 19, (2015) 18 CCLR 5

A person who lacked capacity to consent to care arrangements was deprived of their liberty if they were under continuous supervision and control by those caring for them and were not free to leave.

23.33 *R (SG) v Haringey LBC* [2015] EWHC 2579 (Admin), (2015) 18 CCLR 444

The failure to appoint an independent advocate, under section 67(2) of the Care Act 2014, for a vulnerable adult, who spoke no English and was illiterate, and who suffered from PTSD, insomnia, depression and anxiety, rendered the assessment unlawful

23.34 *North Yorkshire CC and A Clinical Commissioning Group v MAG and GC* [2016] EWCOP 5, (2016) 19 CCLR 169

The MN *principle also applied in the context of alleged deprivations of liberty*

Introduction

23.1 What follows is intended to amount to a brief guide, limited to those aspects of mental capacity law that intersect with adult social care, which occurs most often:

- when local authorities assess needs and make care planning decisions;
- when local authorities discharge their safeguarding functions (see also chapter 24, Safeguarding adults, below); and
- when there is a dispute over ordinary residence (see also chapter 12, 'Ordinary residence/adults lacking capacity', above).

23.2 When local authorities assess needs and make care planning decisions, they are required to take specific steps and, in general, do all they reasonably can to ensure the effective involvement of adults, and on behalf of adults who lack capacity to make decisions about their care, or experience difficulty in so doing, and of persons acting on their behalf: see the statutory provisions at para 23.11 and para 23.12 on assessment and care planning.

23.3 When an adult lacks capacity to decide a certain matter, decisions are taken on behalf of that adult, in their best interests. However, a local authority cannot be compelled to provide all the care and support that it is in the best interests of an adult to receive. For example, if a local authority assesses an adult lacking capacity as not having an 'eligible need' for a particular service, and decides not to exercise its power to provide that service, the adult cannot obtain that service on the ground that it is in his or her 'best interest' to receive it. His or her only remedy is to:

- seek a review of the merits of the decision through the statutory complaints procedure (or the forthcoming appeal procedure – see para 7.97, above); or to
- seek a review of the lawfulness of the decision, in public law terms, through judicial review.[1]

23.4 That applies, even when there is a dispute between a local authority and family members about whether an incapacitated adult should leave the family home and go to live in (for example) supported housing, or a care home. The court is required to decide whether it is in the adult's best interests to live in accordance with the care package proposed by the local authority in the supported housing/care home, rather than in the family home, together with whatever care package may be offered there. The court may (if it considers it to be appropriate) examine, comment, advise or even exhort; but it is not entitled to require the local authority to provide a package that meets the adult's best interests in a better way, either in the proposed supported housing/care home, or in the family home. Only judicial review can achieve that (or use of the complaints process and, in future, any appeal process).[2]

1 *Re MN (An Adult)* [2015] EWCA Civ 411, (2015) 18 CCLR 521.
2 *Re MN (An Adult)* [2015] EWCA Civ 411, (2015) 18 CCLR 521.

23.5 It is difficult to imagine an incapacitated adult having a need for care and support that is *not* an *'eligible need'*, when the care and support in question is needed in order to avoid the adult suffering a deprivation of liberty that it is not in his or her best interests to experience. However, should it come to it, a local authority must always provide care and support so far as necessary to avoid a breach of ECHR rights. Accordingly, hypothetically at least, a local authority may need to provide different/additional care and support services to avoid an adult being deprived of their liberty in breach of Article 5 ECHR in circumstances where, without that care and support, the adult will experience a deprivation of liberty that is assessed to be incompatible with their best interests:

- a deprivation of liberty is justified if, inter alia, 'it is in the best interests of the relevant person to be deprived of liberty', 'it is necessary for them to be deprived of liberty in order to prevent harm to themselves' and 'deprivation of liberty is a proportionate response to the likelihood of the relevant person suffering harm and the seriousness of that harm' (paragraph 4.58 of *The Mental Capacity Act Deprivation of Liberty Safeguards – Code of Practice to supplement the main Mental Capacity Act 2005 Code of Practice* (2008);[3]
- accordingly:

  5.22 ... If the best interests assessor concluded that the proposed or actual deprivation of liberty was not in the relevant person's best interests, the managing authority, in conjunction with the commissioner of the care, will need to consider how the care plan could be changed to avoid deprivation of liberty. (See, for example, the guidance on practical ways to reduce the risk of deprivation of liberty in paragraph 2.7.) They should examine carefully the reasons given in the best interests assessor's report, and may find it helpful to discuss the matter with the best interests assessor. Where appropriate, they should also discuss the matter with family and carers. If the person is not yet a resident in the care home or hospital, the revised care plan may not involve admission to that facility unless the conditions of care are adapted to be less restrictive and deprivation of liberty will not occur.

23.6 It will be, however, very unusual for inadequate accommodation and/or care to result in a breach of rights under the ECHR; even more unusual for that to justify a refusal to authorise a deprivation of liberty and wrong in principle for the court to deploy such considerations in order to pressurise a local authority into reaching different public law decisions.[4]

23.7 When local authorities discharge their safeguarding functions, one option that they may exercise, is to bring proceedings in the Court of Protection aimed safeguarding the incapacitated adult and/or resolving disputes about how the adult should be cared for (see chapter 24, Safeguarding adults, below).

3 http://webarchive.nationalarchives.gov.uk/20130107105354/http:/www.dh.gov.uk/en/Publicationsandstatistics/Publications/PublicationsPolicyAndGuidance/DH_085476).

4 *North Yorkshire CC v MAG and GC* [2016] EWCOP 5.

The statutory mental capacity scheme and resources

23.8 The statutory scheme is set out in:

- the Mental Capacity Act 2005;
- the Court of Protection Rules 2007;
- the Mental Capacity Act 2005 (Transfer of Proceedings) Order 2007;
- the Court of Protection Fees Order 2007;
- the Mental Capacity Act 2005: Code of Practice (2007);[5]
- the Mental Capacity Act Deprivation of Liberty Safeguards – Code of Practice to supplement the main Mental Capacity Act 2005 Code of Practice (2008).[6]

23.9 The following additional resources exist online:

- Court of Protection practice directions and rules;[7]
- Court of Protection forms;[8]
- General government advice and assistance, as well as resources;[9]
- Mentalhealthlawonline, which contains access to legislation, codes, articles and other useful material. It has particularly impressive case-law updates and a case-law database.[10]

23.10 Further information about mental capacity law may be found in *Court of Protection Handbook*.[11]

Critical statutory provisions

23.11 The critical statutory machinery is found in sections 1–4 of the Mental Capacity Act (MCA) 2005 (supplemented by Chapters 1–5 of the Mental Capacity Act 2005 Code of Practice (2007)), which set out general principles and provide, in short, that a person lacks capacity in relation to a matter if, at the material time, they are unable to make a decision for themselves in relation to that matter because of an impairment of, or a disturbance in the functioning of the mind or brain; in such cases, decisions must be made in the person's best interests:

> **The principles**
>
> **1**(1) The following principles apply for the purposes of this Act.
>
> (2) A person must be assumed to have capacity unless it is established that he lacks capacity.

5 www.gov.uk/government/uploads/system/uploads/attachment_data/file/224660/Mental_Capacity_Act_code_of_practice.pdf.

6 http://webarchive.nationalarchives.gov.uk/20130107105354/http:/www.dh.gov.uk/en/Publicationsandstatistics/Publications/PublicationsPolicyAndGuidance/DH_085476.

7 www.judiciary.gov.uk/publications/court-of-protection-practice-directions/.

8 http://hmctsformfinder.justice.gov.uk/HMCTS/GetForms.do?court_forms_category=Court%20of%20Protection.

9 www.gov.uk/courts-tribunals/court-of-protection.

10 www.mentalhealthlaw.co.uk/Main_Page.

11 Ruck Keene, Edwards, Eldergill and Miles, *Court of Protection Handbook* (second edition 2016, LAG).

(3) A person is not to be treated as unable to make a decision unless all practicable steps to help him to do so have been taken without success.
(4) A person is not to be treated as unable to make a decision merely because he makes an unwise decision.
(5) An act done, or decision made, under this Act for or on behalf of a person who lacks capacity must be done, or made, in his best interests.
(6) Before the act is done, or the decision is made, regard must be had to whether the purpose for which it is needed can be as effectively achieved in a way that is less restrictive of the person's rights and freedom of action.

People who lack capacity

2(1) For the purposes of this Act, a person lacks capacity in relation to a matter if at the material time he is unable to make a decision for himself in relation to the matter because of an impairment of, or a disturbance in the functioning of, the mind or brain.
(2) It does not matter whether the impairment or disturbance is permanent or temporary.
(3) A lack of capacity cannot be established merely by reference to–
(a) a person's age or appearance, or
(b) a condition of his, or an aspect of his behaviour, which might lead others to make unjustified assumptions about his capacity.
(4) In proceedings under this Act or any other enactment, any question whether a person lacks capacity within the meaning of this Act must be decided on the balance of probabilities.
(5) No power which a person ('D') may exercise under this Act–
(a) in relation to a person who lacks capacity, or
(b) where D reasonably thinks that a person lacks capacity,
is exercisable in relation to a person under 16.
(6) Subsection (5) is subject to section 18(3).

Inability to make decisions

3(1) For the purposes of section 2, a person is unable to make a decision for himself if he is unable–
(a) to understand the information relevant to the decision,
(b) to retain that information,
(c) to use or weigh that information as part of the process of making the decision, or
(d) to communicate his decision (whether by talking, using sign language or any other means).
(2) A person is not to be regarded as unable to understand the information relevant to a decision if he is able to understand an explanation of it given to him in a way that is appropriate to his circumstances (using simple language, visual aids or any other means).
(3) The fact that a person is able to retain the information relevant to a decision for a short period only does not prevent him from being regarded as able to make the decision.
(4) The information relevant to a decision includes information about the reasonably foreseeable consequences of–
(a) deciding one way or another, or
(b) failing to make the decision.

Best interests

4(1) In determining for the purposes of this Act what is in a person's best interests, the person making the determination must not make it merely on the basis of–
(a) the person's age or appearance, or

(b) a condition of his, or an aspect of his behaviour, which might lead others to make unjustified assumptions about what might be in his best interests.

(2) The person making the determination must consider all the relevant circumstances and, in particular, take the following steps.

(3) He must consider–

(a) whether it is likely that the person will at some time have capacity in relation to the matter in question, and

(b) if it appears likely that he will, when that is likely to be.

(4) He must, so far as reasonably practicable, permit and encourage the person to participate, or to improve his ability to participate, as fully as possible in any act done for him and any decision affecting him.

(5) Where the determination relates to life-sustaining treatment he must not, in considering whether the treatment is in the best interests of the person concerned, be motivated by a desire to bring about his death.

(6) He must consider, so far as is reasonably ascertainable–

(a) the person's past and present wishes and feelings (and, in particular, any relevant written statement made by him when he had capacity),

(b) the beliefs and values that would be likely to influence his decision if he had capacity,

(c) the other factors that he would be likely to consider if he were able to do so.

(7) He must take into account, if it is practicable and appropriate to consult them, the views of–

(a) anyone named by the person as someone to be consulted on the matter in question or on matters of that kind,

(b) anyone engaged in caring for the person or interested in his welfare,

(c) any donee of a lasting power of attorney granted by the person, and

(d) any deputy appointed for the person by the court,

as to what would be in the person's best interests and, in particular, as to the matters mentioned in subsection (6).

(8) The duties imposed by subsections (1)–(7) also apply in relation to the exercise of any powers which–

(a) are exercisable under a lasting power of attorney, or

(b) are exercisable by a person under this Act where he reasonably believes that another person lacks capacity.

(9) In the case of an act done, or a decision made, by a person other than the court, there is sufficient compliance with this section if (having complied with the requirements of subsections (1)–(7)) he reasonably believes that what he does or decides is in the best interests of the person concerned.

(10) 'Life-sustaining treatment' means treatment which in the view of a person providing health care for the person concerned is necessary to sustain life.

(11) 'Relevant circumstances' are those–

(a) of which the person making the determination is aware, and

(b) which it would be reasonable to regard as relevant.

Assessment and care planning

23.12 The Care Act 2014 applies to many adults who lack the mental capacity to make decisions about their care and support and, in certain cases, makes specific provision for such persons.

23.13 In relation to assessment:

- section 9(5) of the Care Act 2014 requires the local authority to involve any person who appears interested in the adult's welfare, when the adult lacks the capacity to ask the local authority to involve a particular individual; section 25(3) makes similar provision in relation to the preparation of care plans; section 27(2) makes similar provision in relation to reviews; section 28(5) makes similar provision in relation to independent personal budgets;
- section 11 provides that a local authority must undertake an assessment even if the adult refuses one, if the adult lacks capacity to refuse the assessment and the local authority is satisfied that an assessment would be in their best interests or they are experiencing, or at risk of, abuse or neglect;
- section 67 can require the provision of 'independent advocates' (see immediately below), as can sections 35–41 of the Mental Capacity Act 2005;
- guidance is at *Care and Support Statutory Guidance*, in Chapters 6 and 10.

23.14 Independent advocacy support is required to be provided by section 67 of the Care Act 2014, in connection with a number of issues that arise under the Act during the assessment and care planning, where an individual 'would experience substantial difficulty' in making decisions and has no 'appropriate person' to assist them: see paras 7.53–7.65 above (section 68 requires local authorities to provide independent advocacy support, in similar circumstances, where there is a safeguarding enquiry or review: see para 24.10 below).

23.15 Also, sections 35–41 of the Mental Capacity Act 2005 can require/allow for the appointment of an independent mental capacity advocate (IMCA) in relation to a care and support assessment process (see 'Involvement/independent advocates/relevance of Mental Capacity Act 2005', above at paras 7.53–7.65).

23.16 Direct payments are subject to a significantly different regime where the adult lacks capacity to request direct payments, by virtue of section 32 of the Care Act 2014 and the Care and Support (Direct Payments) Regulations 2014 (see para 9.53 on 'direct payments', above).

23.17 It follows that, right at the start of the assessment process, and later on, whenever a local authority performs a function under the Care Act 2014, one of the first questions that the local authority will have to ask itself is whether the adult may lack the mental capacity to participate effectively in the process, or may experience substantial difficulty in so doing. Accordingly, as the *Care and Support Statutory Guidance* advises, an assessment of capacity may need to be undertaken at an early stage:

> 6.32 Where there is concern about a person's capacity to make a specific decision, for example as a result of a mental impairment such as dementia,

acquired brain injury or learning disabilities, then an assessment of capacity should be carried out under the Mental Capacity Act (MCA). Those who may lack capacity will need extra support to identify and communicate their needs and make subsequent decisions, and may need an Independent Mental Capacity Advocate. The more serious the needs, the more support people may need to identify their impact and the consequences. Professional qualified staff, such as social workers, can advise and support assessors when they are carrying out an assessment with a person who may lack capacity.

Safeguarding

23.18 The core duty, at section 42 of the Care Act 2014, is to enquire into the possible abuse or neglect of adults with care and support needs and decide what if any action should be taken, under Part 1 of the Care Act 2014 or otherwise: see chapter 24 on 'Safeguarding' below.

23.19 Where the adult in question lacks the capacity to engage, or would experience substantial difficulty in engaging with an enquiry, and does not already have an 'appropriate adult', the local authority must appoint an independent advocate to represent and support the adult: see section 68 of the Act and 'Involvement/independent advocates/relevance of Mental Capacity Act 2005, above at paras 7.53–7.65 and see para 24.10 below.

23.20 As discussed in chapter 24 on safeguarding, there is a range of possible responses to abuse or neglect, ranging from:

- the provision of support services, designed to enable carers to provide better care; to
- removing the adult to care home or other accommodation, prohibiting further contact with the former carers and bringing criminal proceedings against them, either for conventional criminal offences or for the new offences created at section 44 of the Mental Capacity Act 2005, of ill treatment and wilful neglect of a person who lacks capacity to make relevant decisions, on the part of a carer, the done of a lasting or enduring power of attorney, or a court-appointed deputy.

23.21 The critical challenge for the local authority, when undertaking safeguarding functions in the case of an adult whose capacity for involvement is lacking, or undermined, is to fashion a response that protects the adult but, nonetheless, is proportionate, takes reasonable steps to promote as well as support family life and takes full account of the centrality of the wishes and best interests of the adult concerned. Guidance is provided at:

- Chapter 14 of the *Care and Support Statutory Guidance*; and at
- Chapters 6, 8 and 14 of the Mental Capacity Act 2005: Code of Practice (2007).

23.22 Paragraphs 6.12 and 8.28 of the Mental Capacity Act 2005: Code of Practice (2007) advise that local authorities should consider applying to the Court of Protection where, for example, there is a major disagreement about a serious decision (eg about where a person who lacks capacity to decide for themselves should live), or harm or abuse is suspected (when, for example, the court could stop the individual concerned living with, or contacting the adult).

23.23 There is a very useful suite of practice guidance on adult safeguarding, including recourse to the Court of Protection, provided by the Social Care Institute of Excellence.[12] Its practice guidance *Safeguarding adults at risk of harm: a legal guide for practitioners* (2011)[13] is out of date in some respects (it pre-dates the Care Act 2014) but contains a great deal of extremely useful guidance as to law and practice. In outline:

- unless the welfare of the adult requires urgent action, local authorities should attempt to resolve matters, or at least refine the issues, by discussion and agreement;
- local authorities must obtain the authority of the court if they consider it necessary to remove a person lacking capacity to consent from their home or restrict their contact with others.[14] Such consent can be secured if necessary on an urgent basis, although every effort should be made, as far as appears consistent with the welfare of the adult, to give adequate notice to persons likely to be affected and to ensure that the evidence (of real risk) warrants such application;
- local authorities should, as a last resort, obtain a ruling from the court on more finely balanced disputes that relate to important aspects of the incapacitated adult's welfare.

Cases

23.24 *R v North Yorkshire CC ex p William Hargreaves* (1997–8) 1 CCLR 104, QBD

An assessment that failed to take into account the service user's preferences, incompatibly with the statutory guidance, was unlawful, notwithstanding her communication difficulties

Facts: a dispute arose between Mr Hargreaves and North Yorkshire as to what form suitable respite care ought to take for Mr Hargreaves' intellectually impaired sister, Beryl Hargreaves. North Yorkshire had experienced great difficulty in communicating with Ms Hargreaves, exacerbated by Mr Hargreaves' overly protective actions. However, Ms Hargeaves had demonstrated an ability to express preferences and there was some evidence that her preferences were not identical to her brother's.

Judgment: paragraphs 3.15 and 3.25 of the statutory guidance at the time, *The Policy Guidance*, required local authorities to involve the individual service user in the assessment process and take account of their preferences. At 112H, Dyson J held that:

> ... the Respondent made its decision without taking into account the preferences of Miss Hargreaves on the issue in question. It must follow that the decision was unlawful in the sense that it was made in breach of paragraphs 3.16 and 3.25 of the Policy Guidance.

12 www.scie.org.uk/adults/safeguarding/resources/index.asp.

13 www.scie.org.uk/publications/reports/report50.pdf.

14 *Hillingdon LBC v Neary* [2011] EWHC 1377 COP, [2011] 4 All ER 584.

Comment: no doubt, had it been impossible or impracticable to ascertain Ms Hargreaves' preferences, North Yorkshire's failure to do so would have been lawful because it would have had a cogent reason for departure from the statutory guidance. However, under the current statutory scheme, the question would arise as to why the local authority had not appointed an independent advocate, or an IMCA, see:

- Involvement/independent advocates/relevance of Mental Capacity Act 2005, above at paras 7.53–7.65; and
- *R (SG) v Haringey LBC* (below at para 23.33), where an assessment was quashed owing to the local authority's failure to appoint an independent advocate, in breach of section 67 of the Care Act 2014.

23.25 *Z v United Kingdom* Application no 29392/95, (2001) 4 CCLR 310, ECtHR

Article 3 imposes a duty to take reasonable steps to provide effective protection to children and other vulnerable persons whom the state knows, or ought reasonably to know, are being subject to inhuman or degrading treatment

Facts: the applicants were siblings who had suffered personal injury as a result of abuse and neglect whilst living with their parents. The local social services authority had been aware of the situation for a period of years but had failed to take effective action.

Judgment: the treatment meted out by the parents violated the children's rights under Article 3 ECHR; moreover, the State was itself in breach of Article 3, in that it had failed in its duty to take measures to provide effective protection to children and other vulnerable persons, including by taking reasonable steps to prevent ill-treatment of which the authorities knew or ought to have known. The applicants had also been denied a remedy, in breach of Article 13 of the ECHR in that, because the House of Lords had determined that the local authority had not owed the applicants a duty of care in negligence, then, notwithstanding the availability of complaints to the Criminal Injuries Compensation Board and the Local Government Ombudsman (LGO), the applicants had not had available to them an appropriate means of obtaining a determination of their allegation that the local authority had failed to protect them from inhuman and degrading treatment and the possibility of obtaining compensation. The Court awarded the children pecuniary damages (for loss of earnings, the cost of medical treatment etc) of £8,000, £100,000, £80,000 and £4,000 and non-pecuniary damages of £32,000 each.

23.26 *R (A and B) v East Sussex CC* [2003] EWHC 167 (Admin), (2003) 6 CCLR 194

The recognition and protection of human dignity is a core value protected by Article 8 ECHR. Nonetheless the rights of persons with disabilities required to be balanced against those of their carers, where there was a conflict

Facts: A and B were severely disabled sisters who continued to live in the family home, owing to a dispute with Sussex over aspects of the care package, in particular, as to the extent to which Sussex could be required to instruct carers to undertake manual lifting.

Judgment: Munby J held that it was necessary to balance the Article 8 rights of the sisters and their carers. He gave prolonged consideration to the case-law relating to Article 8 ECHR in the adult social care context, including the following:

> 85. In *Botta v Italy* [1998] ECHR 12, (1999) 2 CCLR 53, as we have seen, the court identified a person's 'physical and psychological integrity' as being part of the private life protected by Article 8 and which the State may in principle be under an obligation to take positive steps to protect. In the present type of case this 'physical and psychological integrity' embraces, though it is not of course confined to, two particularly important concepts which for the purposes of proper analysis it is desirable to distinguish and consider separately.
>
> 86. The first is human dignity. True it is that the phrase is not used in the Convention but it is surely immanent in Article 8, indeed in almost every one of the Convention's provisions. The recognition and protection of human dignity is one of the core values – in truth *the* core value – of our society and, indeed, of all the societies which are part of the European family of nations and which have embraced the principles of the Convention. It is a core value of the common law, long pre-dating the Convention and the Charter. The invocation of the dignity of the patient in the form of declaration habitually used when the court is exercising its inherent declaratory jurisdiction in relation to the gravely ill or dying is not some meaningless incantation designed to comfort the living or to assuage the consciences of those involved in making life and death decisions: it is a solemn affirmation of the law's and of society's recognition of our humanity and of human dignity as something fundamental. Not surprisingly, human dignity is extolled in Article 1 of the Charter, just as it is in article 1 of the Universal Declaration. And the latter's call to us to 'act towards one another in a spirit of brotherhood' is nothing new. It reflects the fourth Earl of Chesterfield's injunction, 'Do as you would be done by' and, for the Christian, the biblical call (Matthew ch 7, v 12): 'all things whatsoever ye would that men should do to you, do ye even so to them: for this is the law and the prophets'.
>
> ...
>
> 99. The other important concept embraced in the 'physical and psychological integrity' protected by Article 8 is the right of the disabled to participate in the life of the community and to have what has been described (see below) as 'access to essential economic and social activities and to an appropriate range of recreational and cultural activities'. This is matched by the positive obligation of the State to take appropriate measures designed to ensure to the greatest extent feasible that a disabled person is not 'so circumscribed and so isolated as to be deprived of the possibility of developing his personality'.

23.27 *A Local Authority v A* [2010] EWHC 978 (Fam), (2010) 13 CCLR 404

Article 5 ECHR imposed a duty on local authorities to take reasonable steps to prevent the deprivation of liberty of a child or vulnerable adult that it knows or reasonably ought to know about

Facts: The local authority provided care services to families with seriously disabled children. An issue arose as to whether the (exemplary) care provided to the children had resulted in a deprivation of the children's liberty for which the local authority was directly responsible, or unlawfully had failed to prevent.

Judgment: Munby J held that, on the facts, the children had not been deprived of their liberty; that, in any event, the local authority would not have been directly liable for any deprivation of liberty merely because it was providing care services; that the local authority had been under a duty to investigate the possible deprivation of liberty, but it had discharged that duty. Munby J said this:

> 95. For present purposes I can summarise my conclusions as follows. Where the State – here, a local authority – knows or ought to know that a vulnerable child or adult is subject to restrictions on their liberty by a private individual that arguably give rise to a deprivation of liberty, then its positive obligations under Article 5 will be triggered.
>
> i) These will include the duty to investigate, so as to determine whether there is, in fact, a deprivation of liberty. In this context the local authority will need to consider all the factors relevant to the objective and subjective elements referred to in paragraph [48] above.
>
> ii) If, having carried out its investigation, the local authority is satisfied that the objective element is not present, so there is no deprivation of liberty, the local authority will have discharged its immediate obligations. However, its positive obligations may in an appropriate case require the local authority to continue to monitor the situation in the event that circumstances should change.
>
> iii) If, however, the local authority concludes that the measures imposed do or may constitute a deprivation of liberty, then it will be under a positive obligation, both under Article 5 alone and taken together with Article 14, to take reasonable and proportionate measures to bring that state of affairs to an end. What is reasonable and proportionate in the circumstances will, of course, depend upon the context, but it might for example, Mr Bowen suggests, require the local authority to exercise its statutory powers and duties so as to provide support services for the carers that will enable inappropriate restrictions to be ended, or at least minimised.
>
> iv) If, however, there are no reasonable measures that the local authority can take to bring the deprivation of liberty to an end, or if the measures it proposes are objected to by the individual or his family, then it may be necessary for the local authority to seek the assistance of the court in determining whether there is, in fact, a deprivation of liberty and, if there is, obtaining authorisation for its continuance.
>
> 96. What emerges from this is that, whatever the extent of a local authority's positive obligations under Article 5, its duties, and more important its powers, are limited. In essence, its duties are threefold: a duty in appropriate circumstances to investigate; a duty in appropriate circumstances to provide supporting services; and a duty in appropriate circumstances to refer the matter to the court. But, and this is a key message, whatever the positive obligations of a local authority under Article 5 may be, they do not clothe it with any power to regulate, control, compel, restrain, confine or coerce. A local authority which seeks to do so must either point to specific statutory authority for what it is doing – and, as I have pointed out, such statutory powers are, by and large, lacking in cases such as this – or obtain the appropriate sanction of the court. Of course if there is immediate threat to life or limb a local authority will be justified in taking protective (including compulsory) steps: *R (G) v Nottingham City Council* [2008] EWHC 152 (Admin), [2008] 1 FLR 1660, at para [21]. But it must follow up any such intervention with an immediate application to the court.

...

1. Before passing from this part of the case there are two final points which I should emphasise. In the first place, it is vital that local authorities embark upon the kind of investigations that Hedley J and I have described with sensitivity and with a proper appreciation of the limited extent of their powers. Social workers need to keep their eyes open and their professional antennae alert when meeting or visiting their clients. And if there is real cause for concern they must act quickly and decisively. But they must guard against being seen as prying or snooping on the families who they are there to help and support. Nothing is more destructive of the 'working together' relationship which in this kind of context, as in others, is so vitally important than a perception by family carers that the local authority is being heavy-handed or worse. I repeat in this context what I have already said in paragraphs [51]–[53] above.

2. The other point relates to how local authority applications to the court should be made. Too often, in my experience, local authorities seeking the assistance of the court in removing an incapacitated or vulnerable adult from their home against their wishes or against the wishes of the relatives or friends caring for them, apply ex parte (without notice) and, I have to say, too often such orders have been made by the court without any prior warning to those affected and in circumstances where such seeming heavy-handedness is not easy to justify and can too often turn out to be completely counter-productive: cf *X Council v B (Emergency Protection Orders)* [2004] EWHC 2015 (Fam), [2005] 1 FLR 341, at para [93]. I agree in every respect and would wish to associate myself with what Charles J said in *B Borough Council v S (By the Official Solicitor)* [2006] EWHC 2584 (Fam), [2007] 1 FLR 1600, at paras [37]–[42]. And although I accept that the analogy is not exact, it seems to me that, generally speaking, a local authority will only be justified in seeking a without notice order for the removal of an incapacitated or vulnerable adult in the kind of circumstances which in the case of a child would justify a without notice application for an emergency protection order; as to which see *X Council v B (Emergency Protection Orders)* [2004] EWHC 2015 (Fam), [2005] 1 FLR 341, and *Re X (Emergency Protection Orders)* [2006] EWHC 510 (Fam), [2006] 2 FLR 701. That said, there will, of course, be cases in the adult jurisdiction where, just as in the corresponding children jurisdiction, a without notice application will be justified; indeed (see para [81]), *B Borough Council* was just such a case.

23.28 *AH v Hertfordshire Partnership NHS Foundation Trust* [2011] EWHC 276 (COP), (2011) 14 CCLR 301

It was not in the best interests of a severely learning disabled man to be moved from an NHS facility where he had lived for many years to a flat in London

Facts: AH was a learning disabled adult who had spent most of his life in a long-stay hospital and, when it closed, moved to a specialist facility within the grounds of a former hospital, in a rural location. Pursuant to central government policy, *Valuing People,* that persons with a learning disability should have increased choice and control over their lives, the NHS decided to move AH, contrary to the wishes of all those concerned about him, to a flat in London, to be cared for by an agency and the local authority there. AH himself lacked the relevant capacity to oppose this move.

Judgment: Peter Jackson J held that the proposed move did not entail a single benefit for AH but would cause him significant upset possibly amounting to serious harm:

> **77.** Although the ambition to maximise Alan's opportunities is laudable, it has not been possible to identify a single dependable benefit arising from the proposed move. The thesis is that it would provide him with a greater experience of ordinary life in a local community, and that this would improve his quality of life. Each element of this proposition is incongruous with the realities of Alan's life. His experience is so far from being ordinary that it is not useful to use ordinariness as a yardstick. Ealing is not local for Alan and there is no community there which would be meaningful for him. I also accept the evidence of the clinicians, the experts, and not least of Alan's committed parents, that the prospect of him living a more expansive and fulfilled life following a move is a chimera. It is more likely that it would lead to a deterioration from which he might – or might not – recover. It is not enough to say that *'the benefits of community living may matter to Alan"* if one cannot show that they will. Facing up to these realities does not in any way diminish or demean Alan, but values and respects him for who he is.
>
> 78. I agree that the prospect of a home for life for Alan is attractive and accept that there is no guarantee that an alternative of the quality now offered would be available if he had to move at some point in the future. Nevertheless, only the closure of SRS could justify the turmoil of a move and as this is not expected in the foreseeable future, there is no reason to anticipate it.
>
> ...
>
> 80. This case illustrates the obvious point that guideline policies cannot be treated as universal solutions, nor should initiatives designed to personalise care and promote choice be applied to the opposite effect. The very existence of SRS, after most of the institutional population had been resettled in the community, is perhaps the exception that proves this rule. These residents are not an anomaly simply because they are among the few remaining recipients of this style of social care. They might better be seen as a good example of the kind of personal planning that lies at the heart of the philosophy of care in the community. Otherwise, an unintended consequence of national policy may be to sacrifice the interests of vulnerable and unusual people like Alan.

23.29 *A Local Authority v DL, ML, GRL and JP* [2011] EWHC 1022 (Fam), (2011) 14 CCLR 441

The court retained an inherent jurisdiction to protect persons who, whilst not lacking mental capacity, were incapacitated from making a relevant decision by reason of constraint, coercion, undue influence or other vitiating factors

Facts: GL and ML were an elderly couple, who at the relevant time did not lack the mental capacity, but whose will was said to have been overborne by their adult son, DL, who lived with them and was said to assault them, rendering them unable to make decisions, such as to tell the son to leave, to maintain contact with family and friends and to move to a care home.

Judgment: Theis J, determining a preliminary issue, reviewed a number of authorities and concluded that the court retained jurisdiction to make protective declarations in a case such as this, notwithstanding the enactment of the Mental Capacity Act 2005:

> 53.(4) Each case will, of course, have to be carefully considered on its own facts, but if there is evidence to suggest that an adult who does not suffer from any kind of mental incapacity that comes within the MCA but who is, or reasonably believed to be, incapacitated from making the relevant decision by reason of such things as constraint, coercion, undue influence or other vitiating factors they may be entitled to the protection of the inherent jurisdiction (see: *SA* [[2005] EWHC 2942 (Fam)] para [79]). This may, or may not, include a vulnerable adult. I respectfully agree with Munby J in *SA* at para [83] '*The inherent jurisdiction is not confined to those who are vulnerable adults, however that expression is understood, nor is a vulnerable adult amenable as such to the jurisdiction. The significance in this context of the concept of a vulnerable adult is pragmatic and evidential: it is simply that an adult who is vulnerable is more likely to fall into the category of the incapacitated in relation to whom the inherent jurisdiction is exercisable than an adult who is not vulnerable. So it is likely to be easier to persuade the court that there is a case calling for investigation where the adult is apparently vulnerable than where the adult is not on the face of it vulnerable*'. In the cases I have been referred to the term 'vulnerable adult' appears to have been used to include the *SA* definition, whether the adult in question is vulnerable or not. Obviously the facts in *SA* were very different to the case I am concerned with. For example, in this case ML and DL have capacity to litigate but that does not, in my judgment, mean that the inherent jurisdiction should not be available to protect ML, once the court has undertaken the correct balancing exercise.
>
> ...
>
> (8) The mere existence of the jurisdiction does not mean it will always be exercised. Each case will have to be considered on its own facts and a careful balance undertaken by the court of the competing (often powerful) considerations as to whether declarations or other orders should be made. As Miss Lieven QC points out the assumed facts in this case are not accepted by DL and even if they are one of the important considerations for the court to consider are the views of adults concerned; they do not support the orders being sought by the LA. In addition, the terms of the orders being sought in this case are likely to require very careful scrutiny.

23.30 *Re MN (An Adult)* [2015] EWCA Civ 411, (2015) 18 CCLR 521

The Court of Protection has no power to require a public authority to provide different services, only to consider whether services on offer are in P's best interests, so any legal challenge to the sufficiency of services offered must be brought by way of judicial review

Facts: MN was a severely disabled young adult. It was reluctantly conceded by his parents that it was in his best interests to live in a residential placement but they disputed that the package of care on offer was in MN's best interests and asked the Court of Protection (COP) to investigate and make a declaration on that issue. The COP declined to take that course on the basis that its role was limited to determining whether care packages actually on offer were in P's best interests. MN's parents appealed.

Judgment: the Court of Appeal (Sir James Munby, President of the COP, Treacey and Gloster LJJ) dismissed the appeal, holding that that the COP had no power to require a public authority to provide a different care package, only to consider whether what was on offer was in the best interests of P; if P or some other person wanted to secure change in the care package, then they had to bring judicial review proceedings. Accordingly, it was pointless and inappropriate for the COP to embark upon an investigation on whether a different care plan would be in P's best interests:

> 11. The starting point, in my judgment, is the fundamentally important principle identified by the House of Lords in *A v Liverpool City Council* [1982] AC 363 and re-stated by the House in *In re W (A Minor) (Wardship: Jurisdiction)* [1985] AC 791. For present purposes I can go straight to the speech of Lord Scarman in the latter case. Referring to *A v Liverpool City Council*, Lord Scarman said (page 795):
>
> > 'Authoritative speeches were delivered by Lord Wilberforce and Lord Roskill which it was reasonable to hope would put an end to attempts to use the wardship jurisdiction so as to secure a review by the High Court upon the merits of decisions taken by local authorities pursuant to the duties and powers imposed and conferred upon them by the statutory code.'
>
> He continued (page 797):
>
> > 'The High Court cannot exercise its powers, however wide they may be, so as to intervene on the merits in an area of concern entrusted by Parliament to another public authority. It matters not that the chosen public authority is one which acts administratively whereas the court, if seized by the same matter, would act judicially. If Parliament in an area of concern defined by statute (the area in this case being the care of children in need or trouble) prefers power to be exercised administratively instead of judicially, so be it. The courts must be careful in that area to avoid assuming a supervisory role or reviewing power over the merits of decisions taken administratively by the selected public authority.'
>
> 12. Lord Scarman was not of course disputing the High Court's power of judicial review under RSC Ord 53 (now CPR Pt 54) when exercised by what is now the Administrative Court: he was disputing the High Court's powers when exercising in the Family Division the parens patriae or wardship jurisdictions. This is made clear by what he said (page 795):
>
> > 'The ground of decision in *A v Liverpool City Council* [1982] AC 363 was nothing to do with judicial discretion but was an application in this field of the profoundly important rule that where Parliament has by statute entrusted to a public authority an administrative power subject to safeguards which, however, contain no provision that the High Court is to be required to review the merits of decisions taken pursuant to the power, the High Court has no right to intervene. If there is abuse of the power, there can of course be judicial review pursuant to RSC Ord 53: but no abuse of power has been, or could be, suggested in this case.'
>
> It is important to appreciate that Lord Scarman was not referring to a rule going to the exercise of discretion; it is a rule going to jurisdiction
>
> ...
>
> 80. The function of the Court of Protection is to take, on behalf of adults who lack capacity, the decisions which, if they had capacity, they would take themselves. The Court of Protection has no more power, just because it is acting on behalf of an adult who lacks capacity, to obtain resources or facilities from a third party, whether a private individual or a public authority, than the adult if he had capacity would be able to obtain himself. The *A v Liverpool* principle applies as much to the Court of Protection as it applies

to the family court or the Family Division. The analyses in *A v A Health Authority* and in *Holmes-Moorhouse* likewise apply as much in the Court of Protection as in the family court or the Family Division. The Court of Protection is thus confined to choosing between available options, including those which there is good reason to believe will be forthcoming in the foreseeable future.

81. The Court of Protection, like the family court and the Family Division, can explore the care plan being put forward by a public authority and, where appropriate, require the authority to go away and think again. Rigorous probing, searching questions and persuasion are permissible; pressure is not. And in the final analysis the Court of Protection cannot compel a public authority to agree to a care plan which the authority is unwilling to implement.

Comment: the author cannot see any reason why a complaints process, or judicial review proceedings challenging a service provision decision, cannot be run in tandem with COP proceedings or, even, why a High Court judge entitled to sit in the Administrative Court and COP should not determine both the public law and best interests issues, providing that they carefully separated the different functions being exercised. All that this case decides, reflecting earlier case-law, is that one cannot use the best interests jurisdiction to 'get around' the limits of judicial review.

23.31 *RP v United Kingdom* Application no 38245/08, (2013) 16 CCLR 135, ECtHR

Providing there were adequate safeguards, it was compatible with Article 6 ECHR for the Official Solicitor to represent an incapacitated mother in care proceedings relating to her daughter

Facts: RP had a significant learning disability and, when the local authority brought care proceedings in respect of her daughter, the Official Solicitor was appointed to represent RP, on account of her lack of capacity. The court granted the local authority's application for a placement order in respect of the daughter. However, RP complained that she had not been properly informed about the Official Solicitor's role and that he should not have represented her because she had not lacked litigation capacity.

Judgment: the European Court of Human Rights held:

65. In cases involving those with disabilities the court has permitted the domestic courts a certain margin of appreciation to enable them to make the relevant procedural arrangements to secure the good administration of justice and protect the health of the person concerned (see, for example, *Shtukaturov v Russia,* Application no 44009/05, § 68, 27 March 2008). This is in keeping with the United Nations Convention on the Rights of Persons with Disabilities, which requires States to provide appropriate accommodation to facilitate the role of disabled persons in legal proceedings. However, the court has held that such measures should not affect the very essence of an applicant's right to a fair trial as guaranteed by Article 6(1) of the Convention. In assessing whether or not a particular measure was necessary, the court will take into account all relevant factors, including the nature and complexity of the issue before the domestic courts and what was at stake for the applicant (see, for example, *Shtukaturov v Russia,* cited above, § 68).

66. It is clear that in the present case the proceedings were of the utmost importance to RP, who stood to lose both custody of and access to her only child. Moreover, while the issue at stake was relatively straightforward – whether or not RP had the skills necessary to enable her successfully to parent KP – the evidence which would have to be considered before the issue could be addressed was not. In particular, the court notes the significant quantity of expert reports, including expert medical and psychiatric reports, parenting assessment reports, and reports from contact sessions and observes the obvious difficulty an applicant with a learning disability would have in understanding both the content of these reports and the implications of the experts' findings.

67. In light of the above, and bearing in mind the requirement in the UN Convention that State parties provide appropriate accommodation to facilitate disabled persons' effective role in legal proceedings, the court considers that it was not only appropriate but also necessary for theUnited Kingdom to take measures to ensure that RP's best interests were represented in the childcare proceedings. Indeed, in view of its existing case-law the Court considers that a failure to take measures to protect RP's interests might in itself have amounted to a violation of Article 6(1)of the Convention (see, *mutatis mutandis, T v United Kingdom* [GC], Application no 24724/94, §§ 79–89, 16 December 1999).

68. It falls to the court to consider whether the appointment of the Official Solicitor in the present case was proportionate to the legitimate aim pursued or whether it impaired the very essence of RP's right of access to a court. In making this assessment, the court will bear in mind the margin of appreciation afforded to Contracting States in making the necessary procedural arrangements to protect persons who lack litigation capacity (*Shtukaturov v Russia*, cited above, § 68).

69. With regard to the appointment of the Official Solicitor, the court observes that he was only invited to act following the commissioning of an expert report by a consultant clinical psychologist. In assessing RP, the psychologist applied the test set out in *Masterman-Lister v Brutton & Co (Nos 1 and 2)* [2002] EWCA Civ 1889; *Masterman-Lister v Jewell and another* [2003] EWCA Civ 70, namely whether RP was capable of understanding, with the assistance of such proper explanation from legal advisers and experts in other disciplines as the case may require, the issues on which her consent or decision was likely to be necessary in the course of the proceedings. She concluded that RP would find it very difficult to understand the advice given by her solicitor and would not be able to make informed decisions on the basis of that advice, particularly when it involved anticipating possible outcomes. The psychologist produced two more reports in the course of the proceedings, the second of which contained a further assessment of RP's litigation capacity. In that report she noted that RP did not have the capacity to give informed consent to a placement order as she could not really understand the proceedings, except at a very basic level. The court is satisfied that the decision to appoint the Official Solicitor was not taken lightly. Rather, it was taken only after RP had been thoroughly assessed by a consultant clinical psychologist and, while there was no formal review procedure, in practice further assessments were made of RP's litigation capacity in the course of the proceedings.

70. The court considers that in order to safeguard RP's rights under Article 6(1) of the Convention, it was imperative that a means existed whereby it was possible for her to challenge the Official Solicitor's appointment or the continuing need for his services. In this regard, the Court observes that

the letter and leaflet which the Official Solicitor sent to RP informed her that if she was unhappy with the way her case was being conducted, she could speak to either SC or to the Official Solicitor, or she could contact a Complaint's Officer. Moreover, in his statement to the Court of Appeal the Official Solicitor indicated that RP could have applied to the court at any time to have him discharged. Alternatively, he indicated that if it had come to his attention that RP was asserting capacity, then he would have invited her to undergo further assessment. While the court observes that these procedures fall short of a formal right of appeal, in view of the finding that RP lacked litigation capacity, it considers that they would have afforded her an appropriate and effective means by which to challenge the appointment or the continued need for the appointment of the Official Solicitor.

71. The court does not consider that it would have been appropriate for the domestic courts to have carried out periodic reviews of RP's litigation capacity, as such reviews would have caused unnecessary delay and would therefore have been prejudicial to the welfare of KP In any event, as noted above (see paragraph 69), assessments were in fact carried out of RP's litigation capacity in the course of the proceedings. The court would also reject RP's assertion that she should have been encouraged to seek separate legal advice at this juncture. In view of the fact that she had been found to lack the capacity to instruct a solicitor the court does not consider that this would have been a necessary or even an effective means by which to protect her interests.

72. As stated in paragraph 61 above, the Convention is intended to guarantee not rights that are theoretical or illusory but rights that are practical and effective and this is particularly so of the right of access to a court in view of the prominent place held in a democratic society by the right to a fair trial (*Airey v Ireland*, cited above, § 24). Consequently, any means of challenging the appointment of the Official Solicitor, however effective in theory, will only be effective in practice and thus satisfy the requirements of Article 6(1) of the Convention if the fact of his appointment, the implications of his appointment, the existence of a means of challenging his appointment and the procedure for exercising it are clearly explained to the protected person in language appropriate to his or her level of understanding.

73. In this regard, the court recalls that the letter sent to RP indicated that the Official Solicitor would act as her *guardian ad litem* and would instruct her solicitor for her. It further indicated that SC would tell the Official Solicitor how RP felt about things and that he would consider her wishes and views before he filed a statement on her behalf. He would do his best to protect her interests but also had to bear in mind what was best for KP The leaflet accompanying the letter informed RP that the Official Solicitor made decisions about court cases, such as whether to bring, defend or settle a claim. Under the heading 'Will the client be consulted' RP was informed that 'the instructed solicitor will communicate with the client and attend court hearings and will report on the outcome to the case manager'. If she was dissatisfied with the way her case was being conducted, she was informed that she should discuss the matter either with SC or the Official Solicitor's Office. If she remained dissatisfied she could write to the Complaint's Officer. While the court accepts that RP might not have fully understood, on the basis of this information alone, that the Official Solicitor could consent to the making of a placement order regardless of her own personal wishes, it cannot ignore the fact that she was at all times represented by SC and experienced counsel who should have, and by all accounts did, explain to her the exact role of the Official Solicitor and the implications of his

appointment. Indeed, in this regard the court recalls that SC's conduct of the case was commended by the Court of Appeal which found, in its judgment of 8 May 2008, that RP had been fully informed of the involvement of the Official Solicitor and the nature of his role. Nevertheless, she did not seek to complain until ten months after his appointment and two days before the final hearing.

74. Consequently, the court considers that adequate safeguards were in place to ensure that the nature of the proceedings was fully explained to the applicant and, had she sought to challenge the appointment of the Official Solicitor, procedures were in place to enable her to do so (cf. *Stanev v Bulgaria*, [GC], Application no 36760/06, 17 January 2012, where no direct access to court was open to the applicant to have his status as a partially incapacitated person reviewed by a court).

75. With regard to the role of the Official Solicitor in the legal proceedings, the court recalls that he was to act 'for the benefit of the protected party'. The court has taken note of RP's concerns about his focus in the present case on 'what was best for KP'. However, the court accepts that the best interests of KP were the touchstone by which the domestic courts would assess the case. Thus, in determining whether a case was arguable or not, it was necessary for the Official Solicitor to consider what was in KP's best interests. Consequently, the court does not consider that the fact the Official Solicitor 'bore in mind' what was best for KP in deciding how to act amounted to a violation of RP's rights under Article 6(1)of the Convention.

76. Moreover, the court does not consider that 'acting in RP's best interests' required the Official Solicitor to advance any argument RP wished. On the contrary, it would not have been in RP's – or in any party's – best interests for the Official Solicitor to have delayed proceedings by advancing an unarguable case. Nevertheless, in view of what was at stake for RP, the court considers that in order to safeguard her rights under Article 6(1) of the Convention, it was imperative that her views regarding KP's future be made known to the domestic court. It is clear that this did, in fact, occur as RP's views were referenced both by the Official Solicitor in his statement to the court and by RP's counsel at the hearing itself.

77. Moreover, the court recalls that RP was able to appeal to the Court of Appeal. Although she was not legally represented in the appeal proceedings, this was through choice as she refused the assistance of *pro bono* counsel which the Official Solicitor had secured for her. Nevertheless, the court notes that in the course of the appeal proceedings she was afforded ample opportunity to put her views before the court, and her arguments were fully addressed in the court's judgment.

78. Consequently, the court does not consider that the very essence of RP's right of access to a court was impaired. The court therefore finds that there has been no violation of her rights under Article 6(1) of the Convention.

23.32 *P v Cheshire West and Chester Council, P and Q v Surrey County Council* [2014] UKSC 19, [2014] 1 AC 896, (2015) 18 CCLR 5

A person who lacked capacity to consent to care arrangements was deprived of their liberty if they were under continuous supervision and control by those caring for them and were not free to leave.

Facts: two children, and one adult, who lacked the capacity to give valid consent to any arrangements for their care, were placed in local authority care.

Judgment: the Supreme Court (Neuberger, Hale, Kerr, Clarke, Sumption, Carnwath and Hodge JJSC) held that a person who lacked capacity to consent to care arrangements was deprived of their liberty if they were under continuous supervision and control by those caring for them and were not free to leave.

23.33 *R (SG) v Haringey LBC* [2015] EWHC 2579 (Admin), (2015) 18 CCLR 444

The failure to appoint an independent advocate, under section 67(2) of the Care Act 2014, for a vulnerable adult, who spoke no English and was illiterate, and who suffered from PTSD, insomnia, depression and anxiety, rendered the assessment unlawful

Facts: SG was an asylum-seeker provided with asylum support. She spoke no English and was illiterate, and suffered from PTSD, insomnia, depression and anxiety. She needed help with self-care, preparing and eating food, simple tasks and medication. Haringey declined to provide residential accommodation to SG under section 21 of the National Assistance Act 1948 and then, later, under the Care Act 2014.

Judgment: Deputy High Court Judge Bowers held that the assessment under the Care Act 2014 was unlawful because (i) Haringey failed to ensure that SG was offered an independent advocate, under section 67(2) of the Care Act 2014; and (ii) Haringey failed to ask itself the correct question as to whether accommodation was required. On the issue of the independent advocate, the Deputy High Court Judge said this:

> 53. The defendant appears to accept the claimant was entitled to but did not have an independent advocate when she was assessed under the Care Act, but contends nonetheless that this did not 'lead to flawed assessment process' because referral for such an advocate was made at the time of the assessment and since then an independent advocate has been appointed in the form of Mind.
>
> 54. Section 67(2) of the Act could not be clearer:
>
> > *i. 'The authority must ... arrange for a person who is independent of the authority (an 'independent advocate') to be available to represent and support the individual for the purpose of facilitating the individual's involvement.'*
>
> 55. There are detailed criteria for being an independent advocate, as set out in the Care and Support (Independent Advocacy Support) No 2 Regulations 2014 No 2889, together with the manner in which they are to carry out their functions. This testifies to the importance of this protection for essentially vulnerable persons.
>
> 56. Ms Okafor points to the fact that Mind has now accepted a referral and she contends that as a result of the new Care Act 'demand currently outstrips supply.' She says the claimant's services have not been prejudiced as a result concerning the outcome of the assessment, but I agree with Mr Burton that we simply do not know that. I do accept the defendant's submission that there may be cases in which it is unlikely the presence of an independent advocate would make any difference to the outcome. This is not one of them, because this appears to me the paradigm case where such an advocate was required, as in the absence of one the claimant was in no position to influence matters. I keep particularly in mind the account

given by Ms Mohr-Pietsch. I think the assessment was flawed as a result and must be redone. This is the first of only two grounds of unlawfulness which I find in this case.

23.34 *North Yorkshire CC and A Clinical Commissioning Group v MAG and GC* [2016] EWCOP 5, (2016) 19 CCLR 169

The MN *principle also applied in the context of alleged deprivations of liberty*

Facts: MAG was a severely disabled 35-year-old man who lacked capacity and whose flat, provided by North Yorkshire and the local Clinical Commissioning Group, was grossly unsuited to his needs, such that his residence there amounted to a deprivation of MAG's liberty. DJ Glentworth refused to authorise this deprivation of liberty, pending the authorities re-locating MAG to more suitable accommodation where his occupation would not result in a deprivation of liberty.

Judgment: Cobb J allowed the authorities' appeal and held that (i) it was in MAG's best interests to live in his flat for the time being, in the absence of any other residence being available that offered less restriction; (ii) MAG's flat and care provision did not breach his rights under Article 5 of the ECHR, therefore he was not being deprived of his liberty unlawfully; (iii) MAG may well have had a public law claim against North Yorkshire, but it had been illegitimate of the DJ to decline to authorise MAG's deprivation of liberty in order to pressurise North Yorkshire into providing more suitable accommodation. Cobb J held that the approach in *Re MN (An Adult)*[15] (see para 23.30 above) applied equally to cases where personal liberty and Article 5 of the ECHR were at stake:

> 37. The passage quoted in full above from the supplementary judgment does not, in my view, explain paragraph 28 of the principal judgment. DJ Glentworth sought to make a distinction between welfare decisions (as in *Re MN*) and decisions involving deprivation of liberty (as here), but I find her reasoning unconvincing. She identifies no passage in the judgment in Re MN which purports to limit its scope, nor does she identify any proper basis for asserting that the guidance in *Re MN* as to the limits of the court of Protection's role is irrelevant where Article 5 is engaged. Her reasoning and conclusion is the more surprising given that deprivation of liberty issues which arise in these circumstances (under section 4A(4) and section 16(2)(a) of the MCA 2005) arise specifically in the context of the court's consideration of welfare and proportionality which in turn specifically engage the fundamental principles confirmed and discussed at length in *Re MN* (see also Charles J in *Re NRA & Others* (above: [25]) at [41(i)]: 'the determinative test on an application for a welfare order to authorise a deprivation of liberty is a best interests test'). If there is any doubt (which in my view there is not) it is useful, as Ms Morris argued, to check this against the directly analogous situation if MAG had been resident in residential care. In such circumstances, NYCC would have had to apply for standard authorisation under Schedule A1 of the MCA 2005; standard authorisation would have to be in P's best interests (para 12 and 16(3)), and a 'proportionate response' to the likelihood of 'the relevant person suffering harm and the seriousness of that harm' (para 16(5) of Schedule A1 of the MCA 2005). Ms Morris makes good her submission that the requirement of proportionality must

15 [2015] EWCA Civ 411, (2015) 18 CCLR 521.

similarly apply to a determination under section 4A and section 16 and that *Re MN* applies across all welfare determinations, including those which involve deprivation of liberty.

CHAPTER 24

Safeguarding

24.1 The Care Act 2014:

- imposes a new safeguarding duty on local authorities, to safeguard adults who have needs for care and support, are experiencing or at risk of abuse or neglect and are unable to protect themselves (section 42);
- sets up Safeguarding Adults Boards to help and protect adults at risk of abuse or neglect by co-ordinating the work of agencies, strategic and monitoring work (sections 43–45).

24.2 The *Care and Support Statutory Guidance* provides guidance on these functions at Chapter 14, which replaces the *No Secrets* guidance.

24.3 In addition, the Office of the Public Guardian has made public its Safeguarding Policy,[1] outlining the approach it adopts to investigating suspected abuse by deputies and attorneys. It contains much useful guidance.

See also:

- the useful safeguarding material produced by the Social Care Institute for Excellence;[2]
- NHS England's Safeguarding Policy;[3] and
- Safeguarding Adults published by Skills for Care.[4]

Safeguarding individual adults

24.4 Safeguarding raises particular issues in relation to adults lacking mental capacity, who are at risk of abuse or neglect and those issues are considered above in chapter 23 at para 23.18 onwards. This chapter considers safeguarding issues more generally.

24.5 The core duty, at section 42 of the Care Act 2014, is to enquire into possible abuse or neglect and decide what if any action should be taken, under Part 1 of the Care Act 2014 or otherwise. The threshold for action is at section 42(1):

Enquiry by local authority

42(1) This section applies where a local authority has reasonable cause to suspect that an adult in its area (whether or not ordinarily resident there)–
(a) has needs for care and support (whether or not the authority is meeting any of those needs),
(b) is experiencing, or is at risk of, abuse or neglect, and
(c) as a result of those needs is unable to protect himself or herself against the abuse or neglect or the risk of it.

24.6 One should note the following particular features of section 42 which, in addition to being of individual note, lead to the conclusion that Parliament has set a very low threshold for the enquiry duty to arise:

1 www.gov.uk/government/uploads/system/uploads/attachment_data/file/481414/01.12.15_-_safeguarding_policy_2015_v4_FINAL.pdf.

2 http://www.scie.org.uk/care-act-2014/safeguarding-adults/.

3 https://www.england.nhs.uk/wp-content/uploads/2015/07/safeguard-policy.pdf.

4 www.skillsforcare.org.uk/Document-library/Standards/Care-Certificate/Standard-10-Updated-7-7-15.pdf.

- the duty is owed to any adult physically present '*in*' the local authority's area, which will include any adult who is physically present only fleetingly;
- the threshold requires that an adult has needs for care and support, but not that they are 'eligible needs', or being met by the local authority or, indeed, any authority;
- 'abuse' includes 'financial abuse', which is defined widely, at section 42(3) as including having money or other property stolen, being defrauded, being put under pressure in relation to money or other property and having money or other property misused;
- while the local authority is the lead agency (paragraph 14.100 of the *Care and Support Statutory Guidance*), multi-agency working, information-sharing and co-operation is vital (section 6(7) and paragraphs 14.62–14.67, 14.76–14.82 of the *Care and Support Statutory Guidance*);
- paragraphs 14.16–14.32 of the *Care and Support Statutory Guidance* give further examples of abuse and neglect, emphasising the breadth of the duty, which applies to cases of physical abuse, domestic violence and so-called '*honour*'-based violence, sexual abuse, psychological abuse, financial/material abuse, modern slavery, discriminatory abuse, organisational abuse, neglect and acts of omission and self-neglect;
- guidance as the meaning of domestic abuse, at paragraph 14.20, may be of particular interest:

> 14.20 The cross-government definition of domestic violence and abuse is: any incident or pattern of incidents of controlling, coercive, threatening behaviour, violence or abuse between those aged 16 or over who are, or have been, intimate partners or family members regardless of gender or sexuality. The abuse can encompass, but is not limited to:
> - psychological
> - sexual
> - financial
> - emotional.

24.7 The Guidance also sets out (at paragraphs 14.13 and 14.14) the key principles that should underpin all adult safeguarding:

> **Six key principles underpin all adult safeguarding work**
>
> **Empowerment**
> People being supported and encouraged to make their own decisions and informed consent.
>
> 'I am asked what I want as the outcomes from the safeguarding process and these directly inform what happens.'
>
> **Prevention**
> It is better to take action before harm occurs.
>
> 'I receive clear and simple information about what abuse is, how to recognise the signs and what I can do to seek help.'
>
> **Proportionality**
> The least intrusive response appropriate to the risk presented.
>
> 'I am sure that the professionals will work in my interest, as I see them and they will only get involved as much as needed.'

Protection
Support and representation for those in greatest need.

'I get help and support to report abuse and neglect. I get help so that I am able to take part in the safeguarding process to the extent to which I want.'

Partnership
Local solutions through services working with their communities. Communities have a part to play in preventing, detecting and reporting neglect and abuse.

'I know that staff treat any personal and sensitive information in confidence, only sharing what is helpful and necessary. I am confident that professionals will work together and with me to get the best result for me.'

Accountability
Accountability and transparency in delivering safeguarding.

'I understand the role of everyone involved in my life and so do they.'

Making safeguarding personal

14.14 In addition to these principles, it is also important that all safeguarding partners take a broad community approach to establishing safeguarding arrangements. It is vital that all organisations recognise that adult safeguarding arrangements are there to protect individuals. We all have different preferences, histories, circumstances and life-styles, so it is unhelpful to prescribe a process that must be followed whenever a concern is raised; and the case study below helps illustrate this.

24.8 As to what can be done, this can range from and include (but may well go beyond):

- providing care and support/support, mediation, therapy or other family support work, for example, to improve an abusive relationship and sustain family links;
- a referral to the police for a criminal investigation;
- an employer-led disciplinary response or action by the Care Quality Commission;
- protective proceedings under the Mental Capacity Act 2005 (see chapter 23 on Mental Capacity, above).

24.9 Further advice is provided in the *Care and Support Statutory Guidance*, which:

- at paragraphs 14.52–14.54, emphasises the importance of local authorities publishing and keeping up-to-date adult safeguarding policies and procedures, that ensure that individuals involved in the process understand their role and that set out procedures and guidelines for proportionate responses;
- at paragraphs 14.96–14.99, which emphasise the importance of placing the adult concerned, and their views and wishes, at the centre of the process (for example, 'The wishes of the adult are important, particularly where they have capacity to make decisions about their safeguarding. The wishes of those who lack capacity are of equal importance' although 'Wishes need to be balanced alongside wider considerations such as the level of risk or risk to others including any children affected').

24.10 Often critical to achieving that, will be the involvement of an independent advocate. Section 68 of the Care Act 2014 provides that:

- where there is to be a safeguarding enquiring under section 42(2); and
- the local authority considers that, without an independent advocate, the individual would experience substantial difficulty in understanding relevant information, retaining that information, using or weighing that information as part of the process of being involve or communicating their views, wishes or feelings; and
- there is no appropriate person (not engaged in providing care or treatment for the individual in a professional or paid capacity) who would be an appropriate person to undertake the 'independent advocate' function; then
- except insofar as it is necessary to take urgent steps, the local authority must arrange for an 'independent advocate' to 'represent and support the adult to whose case the enquiry ... relates for the purpose of facilitating his or her involvement in the enquiry...'; unless
- the local authority is satisfied that there is an appropriate person (not engaged in providing care or treatment for the individual in a professional or paid capacity) who would be an appropriate person to undertake the 'independent advocate' function. However, this exception is itself dis-applied by regulation 4 of the Care and Support (Independent Advocacy Support) (No 2) Regulations 2014[5] when either (i) the NHS is likely to accommodate the individual in hospital for at least 28 days or in a care home for least eight weeks, or (ii) the local authority and the potentially appropriate person disagree on a material issue but agree that the individual should have an 'independent advocate': (see 'Involvement/independent advocates/relevance of Mental Capacity Act 2005' in chapter 7, paras 7.53–7.65 above).

24.11 Finally, section 73(7)–(10) of the Care Act 2014 largely disapply the safeguarding provisions in the case of prisoners and adults resident on approved premises, except that a Safeguarding Adults Board may provide advice or assistance to adults in prisons or approved premises in their area with needs for care and support, who are at risk of abuse or neglect.

24.12 On a practical note, whilst everyone understands how extremely difficult it can be for social workers to balance (i) the need to intervene to protect vulnerable adults; (ii) the importance of preserving family life; (iii) the importance of respecting the wishes of the vulnerable adult; and (iv) other relevant factors – often in circumstances where reliable information is thin on the ground and hard to come by – there has been a run of cases (which may possibly betoken a more generalised failure of approach) where local authorities have been criticised for being too precipitate and heavy-handed: *Somerset CC v MK*,[6] *Milton Keynes Council v RR*[7] and *Essex CC v RF*.[8]

5 SI No 2889.
6 [2014] EWCOP B25.
7 [2014] EWCOP 34.
8 [2015] EWCOP 1.

Safeguarding Adults Boards

24.13 Safeguarding Adults Boards mirror Local Safeguarding Children Boards, with which local authorities, their Board partners and others are already familiar.

24.14 The statutory provisions are at sections 43–45 of the Care Act 2014 and *The Care and Support Statutory Guidance* provides guidance at paragraphs 14.133–14.161, setting out the core duties as follows:

> **Safeguarding Adults Boards**
>
> 14.133 Each local authority must set up a Safeguarding Adults Board (SAB). The main objective of a SAB is to assure itself that local safeguarding arrangements and partners act to help and protect adults in its area who meet the criteria set out at paragraph 14.2.
>
> 14.134 The SAB has a strategic role that is greater than the sum of the operational duties of the core partners. It oversees and leads adult safeguarding across the locality and will be interested in a range of matters that contribute to the prevention of abuse and neglect. These will include the safety of patients in its local health services, quality of local care and support services, effectiveness of prisons and approved premises in safeguarding offenders and awareness and responsiveness of further education services. It is important that SAB partners feel able to challenge each other and other organisations where it believes that their actions or inactions are increasing the risk of abuse or neglect. This will include commissioners, as well as providers of services.
>
> 14.135 The SAB can be an important source of advice and assistance, for example in helping others improve their safeguarding mechanisms. It is important that the SAB has effective links with other key partnerships in the locality and share relevant information and work plans. They should consciously cooperate to reduce any duplication and maximise any efficiency, particularly as objectives and membership is likely to overlap.
>
> 14.136 A SAB has 3 core duties:
>
> - It must publish a strategic plan for each financial year that sets how it will meet its main objective and what the members will do to achieve this. The plan must be developed with local community involvement, and the SAB must consult the local Healthwatch organisation. The plan should be evidence based and make use of all available evidence and intelligence from partners to form and develop its plan.
> - It must publish an annual report detailing what the SAB has done during the year to achieve its main objective and implement its strategic plan, and what each member has done to implement the strategy as well as detailing the findings of any Safeguarding Adults Reviews and subsequent action.
> - It must conduct any Safeguarding Adults Review in accordance with Section 44 of the Act.
>
> 14.137 Safeguarding requires collaboration between partners in order to create a framework of inter-agency arrangements. Local authorities and their relevant partners must collaborate and work together as set out in the co-operation duties in the Care Act and, in doing so, must, where appropriate, also consider the wishes and feelings of the adult on whose behalf they are working.

24.15 There are three types of review of individual cases undertaken by the Safeguarding Adults Board, where there is reasonable cause for concern about how the Safeguarding Adults Board, members of it or other persons with 'relevant functions' have worked together to safeguard the adult, and:

- where the adult has died and the Safeguarding Adults Board knows or suspects that the death result from abuse or neglect (in which case it is mandatory to undertake a review);
- where the adult is still alive and the Safeguarding Adults Board knows or suspects that the adult has experienced serious abuse or neglect (in which case it is mandatory to undertake a review);
- in any other case involving an adult in the area with needs for care and support (whether or not met by the local authority)(in which case a review is not mandatory).

24.16 In the second and third of these cases, section 68 of the Care Act 2014 requires the local authority to appoint an 'independent advocate', when

- the local authority considers that, without an independent advocate, the individual would experience substantial difficulty in understanding relevant information, retaining that information, using or weighing that information as part of the process of being involve or communicating their views, wishes or feelings;
- and there is no appropriate person (not engaged in providing care or treatment for the individual in a professional or paid capacity) who would be an appropriate person to undertake the 'independent advocate' function;
- then, except insofar as it is necessary to take urgent steps, the local authority must arrange for an 'independent advocate' to 'represent and support the adult to whose case the ...review relates for the purpose of facilitating his or her involvement in the ... review...'; unless
- the local authority is satisfied that there is an appropriate person (not engaged in providing care or treatment for the individual in a professional or paid capacity) who would be an appropriate person to undertake the 'independent advocate' function. However, this exception is itself dis-applied by regulation 4 of the Care and Support (Independent Advocacy Support) (No 2) Regulations 2014 when either (i) the NHS is likely to accommodate the individual in hospital for at least 28 days or in a care home for least eight weeks, or (ii) the local authority and the potentially appropriate person disagree on a material issue but agree that the individual should have an 'independent advocate'.

24.17 See 'Involvement/independent advocates/relevance of Mental Capacity Act 2005' in chapter 7, para 7.53 for further information about independent advocates.

Cases

24.18 *Z v United Kingdom* Application no 29392/95, (2001) 4 CCLR 310,

Article 3 imposes a duty to take reasonable steps to provide effective protection to children and other vulnerable persons whom the state knows, or ought reasonably to know, are being subject to inhuman or degrading treatment

Facts: the applicants were siblings who had suffered personal injury as a result of abuse and neglect whilst living with their parents. The local social services authority had been aware of the situation for a period of years but had failed to take effective action.

Judgment: the treatment meted out by the parents violated the children's rights under Article 3 ECHR; moreover, the State was itself in breach of Article 3, in that it had failed in its duty to take measures to provide effective protection to children and other vulnerable persons, including by taking reasonable steps to prevent ill-treatment of which the authorities knew or ought to have known. The applicants had also been denied a remedy, in breach of Article 13 of the ECHR in that, because the House of Lords had determined that the local authority had not owed the applicants a duty of care in negligence, then, notwithstanding the availability of complaints to the Criminal Injuries Compensation Board and the Local Government Ombudsman, the applicants had not had available to them an appropriate means of obtaining a determination of their allegation that the local authority had failed to protect them from inhuman and degrading treatment and the possibility of obtaining compensation. The court awarded the children pecuniary damages (for loss of earnings, the cost of medical treatment etc) of £8,000, £100,000, £80,000 and £4,000 and non-pecuniary damages of £32,000 each.

24.19 *Re Z (An Adult: Capacity)* [2004] EWHC 2817 (Fam), (2005) 8 CCLR 146

Local authorities were required to investigate, where it appeared that a vulnerable adult intended to undertake an assisted suicide, to ensure that the adult was competent properly, informed and not improperly influenced; but it had no power to stop an adult with capacity taking that course

Facts: Mrs Z suffered from an incurable condition and was deteriorating; she had eventually persuaded her family to accede to her wish to undertake an assisted suicide in Switzerland. The local authority sought an injunction to prevent Mr Z taking her there, under the Family Division's inherent jurisdiction.

Judgment: Hedley J refused the application, holding that it was not unlawful for a person with the mental capacity to make the choice to take their own life, and that although a family member who assisted them would probably incur criminal liability, it was pre-eminently a matter for the police and the DPP to decide whether to enforce it. However, where a local authority learnt that a vulnerable person in their area intended to undertake assisted suicide, it had a duty to take some action:

19. In my judgment in a case such as this the local authority incurred the following duties: (i) to investigate the position of a vulnerable adult to consider what was her true position and intention; (ii) to consider whether she was legally competent to make and carry out her decision and intention; (iii) to consider whether any other (and if so, what) influence may be operating on her position and intention and to ensure that she has all relevant information and knows all available options; (iv) to consider whether to invoke the inherent jurisdiction of the High Court so that the question of competence could be judicially investigated and determined; (v) in the event of the adult not being competent, to provide all such assistance as may be reasonably required both to determine and give effect to her best interests; (vi) in the event of the adult being competent to allow her in any lawful way to give effect to her decision although that should not preclude the giving of advice or assistance in accordance with what are perceived to be her best interests; (vii) where there are reasonable grounds to suspect that the commission of a criminal offence may be involved, to draw that to the attention of the police; (viii) in very exceptional circumstances, to invoke the jurisdiction of the court under section 222 of the Local Government Act 1972. My view is that their duties do not extend beyond that. In this case, although they have the power to do so under section 222 of the 1972 Act, in my judgment they have no obligation to seek the continuation of the injunction made by Black J. It is clear that the criminal justice agencies have all the necessary powers. Moreover Parliament has committed to the Director of Public Prosecutions the discretion as to whether to permit a prosecution. Both those points militate strongly against the intervention of the civil remedy of an injunction. The local authority have made it clear that if they are under no duty to seek the continuation of the injunction, they do not wish to do so.

24.20 *A Local Authority v A* [2010] EWHC 978 (Fam), (2010) 13 CCLR 404

Article 5 ECHR imposed a duty on local authorities to take reasonable steps to prevent the deprivation of liberty of a child or vulnerable adult that it knows or reasonably ought to know about

Facts: The local authority provided care services to families with seriously disabled children. An issue arose as to whether the (exemplary) care provided to the children had resulted in a deprivation of the children's liberty for which the local authority was directly responsible, or unlawfully had failed to prevent.

Judgment: Munby J held that, on the facts, the children had not been deprived of their liberty; that, in any event, the local authority would not have been directly liable for any deprivation of liberty merely because it was providing care services; that the local authority had been under a duty to investigate the possible deprivation of liberty, but it had discharged that duty. Munby J said this:

95. For present purposes I can summarise my conclusions as follows. Where the State – here, a local authority – knows or ought to know that a vulnerable child or adult is subject to restrictions on their liberty by a private individual that arguably give rise to a deprivation of liberty, then its positive obligations under Article 5 will be triggered.

i) These will include the duty to investigate, so as to determine whether there is, in fact, a deprivation of liberty. In this context the local authority will need to consider all the factors relevant to the objective and subjective elements referred to in paragraph [48] above.

ii) If, having carried out its investigation, the local authority is satisfied that the objective element is not present, so there is no deprivation of liberty, the local authority will have discharged its immediate obligations. However, its positive obligations may in an appropriate case require the local authority to continue to monitor the situation in the event that circumstances should change.

iii) If, however, the local authority concludes that the measures imposed do or may constitute a deprivation of liberty, then it will be under a positive obligation, both under Article 5 alone and taken together with Article 14, to take reasonable and proportionate measures to bring that state of affairs to an end. What is reasonable and proportionate in the circumstances will, of course, depend upon the context, but it might for example, Mr Bowen suggests, require the local authority to exercise its statutory powers and duties so as to provide support services for the carers that will enable inappropriate restrictions to be ended, or at least minimised.

iv) If, however, there are no reasonable measures that the local authority can take to bring the deprivation of liberty to an end, or if the measures it proposes are objected to by the individual or his family, then it may be necessary for the local authority to seek the assistance of the court in determining whether there is, in fact, a deprivation of liberty and, if there is, obtaining authorisation for its continuance.

96. What emerges from this is that, whatever the extent of a local authority's positive obligations under Article 5, its duties, and more important its powers, are limited. In essence, its duties are threefold: a duty in appropriate circumstances to investigate; a duty in appropriate circumstances to provide supporting services; and a duty in appropriate circumstances to refer the matter to the court. But, and this is a key message, whatever the positive obligations of a local authority under Article 5 may be, they do not clothe it with any power to regulate, control, compel, restrain, confine or coerce. A local authority which seeks to do so must either point to specific statutory authority for what it is doing – and, as I have pointed out, such statutory powers are, by and large, lacking in cases such as this – or obtain the appropriate sanction of the court. Of course if there is immediate threat to life or limb a local authority will be justified in taking protective (including compulsory) steps: *R (G) v Nottingham City Council* [2008] EWHC 152 (Admin), [2008] 1 FLR 1660, at para [21]. But it must follow up any such intervention with an immediate application to the court.

...

98. Before passing from this part of the case there are two final points which I should emphasise. In the first place, it is vital that local authorities embark upon the kind of investigations that Hedley J and I have described with sensitivity and with a proper appreciation of the limited extent of their powers. Social workers need to keep their eyes open and their professional antennae alert when meeting or visiting their clients. And if there is real cause for concern they must act quickly and decisively. But they must guard against being seen as prying or snooping on the families who they are there to help and support. Nothing is more destructive of the 'working together' relationship which in this kind of context, as in others, is so vitally important than a perception by family carers that the local authority is being heavy-handed or worse. I repeat in this context what I have already said in paragraphs [51]–[53] above.

99. The other point relates to how local authority applications to the court should be made. Too often, in my experience, local authorities seeking the assistance of the court in removing an incapacitated or vulnerable adult

from their home against their wishes or against the wishes of the relatives or friends caring for them, apply ex parte (without notice) and, I have to say, too often such orders have been made by the court without any prior warning to those affected and in circumstances where such seeming heavy-handedness is not easy to justify and can too often turn out to be completely counter-productive: cf *X Council v B (Emergency Protection Orders)* [2004] EWHC 2015 (Fam), [2005] 1 FLR 341, at para [93]. I agree in every respect and would wish to associate myself with what Charles J said in *B Borough Council v S (By the Official Solicitor)* [2006] EWHC 2584 (Fam), [2007] 1 FLR 1600, at paras [37]–[42]. And although I accept that the analogy is not exact, it seems to me that, generally speaking, a local authority will only be justified in seeking a without notice order for the removal of an incapacitated or vulnerable adult in the kind of circumstances which in the case of a child would justify a without notice application for an emergency protection order; as to which see *X Council v B (Emergency Protection Orders)* [2004] EWHC 2015 (Fam), [2005] 1 FLR 341, and *Re X (Emergency Protection Orders)* [2006] EWHC 510 (Fam), [2006] 2 FLR 701. That said, there will, of course, be cases in the adult jurisdiction where, just as in the corresponding children jurisdiction, a without notice application will be justified; indeed (see para [81]), *B Borough Council* was just such a case.

24.21 *MAK and RK v United Kingdom* Application nos 45901/05 and 40146/06, (2010) 13 CCLR 241

Disproportionate actions by a hospital doctor, resulting in his erroneously concluding that parents had abused their daughter, were incompatible with Article 8 ECHR

Facts: a hospital doctor negligently concluded that the daughter had been abused, resulting in the parents' access to their doctor being blocked, then impeded, for about a week. The English Court of Appeal struck out the parents' action in negligence (*JD v East Berkshire Community Health NHS Trust*).[9]

Judgment: the European Court of Human Rights held that whilst mistaken judgments or assessments by professionals do not in themselves render protection measures incompatible with Article 8 ECHR, in this case, the doctor's actions had been disproportionate: there had been a breach of Article 8 ECHR and, because the Human Rights Act 1998 had not been in force at the relevant time, of Article 13 ECHR.

24.22 *Đorđević v Croatia* Application no 41526/10, (2012) 15 CCLR 657

The authorities had been in breach of Articles 3 and 8 ECHR in failing to prevent children harassing a man with significant disabilities and his mother

Facts: the first applicant, who had significant disabilities, had been subjected to continued harassment by children, as had his mother, who looked after him. The authorities took some steps to protect them, but did not take effective or systematic action.

Judgment: the European Court of Human Rights held that the first applicant's rights under Article 3 ECHR and that the second applicant's rights under Article 8 ECHR had been violated:

9 [2005] 2 AC 373, (2005) 8 CCLR 185.

138. The Court reiterates that, as regards the question whether the State could be held responsible, under Article 3, for ill-treatment inflicted on persons by non-State entities, the obligation on the High Contracting Parties under Article 1 of the Convention to secure to everyone within their jurisdiction the rights and freedoms defined in the Convention, taken together with Article 3, requires States to take measures designed to ensure that individuals within their jurisdiction are not subjected to torture or inhuman or degrading treatment or punishment, including such ill-treatment administered by private individuals (see, *mutatis mutandis, HLR v France,* 29 April 1997, para 40, *Reports* 1997-III). These measures should provide effective protection, in particular, of children and other vulnerable persons, and include reasonable steps to prevent ill-treatment of which the authorities had or ought to have had knowledge (see, *mutatis mutandis, Osman v United Kingdom,* 28 October 1998, para 116, *Reports* 1998-VIII, and *E and Others v United Kingdom,* Application no 33218/96, para 88, 26 November 2002).

139. Bearing in mind the difficulties in policing modern societies, the unpredictability of human conduct and the operational choices which must be made in terms of priorities and resources, the scope of this positive obligation must, however, be interpreted in a way which does not impose an impossible or disproportionate burden on the authorities. Not every claimed risk of ill-treatment, thus, can entail for the authorities a Convention requirement to take operational measures to prevent that risk from materialising. For a positive obligation to arise, it must be established that the authorities knew or ought to have known at the time of the existence of a real and immediate risk of ill-treatment of an identified individual from the criminal acts of a third party and that they failed to take measures within the scope of their powers which, judged reasonably, might have been expected to avoid that risk. Another relevant consideration is the need to ensure that the police exercise their powers to control and prevent crime in a manner which fully respects the due process and other guarantees which legitimately place restraints on the scope of their action to investigate crime and bring offenders to justice, including the guarantees contained in Article 8 of the Convention (see *Mubilanzila Mayeka and Kaniki Mitunga v Belgium,* Application no 13178/03, para 53, ECHR 2006-XI; *Members (97) of the Gldani Congregation of Jehovah's Witnesses v Georgia,* Application no 71156/01, para 96, 3 May 2007; and *Milanović v Serbia,* Application no 44614/07, para 84, 14 December 2010; see also, *mutatis mutandis, Osman,* cited above, para 116).

...

(i) General principles

151. While the essential object of Article 8 is to protect the individual against arbitrary interference by public authorities, it does not merely compel the State to abstain from such interference: in addition to this negative undertaking, there may be positive obligations inherent in effective respect for private or family life. These obligations may involve the adoption of measures designed to secure respect for private life even in the sphere of the relations of individuals between themselves (see *X and Y v The Netherlands,* cited above, para 23; *Botta v Italy,* 24 February 1998, para 33, *Reports* 1998-I; *Mikulić v Croatia,* Application no 53176/99, para 57, ECHR 2002-I; and *Sandra Janković,* cited above, para 44).

152. The court has previously held, in various contexts, that the concept of private life includes a person's psychological integrity. Under Article 8, States have in some circumstances a duty to protect the moral integrity

of an individual from acts of other persons. The court has also held that a positive obligation exists upon States to ensure respect for human dignity and the quality of life in certain respects (see *L v Lithuania*, Application no 27527/03, para 56, ECHR 2007-IV, and, *mutatis mutandis, Pretty v United Kingdom*, Application no 2346/02, para 65, ECHR 2002-III).

(ii) Application of these principles to the present case

153. The court considers that the acts of ongoing harassment have also affected the private and family life of the second applicant. It has found that the State authorities have not put in place adequate and relevant measures to prevent further harassment of the first applicant. Likewise, the State authorities have failed to afford adequate protection in that respect to the second applicant. Therefore, there has also been a violation of Article 8 of the Convention in respect of the second applicant.

24.23 *A and S (Children) v Lancashire CC* [2012] EWHC 1689 (Fam), (2012) 15 CCLR 471

A failure properly to place looked after children with a view to securing their adoption breached their rights under Articles 3, 6 and 8 ECHR

Facts: A and S were brothers who came into Lancashire's care as infants but, instead of securing their adoption, Lancashire provided a succession of short-term placements. A and S had been subjected to abuse and neglect and became increasingly unsettled and disturbed. When Lancashire sought to move A (again) from a placement, where he felt settled, A sought legal advice and brought proceedings.

Judgment: Peter Jackson J transferred A and S's damages claims to the QBD and sent a copy of his judgment to the Children's Commissioner, the President of the Family Division and to Designated Family Judges in the North West, in the light of the wider failures identified by him, and granted the following declaration:

IT IS DECLARED THAT:

Lancashire County Council has acted incompatibly with the rights of A and S, as guaranteed by Articles 8, 6 and 3 of the European Convention of Human Rights and Fundamental Freedoms 1950, in that it:

(1) Failed to provide A and S with a proper opportunity of securing a permanent adoptive placement and a settled and secure home life. (Article 8)

(2) Failed to seek revocation of the orders freeing A and S for adoption, made on the 19 March 2001 pursuant to Section 18(1) of the Adoption Act 1976, which effectively deprived them of:

(a) The protection afforded to children under the Children Act 1989;
(b) Contact with their mother and/or other members of their family;
(c) Access to the court and the procedural protection of a Guardian. (Articles 6 and 8)

(3) Permitted A and S to be subjected to degrading treatment and physical assault and failed adequately to protect their physical and sexual safety and their psychological health (Articles 3 and 8).

(4) Failed to provide accurate information concerning A and S's legal status to the Independent Reviewing Officers. (Article 8)

(5) Failed to ensure that there were sufficient procedures in place to give effect to the recommendations of the Looked After Child Reviews. (Article 8)

> (6) Failed to promote the rights of A and S to independent legal advice. (Article 6)
>
> (7) Specifically, failed to act as the 'responsible body' to enable A and S to pursue any potential claims for criminal injuries compensation, tortious liability and/or breach of Human Rights arising from their treatment by their mother, or by the Hs or by Mrs B. (Article 6)
>
> Mr H, the Independent Reviewing Officer for A and S, has acted incompatibly with the rights of A and S, as guaranteed by Articles 8 and 6 of the European Convention of Human Rights and Fundamental Freedoms 1950, in that he:
>
> (1) Failed to identify that A and S's Human Rights had been and were being infringed. (Articles 6 and 8)
>
> (2) Failed to take effective action to ensure that LCC acted upon the recommendations of Looked After Child Reviews. (Article 8)
>
> (3) Failed to refer the circumstances of A and S to CAFCASS Legal. (Article 8)

24.24 *Somerset CC v MK* [2014] EWCOP B25

Serious breaches of proper safeguarding procedures and the DOLS resulted in a deprivation of liberty in breach of Articles 5 and 8 ECHR

Facts: P was a young woman aged 19, with severe learning disabilities and autism, who had lived with her family all her life. During a school trip, bruising was noticed to P's chest and safeguarding procedures were initiated, which resulted in P being deprived of her liberty in a placement, against the wishes of her family, and prescribed unnecessary medication.

Judgment: HHJ Nicholas Marston held that a key failure was the failure of those involved in the safeguarding process to obtain the '*easily discoverable*' information that P had been seen to hit herself heavily on the chest during the school trip, but there followed a wholesale failure to follow proper safeguarding procedures:

> 75. In its position statement of 22 April 2014 the LA concede that P was deprived of liberty and that there was a period where that deprivation was unlawful. Its case is that was from the end of the respite care in early June to the urgent authorisation on 28 November 2013. It further concedes that the deprivation of liberty and loss of her society to the family amounted to an interference with respect to their right to a private and family life contrary to Article 8 ECHR and that interference was not in accordance with the law. It argues that if a lawful process had been followed it is likely that P would have remained away from home while the LA pursued its concerns over safeguarding (the bruising issue) and in due course of time P would have moved to a residential home as they now suggest. It is conceded that if I do not think the residential home is in P's best interests P should have been returned home at a significantly earlier date.
>
> 76. There is no question here that P was removed unlawfully from her family, she went into Selwyn for respite care and it is from the date of her mother's return from holiday that the breach flows. I further accept that the LA had a duty to investigate the bruising but I find that a competently conducted investigation would have swiftly come to the conclusion that no or no sufficient evidence existed to be able to conclude P's safety was at risk by returning her home. This conclusion should have been reached within a

week or so after the family asked for her back. If the LA came to a different conclusion, as they did, they should have applied to the CoP by early June for a hearing. Not doing so is a further breach. Having not done so they should have told the family they could make an application, not doing that is a further breach. After the Police investigation ended in September P should again have been returned but was not nor was an application made to CoP as it should have been. The limitations and conditions placed on contact between the family and P constitute another breach.

77. The LA seeks to rely on the DOL urgent authorisation it obtained on 28 November 2013 to close off the period of unlawful deprivation of liberty. In the case of *London Borough of Hillingdon v Neary* (2011) EWHC 1377 (COP), a case that has many depressing similarities to this one, Mr Justice Peter Jackson said at paragraph 33:

> 'The DOL scheme is an important safeguard against arbitrary detention. Where stringent conditions are met it allows a managing authority to deprive a person of liberty at a particular place. It is not to be used by a local authority as a means of getting its own way on the question of whether it is in the person's best interests to be in that place at all. Using the DOL regime in that way turns the whole spirit of the MCA on its head, with a code designed to protect the liberty of vulnerable people being used instead as an instrument of confinement. In this case far from being a safeguard the way in which the DOL process was used to mask the real deprivation of liberty which was the refusal to allow Stephen to go home.'

I find that is also precisely what has happened here and the breach of Article 8 rights continues up to now.

78. These findings illustrate a blatant disregard of the process of the MCA and a failure to respect the rights of both P and her family under the ECHR. In fact it seems to me that it is worse than that, because here the workers on the ground did not just disregard the process of the MCA they did not know what the process was and no one higher up the structure seems to have advised them correctly about it.

HHJ Nicholas Marston also said this about some of the allegations that, nonetheless, it was not in P's best interests to return home because of her mother's parenting style and relationship with professionals:

35. Finding 22, inability to accept advice on M's part, and finding 23 M's rigid style both of parenting and of dealing with professionals, are important issues when considering if returning home is an appropriate option because they directly relate to issues about the care P would be getting at home. Three points need to be made first. As I have already said, given the longevity of the relationship between M and the social workers and the number of social workers involved, there are bound to be some people who don't get on and some who do. In her evidence M told me of social workers she had had good relationships with and others (the majority it has to be said) she did not. Second, M has a strong personality, otherwise she would have sunk under the weight of cares and problems in the last 20 years and she perceives herself as having to fight for a good deal for in particular P and A. Third, as will become clear in the later parts of this judgment when I examine the conduct of the LA over the last 13 months, she and her family have had a lot to put up with. In his evidence the senior manager for social services conceded LA failures across the board and the damage that has done to the family and its relationship with the LA. Having said all of that there have in the past, prior to May 2013, been real clashes of personality

and failures in communication but I cannot find that it has been proved on the balance of probabilities there has been an irrational refusal to co-operate from the family with the statutory authorities. The best evidence for that is that there was never, in the whole of Ps minority, an application in public law proceedings and no doubt if the LA had had evidence at the time of failure to co-operate on a scale which was causing P or any of the children significant harm such an application would have been made.

Comment: see also *Milton Keynes Council v RR*[10] and *Essex CC v RF*[11] which are to similar effect.

10 [2014] EWCOP 34.
11 [2015] EWCOP 1.

CHAPTER 25

Human rights

continued

25.57 *Z v United Kingdom* Application no 29392/95, [2001] ECHR 333, (2001) 4 CCLR 310

Article 3 imposes a duty to take reasonable steps to provide effective protection to children and other vulnerable persons whom the state knows, or ought reasonably to know, are being subjected to inhuman or degrading treatment

25.58 *TP and KM v United Kingdom* Application no 28945/95, [2001] ECHR 332, (2001) 4 CCLR 398

The failure to disclose to material that undermined the local authority case of child abuse against a male carer had been incompatible with Article 8 ECHR; as had the failure to promote contact between the child and her family

25.59 *Price v United Kingdom* Application no 33394/96, [2001] ECHR 458, (2002) 5 CCLR 306

It had been a breach of Article 3 ECHR to detain a severely disabled woman in grossly unsuitable conditions

25.60 *Passannante v Italy* Application no 32647/96, (2002) 5 CCLR 340

A delay in providing healthcare to which a person was entitled by virtue of contributions might raise an issue under Article 8 ECHR if there was a serious risk to health

25.61 *R (Bernard) v Enfield LBC* [2002] EWHC 2282 (Admin), (2002) 5 CCLR 577

A serious failure to provide the services required under section of the National Assistance Act 1948, which had severe repercussion on Ms Bernard's family and private law, breached Article 8 ECHR

25.62 *R (S) v Plymouth CC* [2002] EWCA Civ 388, (2002) 5 CCLR 251

Fairness and the ECHR required disclosure of the son's mental health records to his mother, in nearest relative displacement proceedings

25.63 *R (Beeson) v Dorset CC and Secretary of State for Health* [2002] EWCA Civ 1812, (2003) 6 CCLR 5

It was compatible with Article 6 ECHR for disputes about social care charges to be determined by local authorities subject to judicial review, rather than a merits appeal

25.64 *R (A and B) v East Sussex CC* [2003] EWHC 167 (Admin), (2003) 6 CCLR 194

The recognition and protection of human dignity is a core value protected by Article 8 ECHR. Nonetheless the rights of persons with disabilities required to be balanced against those of their carers, where there was a conflict

25.65 *Collins v United Kingdom* Application no 11909/02, (2003) 6 CCLR 388

It was lawful in national law to resile from a 'home for life' promise and in this case is had been proportionate and compatible with Article 8 ECHR

25.66 *R (Anufrijeva) v Southwark LBC* [2003] EWCA Civ 1406, (2003) 6 CCLR 415

A failure to provide a statutory service will usually only breach Article 8 ECHR where there is a level of culpability on the part of the authority and where the consequences are so serious as to be comparable with cases of violations of Article 3 ECHR although a lower threshold could apply in the case of children

25.67 *Sentges v Netherlands* Application No 27677/02, (2004) 7 CCLR 400

The margin of appreciation was, especially in relation to the allocation of scarce healthcare resources, that it could not be said that the refusal to supply a robotic arm, in the context of the provision of other services, was incompatible with Article 8 ECHR

25.68 *Autism-Europe v France* (complaint 13/2002) (2004) 38 EHRR CD265
The European Committee of Social Rights declared admissible a complaint that France was in breach of the revised European Social Charter by failing to ensure that children and adults were entitled to education in mainstream schools in sufficient numbers

25.69 *van Kuck v Germany* Application no 35968/97, (2005) 8 CCLR 121
It was incompatible with Articles 6 and 8 ECHR to decline to fund gender re-assignment surgery on the basis of an incorrect understanding of the medical evidence

25.70 *Re Z (An Adult: Capacity)* [2004] EWHC 2817 Fam, (2005) 8 CCLR 146
Local authorities were required to investigate, where it appeared that a vulnerable adult intended to undertake an assisted suicide, to ensure that the adult was competent properly, informed and not improperly influenced; but it had no power to stop an adult with capacity taking that course

25.71 *Pentiacova v Moldova* Application no 14462/03, (2005) 40 EHRR SE23
It was not a breach of the ECHR radically to reduce haemodialysis provision, notwithstanding the suffering occasioned

25.72 *R (Hughes) v Liverpool CC* [2005] EWHC 428 (Admin), (2005) 8 CCLR 243
A breach of duty to provide social care did not inevitably result in a breach of the ECHR, for which the threshold was high

25.73 *R (Limbuela) v Secretary of State for the Home Department* [2005] UKHL 66, (2006) 9 CCLR 30
It was necessary to provide accommodation and support to asylum-seekers who were destitute or faced imminent destitution, to avoid a breach of Article 3 ECHR

25.74 *R (YL) v Birmingham CC* [2007] UKHL 27, (2007) 10 CCLR 505
A privately run care home was not discharging functions of a public nature

25.75 *R (Weaver) v London and Quadrant Housing Trust* [2009] EWCA Civ 587, [2010] 1 WLR 363
On the assumption that some functions of an RSL were public functions, it was a public body for the purposes of the Human Rights Act 1998 and for the purposes of judicial review proceedings, because its termination of a social tenancy was not a private act

25.76 *Tysiac v Poland* Application No 5410/03, (2007) 45 EHRR 42
The absence of clear procedures for determining eligibility for an abortion and resolving disputes was incompatible with Article 8 ECHR

25.77 *R (Wilson) v Coventry CC; R (Thomas) v Havering LBC* [2008] EWHC 2300 (Admin), (2009) 12 CCLR 7
Care home closures did not in general breach Article 2 ECHR

25.78 *Re E (A Child) (Northern Ireland)* [2008] UKHL 66, [2009] 1 AC 536
Children and other vulnerable persons require special protection under the ECHR

25.79 *MAK and RK v United Kingdom* Application nos 45901/05 and 40146/06, [2010] ECHR 363, (2010) 13 CCLR 241
Disproportionate actions by a hospital doctor, resulting in his erroneously concluding that parents had abused their daughter, were incompatible with Article 8 ECHR

25.80 *Watts v United Kingdom* Application no 53586/09, [2010] ECHR 793, (2010) 51 EHRR SE5
A carefully managed process of care home closure did not violate rights under Articles 2, 3 or 8 ECHR

continued

25.81 *Stanev v Bulgaria* Application No 36760/06, (2012) 55 EHRR 22
Very poor living conditions in a care home for seven years amounted to inhuman and degrading treatment

25.82 *Đorđević v Croatia* Application no 41526/10, [2012] ECHR 1640, (2012) 15 CCLR 657
The authorities were in breach of Articles 3 and 8 ECHR by failing to protect a disabled man and his mother from harassment by local ragamuffins

25.83 *Nencheva v Bulgaria* Application no 48609/06, [2013] ECHR 554
Public authorities are under a duty to take reasonable steps to prevent the death of vulnerable individuals in state care and to undertake an effective investigation into deaths where the state was involved

25.84 *Commissioner of Police for the Metropolis v ZH* [2013] EWCA Civ 69, (2013) 16 CCLR 109
Callous restraint of a young autistic male by the police violated his rights under Articles 3, 5 and 8 ECHR

25.85 *McDonald v United Kingdom* Application no 4241/12, [2014] ECHR 492, (2014) 17 CCLR 187
It had been proportionate and compatible with Article 8 ECHR radically to reduce a person's social care provision

25.86 *Campeanu v Romania* Application no 47848/08, [2014] ECHR 789
Exceptionally, an NGO was permitted to bring a complaint under the ECHR on behalf of a deceased individual

25.87 *European Committee for Home-Based Priority Action for the Child and the Family (EUROCEF) v France* Complaint No 114/2015
The European Committee of Social Rights upheld as admissible EUROCEF's complaint that France was failing to discharge its duty under the revised European Social Charter to provide housing, social and medical assistance, social welfare and other benefits to unaccompanied minors, seeking asylum in France or living irregularly in France

25.88 *R (SG and NS) v Secretary of State for Work and Pensions* [2015] UKSC 16, (2015) 18 CCLR 215
It was not a breach of Article 14 ECHR to treat women more harshly than men in the benefits regime and the best interests of their children were irrelevant

25.89 *Williams v Hackney LBC* [2015] EWHC 2629 (QB)
It had been a breach of the parents' rights under the ECHR to elicit their uninformed consent to the accommodation of their children under section 20 of the Children Act 1989

25.90 *Matheison v Secretary of State for Work and Pensions* [2015] UKSC 47, [2015] 1 WLR 3250
It was incompatible with Articles 8 and 14 ECHR, construed harmoniously with the UN Convention on the Rights of Persons with Disabilities, not to provide Disability Living Allowance to children after 84 days of hospital in-patient treatment

25.91 *Di Trizio v Switzerland* Application no 7186/09, [2016] ECHR 143
Invalidity benefit was capable of falling within the ambit of Article 8 ECHR

25.92 *Guberina v Croatia* Application no 23682/13, [2016] ECHR 287
Article 14 ECHR applies where a person is treated differently because of the status of another person and the UN Convention on the Rights of Persons with Disabilities was relevant to the proper construction of the scope of Article 14 ECHR

Introduction

25.1 National legislation, and the common law, often afford the strongest protection for human rights and are all too often neglected as remedies for breaches of fundamental rights. In particular, the common law is often able to engage with the detail of the lawfulness or otherwise of the process by which state action threatens to infringe fundamental rights, in ways that more broadly expressed treaty-based principles cannot.[1]

25.2 Nonetheless, international law plays an increasingly important role:

- when it has not been incorporated into national law it may inform the proper construction of legislation within its scope;[2]
- when it has been incorporated into national law it will generally prevail unless the situation is governed by national primary legislation but even then, international law may override primary legislation (in the case of EU law), or require it to be construed as far as possible so that it is compliant with the incorporated treaty (ECHR law);
- in addition, the general principles of international law, and international instruments, such as the UN Convention on the Rights of the Child (UNCRC) and the UN Convention on the Rights of Persons with Disabilities (UNCRPD), can percolate indirectly into national law[3] as a result of the principle that the ECHR, and EU law, should in general be construed harmoniously with other relevant provisions of international law.[4]

25.3 When it comes to challenges to decisions involving the allocation of 'scarce' national resources, such as health or social care, the claimant is often better off relying on the common law, and public law supervision, in order to question the legality of the decision-making process. The European Court of Human Rights (ECtHR) does monitor procedures to some extent, in some cases,[5] but its tendency is generally to shy away from interfering with the allocation of health or social care resources.[6] The common law seems more adept at examining whether, for example: (i) resources have been allocated in accordance with a published policy;[7] (ii) such a policy is vitiated by legal error, breach of the PSED or illogicality;[8] (iii) the decision-maker has failed properly to understand or implement such policy, or consider making an exception to it[9] – and so forth.

25.4 International law has, however, been very effective in protecting core fundamental rights such as the right to personal liberty and freedom from

1 *Re Reilly's Application for Judicial Review* [2013] UKSC 61, [2014] AC 11115.

2 *Assange v Swedish Prosecution Authority* [2012] UKSC 22, [2012] 2 WLR 1275.

3 In addition, some rules of customary international law are treated as forming part of the common law: *Trendtex Trading v Bank of Nigeria* [1977] 1 QB 529 at 553B–554H, 576G–H.

4 *A v Secretary of State for the Home Department* [2005] UKHL 71, [2006] 2 AC 221 at paras 27–29.

5 *Tysiac v Poland* (2007) 45 EHRR 42.

6 *Pentiacova v Moldova* (2005) 40 EHRR SE23.

7 *R v North West Lancashire HA ex p A, D and G* (1999) 2 CCLR 419.

8 *R v North West Lancashire HA ex p A, D and G* (1999) 2 CCLR 419.

9 *R v North West Lancashire HA ex p A, D and G* (1999) 2 CCLR 419; *R v North Derbyshire HA ex p Fisher* (1997–8) 1 CCLR 150.

inhuman and degrading treatment;[10] aiding challenges to the provision of health or social care that is discriminatory;[11] and in changing the context of decision-making about vulnerable groups, such as children or disabled adults, so that their welfare is treated as a very important consideration throughout the process.[12]

There is a range of material on human rights in health and social care published by, among others:

- the Equality and Human Rights Commission;[13]
- Citizens' Advice;[14]
- the Social Care Institute for Excellence;[15]
- Age UK;[16] and
- the Care Quality Commission.[17]

European Union law

The basic framework of European law

25.5 European Union law is founded on the Treaty on European Union (TEU) and the Treaty on the Functioning of the European Union (TFEU). Article 6 of the TEU gives treaty effect to the Charter of Fundamental Rights (CFR).

25.6 The EU enjoys exclusive competence in the areas of customs union, the functioning of the internal market, monetary policy, the conservation of marine biological resources and common commercial policy.[18] It shares competence with Member States in the following areas:[19]

> 4(2) Shared competence between the Union and the Member States applies in the following principal areas:
> (a) internal market;
> (b) social policy, for the aspects defined in this Treaty;
> (c) economic, social and territorial cohesion;
> (d) agriculture and fisheries, excluding the conservation of marine biological resources;
> (e) environment;
> (f) consumer protection;
> (g) transport;
> (h) trans-European networks;

10 *Z v United Kingdom* (2001) 4 CCLR 310.

11 *Van Kuck v Germany* (2005) 8 CCLR 121.

12 *E v Chief Constable of the Royal Ulster Constabulary* [2008] UKHL 66, [1009] 1 AC 536.

13 www.equalityhumanrights.com/en/advice-and-guidance/human-rights-health-and-social-care.

14 www.citizensadvice.org.uk/healthcare/discrimination-in-health-and-care-services/taking-action-about-discrimination-in-health-and-care-services/protecting-your-human-rights-when-using-health-and-care-services/.

15 www.scie.org.uk/publications/guides/guide15/legislation/humanrightsact/.

16 www.ageuk.org.uk/documents/en-gb/for-professionals/equality-and-human-rights/older_people_human_rights__expert_series_pro.pdf?dtrk=true.

17 www.cqc.org.uk/sites/default/files/20140406_our_human_rights_approach_public_consultation_final.pdf.

18 TFEU Article 2.

19 TFEU Article 4(2)

(i) energy;
(j) area of freedom, security and justice;
(k) common safety concerns in public health matters, for the aspects defined in this Treaty.

The primacy of EU Law

25.7 All rules of EU law prevail over any inconsistent national law, whether that be common law or primary legislation, such that every tribunal, however lowly, is required to override any type of national law insofar as it may be inconsistent with rules of EU law.[20] An EU rule can be relied on directly by litigants in national law:

- against the State ('vertically') and against other persons ('horizontally'), when it is in a Treaty and creates rights and obligations that are sufficiently complete, unconditional, clear and precise;[21]
- against the State and against other persons, when it is in a regulation;[22]
- against the State, when it is in a directive, providing that (i) time for implementing the directive into national law has expired; (ii) the Member State has failed to implement the directive properly, or at all; and (iii) the rule creates justiciable rights and obligations that are unconditional and sufficiently precise;[23]
- against the State and other persons, when it is a decision of the Court of Justice of the European Union (CJEU);[24]
- where binding decisions are made, authorised by the TFEU or subordinate EU legislation, in terms that are sufficiently clear and precise so as to confer directly effective rights.[25]

25.8 Even where EU law is not directly effective in a Member State, the courts are required to construe national law consistently with it as far as possible.[26]

Important principles of EU law

25.9 The most important principles, in the present context, are as follows:

- national courts must construe national legislation, dealing with the same subject matter as EU law, consistently with EU law, as far as possible, so as to give effect to EU law:[27] no ambiguity is needed and bold departures from the ordinary meaning of words are required, so long as the process does not exceed one of reasonable construction;[28]

20 *Costa v ENEL* [1964] ECR 585; *Simmenthal* [1978] ECR 629 at para 22.
21 *Van Gend en Loos* [1963] ECR 1.
22 TFEU Article 288.
23 *Van Duyn v Home Office* [1974] ECR 1337.
24 TFEU Article 267.
25 TFEU Article 288.
26 *Marleasing SA v La Commercial Internacional de Alimentacion SA* [1990] ECR 1–4135.
27 TEU Article 4(3); *Marleasing SA v La Commercial Internacional de Alimentacion SA* [1990] ECR 1–4135.
28 *R (Equal Opportunities Commission) v Secretary of State for Communities and Local Government* [2007] EWHC 483 (Admin), [2007] 2 CMLR 49.

- Where EU law vests rights in persons without prescribing any process whereby those persons may enforce those rights, it is for the national legal system to decide on the most appropriate process[29] providing that (i) the process is just as favourable as the procedures for the enforcement of similar national rights ('the principle of equivalence');[30] and (ii) the process does not make it impossible or excessively difficult to enforce the EU right ('the principle of effectiveness');[31]
- Member States must provide effective remedies, including for financial compensation for harm caused by breaches of EU law for which the Member State is responsible;[32]
- any national court or tribunal is entitled to refer a question on the interpretation of EU law to the CJEU[33] and ought to refer an issue that is critical to its decision, unless it can with complete confidence determine the issue for itself, notwithstanding the wider perspective and expertise of the CJEU;[34]
- in the absence of any specific requirement of equal treatment, in principle all comparable situations must be treated the same unless the difference is objectively justified[35] and different situations must not be treated in the same way unless each treatment is objectively justified;[36]
- proportionality is a general principle of EU law,[37] accordingly, all actions and decision of the EU and its various agencies, and of national authorities acting within the scope of EU law, must be proportionate, in the sense that the means employed to achieve the aim must be suitable or appropriate to achieve the aim; must be necessary for its achievement such that there is no less onerous method of achieving the aim; and must not impose a burden that is disproportionate to the aimed for benefits;[38]
- there must be legal certainty and the protection of legitimate expectations – the effect of EU legislation must be clear and predictable;[39]
- notwithstanding the existence of the CFR, general fundamental rights principles remain principles of EU law.[40]

29 *Comet BV v Produktschap voor Siergewassen* [1976] ECR 2043 at para 13.

30 *R v Secretary of State for Transport ex p Factortame* [1990] ECR 1–2433 at para 20; *Danske Slagterier v Bundesrepublik Deutschland* [2009] ECR 1–2110 at para 48.

31 *FA (Iraq) v Secretary of State for the Home Department* [2011] UKSC 22, [2011] 3 CMLR 23 at para 35; *Danske Slagterier v Bundesrepublik Deutschland* [2009] ECR 1–2110 at para 48.

32 *Francovich v Italy* [1991] ECR 1–5357.

33 TFEU Article 276.

34 *R v International Stock Exchange ex p Else Ltd* [1993] QB 534 at 545; *CILFIT v Ministry of Health* [1982] ECR 3415 at para 16.

35 *Uberschar v Bundesversichorunganstalt fur Angestellete* [1980] ECR 2747 at para 16.

36 *R (Novartis) v Licensing Authority* [2004] ECR 1–4403 at para 69.

37 TEU Article 5(4); *Lumsdon v Legal Services Board* [2015] UKSC 41, [2015] 3 WLR 121 at paras 23–32.

38 *Internationale Handelsgesellschaft v Einfuhr und Vorratstelle Getreide* [1970] ECR 1125; *Lumsdon v Legal Services Board* [2015] UKSC 41, [2015] 3 WLR 121 at paras 33–39.

39 *Duff v MAF* [1996] ECR 1–569 at para 20.

40 *Stauder v City of Ulm* [1969] ECR 419; *Internationale Handelsgesellschaft v Einfuhr und Vorratstelle Getreide* [1970] ECR 1125.

The Charter of Fundamental Rights

25.10 The Charter of Fundamental Rights (CFR) became legally binding on 1 December 2009.[41]

25.11 According to the CFR, it is binding on EU institutions and Member States 'when they are implementing Union law'.[42] This has been construed by the CJEU broadly, as meaning that Member States must abide by the fundamental rights in the CFR when they are 'acting within the scope of EU law'.[43] Notably, Member States are 'acting within the scope of EU law' when they process claims for international protection and provide reception conditions for such claimants.[44]

25.12 The CFR contains a Protocol that appears intended to limit the impact of the CFR on the UK (and Poland) but in fact seems to have no real meaning.[45]

25.13 The CFR essentially comprises:

- a statement of fundamental rights, drawing from the ECHR, EU law and the human rights traditions of the Member States, in six chapters covering dignity, freedoms, equality, solidarity, citizen's rights and justice;
- a set of principles, which may be implemented in EU or national law.

25.14 The CFR provides that the rights set out therein, which correspond to rights in the ECHR, are in general to have the same meaning and scope as the ECHR rights;[46] but case-law suggests that such rights will not be so limited when they already have a wider EU meaning.[47]

25.15 Any limitation on a right in the CFR must be provided for by law, respect the essence of the right and be proportionate.[48]

25.16 The EU has published a useful explanatory document called *Explanations Relating to the Charter of Fundamental Rights* (2007/C 303/02),[49] which the CFR requires to be taken into account when construing the CFR.[50]

25.17 There is also an illuminating Commentary of the Charter of Fundamental Rights of the European Union, published by the EU Network of Independent Experts on Fundamental Rights.[51]

41 The CFR has its own website at http://ec.europa.eu/justice/fundamental-rights/charter/index_en.htm.

42 CFR Article 51(1).

43 *ERT v DEP and Kouvelas* [1991] ECR 2925; *Dereci v Bundesministerium fur Inneres* [2012] 1 CMLR 22 at para 58.

44 *NS v Secretary of State for the Home Department* [2013] QB 102.

45 *NS v Secretary of State for the Home Department* [2013] QB 102.

46 CFR Article 52(3).

47 *Diouf v Ministre du Travail* [2012] 1 CMLR 8 at para 39.

48 CFR Article 52(1).

49 http://eur-lex.europa.eu/LexUriServ/LexUriServ.do?uri=OJ:C:2007:303:0017:0035:en:PDF.

50 CFR Article 52(7).

51 http://ec.europa.eu/justice/fundamental-rights/files/networkcommentaryfinal_en.pdf, referred to with approval, as a useful guide at para 30 of *Adebayo Abdul v Secretary of State for the Home Department* (ref to be supplied when reported).

25.18 As stated by Munby J in *R (Howard League for Penal Reform) v Secretary of State for the Home Department and another*:[52]

> ... the UN [Child] Convention [and] the European Charter ... can ... properly be consulted insofar as they proclaim, reaffirm or elucidate the content of those human rights that are generally recognised throughout the European family of nations, in particular the nature and scope of those fundamental rights that are guaranteed by the European Convention.

25.19 In addition, the European Social Charter of 1961 (ratified by the UK) and the Revised European Social Charter of 1996 (not ratified by the UK) contain a number of human rights, implementation of which is monitored by the European Committee of Social Rights, whose case-law (based on a collective complaint procedure in the Revised European Social Charter of 1996) is of great interest.[53]

25.20 A recent decision on the website in fact gives a good flavour of the Committee's approach and the subject matter of its cases: in *European Committee for Home-Based Priority Action for the Child and the Family (EUROCEF) v France* (Complaint No 114/2015),[54] the Committee accepted as admissible a complaint that France was failing to discharge its obligations under the Revised European Social Charter of 1996 to provide housing, social and medical assistance, social welfare and other benefits to unaccompanied minors, living irregularly in France, or seeking asylum.

25.21 The most useful CFR rights in this context are as follows:

Article 3: Right to the integrity of the person

1. Everyone has the right to respect for his or her physical and mental integrity.

2. In the fields of medicine and biology, the following must be respected in particular:

- the free and informed consent of the person concerned, according to the procedures laid down by law,
- the prohibition of eugenic practices, in particular those aiming at the selection of persons, t
- the prohibition on making the human body and its parts as such a source of financial gain,
- the prohibition of the reproductive cloning of human beings.

Article 4: Prohibition of torture and inhuman or degrading treatment or punishment

No one shall be subjected to torture or to inhuman or degrading treatment or punishment.

Article 7: Respect for private and family life

Everyone has the right to respect for his or her private and family life, home and communications.

Article 8: Protection of personal data

1. Everyone has the right to the protection of personal data concerning him or her.

2. Such data must be processed fairly for specified purposes and on the basis of the consent of the person concerned or some other legitimate basis

52 [2002] EWHC 2497 (Admin) at [51].

53 www.coe.int/t/dghl/monitoring/socialcharter/ECSR/ECSRdefault_en.asp.

54 http://hudoc.esc.coe.int/eng.

laid down by law. Everyone has the right of access to data which has been collected concerning him or her, and the right to have it rectified.

3. Compliance with these rules shall be subject to control by an independent authority

Article 20: Equality before the law

Everyone is equal before the law.

Article 21: Non-discrimination

1. Any discrimination based on any ground such as sex, race, colour, ethnic or social origin, genetic features, language, religion or belief, political or any other opinion, membership of a national minority, property, birth, disability, age or sexual orientation shall be prohibited.

2. Within the scope of application of the Treaties and without prejudice to any of their specific provisions, any discrimination on grounds of nationality shall be prohibited.

Article 22: Cultural, religious and linguistic diversity

The Union shall respect cultural, religious and linguistic diversity.

Article 23: Equality between women and men

Equality between women and men must be ensured in all areas, including employment, work and pay.

The principle of equality shall not prevent the maintenance or adoption of measures providing for specific advantages in favour of the under-represented sex.

Article 24: The rights of the child

1. Children shall have the right to such protection and care as is necessary for their well-being. They may express their views freely. Such views shall be taken into consideration on matters which concern them in accordance with their age and maturity.

2. In all actions relating to children, whether taken by public authorities or private institutions, the child's best interests must be a primary consideration.

3. Every child shall have the right to maintain on a regular basis a personal relationship and direct contact with both his or her parents, unless that is contrary to his or her interests.

Article 25: The rights of the elderly

The Union recognises and respects the rights of the elderly to lead a life of dignity and independence and to participate in social and cultural life.

Article 26: Integration of persons with disabilities

The Union recognises and respects the right of persons with disabilities to benefit from measures designed to ensure their independence, social and occupational integration and participation in the life of the community.

Article 34: Social security and social assistance

1. The Union recognises and respects the entitlement to social security benefits and social services providing protection in cases such as maternity, illness, industrial accidents, dependency or old age, and in the case of loss of employment, in accordance with the rules laid down by Union law and national laws and practices.

2. Everyone residing and moving legally within the European Union is entitled to social security benefits and social advantages in accordance with Union law and national laws and practices.

3. In order to combat social exclusion and poverty, the Union recognises and respects the right to social and housing assistance so as to ensure a decent existence for all those who lack sufficient resources, in accordance with the rules laid down by Union law and national laws and practices.

Article 35: Health care

Everyone has the right of access to preventive health care and the right to benefit from medical treatment under the conditions established by national laws and practices. A high level of human health protection shall be ensured in the definition and implementation of all the Union's policies and activities.

Article 41: Right to good administration

1. Every person has the right to have his or her affairs handled impartially, fairly and within a reasonable time by the institutions, bodies, offices and agencies of the Union.

2. This right includes:

(a) the right of every person to be heard, before any individual measure which would affect him or her adversely is taken;

(b) the right of every person to have access to his or her file, while respecting the legitimate interests of confidentiality and of professional and business secrecy;

(c) the obligation of the administration to give reasons for its decisions.

3. Every person has the right to have the Union make good any damage caused by its institutions or by its servants in the performance of their duties, in accordance with the general principles common to the laws of the Member States.

4. Every person may write to the institutions of the Union in one of the languages of the Treaties and must have an answer in the same language.

Article 42: Right of access to documents

Any citizen of the Union, and any natural or legal person residing or having its registered office in a Member State, has a right of access to documents of the institutions, bodies, offices and agencies of the Union, whatever their medium.

Article 47: Right to an effective remedy and to a fair trial

Everyone whose rights and freedoms guaranteed by the law of the Union are violated has the right to an effective remedy before a tribunal in compliance with the conditions laid down in this Article.

Everyone is entitled to a fair and public hearing within a reasonable time by an independent and impartial tribunal previously established by law. Everyone shall have the possibility of being advised, defended and represented.

Legal aid shall be made available to those who lack sufficient resources in so far as such aid is necessary to ensure effective access to justice.

Human Rights Act 1998

25.22 Section 1 of the Human Rights Act (HRA) 1998 provides that most of the European Convention on Human Rights is to have effect in the UK:

- Articles 2–12 and 14 of the ECHR;
- Articles 1–3 of the First Protocol; and
- Articles 1 and 2 of the Sixth Protocol.

25.23 Provision is made for the UK to enter reservations or derogations, but none such exist at the present time.

The main ECHR provisions

25.24 The ECHR provisions relied on in social care cases are as follows:

Right to life

Article 2

1. Everyone's right to life shall be protected by law. No one shall be deprived of his life intentionally save in the execution of a sentence of a court following his conviction of a crime for which this penalty is provided by law.

2. Deprivation of life shall not be regarded as inflicted in contravention of this Article when it results from the use of force which is no more than absolutely necessary:

(a) in defence of any person from unlawful violence;

(b) in order to effect a lawful arrest or to prevent the escape of a person lawfully detained;

(c) in action lawfully taken for the purpose of quelling a riot or insurrection.

Prohibition of torture

Article 3

No one shall be subjected to torture or to inhuman or degrading treatment or punishment.

Right to liberty and security

Article 5

1. Everyone has the right to liberty and security of person. No one shall be deprived of his liberty save in the following cases and in accordance with a procedure prescribed by law:

(a) the lawful detention of a person after conviction by a competent court;

(b) the lawful arrest or detention of a person for non-compliance with the lawful order of a court or in order to secure the fulfilment of any obligation prescribed by law;

(c) the lawful arrest or detention of a person effected for the purpose of bringing him before the competent legal authority on reasonable suspicion of having committed an offence or when it is reasonably considered necessary to prevent his committing an offence or fleeing after having done so;

(d) the detention of a minor by lawful order for the purpose of educational supervision or his lawful detention for the purpose of bringing him before the competent legal authority;

(e) the lawful detention of persons for the prevention of the spreading of infectious diseases, of persons of unsound mind, alcoholics or drug addicts or vagrants;

(f) the lawful arrest or detention of a person to prevent his effecting an unauthorised entry into the country or of a person against whom action is being taken with a view to deportation or extradition.

2. Everyone who is arrested shall be informed promptly, in a language which he understands, of the reasons for his arrest and of any charge against him.

3. Everyone arrested or detained in accordance with the provisions of paragraph 1(c) of this Article shall be brought promptly before a judge or other officer authorised by law to exercise judicial power and shall be entitled to trial within a reasonable time or to release pending trial. Release may be conditioned by guarantees to appear for trial.

4. Everyone who is deprived of his liberty by arrest or detention shall be entitled to take proceedings by which the lawfulness of his detention shall be decided speedily by a court and his release ordered if the detention is not lawful.

5. Everyone who has been the victim of arrest or detention in contravention of the provisions of this Article shall have an enforceable right to compensation.

Right to a fair trial

Article 6

1. In the determination of his civil rights and obligations or of any criminal charge against him, everyone is entitled to a fair and public hearing within a reasonable time by an independent and impartial tribunal established by law. Judgment shall be pronounced publicly but the press and public may be excluded from all or part of the trial in the interest of morals, public order or national security in a democratic society, where the interests of juveniles or the protection of the private life of the parties so require, or to the extent strictly necessary in the opinion of the court in special circumstances where publicity would prejudice the interests of justice.

2. Everyone charged with a criminal offence shall be presumed innocent until proved guilty according to law.

3. Everyone charged with a criminal offence has the following minimum rights:

(a) to be informed promptly, in a language which he understands and in detail, of the nature and cause of the accusation against him;

(b) to have adequate time and facilities for the preparation of his defence;

(c) to defend himself in person or through legal assistance of his own choosing or, if he has not sufficient means to pay for legal assistance, to be given it free when the interests of justice so require;

(d) to examine or have examined witnesses against him and to obtain the attendance and examination of witnesses on his behalf under the same conditions as witnesses against him;

(e) to have the free assistance of an interpreter if he cannot understand or speak the language used in court.

Right to respect for private and family life

Article 8

1. Everyone has the right to respect for his private and family life, his home and his correspondence.

2. There shall be no interference by a public authority with the exercise of this right except such as is in accordance with the law and is necessary in a democratic society in the interests of national security, public safety or the economic well-being of the country, for the prevention of disorder or crime, for the protection of health or morals, or for the protection of the rights and freedoms of others.

Public authorities and unlawful acts

25.25 The principle mechanism whereby the Human Rights Act 1998 gives effect to the ECHR rights that now take effect in UK law (from now on, 'ECHR rights') is in sections 6–8, by virtue of which:

- it is unlawful for a 'public authority' to act, or to fail to act, in a way which is incompatible with ECHR rights unless the 'public authority' could not have acted differently as a result of primary legislation/provisions made under primary legislation that cannot be read or given effect in a way that is compatible with ECHR rights;
- a 'public authority' includes a court or tribunal and any person certain of whose functions are of a public nature except in relation to their actions or failures to act that are private in nature;
- a person who is, or would be, a victim of an unlawful act under section 6 can bring proceedings against the 'public authority' in an appropriate court or tribunal, in reliance on their ECHR rights, within one year (or longer, if the court grants an extension);
- if the court or tribunal decides that the 'public authority' has acted, or proposes to act, incompatibly with the claimant's ECHR rights, it may grant any form of remedy that falls within its usual powers and that it considers appropriate, including damages where damages are necessary to accord the victim 'just satisfaction'.

25.26 As discussed in chapter 15 'Status of care home and care providers', the courts tended to the view that care home and home care operators, providing services under contract with local authorities, were exercising any functions of a public nature so as to make the operators liable under the Human Rights Act 1998. However, Parliament has now stepped in to reverse that. Section 73 of the Care Act 2014 provides that a person is to be taken as exercising a function of a public nature, for the purposes of section 6(3)(b) of the Human Rights Act 1998 in providing care or support if:

- the care or support is arranged by an English local authority, or paid for (directly or indirectly, in whole or in part); if that is done
- under sections 2, 18, 19, 20, 38 or 48 of the Care Act 2014; and
- the care provider is registered and provides care and support to an adult in the course of providing personal care in the place where the adult is residing, or residential accommodation together with nursing or personal care.

25.27 Similar provision is made in respect of Wales, Scotland and Northern Ireland in section 73(1)(b)–(d).

25.28 In addition:

- private hospitals discharging functions under the Mental Health Act 1983 are 'public authorities' for these purposes: *R (A) v Partnerships in Care Limited*;[55] and
- registered social landlords are discharging a public function for the purposes of the Human Rights Act 1998 when they manage their social

55 [2002] EWHC 529 (Admin), (2002) 5 CCLR 330.

housing stock and may also be amenable to judicial review in such cases, including when they are, at the same time, providing a form of social care: *R (Weaver) v London and Quadrant Housing Trust*.[56]

Positive obligations

25.29 A recurrent issue in social and health care cases is the extent to which the ECHR, in particular Article 8 ECHR, imposes a positive duty to provide a social or health care service.

25.30 Article 8 ECHR confers on persons a *'right to respect'* for their existing private and family lives and their home and protects persons from any unnecessary and unjustified State *'interference'* in these areas. Thus, it is said, Article 8 ECHR contains a *'negative obligation'* or *'prohibition'* and aims at preventing interference by the State: the knock on the door at night, for example.

25.31 The primary focus of Article 8 ECHR is, indeed, negative in this sense but it has been clear since the earliest case-law of the ECtHR that 'Article 8 does not merely compel the state to abstain from interference. In addition to this, there may be positive obligations inherent in any effective respect for private and family life even in the sphere of the relations of individuals between themselves'.[57]

25.32 In the final analysis, whether Article 8 imposes a positive obligation to provide a service, and whether Article 8 prevents state interference, both depend on the *'fair balance'* that has to be struck between the competing interests of the individual and the community.[58]

25.33 It often seems relatively easy for a court to determine whether State *interference* strikes a fair balance between the competing interests of the individual and society, in the light of the test in Article 8, which requires that any interference is 'necessary in a democratic society in the interests of national security, public safety or the economic well-being of the country, for the prevention of disorder or crime, for the protection of health or morals, or for the protection of the rights and freedoms of other'.

25.34 It often seems much harder for a court to determine, with confidence, that a State failure to take positive action fails to strike a fair balance between the individual and the community. The case-law reveals (i) relevant factors, (ii) the types of case that have succeeded.

25.35 Relevant factors are: (i) the extent to which *'fundamental values'* and *'essential aspects of private life'*[59] or a *'vital interest'*[60] protected by the ECHR are in issue; (ii) the degree of harm that the individual will suffer unless positively assisted;[61] (iii) the breadth and clarity of the positive obligation sought to be imposed;[62] (iv) the extent of consensus on the issue amongst

56 [2009] EWCA Civ 587, [2010] 1 WLR 363.

57 *Marckz v Belgium* (1979) 2 EHRR 330 at para 31.

58 *R (Quila) v Secretary of State for the Home Department* [2011] UKSC 45, [2012] 1 AC 621 at para 69.

59 *X & Y v Netherlands* (1985) 8 EHRR 235 at para 27.

60 *Gaskin v United Kingdom* (1989) 12 EHRR 36 at para 42.

61 *Stjerna v Finland* (1994) 24 EHRR 194 at para 42.

62 *Botta v Italy* (1998) 26 EHRR 241 at para 35.

Council of Europe State or internationally;[63] (v) the extent to which imposing a positive obligation would require the State to change the way in which it allocates scarce financial resources or, otherwise, impinge on matters of political, social or economic policy judgment.[64]

25.36 Consequently, a State may well be under a positive obligation to take relatively inexpensive steps where fundamental interests are at stake, such as (i) officially to recognise a person's changed gender[65] or choice of name;[66] (ii) to determine paternity;[67] and to (iii) to provide access to vital personal information.[68] In general, however, something very special is needed, and the ECHR will not generally require the State to make positive provision of housing,[69] disabled facilities[70] or healthcare.[71]

25.37 It has been suggested that it is more likely that positive provision will be required where such is necessary to preserve family life involving children or to ameliorate suffering so severe as to be comparable with inhuman and degrading treatment;[72] and a discriminatory failure to make positive provision seems well within the scope of ECHR redress.[73]

25.38 Article 8 ECHR may require a public authority to provide services where a failure to do so fails to strike a proportionate balance between the public and private interests at stake and where, otherwise:

- an individual, especially a vulnerable individual, will experience damage to their private life so serious as to be at or around the inhuman or degrading level;[74]
- the health or welfare of a child will be very seriously damaged;[75]
- there will be very serious damage to family life, especially if it involves humiliating or very distressing episodes;[76]
- an individual, or family, will be required to leave the UK before proper consideration has been given to their application for leave to remain on ECHR grounds, providing that the application is not manifestly abusive.[77]

25.39 Article 3 ECHR will require public authorities to provide services in the following circumstances:

- a public authority is under an absolute duty to provide services so far as necessary to alleviate inhuman or degrading suffering caused by its own treatment of the individual, whether that treatment is obvious and

63 *Goodwin v United Kingdom* (2002) 35 EHRR 18 at paras 84–85.
64 *Pentiacova v Moldova* (2005) 40 EHRR SE23.
65 *Goodwin v United Kingdom* (2002) 35 EHRR 53.
66 *Bulgakov v Ukraine* (59894/00, 11 September 2007) at para 43.
67 *Znamenskaya v Russia* (2007) 44 EHRR 15.
68 *Gaskin v United Kingdom* (1989) 12 EHRR 36.
69 *Marzari v Italy* (2000) 30 EHRR CD.
70 *Botta v Italy (*1998) 26 EHRR 241.
71 *Pentiacova v Moldova* (2005) 40 EHRR SE23.
72 *R (Anufrijeva) v Southwark LBC* [2003] EWHC Civ 1406, (2003) 6 CCLR 415.
73 *van Kuck v Germany* (2005) 8 CCLR 121.
74 *R (Anufrijeva) v Southwark LBC* [2003] EWCA Civ 1406, (2003) 6 CCLR 415.
75 *R (Anufrijeva) v Southwark LBC* [2003] EWCA Civ 1406, (2003) 6 CCLR 415.
76 *R (Bernard) v Enfield LBC* [2002] EWHC 2282 (Admin), (2002) 5 CCLR 577.
77 *R (Clue) v Birmingham CC* [2010] EWCA Civ 460, (2010) 13 CCLR 276.

direct (eg sentencing a disabled person to prison when conditions at the prison turn out to be grossly unsuitable[78]) or less obvious but in substance still direct (eg excluding an asylum-seeker from support whilst also barring them from mainstream benefits and employment[79]);

- a public authority is under a duty to take reasonable steps to prevent the inhuman or degrading treatment of individuals, in particular vulnerable individuals, that it knows about, or ought reasonably to know about (eg abuse perpetrated on children or vulnerable adults by their carers);[80]
- a public authority may sometimes be under a positive duty to alleviate inhuman or degrading suffering, whatever the cause, for example, where the individual concerned is especially vulnerable and/or where the public authority is already under an obligation in national law to take positive steps.[81]

25.40 In addition, Articles 3 and 8 ECHR require that laws, procedures and decisions relating to the provision of medical and social care are (i) published; (ii) reasonably clear and functional; and (iii) manifest an understanding of and due regard for the issues at stake for the individual.[82]

The application of ECHR law

25.41 Sections 2–4 of the Human Rights Act 1998 regulate the ways in which ECHR law meshes with existing national law and court procedures.

Section 2

25.42 By virtue of section 2, courts and tribunals 'must take into account' judgments of the European Court of Human Rights (and other specified material) when determining questions that have arisen in connection with ECHR rights. This means that:

- a UK court will usually apply principles that are clearly established in the European Court of Human Rights;
- where a UK court considers that, exceptionally, the European Court of Human Rights may not have adequately taken into account important features of the national scene, it may decline to follow decisions of the European Court of Human Rights, on the basis that this will enable the European Court of Human Rights to reconsider the position ('judicial dialogue');
- however, once an issue has been considered by the Grand Chamber of the European Court of Human Rights, in particular if that has occurred on more than one occasion, there would have to be some truly fundamental affront to the principles of UK law or some most egregious oversight or misunderstanding before a UK court could contemplate

78 *Price v United Kingdom* (2002) 35 EHRR CD 316, (2002) 5 CCLR 306.
79 *R (Limbuela) v Secretary of State for the Home Department* [2005] UKHL 66, [2006] 1 AC 396, (2006) 9 CCLR 30.
80 *E v Chief Constable of the Royal Ulster Constabulary* [2008] UKHL 66, [2009] 1 AC 536.
81 *R (Anufrijeva) v Southwark LBC* [2003] EWCA Civ 1406, (2003) 6 CCLR 415.
82 *Tysiac v Poland* (2007) 45 EHRR 42.

an outright refusal to follow Strasbourg authority (*R (Chester) v Secretary of State for Justice*[83]);

- a lower court should not overrule a higher court in the light of new authority from the European Court of Human Rights, but grant permission to appeal to enable the higher court to consider the matter: *Kay v Lambeth LBC*.[84]

Section 3

25.43 In addition, by virtue of section 3, 'so far as it is possible to do so, primary and subordinate legislation must be read and given effect to in a way which is compatible with the Convention rights'. This accords courts and tribunals a far reaching responsibility:[85]

> 30. From this it follows that the interpretative obligation decreed by section 3 is of an unusual and far-reaching character. Section 3 may require a court to depart from the unambiguous meaning the legislation would otherwise bear. In the ordinary course the interpretation of legislation involves seeking the intention reasonably to be attributed to Parliament in using the language in question. Section 3 may require the court to depart from this legislative intention, that is, depart from the intention of the Parliament which enacted the legislation. The question of difficulty is how far, and in what circumstances, section 3 requires a court to depart from the intention of the enacting Parliament. The answer to this question depends upon the intention reasonably to be attributed to Parliament in enacting section 3.
>
> 31. On this the first point to be considered is how far, when enacting section 3, Parliament intended that the actual language of a statute, as distinct from the concept expressed in that language, should be determinative. Since section 3 relates to the 'interpretation' of legislation, it is natural to focus attention initially on the language used in the legislative provision being considered. But once it is accepted that section 3 may require legislation to bear a meaning which departs from the unambiguous meaning the legislation would otherwise bear, it becomes impossible to suppose Parliament intended that the operation of section 3 should depend critically upon the particular form of words adopted by the parliamentary draftsman in the statutory provision under consideration. That would make the application of section 3 something of a semantic lottery. If the draftsman chose to express the concept being enacted in one form of words, section 3 would be available to achieve Convention-compliance. If he chose a different form of words, section 3 would be impotent.
>
> 32. From this the conclusion which seems inescapable is that the mere fact the language under consideration is inconsistent with a Convention-compliant meaning does not of itself make a Convention-compliant interpretation under section 3 impossible. Section 3 enables language to be interpreted restrictively or expansively. But section 3 goes further than this. It is also apt to require a court to read in words which change the meaning of the enacted legislation, so as to make it Convention-compliant. In other words, the intention of Parliament in enacting section 3 was that, to an extent bounded only by what is 'possible', a court can modify the meaning, and hence the effect, of primary and secondary legislation.

83 [2013] UKSC 63, [2014] AC 271.

84 [2006] UKHL 10, [2006] 2 AC 465.

85 *Ghaidan v Godin-Mendoza* [2004] UKHL 30, [2004] 2 AC 557.

33. Parliament, however, cannot have intended that in the discharge of this extended interpretative function the courts should adopt a meaning inconsistent with a fundamental feature of legislation. That would be to cross the constitutional boundary section 3 seeks to demarcate and preserve. Parliament has retained the right to enact legislation in terms which are not Convention-compliant. The meaning imported by application of section 3 must be compatible with the underlying thrust of the legislation being construed. Words implied must, in the phrase of my noble and learned friend, Lord Rodger of Earlsferry, 'go with the grain of the legislation'. Nor can Parliament have intended that section 3 should require courts to make decisions for which they are not equipped. There may be several ways of making a provision Convention-compliant, and the choice may involve issues calling for legislative deliberation.

34. Both these features were present in *In re S (Minors) (Care Order: Implementation of Care Plan)* [2002] 2 AC 291. There the proposed 'starring system' was inconsistent in an important respect with the scheme of the Children Act 1989, and the proposed system had far-reaching practical ramifications for local authorities. Again, in *R (Anderson) v Secretary of State for the Home Department* [2003] 1 AC 837 section 29 of the Crime (Sentences) Act 1997 could not be read in a Convention-compliant way without giving the section a meaning inconsistent with an important feature expressed clearly in the legislation. In *Bellinger v Bellinger* (Lord Chancellor intervening) [2003] 2 AC 467 recognition of Mrs Bellinger as female for the purposes of section 11(c) of the Matrimonial Causes Act 1973 would have had exceedingly wide ramifications, raising issues ill-suited for determination by the courts or court procedures.

Section 4

25.44 Finally, by virtue of section 4, where primary legislation simply cannot be construed compatibly with ECHR rights, and an individual has suffered a breach of their ECHR rights,[86] as a last resort, the High Court and above may make a 'declaration of incompatibility', which allows a Minister of the Crown to amend the legislation (section 10):

- this leaves Parliament free to examine the situation and determine the best means of resolving the incompatibility[87]; however,
- it does not impose a legal obligation on the Secretary of State to introduce remedial or amending legislation, or any obligation on Parliament;[88] and
- meanwhile, the incompatible legislation continues in effect;[89] so that
- alternative legal routes have to be considered if the individual concerned is to secure action that respects their ECHR rights. Often, there will be no alternative legal route. Where there is, it cannot be used

86 *Secretary of State for Defence v Nicholas* [2015] EWCA Civ 53, [2015] 1 WLR 2116 at paras 17–24.

87 *R (Hooper) v Secretary of State for Work and Pensions* [2003] EWCA Civ 813, [2003] 1 WLR 2623 at para [78]; *R (M) v Secretary of State for Health* [2003] EWHC 1094 (Admin) at para 18.

88 Ibid.

89 Ibid.

simply to circumvent the incompatible legislation but it could be used to provide the individual with a benefit where they qualify under it.[90]

The United Nations Convention on the Rights of Persons with Disabilities

25.45 The United Kingdom ratified the United Nations Convention on the Rights of Persons with Disabilities (UNCRPD) on the 8 June 2009, and its optional protocol on the 7 August 2010.

25.46 The United Nations Convention on the Rights of Persons with Disabilities adopts a *'social model of disability'*, as including 'those who have long-term physical, mental, intellectual or sensory impairments which in interaction with various barriers may hinder their full and effective participation in society on an equal basis with others' (Article 1).

25.47 Article 3 sets out General Principles, as follows:

Article 3 – General principles

The principles of the present Convention shall be:

a) Respect for inherent dignity, individual autonomy including the freedom to make one's own choices, and independence of persons;
b) Non-discrimination;
c) Full and effective participation and inclusion in society;
d) Respect for difference and acceptance of persons with disabilities as part of human diversity and humanity;
e) Equality of opportunity;
f) Accessibility;
g) Equality between men and women;
h) Respect for the evolving capacities of children with disabilities and respect for the right of children with disabilities to preserve their identities.

25.48 The United Nations Convention on the Rights of Persons with Disabilities sets out a number of civil and social rights, the most relevant of which, for present purposes, are at Articles 19, 25, 26 and 28:

Article 19 – Living independently and being included in the community

States Parties to this Convention recognize the equal right of all persons with disabilities to live in the community, with choices equal to others, and shall take effective and appropriate measures to facilitate full enjoyment by persons with disabilities of this right and their full inclusion and participation in the community, including by ensuring that:

a) Persons with disabilities have the opportunity to choose their place of residence and where and with whom they live on an equal basis with others and are not obliged to live in a particular living arrangement;
b) Persons with disabilities have access to a range of in-home, residential and other community support services, including personal assistance necessary to support living and inclusion in the community, and to prevent isolation or segregation from the community;

90 See chapter 17, 'Local authority general powers' and, in particular, *R (Morris) v Westminster CC* [2005] EWCA Civ 1184, [2006] 1 WLR 505.

c) Community services and facilities for the general population are available on an equal basis to persons with disabilities and are responsive to their needs.

Article 25 – Health

States Parties recognize that persons with disabilities have the right to the enjoyment of the highest attainable standard of health without discrimination on the basis of disability. States Parties shall take all appropriate measures to ensure access for persons with disabilities to health services that are gender-sensitive, including health-related rehabilitation. In particular, States Parties shall:

a) Provide persons with disabilities with the same range, quality and standard of free or affordable health care and programmes as provided to other persons, including in the area of sexual and reproductive health and population-based public health programmes;
b) Provide those health services needed by persons with disabilities specifically because of their disabilities, including early identification and intervention as appropriate, and services designed to minimize and prevent further disabilities, including among children and older persons;
c) Provide these health services as close as possible to people's own communities, including in rural areas;
d) Require health professionals to provide care of the same quality to persons with disabilities as to others, including on the basis of free and informed consent by, inter alia, raising awareness of the human rights, dignity, autonomy and needs of persons with disabilities through training and the promulgation of ethical standards for public and private health care;
e) Prohibit discrimination against persons with disabilities in the provision of health insurance, and life insurance where such insurance is permitted by national law, which shall be provided in a fair and reasonable manner;
f) Prevent discriminatory denial of health care or health services or food and fluids on the basis of disability.

Article 26 – Habilitation and rehabilitation

1) States Parties shall take effective and appropriate measures, including through peer support, to enable persons with disabilities to attain and maintain maximum independence, full physical, mental, social and vocational ability, and full inclusion and participation in all aspects of life. To that end, States Parties shall organize, strengthen and extend comprehensive habilitation and rehabilitation services and programmes, particularly in the areas of health, employment, education and social services, in such a way that these services and programmes:

a) Begin at the earliest possible stage, and are based on the multidisciplinary assessment of individual needs and strengths;
b) Support participation and inclusion in the community and all aspects of society, are voluntary, and are available to persons with disabilities as close as possible to their own communities, including in rural areas.

2) States Parties shall promote the development of initial and continuing training for professionals and staff working in habilitation and rehabilitation services.

3) States Parties shall promote the availability, knowledge and use of assistive devices and technologies, designed for persons with disabilities, as they relate to habilitation and rehabilitation.

Article 28 – Adequate standard of living and social protection

1) States Parties recognize the right of persons with disabilities to an adequate standard of living for themselves and their families, including adequate food, clothing and housing, and to the continuous improvement of living conditions, and shall take appropriate steps to safeguard and promote the realization of this right without discrimination on the basis of disability.

2) States Parties recognize the right of persons with disabilities to social protection and to the enjoyment of that right without discrimination on the basis of disability, and shall take appropriate steps to safeguard and promote the realization of this right, including measures:

a) To ensure equal access by persons with disabilities to clean water services, and to ensure access to appropriate and affordable services, devices and other assistance for disability-related needs;
b) To ensure access by persons with disabilities, in particular women and girls with disabilities and older persons with disabilities, to social protection programmes and poverty reduction programmes;
c) To ensure access by persons with disabilities and their families living in situations of poverty to assistance from the State with disability-related expenses, including adequate training, counselling, financial assistance and respite care;
d) To ensure access by persons with disabilities to public housing programmes;
e) To ensure equal access by persons with disabilities to retirement benefits and programmes.

25.49 The optional protocol, ratified by the United Kingdom on the 7 August 2010, recognises the competence of the *Committee on the Rights of Persons with Disabilities* to consider complaints from individuals or groups who claim that their rights under the United Nations Convention on the Rights of Persons with Disabilities have been violated.

25.50 The *Committee on the Rights of Persons with Disabilities* has published a number of General Comments explaining the nature of the Convention rights:[91]

- General Comment No 1 on Article 12: Equal recognition before the Law (11 April 2014);[92]
- General Comment No 2 on Article 9: Accessibility (11 April 2014).[93]

25.51 The jurisprudence of the Committee is currently somewhat limited,[94] and is mainly concerned with employment rights: it is question of '*watch this space*'.

25.52 It seems that the provisions of the ECHR are to be construed '*harmoniously*' with the general principles of international law including,

91 www.ohchr.org/EN/HRBodies/CRPD/Pages/GC.aspx.

92 http://daccess-dds-ny.un.org/doc/UNDOC/GEN/G14/031/20/PDF/G1403120.pdf?OpenElement.

93 http://daccess-dds-ny.un.org/doc/UNDOC/GEN/G14/033/13/PDF/G1403313.pdf?OpenElement.

94 http://tbinternet.ohchr.org/_layouts/treatybodyexternal/TBSearch.aspx?Lang=en&TreatyID=4&DocTypeCategoryID=6.

specifically, the UNCRPD: *Matheison v Secretary of State for Work and Pensions*;[95] and *SHH v United Kingdom*.[96] Any search of a case-law website will show that reference is being made to the United Nations Convention on the Rights of Persons with Disabilities in a large number of cases, in the Court of Protection as well as in judicial review cases.

Cases

Mental health/capacity

25.53 Please see chapter 19 'Mental health' and chapter 23 'Mental capacity' above for cases which evaluate the compatibility of national mental health law with the ECHR, in particular Article 5 ECHR.

Social care

25.54 *Botta v Italy* Application no 21439/93, [1998] ECHR 12, (1999) 2 CCLR 53

Article 8 ECHR might impose a positive obligation to provide services to a disabled person, but only where there was a direct and immediate connection between the service requested and the disabled person's private life

Facts: Mr Botta, who was a physically disabled wheelchair user, had been unable to gain access to a beach in Italy whilst on holiday, because it lacked access ramps and adapted toilets and washrooms.

Judgment: the Italian state was not in breach of a positive obligation to provide disabled facilities on the beach because there was no 'direct and immediate link between the measures sought and.... [Mr Botta's] private and/or family life'; indeed, in this case, Mr Botta's desire to gain access to a beach distant from his home area 'concerns interpersonal relationships of such broad and indeterminate scope that there can be no conceivable direct link between the measures the State was urged to take in order to make good the omissions of the private bathing establishments and the applicant's private life':

> 32. Private life, in the court's view, includes a person's physical and psychological integrity; the guarantee afforded by Article 8 of the Convention is primarily intended to ensure the development, without outside interference, of the personality of each individual in his relations with other human beings (see, *mutatis mutandis*, the *Niemietz v Germany* judgment of 16 December 1992, Series A no 251-B, p33, para 29).
>
> 33. In the instant case the applicant complained in substance not of action but of a lack of action by the State. While the essential object of Article 8 is to protect the individual against arbitrary interference by the public authorities, it does not merely compel the State to abstain from such interference: in addition to this negative undertaking, there may be positive obligations inherent in effective respect for private or family life. These obligations may involve the adoption of measures designed to secure respect for private

95 [2015] UKSC 47, [2015] 1 ELT 3250 at paras 42–45.
96 (2013) 57 EHRR 18 at para 94.

life even in the sphere of the relations of individuals between themselves (see the *X and Y v The Netherlands* judgment of 26 March 1985, Series A no 91, p1, para 23, and the *Stjerna v Finland* judgment of 25 November 1994, Series A no 299-B, p61, para 38). However, the concept of respect is not precisely defined. In order to determine whether such obligations exist, regard must be had to the fair balance that has to be struck between the general interest and the interests of the individual, while the State has, in any event, a margin of appreciation.

34. The court has held that a State has obligations of this type where it has found a direct and immediate link between the measures sought by an applicant and the latter's private and/or family life.

Thus, in the case of *Airey v Ireland* (judgment of 9 October 1979, Series A no 32), the court held that the applicant had been the victim of a violation of Article 8 on the ground that under domestic law there was no system of legal aid in separation proceedings, which by denying access to court directly affected her private and family life.

In the above-mentioned *X and Y v The Netherlands* case, which concerned the rape of a mentally handicapped person and accordingly related to her physical and psychological integrity, the Court found that because of its shortcomings the Netherlands Criminal Code had not provided the person concerned with practical and effective protection (p14, para 30).

More recently, in the *López Ostra v Spain* judgment (*mutatis mutandis*, 9 December 1994, Series A no 303-C), in connection with the harmful effects of pollution caused by the activity of a waste-water treatment plant situated near the applicant's home, the court held that the respondent State had not succeeded in striking a fair balance between the interest of the town of Lorca's economic well-being – that of having a waste-treatment plant – and the applicant's effective enjoyment of her right to respect for her home and her private and family life (p56, para 58).

Lastly, in the *Guerra and Others v Italy* judgment of 19 February 1998 (*mutatis mutandis, Reports of Judgments and Decisions* 1998-I), the court held that the direct effect of the toxic emissions from the Enichem factory on the applicants' right to respect for their private and family life meant that Article 8 was applicable (p227, para 57). It decided that Italy had breached that provision in that it had not communicated to the applicants essential information that would have enabled them to assess the risks they and their families might run if they continued to live in Manfredonia, a town particularly exposed to danger in the event of an accident within the confines of the factory (p228, para 60).

35. In the instant case, however, the right asserted by Mr Botta, namely the right to gain access to the beach and the sea at a place distant from his normal place of residence during his holidays, concerns interpersonal relations of such broad and indeterminate scope that there can be no conceivable direct link between the measures the State was urged to take in order to make good the omissions of the private bathing establishments and the applicant's private life.

Comment: see, to similar effect, *Zehnalova v The Czech Republic* Application no 38621/97 (judgment the 14 May 2002), *Farcas and Romania* Application no 67020/01 (judgment the 10 November 2005) and *Molka v Poland* Application no 56550/00 (judgment the 11 April 2006).

25.55 *R v North and East Devon Health Authority ex p Coughlan* [2001] QB 213, (1999) 2 CCLR 285, CA

Removing a person from their home, unjustifiably breaching a promise they could stay there for life, was incompatible with Article 8 ECHR

Facts: Ms Coughlan was rendered very severely disabled by a road traffic accident. After a period of treatment at Newcourt Hospital, which the health authority then wished to close, she and seven other patients were moved to Mardon House hospital, with an assurance that it would be their 'home for life'. However, the health authority then resolved to close Mardon House. In addition, it determined that Ms Coughlan no longer met the criteria for NHS continuing healthcare, so that she had to resort to local authority residential accommodation. Ms Coughlan submitted that it was beyond the powers of a local authority to provide her with the nursing care she needed and that it was unlawful for the health authority to resile from its 'home for life' promise; and a breach of Article 8 ECHR.

Judgment: the Court of Appeal (Lord Woolf MR, Mummery,Sedley LJJ) held, on the ECHR point:

> 93. The judge was entitled to treat this as a case where the Health Authority's conduct was in breach of Article 8 and was not justified by the provisions of Article 8(2). Mardon House is, in the circumstances described, Miss Coughlan's home. It has been that since 1993. It was promised to be just that for the rest of her life. It is not suggested that it is not her home or that she has a home elsewhere or that she has done anything to justify depriving her of her home at Mardon House. By closure of Mardon House the Health Authority will interfere with what will soon be her right to her home. For the reasons explained, the Health Authority would not be justified in law in doing so without providing accommodation which meets her needs.. As Sir Thomas Bingham MR said in *R v Ministry of Defence ex p Smith* [1996] QB 517 at 554E:
>
> > 'The more substantial the interference with human rights, the more the court will require by way of justification before it is satisfied that the decision is reasonable ...'
>
> or, we would add, in a case such as the present, fair.

25.56 *Marzari v Italy* Application no 36448/97, (1999) 28 EHRR CD 175

Article 8 ECHR could impose a positive obligation to provide housing assistance in the case of a severely disabled man, where there was a direct and immediate serious adverse impact on his private life

Facts: Mr Marzari claimed that a number of housing-related difficulties experienced by him, connected with his serious disability, resulted from violations of his rights under Article 8 ECHR.

Judgment: the European Court of Human Rights declared the application inadmissible on its facts, but did accept that a positive obligation could arise under Article 8 ECHR, to provide housing assistance to a disabled person:

> The court considers that, although Article 8 does not guarantee the right to have one's housing problem solved by the authorities, a refusal of the authorities to provide assistance in his respect to an individual suffering

from a severe disease might in certain circumstances raise an issue under Article 8 of the Convention because of the impact of such refusal on the private life of the individual. The court recalls in his respect that, while the essential object of Article 8 is to protect the individual against arbitrary interference by public authorities, this provision does not merely compel the State to abstain from such interference: in addition to this negative undertaking, there may be positive obligations inherent in effective respect for private life. A State has obligations of his type where there is a direct and immediate link between the measures sought by an applicant and the latter's private life (*Botta v Italy* (1998) 26 EHRR 241, paras 33–34).

25.57 *Z v United Kingdom* Application no 29392/95, [2001] ECHR 333, (2001) 4 CCLR 310

Article 3 imposes a duty to take reasonable steps to provide effective protection to children and other vulnerable persons whom the state knows, or ought reasonably to know, are being subjected to inhuman or degrading treatment

Facts: the applicants were siblings who had suffered personal injury as a result of abuse and neglect while living with their parents. The local social services authority had been aware of the situation for a period of years but had failed to take effective action.

Judgment: the treatment meted out by the parents violated the children's rights under Article 3 ECHR; moreover, the State was itself in breach of Article 3, in that it had failed in its duty to take measures to provide effective protection to children and other vulnerable persons, including by taking reasonable steps to prevent ill-treatment of which the authorities knew or ought to have known. The applicants had also been denied a remedy, in breach of Article 13 of the ECHR in that, because the House of Lords had determined that the local authority had not owed the applicants a duty of care in negligence, then, notwithstanding the availability of complaints to the CICB and the LGO, the applicants had not had available to them an appropriate means of obtaining a determination of their allegation that the local authority had failed to protect them from inhuman and degrading treatment and the possibility of obtaining compensation. The court awarded the children pecuniary damages (for loss of earnings, the cost of medical treatment etc) of £8,000, £100,000, £80,000 and £4,000 and non-pecuniary damages of £32,000 each.

25.58 *TP and KM v United Kingdom* Application no 28945/95, [2001] ECHR 332, (2001) 4 CCLR 398

The failure to disclose to material that undermined the local authority case of child abuse against a male carer had been incompatible with Article 8 ECHR; as had the failure to promote contact between the child and her family

Facts: Newham LBC took child protection proceedings, on the basis of suspected sexual abuse of a child, KM, by XY, a male who lived with KM's mother, TP. Newham interviewed KM on video and KM asserted that she had been abused, but not by XY, rather, by another male, X. Newham made KM a ward of court, without disclosing the video. The existence of the video eventually came to light and mother and child were re-united, but only after having been separated for about a year. Mother and child sued Newham in negligence but the proceedings were struck out, ultimately by the House of Lords, on the basis that Newham had not owed either a duty of care.

Judgment: the European Court of Human Rights held that the United Kingdom had violated TP's and KM's rights under Articles 8 and 13 ECHR:

> 70. In determining whether the impugned measures were 'necessary in a democratic society', the court will consider whether, in the light of the case as a whole, the reasons adduced to justify them were relevant and sufficient for the purposes of paragraph 2 of Article 8 of the Convention. Undoubtedly, consideration of what lies in the best interest of the child is of crucial importance in every case of this kind. Moreover, it must be borne in mind that the national authorities have the benefit of direct contact with all the persons concerned. It follows from these considerations that the court's task is not to substitute itself for the domestic authorities in the exercise of their responsibilities regarding custody and access issues, but rather to review, in the light of the Convention, the decisions taken by those authorities in the exercise of their power of appreciation (see the *Hokkanen v Finland* judgment of 23 September 1994, Series A no 299-A, p20, para 55, and, *mutatis mutandis*, the *Bronda v Italy* judgment of 9 June 1998, *Reports of Judgments and Decisions* 1998-IV, p1491, para 59).
>
> 71. The margin of appreciation to be accorded to the competent national authorities will vary in accordance with the nature of the issues and the importance of the interests at stake. Thus, the court recognises that the authorities enjoy a wide margin of appreciation, in particular when assessing the necessity of taking a child into care. However, a stricter scrutiny is called for in respect of any further limitations, such as restrictions placed by those authorities on parental rights of access, and of any legal safeguards designed to secure an effective protection of the right of parents and children to respect for their family life. Such further limitations entail the danger that the family relations between the parents and a young child would be effectively curtailed (see, amongst other authorities, the *Johansen v Norway* judgment of 7 August 1996, *Reports* 1996-III, p1003, para 64).
>
> 72. The court further recalls that whilst Article 8 contains no explicit procedural requirements, the decision-making process involved in measures of interference must be fair and such as to afford due respect to the interests safeguarded by Article 8:
>
>> '[W]hat has to be determined is whether, having regard to the particular circumstances of the case and notably the serious nature of the decisions to be taken, the parents have been involved in the decision-making process, seen as a whole, to a degree sufficient to provide them with the requisite protection of their interests. If they have not, there will have been a failure to respect their family life and the interference resulting from the decision will not be capable of being regarded as 'necessary' within the meaning of Article 8.' (see the *W v United Kingdom* judgment of 8 July 1987, Series A no. 121-A, pp. 28–29, paras 62 and 64).
>
> 73. It has previously found that the failure to disclose relevant documents to parents during the procedures instituted by the authorities in placing and maintaining a child in care meant that the decision-making process determining the custody and access arrangements did not afford the requisite protection of the parents' interests as safeguarded by Article 8 (see the *McMichael v United Kingdom* judgment of 24 February 1995, Series A no 307-B, p57, para 92).

> …
>
> 83. The court concludes that the question whether to disclose the video of the interview and its transcript should have been determined promptly to allow the first applicant an effective opportunity to deal with the allegations that her daughter could not be returned safely to her care. The local authority's failure to submit the issue to the court for determination deprived her of an adequate involvement in the decision-making process concerning the care of her daughter and thereby of the requisite protection of their interests. There was in this respect a failure to respect their family life and a breach of Article 8 of the Convention.

25.59 *Price v United Kingdom* Application no 33394/96, [2001] ECHR 458, (2002) 5 CCLR 306

It had been a breach of Article 3 ECHR to detain a severely disabled woman in grossly unsuitable conditions

Facts: Ms Price, who was severely disabled as a result of Thalidomide, was imprisoned for three nights and four days in wholly unsuitable conditions.

Judgment: the European Court of Human Rights held that Ms Price had been subjected to inhuman and degrading treatment in breach of Article 3 ECHR and was awarded £4,500 damages:

> 24. The court recalls that ill-treatment must attain a minimum level of severity if it is to fall within the scope of Article 3. The assessment of this minimum level of severity is relative; it depends on all the circumstances of the case, such as the duration of the treatment, its physical and mental effects and, in some cases, the sex, age and state of health of the victim.
>
> In considering whether treatment is 'degrading' within the meaning of Article 3, one of the factors which the court will take into account is the question whether its object was to humiliate and debase the person concerned, although the absence of any such purpose cannot conclusively rule out a finding of violation of Article 3 (see the *Peers v Greece* judgment of 19 April 2001, paragraphs 67–68 and 74).
>
> …
>
> 30. There is no evidence in this case of any positive intention to humiliate or debase the applicant. However, the court considers that to detain a severely disabled person in conditions where she is dangerously cold, risks developing sores because her bed is too hard or unreachable, and is unable to go to the toilet or keep clean without the greatest of difficulty, constitutes degrading treatment contrary to Article 3 of the Convention. It therefore finds a violation of this provision in the present case.

Comment: there have been many subsequent cases where the European Court has decided that prison conditions have amounted to inhuman and degrading treatment for disabled prisoners: *Vincent v France* Application no 6253/03 (judgment 24 October 2006); *ZH v Hungary* Application no 28973/11 (judgment 6 November 2011); *Arutyunyan v Russia* Application no 48977/09 (judgment 10 January 2012); *Zarzycki v Poland* Application no 15351/03 (judgment 12 March 2013) (no breach); *Grimailovs v Latvia* Application no 6087/03 (judgment 25 June 2013); *Semikhvostov v Russia* Application no 2689/12 (judgment 6 February 2014); *Asalya v Turkey* Application no 43875/09 (judgment 15 April 2014); *Helhal v France* Application no 1040/12 (judgment 19 February 2015).

25.60 *Passannante v Italy* Application no 32647/96, (2002) 5 CCLR 340

A delay in providing healthcare to which a person was entitled by virtue of contributions might raise an issue under Article 8 ECHR if there was a serious risk to health

Facts: Ms Passannate was told she would have to wait five months to see a consultant at public expense but could see him in four days on a private paying basis. She declined to see the consultant at all and claimed that her rights under Article 8 ECHR had been breached.

Judgment: the Commission declared the complaint inadmissible but held the door ajar for stronger cases:

> The Commission recalls that, while the essential object of Article 8 is to protect the individual against arbitrary interference by the public authorities, it does not merely compel the State to abstain from such interference: in addition to this negative undertaking, there may be positive obligations inherent in effective respect for private life (see ECtHR, *Stjerna v Finland* judgment of 25 November 1994, Series A No 299-B, p 61, para 38 and ECtHR, *Botta* judgment of 24 February 1998, para 33, cited above).
>
> The Commission notes the Italian public health service is based on compulsory contributions which entitle those who pay them to certain services, among which medical examinations within public hospitals. Therefore, the Commission considers that, in such circumstances where the State has an obligation to provide medical care, an excessive delay of the public health service in providing a medical service to which the patient is entitled and the fact that such delay has, or is likely to have, a serious impact on the patient's health could raise an issue under Article 8 para 1 of the Convention.
>
> The Commission notes the absence under domestic law of time-limits within which a person should be granted the required medical service. However, although the applicant submits that she had to wait five months in order merely to book the medical examination, she did not prove nor even allege that the above delay had a serious impact on her physical or psychological conditions.
>
> The Commission further notes that the applicant, after the telephone conversation with the hospital's operator, apparently renounced from seeing the doctor which indicates, in the Commission's opinion, that she did not consider the medical visit crucial for her health.
>
> Therefore the Commission considers that the circumstances of the present case are not such as to warrant the conclusion that the delay of the public authorities raises a serious issue under Article 8 of the Convention and that the present application is manifestly ill-founded within the meaning of Article 27 para 2 of the Convention.
>
> For these reasons, the Commission, unanimously, declares the application inadmissible.

25.61 *R (Bernard) v Enfield LBC* [2002] EWHC 2282 (Admin), (2002) 5 CCLR 577

A serious failure to provide the services required under section 21 of the National Assistance Act 1948, which had severe repercussion on Ms Bernard's family and private law, breached Article 8 ECHR

Facts: Mrs Bernard and her family had become intentionally homeless but meanwhile occupied temporary accommodation provided under the Housing Act 1996. Being unable to secure suitable, alternative accommodation, because of Mrs Bernard's disability, they sought a community care assessment from Enfield. Enfield assessed Mrs Bernard as being wholly wheelchair dependent, but as being unable to use her wheelchair in her home, confining her to the living room, where she had no privacy and was in discomfort, as being wholly dependent on her husband and as being unable to gain access to the bathroom without great difficulty, although she was doubly incontinent: it concluded that the family needed assistance to move to suitable adapted accommodation. Enfield failed to secure the family's re-housing and meanwhile Mrs Bernard's circumstances remained dire: not only did she lack privacy, and any ability to mobilise within the home, she was incontinent in the living room several times a day, so that her husband had to clean her and her clothes/bedding and the carpets.

Judgment: Sullivan J noted that Enfield accepted that, in substance, it had assessed Mrs Bernard as requiring to be moved to suitable, adapted accommodation so as to trigger the duty to provide residential accommodation in section 21 of the National Assistance Act 1948. He held that Enfield's failure to discharge that duty, for about 20 months, did not quite reach the threshold of inhuman or degrading treatment in breach of Article 3 ECHR, but that it was an unjustified breach of Mrs Bernard's rights under Article 8, for which damages would be awarded of £10,000 (£8,000 for Mrs Bernard and £2,000 for her husband):

> 32. I accept the defendant's submission that not every breach of duty under section 21 of the 1948 Act will result in a breach of Article 8. Respect for private and family life does not require the state to provide every one of its citizens with a house: see the decision of Jackson J in *Morris v Newham LBC* [2002] EWHC 1262 (Admin) paras 59–62. However, those entitled to care under section 21 are a particularly vulnerable group. Positive measures have to be taken (by way of community care facilities) to enable them to enjoy, so far as possible, a normal private and family life. In *Morris* Jackson J was concerned with an unlawful failure to provide accommodation under Part VII of the Housing Act 1996, but the same approach is equally applicable to the duty to provide suitably adapted accommodation under the 1948 Act. Whether the breach of statutory duty has also resulted in an infringement of the claimants' Article 8 rights will depend upon all the circumstances of the case. Just what was the effect of the breach in practical terms on the claimants' family and private life?
>
> 33. Following the assessments in September 2000 the defendant was under an obligation not merely to refrain from unwarranted interference in the claimants' family life, but also to take positive steps, including the provision of suitably adapted accommodation, to enable the claimants and their children to lead as normal a family life as possible, bearing in mind the second claimant's severe disabilities. Suitably adapted accommodation would not merely have facilitated the normal incidents of family life, for example the second claimant would have been able to move around her home to some extent and would have been able to play some part, together with the first claimant, in looking after their children. It would also have secured her 'physical and psychological integrity'. She would no longer have been

> housebound, confined to a shower chair for most of the day, lacking privacy in the most undignified of circumstances, but would have been able to operate again as part of her family and as a person in her own right, rather than being a burden, wholly dependent upon the rest of her family. In short, it would have restored her dignity as a human being.
>
> 34. The Council's failure to act on the September 2000 assessments showed a singular lack of respect for the claimants' private and family life. It condemned the claimants to living conditions which made it virtually impossible for them to have any meaningful private or family life for the purposes of Article 8. Accordingly, I have no doubt that the defendant was not merely in breach of its statutory duty under the 1948 Act. Its failure to act on the September 2000 assessments over a period of 20 months was also incompatible with the claimants' rights under Article 8 of the Convention.

Comment: this is a rare, extreme case where a failure to provide services (in breach of a statutory obligation) violated ECHR rights (although Article 8, still not Article 3) and resulted in an award of financial compensation.

25.62 *R (S) v Plymouth CC* [2002] EWCA Civ 388, (2002) 5 CCLR 251

Fairness and the ECHR required disclosure of the son's mental health records to his mother, in nearest relative displacement proceedings

Facts: C suffered from a mental disorder and mental impairment. His mother, who was his nearest relative, opposed his being made subject to a guardianship order but, despite requests by her, she had not been shown the material on which that proposed application would be based, on the ground that it was confidential and C lacked capacity to consent to its disclosure to his mother.

Judgment: the Court of Appeal (Kennedy (dissenting in part), Clarke and Hale LJJ) held that such material would have to be disclosed in any proceedings to displace the nearest relative and that such proceedings were likely if the mother continued to object. For that reason, and because of the importance under the ECHR of involving the mother, disclosure would be ordered – not just to the mother's lawyers and expert, but also (Kennedy LJ dissenting) to the mother personally. Hale LJ said this:

> 48. Hence both the common law and the Convention require that a balance be struck between the various interests involved. These are the confidentiality of the information sought; the proper administration of justice; the mother's right of access to legal advice to enable her to decide whether or not to exercise a right which is likely to lead to legal proceedings against her if she does so; the rights of both C and his mother to respect for their family life and adequate involvement in decision-making processes about it; C's right to respect for his private life; and the protection of C's health and welfare. In some cases there might also be an interest in the protection of other people, but that has not been seriously suggested here.
>
> 49. C's interest in protecting the confidentiality of personal information about himself must not be underestimated. It is all too easy for professionals and parents to regard children and incapacitated adults as having no independent interests of their own: as objects rather than subjects. But we are not concerned here with the publication of information to the whole wide world. There is a clear distinction between disclosure to the media with a view to publication to all and sundry and disclosure in confidence

to those with a proper interest in having the information in question. We are concerned here only with the latter. The issue is only whether the circle should be widened from those professionals with whom this information has already been shared (possibly without much conscious thought being given to the balance of interests involved) to include the person who is probably closest to him in fact as well as in law and who has a statutory role in his future and to those professionally advising her. C also has an interest in having his own wishes and feelings respected. It would be different in this case if he had the capacity to give or withhold consent to the disclosure: any objection from him would have to be weighed in the balance against the other interests, although as *W v Egdell* [1990] Ch 359 shows, it would not be decisive. C also has an interest in being protected from a risk of harm to his health or welfare which would stem from disclosure; but it is important not to confuse a possible risk of harm to his health or welfare from being discharged from guardianship with a possible risk of harm from disclosing the information sought. As *In re D (Minors) (Adoption Reports: Confidentiality)* [1996] AC 593 shows, he also has an interest in decisions about his future being properly informed.

50. That balance would not lead in every case to the disclosure of all the information a relative might possibly want, still less to a fishing exercise amongst the local authority's files. But in most cases it would lead to the disclosure of the basic statutory guardianship documentation. In this case it must also lead to the particular disclosure sought. There is no suggestion that C has any objection to his mother and her advisers being properly informed about his health and welfare. There is no suggestion of any risk to his health and welfare arising from this. The mother and her advisers have sought access to the information which her own psychiatric and social work experts need in order properly to advise her. That limits both the context and the content of disclosure in a way which strikes a proper balance between the competing interests.

25.63 *R (Beeson) v Dorset CC and Secretary of State for Health* [2002] EWCA Civ 1812, (2003) 6 CCLR 5

It was compatible with Article 6 ECHR for disputes about social care charges to be determined by local authorities subject to judicial review, rather than a merits appeal

Facts: after having suffered a stroke, but before going into residential care, Mr Beeson transferred his home to his son, by deed of gift. Dorset concluded that Mr Beeson had deprived himself of capital for the purpose of decreasing the amount that he might become liable to pay for residential accommodation and treated the value of the home as notional capital.

Judgment: the Court of Appeal (The President, Waller and Laws LJJ) held that the decision-making process involved a determination of Mr Beeson's civil rights and obligations, for the purposes of Article 6 ECHR because the question of what accommodation Mr Beeson would occupy, and on what terms, affected his rights in private law. However, Mr Beeson had had 'a fair and public hearing within a reasonable time by an independent and impartial tribunal established by law', in that he had utilised Dorset's complaints procedure (culminating in a hearing before a panel comprising two councillors and an independent chair) and then judicial review. Although the issues were fact-laden and turned on credibility, the context was a statutory scheme instituted by Parliament for the allocation of public resources by a local authority and in that context the availability of judicial review as an ultimate recourse, notwithstanding its restricted ambit, satisfied the requirements of Article 6 ECHR.

25.64 *R (A and B) v East Sussex CC* [2003] EWHC 167 (Admin), (2003) 6 CCLR 194

The recognition and protection of human dignity is a core value protected by Article 8 ECHR. Nonetheless the rights of persons with disabilities required to be balanced against those of their carers, where there was a conflict

Facts: A and B were severely disabled sisters who continued to live in the family home, owing to a dispute with Sussex over aspects of the care package, in particular, as to the extent to which Sussex could be required to instruct carers to undertake manual lifting.

Judgment: Munby J held that it was necessary to balance the Article 8 rights of the sisters and their carers. He gave prolonged consideration to the case-law relating to Article 8 ECHR in the adult social care context, including the following:

> 85. In *Botta*, as we have seen, the court identified a person's 'physical and psychological integrity' as being part of the private life protected by Article 8 and which the State may in principle be under an obligation to take positive steps to protect. In the present type of case this 'physical and psychological integrity' embraces, though it is not of course confined to, two particularly important concepts which for the purposes of proper analysis it is desirable to distinguish and consider separately.
>
> 86. The first is human dignity. True it is that the phrase is not used in the Convention but it is surely immanent in Article 8, indeed in almost every one of the Convention's provisions. The recognition and protection of human dignity is one of the core values – in truth *the* core value – of our society and, indeed, of all the societies which are part of the European family of nations and which have embraced the principles of the Convention. It is a core value of the common law, long pre-dating the Convention and the Charter. The invocation of the dignity of the patient in the form of declaration habitually used when the court is exercising its inherent declaratory jurisdiction in relation to the gravely ill or dying is not some meaningless incantation designed to comfort the living or to assuage the consciences of those involved in making life and death decisions: it is a solemn affirmation of the law's and of society's recognition of our humanity and of human dignity as something fundamental. Not surprisingly, human dignity is extolled in Article 1 of the Charter, just as it is in Article 1 of the Universal Declaration. And the latter's call to us to 'act towards one another in a spirit of brotherhood' is nothing new. It reflects the fourth Earl of Chesterfield's injunction, 'Do as you would be done by' and, for the Christian, the biblical call (Matthew ch 7, v 12): 'all things whatsoever ye would that men should do to you, do ye even so to them: for this is the law and the prophets'.
>
> ...
>
> 99. The other important concept embraced in the 'physical and psychological integrity' protected by Article 8 is the right of the disabled to participate in the life of the community and to have what has been described (see below) as 'access to essential economic and social activities and to an appropriate range of recreational and cultural activities'. This is matched by the

> positive obligation of the State to take appropriate measures designed to ensure to the greatest extent feasible that a disabled person is not 'so circumscribed and so isolated as to be deprived of the possibility of developing his personality'.

25.65 *Collins v United Kingdom* Application no 11909/02, (2003) 6 CCLR 388

It was lawful in national law to resile from a 'home for life' promise and in this case is had been proportionate and compatible with Article 8 ECHR

Facts: Ms Collins had been promised a 'home for life' at a bungalow in the hospital grounds, where she was a long-term resident. She sought to resist a proposal to re-locate her in a community setting on the ground that it was incompatible with her rights under Article 8 ECHR.

Judgment: the application was declared inadmissible: the local authority decision had been lawful as a matter of national law and, also, proportionate:

> As regards the necessity of the decision, the court observes that the applicant's principal objections to the decision are that it runs counter to her own wishes to remain where she is and to the promise made by the LHA that Long Leys would be a 'home for life'. Though the applicant's family sought to argue that a move would be harmful as the applicant disliked and reacted badly to a change in routine, the consultant psychiatrist who gave evidence to the court and who had experience of such moves took the view that the impact on the residents of the move would be beneficial in a wide range of areas. While it was noted that residents and their carers could often be resistant to change for understandable reasons, it was envisaged that with proper care and support the applicant would be able to cope with the move.
>
> The court further notes that in reaching the decision to move the applicant and the other residents the LHA consulted the concerned parties and was careful to obtain legal advice as to the status of the promise of a 'home for life'. It cannot therefore be said that the LHA did not give weight to the applicant's wishes or the assurance given many years before. The propriety of the decision-making procedure was, in addition, subject to the scrutiny of the High Court which found that the LHA had acted with due regard to all the relevant factors.
>
> Though the court considers that it was highly regrettable that a promise was apparently made that misled the applicant and her family into the belief that she would be able to remain at Long Leys indefinitely, this assurance was not, in the event, found to amount to a legally binding obligation on the LHA to comply with the applicant's personal preferences. The court does not find that this an unreasonable or arbitrary conclusion, since, given the vagaries of future circumstances, a statement made in 1990 could not realistically have been expected to guarantee the continued suitability of Long Leys as a placement for the applicant, whether for practical, medical or other reasons.
>
> In conclusion, the court finds that the decision to move the applicant from Long Leys into alternative social care was not disproportionate, gave proper consideration to her interests and was supported by relevant and sufficient reasons relative to her welfare. It may therefore be regarded as 'necessary in a democratic society' in the pursuit of protecting her rights.

It follows that the application must be rejected as manifestly ill-founded pursuant to Article 35(3) and (4) of the Convention.

For these reasons, the court unanimously declares the application inadmissible.

25.66 *R (Anufrijeva) v Southwark LBC* [2003] EWCA Civ 1406, (2003) 6 CCLR 415

A failure to provide a statutory service will usually only breach Article 8 ECHR where there is a level of culpability on the part of the authority and where the consequences are so serious as to be comparable with cases of violations of Article 3 ECHR although a lower threshold could apply in the case of children

Facts: Southwark was under a duty to secure suitable residential accommodation for Mrs Anufrijeva, under section 21 of the National Assistance Act 1948.

Judgment: on the facts, Southwark had made reasonable efforts to provide appropriate accommodation and it could not be said that Southwark had departed so far from what section 21 required as to amount to a breach of Article 8 ECHR:

> 45. In so far as Article 8 imposes positive obligations, these are not absolute. Before inaction can amount to a lack of respect for private and family life, there must be some ground for criticising the failure to act. There must be an element of culpability. At the very least there must be knowledge that the claimant's private and family life were at risk – see the approach of the ECtHR to the positive obligation in relation to Article 2 in *Osman v United Kingdom* (1998) 29 EHRR 245 and the discussion of Silber J in *N* at paragraphs 126 to 148. Where the domestic law of a State imposes positive obligations in relation to the provision of welfare support, breach of those positive obligations of domestic law may suffice to provide the element of culpability necessary to establish a breach of Article 8, provided that the impact on private or family life is sufficiently serious and was foreseeable.
>
> 46. Where the complaint is that there has been culpable delay in the administrative processes necessary to determine and to give effect to an Article 8 right, the approach of both the Strasbourg Court and the Commission has been not to find an infringement of Article 8 unless substantial prejudice has been caused to the applicant. In cases involving custody of children, procedural delay has been held to amount to a breach of Article 8 because of the prejudice such delay can have on the ultimate decision – thus in *H v United Kingdom* (1987) 10 EHRR 95 the court held Article 8 infringed by delay in the conduct of access and adoption proceedings because the proceedings 'lay within an area in which procedural delay may lead to a *de facto*determination of the matter in issue', which was precisely what had occurred. The ECtHR had adopted similar reasoning in *W v United Kingdom* (1987) 10 EHRR 29. In contrast, in *Askar v United Kingdom* (application no. 26373/95) the Commission held inadmissible a complaint of substantial delay in granting permission for the family of a refugee to join him in this country, observing:
>
>> 'The Commission recalls that delay in proceedings concerning matters of 'family life' may raise issues under Article 8 of the Convention. In the case of *H v United Kingdom,* the court found a violation of Article 8 in respect of proceedings concerning the mother's access to her child which lasted two years and seven months. However, the court had

regard in reaching that conclusion that the proceedings concerned a fundamental element of family life (whether a mother would be able to see her child again) and that they had a quality of irreversibility, lying within an area in which delay might lead to a de facto determination of the matter, whereas an effective respect for the mother's family life required that the question be determined solely in the light of all relevant considerations and not by mere effluxion of time.'

H, *W* and a third case were then cited. The Commission continued:

'The Commission finds that the present case is not comparable. The subject-matter of the proceedings concerns the granting of permission to enter the United Kingdom for members of the applicant's family, whom the applicant had not seen for at least six years and with some of whom the nature of his ties has not been specified beyond the fact that, pursuant to Somali tradition, the applicant has on the death of his father become head of the extended family group. Further, it is not apparent that the delay in the proceedings has any prejudicial effect on their eventual determination or that the effect of the passage of time is such as to prevent the proper and fair examination of the merits of the case.'

47. We consider that there is sound sense in this approach at Strasbourg, particularly in cases where what is in issue is the grant of some form of welfare support. The Strasbourg Court has rightly emphasised the need to have regard to resources when considering the obligations imposed on a State by Article 8. The demands on resources would be significantly increased if States were to be faced with claims for breaches of Article 8 simply on the ground of administrative delays. Maladministration of the type that we are considering will only infringe Article 8 where the consequence is serious.

The judgment also contains detailed consideration of the basis on which damages should be awarded for breaches of the ECHR:

1) Awards of damages have a less prominent role to play in actions based on breaches of the ECHR than in relation to alleged breaches of private law rights. In relation to breaches of human rights, the primary concern is to bring the infringement to an end. The consequences of administrative delay must amount to more than distress and frustration before Article 8 is even engaged.

2) In terms of an entitlement to an award of damages, the scale and manner of the violation should be taken into account, in the context of whether it is just and appropriate or necessary to afford just satisfaction, as is the manner in which the violation has taken place.

3) The court should take a summary, broad brush approach to damages. If damages are to be awarded for maladministration, the awards of the Judicial Studies Board, the Criminal Injuries Compensation Authority and the relevant ombudsman are likely to provide rough guidance.

4) In order to prevent disproportionate costs in claims for damages under the Human Rights Act 1998 for maladministration, courts should look carefully at attempts to recover damages for maladministration. Such claims should be brought in the Administrative Court, which should control the evidence and procedure to be followed, with an emphasis on summary determination of the damages aspect of the claim. Before giving permission to apply for judicial review the judge should require the claimant to

explain why it would not be more appropriate to use any available internal complaints procedure, or to make a complaint to the Parliamentary Commissioner for Administration or the Local Government Ombudsman.

Comment: like the *Bernard* case, this case illustrates how extreme the facts must be, for a failure to provide a social welfare service, to amount to a breach of the ECHR: unless children or family life is involved, the consequences must be equivalent to the type of consequences that trigger the core duty of the court to protect individuals from serious harm perpetrated by the State, incompatibly with Article 3 ECHR. A classic example, is *R (Limbuela) v Secretary of State for the Home Department*,[97] in which the House of Lords held that it was incompatible with Article 3 ECHR to decline to provide asylum support to destitute asylum-seekers. In *R (Greenfield) v Secretary of State for the Home Department*,[98] the House of Lords endorsed a restrictive approach to the award of financial compensation in ECHR cases, pointing out that declaratory relief will often amount of 'just satisfaction'.

25.67 *Sentges v Netherlands* Application No 27677/02, (2004) 7 CCLR 400

The margin of appreciation was, especially in relation to the allocation of scarce healthcare resources, that it could not be said that the refusal to supply a robotic arm, in the context of the provision of other services, was incompatible with Article 8 ECHR

Facts: Mr Sentges suffered from Duchenne Muscular Dystrophy, which left him unable to stand, walk or lift his arms and with minimal manual or digital function. He had an electric wheelchair with an adapted joystick and he applied to the Dutch health insurance fund for a robotic arm that would enable him to perform many tasks unassisted (he was otherwise entirely dependent on others for every act of day-to-day living).

Judgment: the ECtHR held that the refusal to provide a robotic arm was not incompatible with Article 8 ECHR:

> In the instant case the applicant complained in substance not of action but of a lack of action by the State. While the essential object of Article 8 is to protect the individual against arbitrary interference by the public authorities, it does not merely compel the State to abstain from such interference: in addition to this negative undertaking, there may be positive obligations inherent in effective respect for private or family life. These obligations may involve the adoption of measures designed to secure respect for private life even in the sphere of the relations of individuals between themselves (see, *inter alia*, *X and Y v The Netherlands*, judgment of 26 March 1985, para 23), *Stubbings and Others v The United Kingdom*, judgment of 22 October 1996, *Reports* 1996-IV, p1505, para 62).
>
> The court has held that Article 8 may impose such positive obligations on a State where there is a direct and immediate link between the measures sought by an applicant and the latter's private life (see *Botta v Italy*, cited above, para 34). However, Article 8 does not apply to situations concerning interpersonal relations of such broad and indeterminate scope that there can be no conceivable link between the measures the State is urged to take

97 [2005] UKHL 66, (2006) 9 CCLR 30.

98 [2005] UKHL 14, [2005] 1 WLR 673.

and an individual's private life (see *Botta*, cited above, para 35). The court has also held that Article 8 cannot be considered applicable each time an individual's everyday life is disrupted, but only in the exceptional cases where the State's failure to adopt measures interferes with that individual's right to personal development and his or her right to establish and maintain relations with other human beings and the outside world. It is incumbent on the individual concerned to demonstrate the existence of a special link between the situation complained of and the particular needs of his or her private life (see *Zehnalovà and Zehnal v The Czech Republic* (dec.), Application no 38621/97, ECHR 2002-V).

Even assuming that in the present case such a special link indeed exists – as was accepted by the Central Appeals Tribunal –, regard must be had to the fair balance that has to be struck between the competing interests of the individual and of the community as a whole and to the wide margin of appreciation enjoyed by States in this respect in determining the steps to be taken to ensure compliance with the Convention (see *Zehnalovà and Zehnal*, cited above).

This margin of appreciation is even wider when, as in the present case, the issues involve an assessment of the priorities in the context of the allocation of limited State resources (see, *mutatis mutandis, Osman v the United Kingdom*, judgment of 28 October 1998, *Reports* 1998-VIII, p. 3159, para 116, *O'Reilly and Others v Ireland* (dec.), Application no 54725/00, 28 February 2002, unreported). In view of their familiarity with the demands made on the health care system as well as with the funds available to meet those demands, the national authorities are in a better position to carry out this assessment than an international court. In addition, the court should also be mindful of the fact that, while it will apply the Convention to the concrete facts of this particular case in accordance with Article 34, a decision issued in an individual case will nevertheless at least to some extent establish a precedent (see *Pretty*, cited above, para 75), valid for all Contracting States.

In the present case the court notes that the applicant has access to the standard of health care offered to all persons insured under the Health Insurance Act and the Exceptional Medical Expenses Act (see *Nitecki v Poland* (dec.), Application no 65653/01, 21 March 2002, unreported). It thus appears that he has been provided with an electric wheelchair with an adapted joystick. The court by no means wishes to underestimate the difficulties encountered by the applicant and appreciates the very real improvement which a robotic arm would entail for his personal autonomy and his ability to establish and develop relationships with other human beings of his choice. Nevertheless the court is of the opinion that in the circumstances of the present case it cannot be said that the respondent State exceeded the margin of appreciation afforded to it.

25.68 *Autism-Europe v France* (complaint 13/2002) (2004) 38 EHRR CD 265

The European Committee of Social Rights declared admissible a complaint that France was in breach of the revised European Social Charter by failing to ensure that children and adults were entitled to education in mainstream schools in sufficient numbers

Facts: Autism-Europe brought proceedings against France in reliance on Articles 15, 17 and E of the revised European Social Charter, which provide as follows:

Article 15 — The right of persons with disabilities to independence, social integration and participation in the life of the community
With a view to ensuring to persons with disabilities, irrespective of age and the nature and origin of their disabilities, the effective exercise of the right to independence, social integration and participation in the life of the community, the Parties undertake, in particular:

1. to take the necessary measures to provide persons with disabilities with guidance, education and vocational training in the framework of general schemes wherever possible or, where this is not possible, through specialised bodies, public or private;

...

Article 17 — The right of children and young persons to social, legal and economic protection
With a view to ensuring the effective exercise of the right of children and young persons to grow up in an environment which encourages the full development of their personality and of their physical and mental capacities, the Parties undertake, either directly or in co-operation with public and private organisations, to take all appropriate and necessary measures designed:

1. a) to ensure that children and young persons, taking account of the rights and duties of their parents, have the care, the assistance, the education and the training they need, in particular by providing for the establishment or maintenance of institutions and services sufficient and adequate for this purpose;

...

Article E — Non-discrimination
The enjoyment of the rights set forth in this Charter shall be secured without discrimination on any ground such as race, colour, sex, language, religion, political or other opinion, national extraction or social origin, health, association with a national minority, birth or other status.

Judgment: the Committee held as follows:

48. As emphasised in the General Introduction to its Conclusions of 2003 (p10), the Committee views Article 15 of the Revised Charter as both reflecting and advancing a profound shift of values in all European countries over the past decade away from treating them as objects of pity and towards respecting them as equal citizens – an approach that the Council of Europe contributed to promote, with the adoption by the Committee of Ministers of Recommendation (92) 6 of 1992 on a coherent policy for people with disabilities. The underlying vision of Article 15 is one of equal citizenship for persons with disabilities and, fittingly, the primary rights are those of 'independence, social integration and participation in the life of the community'. Securing a right to education for children and others with disabilities plays an obviously important role in advancing these citizenship rights. This explains why education is now specifically mentioned in the revised Article 15 and why such an emphasis is placed on achieving that education 'in the framework of general schemes, wherever possible'. It should be noted that Article 15 applies to all persons with disabilities regardless of the nature and origin of their disability and irrespective of their age. It thus clearly covers both children and adults with autism.

49. Article 17 is predicated on the need to ensure that children and young persons grow up in an environment which encourages the 'full development of their personality and of their physical and mental capacities'. This

approach is just as important for children with disabilities as it is for others and arguably more in circumstances where the effects of ineffective or untimely intervention are ever likely to be undone. The Committee views Article 17, which deals more generally, *inter alia*, with the right to education for all, as also embodying the modern approach of mainstreaming. Article 17(1), in particular, requires the establishment and maintenance of sufficient and adequate institutions and services for the purpose of education. Since Article 17(1) deals only with children and young persons it is important to read it in conjunction with Article 15(1) as far as adults are concerned...

51. The Committee considers that the insertion of Article E into a separate Article in the Revised Charter indicates the heightened importance the drafters paid to the principle of non-discrimination with respect to the achievement of the various substantive rights contained therein. It further considers that its function is to help secure the equal effective enjoyment of all the rights concerned regardless of difference. Therefore, it does not constitute an autonomous right which could in itself provide independent grounds for a complaint. It follows that the Committee understands the arguments of the complainant as implying that the situation as alleged violates Arts 15(1) and 17(1) when read in combination with Article E of the Revised Charter. Although disability is not explicitly listed as a prohibited ground of discrimination under Art.E, the Committee considers that it is adequately covered by the reference to 'other status'. Such an interpretative approach, which is justified in its own rights, is fully consistent with both the letter and the spirit of the Political Declaration adopted by the 2nd European conference of ministers responsible for integration policies for people with disabilities (Malaga, April, 2003), which reaffirmed the anti-discriminatory and human rights framework as the appropriate one for development of European policy in this field.

52. The Committee observes further that the wording of Article E is almost identical to the wording of Article 14 of the European Convention on Human Rights. As the European Court of Human Rights has repeatedly stressed in interpreting Article 14 and most recently in the *Thlimmenos* case [(2001) 31 EHRR 15, para [44]], the principle of equality that is reflected therein means treating equals equally and unequals unequally. In particular it is said in the above-mentioned case:

> 'The right not to be discriminated against in the enjoyment of the rights guaranteed under the Convention is also violated when States without an objective and reasonable justification fail to treat differently persons whose situations are significantly different'.

In other words, human difference in a democratic society should not only be viewed positively but should be responded to with discernment in order to ensure real and effective equality.

In this regard, the Committee considers that Article E not only prohibits direct discrimination but also all forms of indirect discrimination. Such indirect discrimination may arise by failing to take due and positive account of all relevant differences or by failing to take adequate steps to ensure that the rights and collective advantages that are open to all are genuinely accessible by and to all.

53. The Committee recalls, as stated in its decision relative to Complaint No 1/1998 (*International Commission of Jurist v Portugal,* para [32]), that the implementation of the Charter requires the State Parties to take not merely legal action but also practical action to give full effect to the rights recognised in the Charter. When the achievement of one of the rights in

question is exceptionally complex and particularly expensive to resolve, a State Party must take measures that allows it to achieve the objectives of the Charter within a reasonable time, with measurable progress and to an extent consistent with the maximum use of available resources. States Parties must be particularly mindful of the impact that their choices will have for groups with heightened vulnerabilities as well as for others persons affected including, especially, their families on whom falls the heaviest burden in the event of institutional shortcomings.

54. In the light of the afore-mentioned, the Committee notes that in the case of autistic children and adults, notwithstanding a national debate going back more than 20 years about the number of persons concerned and the relevant strategies required, and even after the enactment of the Disabled Persons Policy Act of June 30, 1975, France has failed to achieve sufficient progress in advancing the provision of education for persons with autism. It specifically notes that most of the French official documents, in particular those submitted during the procedure, still use a more restrictive definition of autism than that adopted by the World Heath Organisation and that there are still insufficient official statistics with which to rationally measure progress through time. The Committee considers that the fact that the establishments specialising in the education and care of disabled children (particularly those with autism) are not in general financed from the same budget as normal schools, does not in itself amount to discrimination, since it is primarily for States themselves to decide on the modalities of funding.

Nevertheless, it considers, as the authorities themselves acknowledge, and whether a broad or narrow definition of autism is adopted, that the proportion of children with autism being educated in either general or specialist schools is much lower than in the case of other children, whether or not disabled. It is also established, and not contested by the authorities, that there is a chronic shortage of care and support facilities for autistic adults.

Conclusion

For these reasons, the Committee concludes by 11 votes to 2 that the situation constitutes a violation of Arts 15(1) and 17(1) whether alone or read in combination with Article E of the revised European Social Charter.

25.69 *van Kuck v Germany* Application no 35968/97, (2005) 8 CCLR 121

It was incompatible with Articles 6 and 8 ECHR to decline to fund gender re-assignment surgery on the basis of an incorrect understanding of the medical evidence

Facts: Ms van Kuck was a transsexual, who had been born male but had changed her forename to a woman's name and received hormone treatment; she now applied for funding for gender re-assignment surgery, from her insurance company, which refused to pay. The German courts heard expert evidence, which recommended surgery, but had nonetheless concluded that she had a disease which it was appropriate to endeavour to cure through psychotherapy.

Judgment: the German courts had failed to properly understand and taken into account the medical evidence, rendering the trial incompatible with Article 6 ECHR and the refusal to surgery incompatible with Article 8 ECHR, in that a fair balance had not been struck between the interests of Ms van Kuck and the German insurance company.

25.70 *Re Z (An Adult: Capacity)* [2004] EWHC 2817 Fam, (2005) 8 CCLR 146

Local authorities were required to investigate, where it appeared that a vulnerable adult intended to undertake an assisted suicide, to ensure that the adult was competent properly, informed and not improperly influenced; but it had no power to stop an adult with capacity taking that course

Facts: Mrs Z suffered from an incurable condition and was deteriorating; she had eventually persuaded her family to accede to her wish to undertake an assisted suicide in Switzerland. The local authority sought an injunction to prevent Mr Z taking her there, under the Family Division's inherent jurisdiction.

Judgment: Hedley J refused the application, holding that it was not unlawful for a person with the mental capacity to make the choice to take their own life, and that although a family member who assisted them would probably incur criminal liability, it was pre-eminently a matter for the police and the DPP to decide whether to enforce that. However, where a local authority learnt that a vulnerable person in their area intended to undertake assisted suicide, it had a duty to take some action:

> 19. In my judgment in a case such as this the local authority incurred the following duties: (i) to investigate the position of a vulnerable adult to consider what was her true position and intention; (ii) to consider whether she was legally competent to make and carry out her decision and intention; (iii) to consider whether any other (and if so, what) influence may be operating on her position and intention and to ensure that she has all relevant information and knows all available options; (iv) to consider whether to invoke the inherent jurisdiction of the High Court so that the question of competence could be judicially investigated and determined; (v) in the event of the adult not being competent, to provide all such assistance as may be reasonably required both to determine and give effect to her best interests; (vi) in the event of the adult being competent to allow her in any lawful way to give effect to her decision although that should not preclude the giving of advice or assistance in accordance with what are perceived to be her best interests; (vii) where there are reasonable grounds to suspect that the commission of a criminal offence may be involved, to draw that to the attention of the police; (viii) in very exceptional circumstances, to invoke the jurisdiction of the court under section 222 of the Local Government Act 1972. My view is that their duties do not extend beyond that. In this case, although they have the power to do so under section 222 of the 1972 Act, in my judgment they have no obligation to seek the continuation of the injunction made by Black J. It is clear that the criminal justice agencies have all the necessary powers. Moreover Parliament has committed to the Director of Public Prosecutions the discretion as to whether to permit a prosecution. Both those points militate strongly against the intervention of the civil remedy of an injunction. The local authority have made it clear that if they are under no duty to seek the continuation of the injunction, they do not wish to do so.

25.71 *Pentiacova v Moldova* Application no 14462/03, (2005) 40 EHRR SE23

It was not a breach of the ECHR radically to reduce haemodialysis provision, notwithstanding the suffering occasioned

Facts: for a period of years, for budgetary reasons, Moldova significantly reduced the amount of publicly-funded haemodialysis that it provided to patients with chronic renal failure, and the level of ancillary medication provided, resulting in many patients suffering a range of distressing symptoms.

Judgment: the European Court of Human Rights dismissed the application as being 'manifestly unfounded', both under Article 8 and 2 ECHR:

> Although the object of Article 8 is essentially that of protecting the individual against arbitrary interference by the public authorities, it does not merely compel the State to abstain from such interference since it may also give rise to positive obligations inherent in effective 'respect' for private and family life. While the boundaries between the State's positive and negative obligations under this provision do not always lend themselves to precise definition, the applicable principles are similar. In both contexts regard must be had to the fair balance that has to be struck between the competing interests of the individual and the community as a whole, and in both contexts the State enjoys a certain margin of appreciation (*Zehnalová and Zehnal v Czech Republic,* App no 38621/97).
>
> The court has previously held that private life includes a person's physical and psychological integrity (*Niemietz v Germany* (1993) 16 EHRR 97 at [29]). While the Convention does not guarantee as such a right to free medical care, in a number of cases the Court has held that Article 8 is relevant to complaints about public funding to facilitate the mobility and quality of life of disabled applicants (see, *Zehnalová and Zehnal,* cited above, and *Sentges v Netherlands,* App no 27677/02). The court is therefore prepared to assume for the purposes of this application, that Article 8 is applicable to the applicants' complaints about lack of sufficient funding of their treatment.
>
> The margin of appreciation referred to above is even wider when, as in the present case, the issues involve an assessment of the priorities in the context of the allocation of limited State resources (see, mutatis mutandis, *Osman v United Kingdom* (2000) 29 EHRR 245 at [116], App no 54725/00, *O'Reilly v Ireland,* App no 54725/00 (2002)). In view of their familiarity with the demands made on the health care system as well as with the funds available to meet those demands, the national authorities are in a better position to carry out this assessment than an international court. In addition, the court should also be mindful of the fact that, while it will apply the Convention to the concrete facts of this particular case in accordance with Article 34, a decision issued in an individual case will nevertheless at least to some extent establish a precedent, valid for all Contracting States (*Sentges v Netherlands,* cited above).
>
> The court considers that the core problem in the present case reflected in the numerous complaints is the alleged insufficient public funding for the treatment of their disease. In support of their claims the applicants compare the amount of public expenditure on renal failure treatment in Moldova to that in some industrialised countries like the United States of America, the United Kingdom, Australia and Israel. The court sees no reason to question the applicants' assertion that they have no means to pay for the cost of the medication not provided free by the State and that the medication and in some cases a third haemodialysis session per week is of great importance for their fight with the disease. However, it notes that the applicants' claim amounts to a call on public funds which, in view of the scarce resources, would have to be directed from other worthy needs funded by the taxpayer.

While it is clearly desirable that everyone has access to a full range of medical treatment, including life-saving medical procedures and drugs, the lack of resources means that there are, unfortunately, in the Contracting States many individuals who do not enjoy them, especially in cases of permanent and expensive treatment.

In the present case the court notes that the applicants had access to the standard of health care offered to the general public both before the implementation of the medical care system reform, and after the implementation thereof. It thus appears that they were provided with basic medical care and basic medication before January 1, 2004, and have been provided with almost full medical care after that date. The Court by no means wishes to underestimate the difficulties apparently encountered by the applicants and appreciates the very real improvement which a total haemodialysis coverage would entail for their private and family lives. Nevertheless, the Court is of the opinion that in the circumstances of the present case it cannot be said that the respondent State failed to strike a fair balance between the competing interests of the applicants and the community as a whole.

Bearing in mind the medical treatment and the facilities provided to the applicants and the fact that the applicants' situation has considerably improved after the implementation of the medical care system reform in January 2004, the Court considers that the respondent State cannot be said, in the special circumstances of the present case, to have failed to discharge its positive obligations under Article 8 of the Convention. As to the problem concerning the non-reimbursement of all the transportation expenses, the court, assuming that the applicants exhausted domestic remedies, notes that the Government produced copies of payment rolls recording the payment of those expenses to all the applicants and that the applicants failed to make any comment on them. Moreover, the applicants sent the court a copy of a judgment of the Briceni District Court, by which Eduard Pritula was awarded money for his travel expenses, to be paid by the local authorities.

It follows that the complaint under Article 8 of the Convention is manifestly ill-founded and must be rejected in accordance with Article 35(3) and (4) of the Convention.

C Alleged violation of Article 2 of the Convention

The applicants complain that the failure of the State to cover the cost of all the medication necessary for their haemodialysis, and the poor financing of the haemodialysis section of the SCR, violated their right to life guaranteed by Article 2 of the Convention.

The court recalls that the first sentence of Article 2 enjoins the State not only to refrain from the intentional and unlawful taking of life, but also to take appropriate steps to safeguard the lives of those within its jurisdiction (see *LCB v United Kingdom* (1999) 27 EHRR 212 at [36]). It cannot be excluded that the acts and omissions of the authorities in the field of health care policy may in certain circumstances engage their responsibility under Article 2 (see *Powell v United Kingdom* (2000) 30 EHRR CD362).

Moreover, an issue may arise under Article 2 where it is shown that the authorities of a Contracting State put an individual's life at risk through the denial of health care which they have undertaken to make available to the population generally (see *Cyprus v Turkey* [GC] (2002) 35 EHRR 30 at [219] and *Nitecki v Poland,* App no 65653/01 (2002)).

Turning to the facts of the instant case, the court notes that the applicants have failed to adduce any evidence that their lives have been put at risk. They claim that a few patients have died in recent years and rely on the

> example of Gheorghe Lungu, but they have not adduced any evidence that the cause of death was the lack of any specific drug or the lack of appropriate medical care. The court notes that chronic renal failure is a very serious progressive disease with a high rate of mortality, not only in Moldova but throughout the world. The fact that a person has died of this disease is not, therefore, proof in itself that the death was caused by shortcomings in the medical care system.
>
> In any event, as regards the issue of the State's positive obligations, the Court has examined the issue under Article 8 of the Convention and sees no reason to reach any different conclusion under Article 2 of the Convention.
>
> Accordingly, the Court concludes that the complaint under Article 2 of the Convention is manifestly ill-founded within the meaning of Article 35(3) of the Convention.

25.72 *R (Hughes) v Liverpool CC* [2005] EWHC 428 (Admin), (2005) 8 CCLR 243

A breach of duty to provide social care did not inevitably result in a breach of the ECHR, for which the threshold was high

Facts: Mr Hughes was a young man who was severely disabled, mentally and physically. He was cared for at home by his mother, with help from outside agencies. Liverpool acknowledged, however, that his mother's accommodation was wholly unsuitable for him. An assessment concluded that he needed suitable accommodation and, also, respite care. However, none was provided.

Judgment: Mitting J held that Liverpool was in breach of section 21 and 29 of the National Assistance Act 1948, by failing to meet Mr Hughes' assessed needs. He ordered respite care to be provided each weekend, and a re-assessment of the mother's needs. He rejected, however, a claim for damages under the ECHR:

> 36. Accepting, without deciding, that Article 6 imposed on Liverpool a positive duty to promote the claimant's private and family life, I am not satisfied that it has acted so as to be in breach of that right. The claimant's private and family life have been protected and promoted by the efforts principally of his mother, but supplemented by carers paid for by Liverpool. Subject to the limitations necessarily imposed upon the claimant by his disabilities, he has been able to enjoy his private and family life. It is true that his mother has identified respects in which protection of his dignity and personal integrity would be improved were suitable accommodation to be provided. But in all other respects, as far as I can tell from the documents that I have read and the submissions that have been made to me, the limitations imposed upon his enjoyment of private and family life stem from his own condition.
>
> 37. The burden imposed on his mother has been very great, even intolerable. But it is not she who is the claimant. As a result of her efforts, the impact upon the claimant's private and family life of Liverpool's shortcomings in fulfilment of its statutory duties has been reduced to a level at which his rights have not been infringed. In any event, I am not satisfied that the high threshold identified by Lord Woolf LCJ in *R (Anufrijeva) v Southwark LBC* [2004] QB 1124 at para 43 has been crossed. Nor do I think it is necessary to achieve just satisfaction of the claimant's claim that damages should

be awarded. I refer to Lord Woolf's analysis of the circumstances in which damages may be awarded in paragraph 55 of that decision.

25.73 *R (Limbuela) v Secretary of State for the Home Department* [2005] UKHL 66, (2006) 9 CCLR 30

It was necessary to provide accommodation and support to asylum-seekers who were destitute or faced imminent destitution, to avoid a breach of Article 3 ECHR

Facts: Four healthy, able-bodied asylum-seekers faced destitution because they claimed asylum late, by virtue of section 55 of the Nationality, Immigration and Asylum Act 2002.

Judgment: the House of Lords (Lords Bingham, Hope, Scott, Lady Hale and Lord Brown) held that a decision to exclude certain asylum-seekers from asylum support was an intentionally inflicted act for which the Secretary of State was responsible and it amounted to 'treatment' for the purposes of Article 3 ECHR. That treatment would be 'inhuman or degrading' when a person was obliged to sleep in the street or go seriously hungry or became unable to satisfy the most basic requirements of hygiene. The duty to avoid inhuman or degrading treatment required the Secretary of State to provide support to avert imminent destitution.

25.74 *R (YL) v Birmingham CC* [2007] UKHL 27, (2007) 10 CCLR 505

A privately run care home was not discharging functions of a public nature

Facts: YL submitted that a privately run care home, that had given her notice to quit, had acted incompatibly with her rights under Article 8 ECHR.

Judgment: the House of Lords (Lords Bingham, Scott, Mance, Neuberger and Lady Hale, Lord Bingham and Lady Hale dissenting) held that the care home provider was not exercising functions of a public nature for the purposes of section 6 of the Human Rights Act 1998: this was not a case where the statutory function itself had been delegated and the provision of care home accommodation was not intrinsically governmental.

Comment: now, by virtue of section 73 of the Care Act 2014, most registered care providers, providing personal care in residential or domestic settings, must be treated as exercising a function of a public nature for the purposes of section 6(3)(b) of the Human Rights Act 1998.

25.75 *R (Weaver) v London and Quadrant Housing Trust* [2009] EWCA Civ 587, [2010] 1 WLR 363

On the assumption that some functions of an RSL were public functions, it was a public body for the purposes of the Human Rights Act 1998 and for the purposes of judicial review proceedings, because its termination of a social tenancy was not a private act

Facts: London and Quadrant, a registered social landlord, served a notice seeking possession on Ms Weaver, who claimed that it infringed her rights under Article 8 ECHR.

Judgment: the Court of Appeal (Lord Collins, Rix and Elias LJJ, Rix LJ dissenting) held that it conceded that some of London and Quadrant's functions were public functions, so the only question was whether the termination of a social tenancy by a social landlord was a private act: viewing all the circumstances in the round, it was not. There was no warrant for applying a different approach to the question whether London and Quadrant was amenable to judicial review:

> *Judicial review*
>
> 83. Both the *Aston Cantlow* case [2004] 1 AC 546 and *YL's* case [2008] AC 95 emphasised that it does not necessarily follow that because a body is a public body for the purposes of section 6, it is therefore subject to public law principles. The Divisional Court held, however, that in this case the two questions had to be determined the same way. Mr Arden does not now seek to contend otherwise. In my judgment, he was right not to do so.

25.76 *Tysiac v Poland* Application No 5410/03, (2007) 45 EHRR 42

The absence of clear procedures for determining eligibility for an abortion and resolving disputes was incompatible with Article 8 ECHR

Facts: the state hospital refused Ms Tysiac an abortion, notwithstanding medical evidence that otherwise her health was at risk (the criteria for a legal abortion in Poland).

Judgment: the European Court of Human Rights held that whilst it was not its task to examine whether the ECHR guarantees the right to have an abortion, the regulation of pregnancy touched upon the sphere of private life such that the authorities were under a positive duty to secure to their citizens their right to effective respect for their physical and psychological integrity and, relevant to the present case, that required clear procedures for determining eligibility and resolving disputes, which had been absent in the present case.

25.77 *R (Wilson) v Coventry CC; R (Thomas) v Havering LBC* [2008] EWHC 2300 (Admin), (2009) 12 CCLR 7

Care home closures did not in general breach Article 2 ECHR

Facts: Coventry and Havering resolved to close a number of care homes, occupied by elderly residents who suffered from dementia or were physically disabled. The claimants sought a judicial review on the basis that officers had failed adequately to communicate to decision-makers the risk of serious injury or death resulting from such closures, failed to undertake adequate assessments of individual residents prior to the decisions to close, (in the case of Havering) failed to communicate to decision-makers a fair assessment of the financial implications. The claimants also submitted that the decisions were incompatible with Article 2 ECHR.

Judgment: Deputy High Court Judge Pelling QC held that there was no requirement to undertake individual assessments before deciding to close a care home, that officers had fairly communicated to decision-makers the risks involved and the financial implications and that, having regard to the broad measure of judgment accorded to public authorities, there had not been any breach of Article 2 ECHR.

25.78 *Re E (A Child) (Northern Ireland)* [2008] UKHL 66, [2009] 1 AC 536

Children and other vulnerable persons require special protection under the ECHR

Facts: the police failed to do more to protect parents and child walking to school from abusive protesters because the police were concerned that further action by them might escalate tensions in the wider community.

Judgment: the House of Lords (Lords Hoffman and Scott, Lady Hale, Lords Carswell and Brown) held that the police had not treated the children incompatibly with Article 3 ECHR because, although children and other vulnerable individuals required special care and protection, they had taken all reasonable steps to protect the families from the actions of third parties. The leading judgment is by Lord Carswell but Lady Hale's judgment may be of particular interest in this context:

> 7. The European Court of Human Rights has taken particular note of the vulnerability of children in its judgments on the obligations of the state to protect people from inhuman or degrading treatment. It is noteworthy that the landmark rulings in which the state has been found responsible for failing to protect victims from serious ill-treatment meted out by private individuals have concerned children. *A v United Kingdom* (1998) 27 EHRR 611 was decided shortly before the leading case of *Osman v United Kingdom* (2000) 29 EHRR 245. *A v United Kingdom* established the principle that the state was obliged to take measures designed to ensure that people were not subjected to ill-treatment by private individuals. Vulnerable people were entitled to be protected by effective deterrent measures. The existence of the defence of reasonable chastisement failed to afford children such protection. Osman took the matter further by establishing a duty to take more pro-active protective measures to guard against real and immediate risk of which the authorities knew or ought to have known. There was no breach in Osman itself; but breaches were found in both *Z v United Kingdom* (2001) 34 EHRR 97 and *E v United Kingdom* (2002) 36 EHRR 519. In *Z*, the authorities had failed to protect children from prolonged abuse and neglect which they knew all about. In *E*, they had failed to monitor the situation after a stepfather had been convicted of sexual abuse, and so it was held that they should have found out that he was abusing the children and done something to protect them. The court said, at para 99:
>
> > 'The test under Article 3 however does not require it to be shown that 'but for' the failing or omission of the public authority ill-treatment would not have happened. A failure to take reasonably available measures which could have had a real prospect of altering the outcome or mitigating the harm is sufficient to engage the responsibility of the state.'
>
> 8. These and later cases show that the special vulnerability of children is relevant in two ways. First, it is a factor in assessing whether the treatment to which they have been subjected reaches the 'minimum level of severity'– that is, the high level of severity–needed to attract the protection of Article 3. As the court recently reiterated in the instructive case of *Mubilanzila Mayeka and Kaniki Mitunga v Belgium* (2006) 46 EHRR 449, para 48:
>
> > 'In order to fall within the scope of Article 3, the ill-treatment must attain a minimum level of severity, the assessment of which depends on all the circumstances of the case, such as the duration of the treatment,

> its physical or mental effects and, in some cases, the sex, age and state of health of the victim.'

Detaining a Congolese child of five, who had been separated from her family, for two months in an immigration detention facility designed for adults met that high threshold even though the staff had done their best to be kind to her.

9. The special vulnerability of children is also relevant to the scope of the obligations of the state to protect them from such treatment. Again, in *Mubilanzila Mayeka and Kaniki Mitunga v Belgium*, at para 53, the court reiterated, citing *Z*, *A* and *Osman*, that:

> 'the obligation on high contracting parties under Article 1 of the Convention to secure to everyone within their jurisdiction the rights and freedoms defined in the Convention, taken in conjunction with Article 3, requires states to take measures designed to ensure that individuals within their jurisdiction are not subjected to torture or inhuman or degrading treatment, including such ill-treatment administered by private individuals. Steps should be taken to enable effective protection to be provided, *particularly to children and other vulnerable members of society*, and should include reasonable measures to prevent ill-treatment of which the authorities have or ought to have knowledge.' (Emphasis supplied.)

Despite the fact that the state had detained the little girl, the court treated the case, not as a breach of its negative obligation, but as a breach of its positive obligation to look after her properly. She:

> 'indisputably came within the class of highly vulnerable members of society to whom the Belgian State owed a duty to take adequate measures to provide care and protection as part of its positive obligations under Article 3 of the Convention': para 55.

This they had failed to do: para 58. The court also found a breach of the state's obligations towards the child's mother, because of the distress she must have suffered at her daughter's treatment, even though it could be said that she had to some extent brought it on herself by arranging for the child to travel through Belgium without a visa: para 62.

10. That case demonstrates the wisdom of what was said by my noble and learned friend, Lord Brown of Eaton-under-Heywood, in *R (Limbuela) v Secretary of State for the Home Department* [2006] 1 AC 396, para 92:

> 'it seems to me generally unhelpful to attempt to analyse obligations arising under Article 3 as negative or positive, and the state's conduct as active or passive. Time and again these are shown to be false dichotomies. The real issue in all these cases is whether the state is properly to be regarded as responsible for the harm inflicted (or threatened) upon the victim.'

Nevertheless, there must be some distinction between the scope of the state's duty not to take life or ill-treat people in a way which falls foul of Article 3 and its duty to protect people from the harm which others may do to them. In the one case, there is an absolute duty not to do it. In the other, there is a duty to do what is reasonable in all the circumstances to protect people from a real and immediate risk of harm. Both duties may be described as absolute but their content is different. So once again it may be a false dichotomy between the absolute negative duty and a qualified positive one. In another recent case about children, *Kontrová v Slovakia* (Application no 7510/04) (unreported) given 31 May 2007, the court, at para 50, reiterated the well known passage from *Osman*, para 116:

> 'Bearing in mind the difficulties in policing modern societies, the unpredictability of human conduct and the operational choices which must be made in terms of priorities and resources, the scope of the positive obligation must be interpreted in a way which does not impose an impossible or disproportionate burden on the authorities.'

In *Kontrová*, the state admitted violating the positive obligation to protect life in Article 2. Despite having received allegations of repeated and serious violence against them by the children's father, and that he had a shotgun and threatened to use it to kill himself and the children, they had failed to act upon these allegations, with the direct result that he carried out his threats and the children were killed.

25.79 *MAK and RK v United Kingdom* Application nos 45901/05 and 40146/06, [2010] ECHR 363, (2010) 13 CCLR 241

Disproportionate actions by a hospital doctor, resulting in his erroneously concluding that parents had abused their daughter, were incompatible with Article 8 ECHR

Facts: a hospital doctor negligently concluded that the daughter had been abused, resulting in the parents' access to their doctor being blocked, then impeded, for about a week. The English Court of Appeal struck out the parents' action in negligence: *JD v East Berkshire Community Health NHS Trust.*[99]

Judgment: the European Court of Human Rights held that whilst mistaken judgments or assessments by professionals do not in themselves render protection measures incompatible with Article 8 ECHR, in this case, the doctor's actions had been disproportionate: there had been a breach of Article 8 ECHR and, because the Human Rights Act 1998 had not been in force at the relevant time, of Article 13 ECHR.

25.80 *Watts v United Kingdom* Application no 53586/09, [2010] ECHR 793, (2010) 51 EHRR SE5

A carefully managed process of care home closure did not violate rights under Articles 2, 3 or 8 ECHR

Facts: Wolverhampton decided to close the local authority care home in which Ms Watts resided, because it did not make cost-effective provision. Ms Watts was not successful in opposing her move to alternative residential accommodation in the UK courts so applied to the European Court of Human Rights.

Judgment: the European Court of Human Rights declared the application inadmissible on the basis that (i) while Article 2 ECHR was applicable, because a badly managed transfer of an elderly care home resident could well have a negative impact on their life expectancy, on the facts of this case, including the care planning undertaken by Wolverhampton, the authorities had plainly discharged their positive obligation under Article 2 to safeguard individuals from a real and immediate risk to life; (ii) whilst the court was content to proceed on the basis that the transfer another care home interfered with Ms Watt's private life, that interference had

99 [2005] 2 AC 373, (2005) 8 CCLR 185.

plainly been justified and proportionate in that there had been extensive consultation and consideration of safe management procedures, so as to minimise the adverse effects of any move, whilst there were reasons for closure based on resource allocation which required a wide margin of appreciation to be afforded.

25.81 *Stanev v Bulgaria* Application No 36760/06, (2012) 55 EHRR 22

Very poor living conditions in a care home for seven years amounted to inhuman and degrading treatment

Facts: Mr Stanev had been placed in a psychiatric institution in a remote mountain location for about seven years where the food was insufficient and of poor quality, the building was inadequately heated, there was only one shower a week in an unhygienic and dilapidated bathroom and the toilets were in an execrable state.

Judgment: the European Court of Human Rights held that this had amounted to inhuman and degrading treatment:

> **2. The Court's assessment**
>
> *(a) General principles*
>
> 201. Article 3 enshrines one of the most fundamental values of democratic society. It prohibits in absolute terms torture or inhuman or degrading treatment or punishment, irrespective of the circumstances and the victim's behaviour.
>
> 202. Ill-treatment must attain a minimum level of severity if it is to fall within the scope of Article 3 . The assessment of this minimum is, in the nature of things, relative; it depends on all the circumstances of the case, such as the nature and context of the treatment, the manner and method of its execution, its duration, its physical or mental effects and, in some instances, the sex, age and state of health of the victim.
>
> 203. Treatment has been held by the court to be 'inhuman' because, inter alia, it was premeditated, was applied for hours at a stretch and caused either actual bodily injury or intense physical or mental suffering. Treatment has been considered 'degrading' when it was such as to arouse in its victims feelings of fear, anguish and inferiority capable of humiliating and debasing them and possibly breaking their physical or moral resistance or driving them to act against their will or conscience. In this connection, the question whether such treatment was intended to humiliate or debase the victim is a factor to be taken into account, although the absence of any such purpose does not inevitably lead to a finding that there has been no violation of Article 3.
>
> 204. The suffering and humiliation involved must in any event go beyond that inevitable element of suffering or humiliation connected with a given form of legitimate treatment or punishment. Measures depriving a person of his liberty may often involve such an element. Yet it cannot be said that deprivation of liberty in itself raises an issue under Article 3 of the Convention. Nevertheless, under that article the state must ensure that a person is detained in conditions which are compatible with respect for his human dignity, that the manner and method of the execution of the measure do not subject him to distress or hardship of an intensity exceeding the unavoidable level of suffering inherent in detention and that, given the practical demands of imprisonment, his health and well-being are adequately

secured by, among other things, providing him with the requisite medical assistance.

205. When assessing the conditions of a deprivation of liberty under Article 3 of the Convention, account has to be taken of their cumulative effects and the duration of the measure in question. In this connection, an important factor to take into account, besides the material conditions, is the detention regime. In assessing whether a restrictive regime may amount to treatment contrary to Article 3 in a given case, regard must be had to the particular conditions, the stringency of the regime, its duration, the objective pursued and its effects on the person concerned.

(b) Application of these principles in the present case

206. In the present case the court has found that the applicant's placement in the Pastra Social Care Home–a situation for which the domestic authorities must be held responsible–amounts to a deprivation of liberty within the meaning of Article 5 of the Convention. It follows that Article 3 is applicable to the applicant's situation, seeing that it prohibits the inhuman and degrading treatment of anyone in the care of the authorities. The court would emphasise that the prohibition of ill-treatment in Article 3 applies equally to all forms of deprivation of liberty, and in particular makes no distinction according to the purpose of the measure in issue; it is immaterial whether the measure entails detention ordered in the context of criminal proceedings or admission to an institution with the aim of protecting the life or health of the person concerned.

207. The court notes at the outset that, according to the Government, the building in which the applicant lives was renovated in late 2009, resulting in an improvement in his living conditions; the applicant did not dispute this. The Court therefore considers that the applicant's complaint should be taken to refer to the period between 2002 and 2009. The Government has not denied that during that period the applicant's living conditions corresponded to his description, and have also acknowledged that, for economic reasons, there were certain deficiencies in that regard.

208. The court observes that although the applicant shared a room measuring 16sqm with four other residents, he enjoyed considerable freedom of movement both inside and outside the home, a fact likely to lessen the adverse effects of a limited sleeping area.

209. Nevertheless, other aspects of the applicant's physical living conditions are a considerable cause for concern. In particular, it appears that the food was insufficient and of poor quality. The building was inadequately heated and in winter the applicant had to sleep in his coat. He was able to have a shower once a week in an unhygienic and dilapidated bathroom. The toilets were in an execrable state and access to them was dangerous, according to the findings by the CPT. In addition, the home did not return clothes to the same people after they were washed, which was likely to arouse a feeling of inferiority in the residents.

210. The court cannot overlook the fact that the applicant was exposed to all the abovementioned conditions for a considerable period of approximately seven years. Nor can it ignore the findings of the CPT, which, after visiting the home, concluded that the living conditions there at the relevant time could be said to amount to inhuman and degrading treatment. Despite having been aware of those findings, during the period from 2002–2009 the Government did not act on its undertaking to close down the institution. The court considers that the lack of financial resources cited by the Government is not a relevant argument to justify keeping the applicant in the living conditions described.

211. It would nevertheless emphasise that there is no suggestion that the national authorities deliberately intended to inflict degrading treatment. However, as noted above, the absence of any such purpose cannot conclusively rule out a finding of a violation of Article 3.

212. In conclusion, while noting the improvements apparently made to the Pastra Social Care Home since late 2009, the court considers that, taken as a whole, the living conditions to which the applicant was exposed during a period of approximately seven years amounted to degrading treatment.

213. There has therefore been a violation of Article 3 of the Convention.

25.82 *Đorđević v Croatia* Application no 41526/10, [2012] ECHR 1640, (2012) 15 CCLR 657

The authorities were in breach of Articles 3 and 8 ECHR by failing to protect a disabled man and his mother from harassment by local ragamuffins

Facts: the first applicant, who had significant disabilities, had been subjected to continued harassment by children, as had his mother, who looked after him. The authorities took some steps to protect them, but did not take effective or systematic action.

Judgment: the European Court of Human Rights held that the first applicant's rights under Article 3 ECHR and that the second applicant's rights under Article 8 ECHR had been violated:

138. The court reiterates that, as regards the question whether the State could be held responsible, under Article 3, for ill-treatment inflicted on persons by non-State entities, the obligation on the High Contracting Parties under Article 1 of the Convention to secure to everyone within their jurisdiction the rights and freedoms defined in the Convention, taken together with Article 3, requires States to take measures designed to ensure that individuals within their jurisdiction are not subjected to torture or inhuman or degrading treatment or punishment, including such ill-treatment administered by private individuals (see, *mutatis mutandis, HLR v France,* 29 April 1997, para 40, *Reports* 1997-III). These measures should provide effective protection, in particular, of children and other vulnerable persons, and include reasonable steps to prevent ill-treatment of which the authorities had or ought to have had knowledge (see, *mutatis mutandis, Osman v United Kingdom,* 28 October 1998, para 116, *Reports* 1998-VIII, and *E and Others v the United Kingdom,* App no 33218/96, para 88, 26 November 2002).

139. Bearing in mind the difficulties in policing modern societies, the unpredictability of human conduct and the operational choices which must be made in terms of priorities and resources, the scope of this positive obligation must, however, be interpreted in a way which does not impose an impossible or disproportionate burden on the authorities. Not every claimed risk of ill-treatment, thus, can entail for the authorities a Convention requirement to take operational measures to prevent that risk from materialising. For a positive obligation to arise, it must be established that the authorities knew or ought to have known at the time of the existence of a real and immediate risk of ill-treatment of an identified individual from the criminal acts of a third party and that they failed to take measures within the scope of their powers which, judged reasonably, might have been expected to avoid that risk. Another relevant consideration is the need to ensure that the police exercise their powers to control and prevent crime in a manner which fully respects the due process and other guarantees which legitimately place restraints on the scope of their action to investigate

crime and bring offenders to justice, including the guarantees contained in Article 8 of the Convention (see *Mubilanzila Mayeka and Kaniki Mitunga v Belgium*, App no 13178/03, para 53, ECHR 2006-XI; *Members (97) of the Gldani Congregation of Jehovah's Witnesses v Georgia*, App no 71156/01, para 96, 3 May 2007; and *Milanović v Serbia*, App no 44614/07, para 84, 14 December 2010; see also, *mutatis mutandis*, *Osman*, 28 October 1998, para 116).

...

(i) General principles

151. While the essential object of Article 8 is to protect the individual against arbitrary interference by public authorities, it does not merely compel the State to abstain from such interference: in addition to this negative undertaking, there may be positive obligations inherent in effective respect for private or family life. These obligations may involve the adoption of measures designed to secure respect for private life even in the sphere of the relations of individuals between themselves (see *X and Y v The Netherlands*, 26 March 1985, para 23; *Botta v Italy*, 24 February 1998, para 33, *Reports* 1998-I; *Mikulić v Croatia*, App no 53176/99, para 57, ECHR 2002-I; and *Sandra Janković*, App no 38478/05, 5 March 2009, para 44).

152. The court has previously held, in various contexts, that the concept of private life includes a person's psychological integrity. Under Article 8, States have in some circumstances a duty to protect the moral integrity of an individual from acts of other persons. The court has also held that a positive obligation exists upon States to ensure respect for human dignity and the quality of life in certain respects (see *L v Lithuania*, App No 27527/03, para 56, ECHR 2007-IV, and, *mutatis mutandis*, *Pretty v the United Kingdom*, App No 2346/02, para 65, ECHR 2002-III).

(ii) Application of these principles to the present case

153. The court considers that the acts of ongoing harassment have also affected the private and family life of the second applicant. It has found that the State authorities have not put in place adequate and relevant measures to prevent further harassment of the first applicant. Likewise, the State authorities have failed to afford adequate protection in that respect to the second applicant. Therefore, there has also been a violation of Article 8 of the Convention in respect of the second applicant.

25.83 *Nencheva v Bulgaria* Application no 48609/06, [2013] ECHR 554

Public authorities are under a duty to take reasonable steps to prevent the death of vulnerable individuals in state care and to undertake an effective investigation into deaths where the state was involved

Facts: 15 children and young adults died over a six-month period in a home for physically and mentally disabled young people, from the effects of cold and shortages of food, medicine and other basics. The manager of the home had repeatedly sought assistance from the authorities but without success.

Judgment: the European Court of Human Rights held that the authorities should have known of the real risk to the lives of the residents and had failed to take reasonable preventative steps: they were in breach of Article 2 ECHR by failing to prevent the deaths and, also, by failing to undertake an effective investigation into the causes of the deaths.

25.84 *Commissioner of Police for the Metropolis v ZH* [2013] EWCA Civ 69, (2013) 16 CCLR 109

Callous restraint of a young autistic male by the police violated his rights under Articles 3, 5 and 8 ECHR

Facts: ZH, who suffered from severe autism, epilepsy and learning disabilities, became fixated by the water at a local swimming pool and would not move away from the poolside. His carers knew that if he was touched he might jump into the pool (he was fully clothed at the time). The swimming pool manager called the police who, after a brief conversation with the carers, that established that ZH was autistic, went up to him and touched him. ZH then jumped into the pool. The police then pulled ZH out of the pool and restrained him before taking him, soaking wet and agitated, to the police station. ZH sued.

Judgment: the Court of Appeal (Lord Dyson MR, Richards and Black LJJ) held that the first instance judge had been entitled to conclude that the police had breached ZH's rights under Articles 3, 5 and 8 ECHR, and that they were guilty of assault and false imprisonment and a breach of section 21B of the Disability Discrimination Act 1995. The police defence under the Mental Capacity Act 2005 failed: while sections 4–6 of that Act permitted certain acts to be done in connection with the care and treatment of persons lacking capacity if it is in their best interests, those statutory defences were pervaded by concepts of reasonableness, practicability and appropriateness, which were lacking in this case: the police could and should have consulted with ZH's carers about how best to handle him and could not have had a reasonable belief that their actions were in his best interests.

25.85 *McDonald v United Kingdom* Application no 4241/12, [2014] ECHR 492, (2014) 17 CCLR 187

It had been proportionate and compatible with Article 8 ECHR radically to reduce a person's social care provision

Facts: Ms McDonald had limited mobility and a small, neurogenic bladder, which caused her to have to urinate several times a night. Kensington initially provided Ms McDonald with a commode and a night-time carer. It then assessed her need using different language, as being for incontinence pads and absorbent sheets. Ms McDonald sought a judicial review.

Judgment: the European Court of Human Rights held that Kensington & Chelsea's decision to withdraw its initial provision of night-time care amounted to an interference with Ms McDonald's private life (rather than a failure to make positive provision) and that its initial withdrawal was incompatible with Article 8 ECHR because (as the Supreme Court also held), Kensington & Chelsea had not acted lawfully in national law, since Ms McDonald's assessment had not changed. However, once Kensington & Chelsea had re-assessed Ms McDonald's needs using radically different language and in much lesser terms, its decision to provide only continence aids was compatible with Article 8 ECHR, in the light of 'the wide margin of appreciation afforded to States in issues of general policy, including social, economic and health care policies' (para 54) – indeed, this aspect of the case was 'manifestly ill founded' (para 58):

> 57. The court is satisfied that the national courts adequately balanced the applicant's personal interests against the more general interest of the competent public authority in carrying out its social responsibility of provision of care to the community at large. It cannot, therefore, agree with the applicant that there has been no proper proportionality assessment at domestic level and that any reliance by it on the margin of appreciation would deprive her of such an assessment at any level of jurisdiction. In such cases, it is not for this court to substitute its own assessment of the merits of the contested measure (including, in particular, its own assessment of the factual details of proportionality) for that of the competent national authorities (notably the courts) unless there are shown to be compelling reasons for doing so (see, for example, *X v Latvia* [GC], App no 27853/09, para 102, ECHR 2013). The present applicant has not adduced any such compelling reasons in her pleadings before this court.

Comment: as this case exemplifies, typically the European Court of Human Rights is reluctant to interfere with social welfare/resource allocation decisions (unless some additional element is present, such as discrimination). Its approach is inevitably coloured, to some extent, by its status as a supranational court, but in practice, courts in the UK afford public authorities just as much margin of judgment in such cases, as the decision of the Supreme Court in the *McDonald* case illustrates. The approach of the ECtHR is unsurprising given that its rulings of legal principle must apply throughout Council of Europe States (of varying degrees of affluence) whilst it cannot hope to gain the detailed understanding of local economic and social factors that national institutions have. The approach of national courts in the UK turns on how they perceive their role, constitutionally: staunch protectors of core rights, such as the right to liberty and freedom from similar, serious wrongs perpetrated by the State; but engaging only with the legal parameters of socio-economic decisions, on the basis that the substantive judgment in such cases is for elected persons to take on a political basis.

25.86 *Campeanu v Romania* Application no 47847/08, [2014] ECHR 789

Exceptionally, an NGO was permitted to bring a complaint under the ECHR on behalf of a deceased individual

Facts: Mr Campeanu was a Romanian orphan with HIV+ and a severe mental disability who died at the age of 18 in a psychiatric hospital after having been provided with wholly inadequate care and treatment. An NGO, the Centre for Legal Resources (CLR), brought proceedings as Mr Campeanu's representative.

Judgment: the European Court of Human Rights held that in the very exceptional circumstances of the case, CLR was permitted to act as Mr Campeanu's representative; and it held that the authorities had breached Article 2 ECHR; and that there was a wider problem in Romania, which the authorities were required to address:

> 112. Against the above background, the court is satisfied that in the exceptional circumstances of this case and bearing in mind the serious nature

of the allegations, it should be open to the CLR to act as a representative of Mr Câmpeanu, notwithstanding the fact that it had no power of attorney to act on his behalf and that he died before the application was lodged under the Convention. To find otherwise would amount to preventing such serious allegations of a violation of the Convention from being examined at an international level, with the risk that the respondent State might escape accountability under the Convention as a result of its own failure to appoint a legal representative to act on his behalf as it was required to do under national law (see paragraphs 59 and 60 above; see also, *mutatis mutandis, P, C and S v United Kingdom,* cited above, and *The Arges College of Legal Advisers v Romania,* Application no 2162/05, § 26, 8 March 2011). Allowing the respondent State to escape accountability in this manner would not be consistent with the general spirit of the Convention, nor with the High Contracting Parties' obligation under Article 34 of the Convention not to hinder in any way the effective exercise of the right to bring an application before the Court.

113. Granting standing to the CLR to act as the representative of Mr Câmpeanu is an approach consonant with that applying to the right to judicial review under Article 5(4) of the Convention in the case of 'persons of unsound mind' (Article 5(1)(e)). In this context it may be reiterated that it is essential that the person concerned should have access to a court and the opportunity to be heard either in person or, where necessary, through some form of representation, failing which he will not have been afforded 'the fundamental guarantees of procedure applied in matters of deprivation of liberty' (see *De Wilde, Ooms and Versyp v Belgium,* 18 June 1971, § 76, Series A no 12). Mental illness may entail restricting or modifying the manner of exercise of such a right (see *Golder v United Kingdom,* 21 February 1975, § 39, Series A no 18), but it cannot justify impairing the very essence of the right. Indeed, special procedural safeguards may prove called for in order to protect the interests of persons who, on account of their mental disabilities, are not fully capable of acting for themselves (see *Winterwerp v The Netherlands,* 24 October 1979, § 60, Series A no 33). A hindrance in fact can contravene the Convention just like a legal impediment (see *Golder,* cited above, § 26)

...

2. The Court's assessment

(a) Article 2 of the Convention

(i) General principles

130. The first sentence of Article 2(1) enjoins the State not only to refrain from the intentional and unlawful taking of life, but also to take appropriate steps to safeguard the lives of those within its jurisdiction (see *LCB v United Kingdom,* 9 June 1998, § 36, Reports of Judgments and Decisions 1998-III).

The positive obligations under Article 2 must be construed as applying in the context of any activity, whether public or not, in which the right to life may be at stake. This is the case, for example, in the health-care sector as regards the acts or omissions of health professionals (see *Dodov,* cited above, §§ 70, 79–83 and 87, and *Vo v France* [GC], Application no 53924/00, §§ 89–90, ECHR 2004-VIII, with further references), States being required to make regulations compelling hospitals, whether public or private, to adopt appropriate measures for the protection of their patients' lives (see *Calvelli and Ciglio v Italy* [GC], Application no 32967/96, § 49, ECHR 2002-I). This applies especially where patients' capacity to look after themselves is limited (see *Dodov,* cited above, § 81); in respect of the management of dangerous activities (see *Öneryıldız v Turkey* [GC], Application no 48939/99, § 71, ECHR 2004-XII); in connection with school authorities, which have an obligation to protect the health and well-being of pupils, in particular young children who are especially vulnerable and are under their exclusive control (see *Ilbeyi Kemaloğlu and Meriye Kemaloğlu v Turkey*, Application no 19986/06, § 35, 10 April 2012); or, similarly, regarding the medical care and assistance given to young children institutionalised in State facilities (see *Nencheva and Others*, cited above, §§ 105–116).

Such positive obligations arise where it is known, or ought to have been known to the authorities in view of the circumstances, that the victim was at real and immediate risk from the criminal acts of a third party (see *Nencheva and Others*, cited above, § 108) and, if so, that they failed to take measures within the scope of their powers which, judged reasonably, might have been expected to avoid that risk (see *A and Others v Turkey*, Application no 30015/96, §§ 44–45, 27 July 2004).

131. In the light of the importance of the protection afforded by Article 2, the court must subject deprivations of life to the most careful scrutiny, taking into consideration not only the actions of State agents but also all the surrounding circumstances. Persons in custody are in a vulnerable position and the authorities are under a duty to protect them. Where the authorities decide to place and maintain in detention a person with disabilities, they should demonstrate special care in guaranteeing such conditions as correspond to his special needs resulting from his disability (see *Jasinskis v Latvia*, Application no 45744/08, §59, 21 December 2010, with further references). More broadly, the court has held that States have an obligation to take particular measures to provide effective protection of vulnerable persons from ill-treatment of which the authorities had or ought to have had knowledge (*Z and Others v United Kingdom* [GC], Application no 29392/95, § 73, ECHR 2001-V). Consequently, where an individual is taken into custody in good health but later dies, it is incumbent on the State to provide a satisfactory and convincing explanation of the events leading to his death (see *Carabulea v Romania*, Application no 45661/99, § 108, 13 July 2010) and to produce evidence casting doubt on the veracity of the victim's allegations, particularly if those allegations are backed up by medical reports (see *Selmouni v France* [GC], Application no 25803/94, § 87, ECHR 1999-V, and *Abdülsamet Yaman v Turkey*, Application no 32446/96, § 43, 2 November 2004).

In assessing evidence, the court adopts the standard of proof 'beyond reasonable doubt'. However, such proof may follow from the coexistence of sufficiently strong, clear and concordant inferences or of similar unrebutted presumptions of fact (see *Orhan v Turkey*, Application no 25656/94, § 264, 18 June 2002, § 264, and *Ireland v the United Kingdom*, cited above, § 161).

132. The State's duty to safeguard the right to life must be considered to involve not only the taking of reasonable measures to ensure the safety of individuals in public places but also, in the event of serious injury or death, having in place an effective independent judicial system securing the availability of legal means capable of promptly establishing the facts, holding accountable those at fault and providing appropriate redress to the victim (see *Dodov*, cited above, § 83).

This obligation does not necessarily require the provision of a criminal-law remedy in every case. Where negligence has been shown, for example, the obligation may for instance also be satisfied if the legal system affords victims a remedy in the civil courts, either alone or in conjunction with a remedy in the criminal courts. However, Article 2 of the Convention will not be satisfied if the protection afforded by domestic law exists only in theory: above all, it must also operate effectively in practice (see *Calvelli and Ciglio*, cited above, § 53).

133. On the other hand, the national courts should not permit life-endangering offences to go unpunished. This is essential for maintaining public confidence and ensuring adherence to the rule of law and for preventing any appearance of tolerance of or collusion in unlawful acts (see, *mutatis mutandis, Nikolova and Velichkova v Bulgaria*, Application no 7888/03, § 57, 20 December 2007). The court's task therefore consists in reviewing whether and to what extent the courts, in reaching their conclusion, have carried out the careful scrutiny required by Article 2 of the Convention, so as to maintain the deterrent effect of the judicial system in place and ensure that violations of the right to life are examined and redressed (see *Öneryıldız*, cited above, § 96)

...

b) Article 13 in conjunction with Article 2

(i) General principles

148. Article 13 of the Convention guarantees the availability at the national level of a remedy to enforce the substance of the Convention rights and freedoms in whatever form they might happen to be secured in the domestic legal order.

The effect of Article 13 is thus to require the provision of a domestic remedy to deal with the substance of an 'arguable complaint' under the Convention and to grant appropriate relief, although Contracting States are afforded some discretion as to the manner in which they conform to their Convention obligations under this provision.

The scope of the obligation under Article 13 varies depending on the nature of the applicant's complaint under the Convention. Nevertheless the remedy required by Article 13 must be 'effective' in practice as well as in law. In particular, its exercise must not be unjustifiably hindered by the acts or omissions of the authorities of the respondent State (see *Paul and Audrey Edwards v United Kingdom*, Application no 46477/99, §§ 96-97, ECHR 2002-II).

149. Where a right of such fundamental importance as the right to life or the prohibition against torture, inhuman and degrading treatment is at stake, Article 13 requires, in addition to the payment of compensation where appropriate, a thorough and effective investigation capable of leading to the identification and punishment of those responsible, including effective access for the complainant to the investigation procedure. Where alleged failure by the authorities to protect persons from the acts of others is concerned, Article 13 may not always require the authorities to assume responsibility for investigating the allegations. There should, however, be available to the victim or the victim's family a mechanism for establishing any liability of State officials or bodies for acts or omissions involving the breach of their rights under the Convention (see *Z and Others v the United Kingdom* [GC], cited above, § 109).

In the court's opinion, the authority referred to in Article 13 may not necessarily in all instances be a judicial authority in the strict sense. Nevertheless, the powers and procedural guarantees an authority possesses are relevant in determining whether the remedy before it is effective (see *Klass and Others*, cited above, § 67). The court has held that judicial remedies furnish strong guarantees of independence, access for the victim and family, and enforceability of awards in compliance with the requirements of Article 13 (see *Z and Others v the United Kingdom*, cited above, § 110).

Comment: recently, in *Bulgarian Helsinki Committee v Bulgaria* Application nos 35653/12 and 66172/12 (judgment the 28 June 2016), the European Court of Human Rights declined to permit an NGO to bring proceedings to represent two children with mental disabilities who had died in special homes where the NGO had not been in touch with the children before their death, did not have a procedural status encompassing all the rights enjoyed by parties to criminal proceedings and had become involved in the criminal proceedings in Bulgaria only after a delay. A similar case is pending – *Centre for Legal Resources on behalf of Miorita Malacu v Romania* Application no 55093/09.

25.87 *European Committee for Home-Based Priority Action for the Child and the Family (EUROCEF) v France* Complaint No 114/2015

The European Committee of Social Rights upheld as admissible EUROCEF's complaint that France was failing to discharge its duty under the revised European Social Charter to provide housing, social and medical assistance, social welfare and other benefits to unaccompanied minors, seeking asylum in France or living irregularly in France

Facts: EUROCEF complained about problems in the process of assessing whether unaccompanied young foreigners are minors; shortcomings in initial reception arrangements and very long delays in care provision, which take no account of the vulnerability of young people and the need to satisfy their basic needs and provide them with social and educational support. EUROCEF relied on Articles 7, 11, 13, 14, 17, 30 and 31 of the revised European Social Charter.

Judgment: the Committee declared the complaint admissible

25.88 *R (SG and NS) v Secretary of State for Work and Pensions* [2015] UKSC 16, (2015) 18 CCLR 215

It was not a breach of Article 14 ECHR to treat women more harshly than men in the benefits regime and the best interests of their children were irrelevant

Facts: SG and NS were single mothers with young children. They submitted that the 'benefits cap' was unlawful in that it discriminated against women in breach of Article 14 and Article 1 of the First Protocol ECHR.

Judgment: the Supreme Court (Hale, Kerr, Reed, Carnwath and Hughes JJSC) held that (Hale and Kerr JJSC dissenting) held that it was legitimate to treat women less favourably in order to reduce public expenditure, incentivise work and impose a reasonable limit on benefits. Further, and by a rather complex process of reasoning, the duty to treat the best interests of children as a primary consideration, founded on Article 3 UNCRC but present also in the ECHR, did not bite.

25.89 *Williams v Hackney LBC* [2015] EWHC 2629 (QB)

It had been a breach of the parents' rights under the ECHR to elicit their uninformed consent to the accommodation of their children under section 20 of the Children Act 1989

Facts: Hackney had been entitled to conclude that the children of the family were at risk but, having issued a police protection order, Hackney then failed to provide the parents with full information, but in effect compelled them to sign an agreement whereby Hackney accommodated the children under section 20 of the Children Act 1989. Hackney then continued to accommodate the children, even after parental consent had been explicitly withdrawn.

Judgment: Deputy High Court Judge Robert Francis QC held that whilst the claims in negligence and misfeasance failed, it was equitable to exend time for bringing a claim under the Human Rights Act 1998, despite the length of time that had elapsed, which included protracted proceedings before the ombudsman. He awarded each parent £10,000.00 on account of the interference with their Article 8 ECHR rights.

25.90 *Matheison v Secretary of State for Work and Pensions* [2015] UKSC 47, [2015] 1 WLR 3250

It was incompatible with Articles 8 and 14 ECHR, construed harmoniously with the UN Convention on the Rights of Persons with Disabilities, not to provide Disability Living Allowance to children after 84 days of hospital in-patient treatment

Facts: the claimant was a disabled child whose DLA ceased, pursuant to the relevant regulations, after he had been in hospital for over 84 days, although his parents continued to visit him and care for him in hospital, at considerable expense.

Judgment: the Supreme Court (Hale, Mance, Clarke, Wilson and Reed JJSC) held that the regulations were unlawful in breach of Articles 8 and 14 ECHR, construed harmoniously with the UNCRPD (and the UNCRC):

> 42. In *ZH (Tanzania) v Secretary of State for the Home Department [2011] 2 AC 166* , Baroness Hale JSC at para 21 quoted with approval the observation of the Grand Chamber of the Court of Human Rights in *Neulinger v Switzerland* (2010) 54 EHRR 1087 , para 131, that 'the Convention cannot be interpreted in a vacuum but must be interpreted in harmony with the general principles of international law.' The Court of Appeal concluded, however, that the circumstances of the present case left no room for either of the international Conventions to give a steer to the proper interpretation of Cameron's rights. Consistently with that conclusion, the Secretary of State proceeds to submit that it is in principle illegitimate to have regard to the conventions and in this regard he relies on the recent decision of this court in the *JS* case [2015] 1 WLR 1449...
>
> 43. It is clear that in the *JS case* the Secretary of State submitted that, while an international covenant might inform interpretation of a substantive right conferred by the Convention, it had no role in the interpretation of the parasitic right conferred by Article 14 and thus, specifically, no role in any inquiry into justification for any difference of treatment in the enjoyment of the substantive rights. But his submission was not upheld. While Lord Reed JSC did not expressly rule on it, it was rejected by Lord Carnwath JSC (paras 113–119), by Lord Hughes JSC (paras 142–144), by Baroness Hale DPSC (paras 211–218) and by Lord Kerr of Tonaghmore JSC: paras 258–262. Lord Carnwath JSC, for example, pointed out at paras 117–119 that the Secretary of State's submission ran counter to observations in the Court of Appeal in the *Burnip* case [2013] PTSR 117, cited at para 23 above, and indeed to the decision of the Grand Chamber in *X v Austria* (2013) 57

EHRR 405. The decision of the majority in the *JS* case [2015] 1 WLR 1449 was not that international Conventions were irrelevant to the interpretation of Article 14 but that the UN Convention on the Rights of the Child was irrelevant to the justification of a difference of treatment visited on women rather than directly on children: para 89 (Lord Reed JSC), paras 129–131 (Lord Carnwath JSC) and para 146 (Lord Hughes JSC).

44 The noun adopted by the Grand Chamber in the *Neulinger* case 54 EHRR 1087, cited above, is 'harmony'. A conclusion, reached without reference to international Conventions, that the Secretary of State has failed to establish justification for the difference in his treatment of those severely disabled children who are required to remain in hospital for a lengthy period would harmonise with a conclusion that his different treatment of them violates their rights under two international Conventions.

25.91 *Di Trizio v Switzerland* Application no 7186/09, [2016] ECHR 143

Invalidity benefit was capable of falling within the ambit of Article 8 ECHR

Facts: part-time workers had to forfeit invalidity allowance, whereas full-time workers did not.

Judgment: the European Court of Human Rights held that the legislation in question fell within the scope of Article 8 ECHR (Switzerland not having ratified Article 1 of the 1st Protocol), in that the legislation was capable of having an effect on the way that the applicant and her husband organised their family and working life and divided up time within the family) and that the legislation was incompatible with Articles 8 and 14 ECHR, being indirectly discriminatory against women, who formed the bulk of part-time workers after the birth of children and without any reasonably justification.

25.92 *Guberina v Croatia* Application no 23682/13, [2016] ECHR 287

Article 14 ECHR applies where a person is treated differently because of the status of another person and the UN Convention on the Rights of Persons with Disabilities was relevant to the proper construction of the scope of Article 14 ECHR

Facts: The father purchased a new dwelling on account of his disabled child, in that the previous dwelling was a flat in a block without a life, whereas the child needed a lift. The father claimed, but was refused, tax relief payable when a new dwelling was purchased because the old dwelling lacked certain basic infrastructure requirements.

Judgment: the European Court of Human Rights held that the father was entitled to complain about discriminatory treatment on the ground of his child's disability because Article 14 covers situations where an individual is treated less favourably because of another's status and that there had been a breach of Article 1 of the 1st Protocol and Article 14 because of the authorities' failure to take positive steps to include amongst the reasons for the grant of tax relief on the purchase of dwellings where the previous dwelling failed to meet basic infrastructure requirements, the reason that the previous dwelling failed to meet the infrastructure requirements of a disabled occupier. The court paid particular regard to the UNCRPD:

88. In justifying the decisions of the domestic authorities, the Government advanced two arguments. First, the Government argued that the relevant domestic law provided for objective criteria for establishing the existence of basic infrastructure requirements of adequate housing, which left no discretion for an interpretation to the administrative tax authorities in a particular case; and secondly, that the applicant had not met the financial requirements for a tax exemption given his financial situation.

89. With regard to the first argument the court cannot fail to observe that it is almost tantamount to the Government's concession that the relevant domestic authorities were not empowered to seek a reasonable relationship of proportionality between the means employed and the aim sought to be realised in the applicant's particular case. Hence, contrary to the requirements of Article 14 of the Convention, they were unable to provide objective and reasonable justification for their failure to correct the factual inequality pertinent to the applicant's case (see paragraph 60 above).

90. The court nevertheless notes, being well aware that it is in the first place for the national authorities, notably the courts, to interpret and apply the domestic law (see *Glor*, cited above, § 91), that the relevant provision of the Real Property Transfer Act is couched in rather general terms referring merely to the 'basic infrastructure' and 'hygiene and technical requirements' (see paragraph 24 above, section 11(9.5) of the Real Property Transfer Act).

91. The court further observes that other relevant provisions of the domestic law provide some guidance with regard to the question of basic requirements of accessibility for persons with disabilities. Thus, for instance, the By-law on the accessibility of buildings to persons with disabilities and reduced mobility envisages the existence of a lift as one of the basic elements of accessibility for persons with disabilities (see paragraph 25 above). However, there is nothing to suggest that any of the competent domestic authorities in the case at hand gave any consideration to such enactments in the relevant domestic law capable of complementing the meaning of terms under the Real Property Transfer Act.

92. Moreover, the court notes that by adhering to the requirements set out in the CRPD the respondent State undertook an obligation to take into consideration its relevant principles, such as reasonable accommodation, accessibility and non-discrimination against persons with disabilities with regard to their full and equal participation in all aspects of social life (see paragraph 34-37 above), and in this sphere the domestic authorities have, as asserted by the Government, undertook certain relevant measures (see paragraph 62 above). In the case in question, however, the relevant domestic authorities gave no consideration to these international obligations which the State undertook to respect.

93. It accordingly follows, contrary to what the Government asserted, that the issue in the case at hand is not the one in which the relevant domestic legislation left no room for an individual evaluation of the tax exemption requests of persons in the applicant's situation. The issue in the instant case is rather that the manner in which the legislation was applied in practice failed to sufficiently accommodate the requirements of the specific aspects of the applicant's case related to the disability of his child and, in particular, to the interpretation of the term 'basic infrastructure requirements' for the housing of a disabled person (compare *Topčić-Rosenberg*, cited above, §§ 40–49).

CHAPTER 26

Private law remedies

26.1 Introduction

Cases

26.11 *Clunis v Camden and Islington Health Authority* (1997–8) 1 CCLR 215, QBD
Health and social services authorities do not owe a duty of care to patients, to discharge their duty to provide after-care services in a reasonably careful manner and, in any event, a patient who killed a man knowing that was wrong, would not be permitted to sue

26.12 *Barrett v Enfield LBC* (1999) 2 CCLR 203, HL
It was arguable that a local authority owed a duty to care to children it was looking after, to look after them properly

26.13 *Kent v Griffiths, Roberts and the London Ambulance Service* [2001] QB 36, [2000] 2 All ER 474, CA
The ambulance service owed a duty of care to attend expeditiously

26.14 *Phelps v Hillingdon LBC* (2000) 3 CCLR 158, HL
Persons exercising a profession or skill may owe a duty of care to those they injure notwithstanding a statutory context

26.15 *S v Gloucestershire CC; L v Tower Hamlets LBC* (2000) 3 CCLR 294, CA
It was arguable that a decision by a social worker should be equated with the decisions of other professional persons, involving a duty of care, despite the statutory context

26.16 *Lister v Hesley Hall Ltd* [2001] UKHL 22, [2002] 1 AC 215
An employer is vicariously liable for the acts of an employee that were closely connected with his employment

26.17 *JD and others v East Berkshire CH and others* [2003] EWCA Civ 1151, (2004) 7 CCLR 63
Healthcare professionals owed a duty of care to children, when they were investigating possible abuse, but not parents

26.18 *A and another v Essex CC* [2003] EWCA Civ 1848, (2004) 7 CCLR 98
Adoption agencies owed a duty of care to prospective adopters to give them information about the children that the agencies had decided ought to be communicated

26.19 *JD v East Berkshire Community Health NHS Trust* [2005] UKHL 23, (2005) 8 CCLR 185
Healthcare professionals investigating the suspected of abuse of children did not owe a duty of care to the suspected perpetrators (the parents)

continued

26.20 *Lawrence v Pembrokeshire CC* [2007] EWCA Civ 446, (2007) 10 CCLR 367

Public authorities owe duties towards children not adults suspected of endangering them

26.21 *Sandford and Scherer v Waltham Forest LBC* [2008] EWHC 1106 QB, (2008) 11 CCLR 480

A local authority owed no duty of care to discharge its functions under section 2 of the Chronically Sick and Disabled Persons Act 1970 with reasonable care and skill

26.22 *AK v Central and North West London Mental Health NHS Trust and another* [2008] EWHC 1217 QB, (2008) 11 CCLR 543

A duty of care was arguably owed to an extremely vulnerable man to whom an NHS Trust was providing services, on which the man was known to be reliant

26.23 *Connor v Surrey CC* [2010] EWCA Civ 286, (2010) 13 CCLR 491

A local authority owed a duty of care to a headteacher to take adequate steps to protect her from a campaign against her

26.24 *Jain v Trent Strategic Health Authority* [2009] UKHL 4, (2009) 12 CCLR 194

A health authority did not owe care home owners a duty of care when investigating suspected inadequate care provided to residents and securing an ex parte order cancelling the care home's registration

26.25 *X and Y v Hounslow LBC* [2009] EWCA Civ 286, (2009) 12 CCLR 254

A local authority did not owe a duty of care to protect vulnerable adults from anti-social behaviour

26.26 *MAK and RK v United Kingdom* Application nos 45901/05 and 40146/06, (2010) 13 CCLR 241

Disproportionate actions by a hospital doctor, resulting in his erroneously concluding that parents had abused their daughter, were incompatible with Article 8 ECHR

26.27 *NA v Nottinghamshire CC* [2015] EWCA Civ 1139, [2016] QB 739

In the absence of negligence, a local authority is not liable for abuse perpetrated by foster carers

26.28 *Cox v Ministry of Justice* [2016] UKSC 10, [2016] AC 660

A is vicariously liable for the torts of B who, whilst not being an employee, is undertaking activities as an integral part of A's undertaking and for A's benefit, rather than for an independent business, and where the risk arises out of A assigning B the activity that led to the tortious act

26.29 *A M Mohamud v WM Morrison Supermarkets PLC* [2016] UKSC 11, [2016] AC 677

An employer is vicariously liable for the tortious action of an employee when there is a sufficiently close connection between the tortious action and what the employee had been employed to do, as when an employee abuses the position entrusted to him

26.30 *JR v Secretary of State for Justice* [2016] EW Misc B8 (CC)

The Probation Service was not liable for physical and emotional abuse suffered by a woman who had begun a relationship with a prisoner on licence without knowing that he had murdered his partner

26.31 *London v Southampton CC* [2016] EWHC 2021 (QB)

There had been a breach of the duty of care towards an elderly man by failing to supervise him, as a result of which he had died

Introduction

26.1 In the social and health care context, the critical question is often whether the public authority, a professional or some other person is liable in negligence for personal injury, property damage or, exceptionally, economic loss. Where the answer is 'no', the fall-back question is whether there may be liability under the ECHR.

26.2 The starting point is that:

- a duty of care arises in relationships where case-law has historically recognised a duty of care as arising and, sometimes, in analogous or incremental cases (ie there is no 'general principle', such as foreseeability of harm, that can be applied to create new duty of care relationships);
- a duty of care will only arise if harm is foreseeable, the parties are in a relationship of 'proximity' or 'neighbourhood' and it would be 'just, fair and reasonable' to recognise a duty of care as existing. These factors cannot be precisely defined or distinguished from each other. They describe features of relationships where the case-law has historically recognised a duty of care as existing and function as restraints against anything other than a cautiously incremental extension of liability beyond such relationships;
- where the defendant has acted in accordance with their powers or duties under a statutory scheme, it is relevant to consider the objectives and limits of the statutory scheme when considering whether harm was foreseeable, there was '*proximity*', and whether it would be 'just, fair and reasonable' to recognise a duty of care as existing: *Caparo Industries plc v Dickman.*[1]

26.3 On that latter point, in *Caparo* it was relevant that the auditor who prepared the defective report did so pursuant to legislation, the purpose of which was to enable shareholders to monitor the activities of the company, rather than to assist shareholders to make investment decisions. That was relevant to the decision that the auditor did not owe a duty of care to shareholders who suffered loss as a result of investment decisions based on the auditor's report.

26.4 In adult social care cases involving public authorities there will almost inevitably be a relevant statutory context and, in most cases, public authorities and professionals will be discharging a statutory function. These are factors that, in general, tilt against the existence of a common law duty of care except where the legislation simply causes the coming together of a professional relationship (eg of doctor and patient) (see further below).

26.5 Before exploring in greater detail the circumstances in which a duty of care may arise in such cases one may dispose of two outliers:

- a failure to discharge a statutory duty can, in some cases, give rise to a claim in the tort of breach of statutory duty. However, except where legislation explicitly creates such liability, it is almost impossible to satisfy the criteria for establishing a claim for breach of statutory duty, which are that (i) the duty in question was imposed for the protection of a limited class of the public, and (ii) Parliament intended to confer a

1 [1990] 2 AC 605.

private right of action for breach of that duty.[2] Those criteria would not be satisfied in the case of any adult social care legislation;

- at the other end of the scale, the statutory framework may be such as to indicate that the matter is not justiciable at all, for example, where it involves the weighing of competing public interests or is dictated by considerations that the courts are not fitted to assess[3]. Such cases are uncommon, but do arise from time to time: for example, decisions by local authorities about how much information to provide potential adopters about the children concerned have been held not to be justiciable unless perhaps a particular decision is wholly and utterly unreasonable.[4]

26.6 Otherwise, in general, and bearing in mind that in many cases all of the relevant facts will need to be evaluated before assessing whether or not the criteria for recognising a duty of care exist:

- common law negligence may occur incidentally in the course of exercising a statutory duty or power (eg the gas undertaker who lights a cigarette causing an explosion will be in breach of a duty of care); however,
- the proximity created by a statutory relationship will almost never by itself create a duty of care:[5] those who suffer injury or loss as a result of the incompetent exercise of statutory power should in general (i) use judicial review; or (ii) use complaints procedures and recourse to the Local Government or Parliamentary Ombudsmen to secure redress including financial redress; or (iii) seek to bring a claim under the ECHR, including for damages by way of just satisfaction.

26.7 The courts will recognise a duty of care where, albeit that a person is discharging a statutory function, they are in fact also exercising a particular skill or profession, which has historically been recognised as involving a duty of care to a class of persons to which the claimant belongs (eg the work undertaken by a doctor, psychologist, psychiatrist, teacher, education officer, nurse or social worker).[6]

26.8 Even then it will often be difficult to establish a breach of duty:

- given the competing considerations that such persons generally have to use their judgment to assess, when they are also discharging a statutory function;
- given the *Bolam*[7] test, under which a professional person is only negligent if they fail to act in accordance with a practice accepted at the time as proper by a responsible body of persons of the same profession or skill;[8]
- given the frequent existence of factors that tilt against the courts recognising a duty of care as existing, the most common of which are:

2 *X v Bedfordshire CC* [1995] 2 AC 633 at 731D.
3 *Carty v Croydon LBC* [2005] EWCA Civ 19, [2005] 1 WLR 2312 at paras 20–35.
4 *A v Essex CC* [2003] EWCA Civ 1848, (2004) 7 CCLR 98.
5 *Mohammed v Home Office* [2011] EWCA Civ 351, [2011] 1 WLR 2862 at paras 12–14.
6 *Phelps v Hillingdon LBC* (2000) 3 CCLR 158.
7 *Bolam v Friern Hospital Management Committee* [1957] 1 WLR 582.
8 *Carty v Croydon LBC* [2005] EWCA Civ 19, [2005] 1 WLR 2312 at paras 32–51.

- where the primary focus of legislation is the protection of members of a different class than the class to which the claimant belongs. Thus, for example, no matter how serious the damage is, persons (including doctors, psychiatrists and social workers) investigating whether children have been abused do not owe a duty of care to the parents[9]; and regulators investigating whether residents of a care home have experienced inadequate care owe no duty of care to the home owners[10] (although such persons could be liable under the ECHR[11]);
- where the claimant has been injured by the deliberate wrongdoing or criminal acts of a third party, a public authority will only owe a duty of care to protect an adult claimant,[12] no matter how foreseeable the danger, if it creates the danger, is in a position of control or supervision of the wrongdoer, or goes beyond merely discharging its statutory functions and does something special to undertake a voluntary assumption of responsibility to take care to protect the claimant from such harm[13] (although there could well be a remedy under the ECHR).[14]

26.9 On the other hand, where a public authority has control over a child or vulnerable adult for the purpose of assuming a function for which it had assumed responsibility, which would normally give rise to a duty of care, that duty of care will normally not be delegable (so the public authority will be liable for injury caused by the negligence of an independent contractor).[15]

26.10 A public authority, and any other person, will be vicariously liable for the torts of:

- their employee, when there is a sufficiently close connection between what the employee was employed to do and the torts in question, as where an employee abuses the position entrusted to them;[16]
- an individual who, whilst not being an employee, carries out an activity to further an integral aspect of the undertaking in question, otherwise than for an independent business, where the risk arises out of that individual being assigned to carry out the activity that led to the tortious act.[17]

9 *JD v East Berkshire Community Health NHS Trust* [2005] UKHL 23, (2005) 8 CCLR 185.

10 *Jain v Trent Strategic Health Authority* [2004] UKHL 4, [2009] 1 AC 853 at paras 21–28.

11 *Jain v Trent Strategic Health Authority* [2004] UKHL 4, [2009] 1 AC 853 at paras 21–28; *MAK and RK v United Kingdom (*2010) 13 CCLR 241.

12 A different approach can apply in the case of children: *CN and GN v Poole BC* [2016] EWHC 569 (QB), (2016) 19 CCLR 309.

13 *X v Hounslow LBC* [2009] EWCA Civ 286, [2009] PTSR 1158 at paras 37–61.

14 *Đorđević v Croatia* Application no 41526/10, (2012) 15 CCLR 657.

15 *Woodland v Swimming Teachers Association* [2013] UKSC 66, [2014] AC 537.

16 *Lister v Hesley Hall Ltd* [2001] UKHL 22, [2002] 1 AC 215; *A M Mohamud v WM Morrison Supermarkets PLC* [2016] UKSC 11.

17 *Cox v Ministry of Justice* [2016] UKSC 10.

Cases

26.11 *Clunis v Camden and Islington Health Authority* (1997–8) 1 CCLR 215, QBD

Health and social services authorities do not owe a duty of care to patients, to discharge their duty to provide after-care services in a reasonably careful manner and, in any event, a patient who killed a man knowing that was wrong, would not be permitted to sue

Facts: Mr Clunis relapsed and killed a man not long after being discharged from psychiatric detention and was convicted of manslaughter on the grounds of diminished responsibility. Mr Clunis sued for damages, on the basis that the health authority had negligently failed to provide him with adequate after-care services under the Mental Health Act 1983, in particular so as to monitor his mental state. His claim was struck out and his appeal dismissed.

Judgment: the Court of Appeal (Beldam and Potter LJJ, Bracewell J) held that:

(1) the maxim *ex turpi causa non oritur action* applied, given that Mr Clunis had known that his actions were wrong, so as to attract criminal responsibility:

> In the present case we consider the defendant has made out its plea that the plaintiff's claim is essentially based on his illegal act of manslaughter; he must be taken to have known what he was doing and that it was wrong, notwithstanding that the degree of his culpability was reduced by reason of mental disorder. The court ought not to allow itself to be made an instrument to enforce obligations alleged to arise out of the plaintiff's own criminal act and we would therefore allow the appeal on this ground,

(2) section 117(2) of the Mental Health Act 1983 did not give rise to a common law duty of care in negligence:

> After care services are not defined in the Act. They would normally include social work, support in helping the ex-patient with problems of employment, accommodation or family relationships, the provision of domiciliary services and the use of day centre and residential facilities. No doubt an assessment of the patient's needs would in the first instance be made by the hospital which discharged him. It was for that purpose in this case that the defendant authority sought to arrange appointments with the plaintiff. In that respect, its actions through Dr Sergeant were essentially in the sphere of administrative activities in pursuance of a scheme of social welfare in the community. Bearing in mind the ambit of the obligations under section 117 of the Act and that they affect a wide spectrum of health and social services, including voluntary services, we do not think that Parliament intended so widespread a liability as that asserted by Mr Irwin. The question of whether a common law duty exists in parallel with the authority's statutory obligations is profoundly influenced by the surrounding statutory framework. See per Lord Browne-Wilkinson *in X v Bedfordshire CC* at page 739C, and per Lord Hoffmann in *Stovin v Wise* [1996] AC 923 at 952F–953A. So, too, in this case, the statutory framework must be a major consideration in deciding whether it is fair and reasonable for the local health authority to be held responsible for errors and omissions of the kind alleged. The duties of care are, it seems

> to us, different in nature from those owed by a doctor to a patient whom he is treating and for whose lack of care in the course of such treatment the local health authority may be liable.
>
> Nor do we think that Dr Sergeant should be held liable for a failure to arrange for a mental health assessment more speedily. The suggestion that because local police had reported that the plaintiff was waving screwdrivers and knives about and talking about devils illustrates to our mind the difficulty of holding her responsible in this case. Under section 136 of the Mental Health Act a constable finding a person in a public place who appears to be suffering from a mental disorder and to be in immediate need of care or control may:
>
> > '... if he thinks it necessary to do so in the interests of that person or for the protection of other persons, remove that person to a place of safety ...'
>
> We doubt if even this language, though specifically requiring the constable to act in the interests of a mentally disordered person, creates a duty to take care which gives rise to a claim for damages at the suit of the disordered person. Moreover as Lord Browne-Wilkinson pointed out in *X v Bedfordshire CC* (supra), the question whether a doctor owes a duty of care to a patient in certifying that a patient is fit to be detained under the Mental Health Acts was left undecided in *Everett v Griffiths* [1920] 3 KB 163; [1921] 1 AC 361 and still remains open for decision in an appropriate case. We have no doubt that it would not be right to hold Dr Sergeant or the defendant health authority liable to the plaintiff in damages for failure to arrange the plaintiff's assessment for the purposes of section 117 more speedily than she did.
>
> For these reasons we do not think the plaintiff can establish a cause of action arising from a failure by the defendant health authority or Dr Sergeant to carry out their functions under section 117 of the Mental Health Act. Nor do we think that it would be fair or reasonable to hold the defendant responsible for the consequences of the plaintiff's criminal act.

Comment: Section 117(1) and (2) remain materially the same; consequently the Court of Appeal's description of the nature of after-care services and the absence of any common law duty of care still apply.

26.12 *Barrett v Enfield LBC* (1999) 2 CCLR 203, HL

It was arguable that a local authority owed a duty to care to children it was looking after, to look after them properly

Facts: Mr Barrett sued Enfield in negligence. He alleged that he had suffered personal injury, including a psychiatric illness, as a result of Enfield's failure to look after him, as a child in care, with reasonable care and skill: it had sent him to a succession of residential homes, failed to provide him with properly trained social workers and psychiatric help, failed to make proper arrangements to re-unite him with his mother and failed to arrange for his adoption.

Judgment: it was inappropriate to strike out the claim: the public policy considerations which meant that a local authority was not (at that time) under a duty of care when deciding whether or not to take action in respect of suspected child abuse did not have the same force in respect of decisions taken once the child was already in local authority care; the question whether it was fair, just and reasonable to impose a duty of care was not to be decided in the abstract, on the basis of assumed hypothetical facts, but on the basis of what had been proved; and that, accordingly, the plaintiff was entitled to have his claim heard and the facts investigated: the court applied the test in *Caparo Industries plc v Dickman*:[18] was the damage relied on foreseeable, were the parties proximate and was it reasonable to recognise the existence of a duty of care.

26.13 *Kent v Griffiths, Roberts and the London Ambulance Service* [2001] QB 36, [2000] 2 All ER 474, CA

The ambulance service owed a duty of care to attend expeditiously

Facts: despite having provided assurances that it would send an ambulance straight away, on an emergency basis, the London Ambulance Service failed to do so for 38 minutes resulting in the claimant suffering serious injury. She brought an action in negligence.

Judgment: the Court of Appeal (Lord Woolf MR, Aldous and Laws LJJ) held that the ambulance service should be equated with the health service and a duty of care recognised:

> 45. Here what was being provided was a health service. In the case of health services under the 1977 Act the conventional situation is that there is a duty of care. Why should the position of the ambulance staff be different from that of doctors or nurses? In addition the arguments based on public policy are much weaker in the case of the ambulance service than they are in the case of the police or the fire service. The police and fire services' primary obligation is to the public at large. In protecting a particular victim of crime, the police are performing their more general role of maintaining public order and reducing crime. In the case of fire the fire service will normally be concerned not only to protect a particular property where a fire breaks out but also to prevent fire spreading. In the case of both services, there is therefore a concern to protect the public generally. The emergency services that can be summoned by a 999 call do, in the majority of situations, broadly carry out a similar function. But in reality they can be very different. The ambulance service is part of the health service. Its care function includes transporting patients to and from hospital when the use of an ambulance for this purpose is desirable. It is therefore appropriate to regard the LAS as providing services of the category provided by hospitals and not as providing services equivalent to those rendered by the police or the fire service. Situations could arise where there is a conflict between the interests of a particular individual and the public at large. But, in the case of the ambulance service in this particular case, the only member of the public who could be adversely affected was the claimant. It was the claimant alone for whom the ambulance had been called.
>
> 46. Cases could arise where an ambulance is required to attend a scene of an accident in which a number of people need transporting to hospital. That could be said to be a different situation, but, as the numbers involved would be limited, I would not regard this as necessarily leading to a different result. The result would depend on the facts. I would be resistant to a suggestion that the ambulance service could be regarded as negligent because by an error of judgment a less seriously injured patient was transported to hospital leaving a more seriously injured patient at the scene who, as a

18 [1990] 2 AC 605.

result, suffered further injuries. In such a situation, on the facts, it is most unlikely that there would be conduct which could be properly regarded as negligent. The requirement to establish that there has been a lack of care provides the [London Ambulance Service] with the necessary protection.

47. An important feature of this case is that there is no question of an ambulance not being available or of a conflict in priorities. Again I recognise that where what is being attacked is the allocation of resources, whether in the provision of sufficient ambulances or sufficient drivers or attendants, different considerations could apply. There then could be issues which are not suited for resolution by the courts. However, once there are available, both in the form of an ambulance and in the form of manpower, the resources to provide an ambulance on which there are no alternative demands, the ambulance service would be acting perversely 'in circumstances such as the present', if it did not make those resources available. Having decided to provide an ambulance an explanation is required to justify a failure to attend within reasonable time.

26.14 *Phelps v Hillingdon LBC* (2000) 3 CCLR 158, HL

Persons exercising a profession or skill may owe a duty of care to those they injure notwithstanding a statutory context

Facts: the claimants (three of whom were dyslexic, one of whom suffered from Duchenne Muscular Dystrophy) asserted that they had suffered personal injury as a result of the failure of their local education authority to provide them with appropriate educational services. The issue that arose was whether a local education authority owes a duty of care to pupils.

Judgment: the House of Lords (Lords Slynn, Jauncey, Lloyd, Nicholls, Clyde, Hutton and Millett) held that: (1) notwithstanding the statutory context, a person exercising a particular skill or profession – such as an educational psychologist – might owe a duty of care to those who might foreseeably be injured if due care and skill were not exercised; where an educational psychologist was specifically asked to advise as to the assessment of and future provision for a child and it was clear that the child's parents and teachers would follow that advice a duty of care prima facie arose; that the local education authority was prima facie vicariously liable for a breach of that duty notwithstanding that the breach had occurred in the course of the performance of a statutory duty; (2) a failure to mitigate the adverse consequences of a congenital defect such as dyslexia was capable of constituting 'personal injuries to a person' within section 33(2) of the Senior Courts Act 1981; (3) teachers owed a duty at common law to exercise the skill and care of reasonable teachers in providing education for their pupils in relation to their needs; that the local education authority might be vicariously liable for breach of such duty; (4) it was also arguable that the authorities could be directly liable:

> It does not follow that the local authority can never be liable in common law negligence for damage resulting from acts done in the course of the performance of a statutory duty by the authority or by its servants or agents. This House decided in *Barrett v Enfield London Borough Council* [2001] 2 AC 550 that the fact that acts which are claimed to be negligent are carried out within the ambit of a statutory discretion is not in itself a reason why it should be held that no claim for negligence can be brought in respect

of them. It is only where what is done has involved the weighing of competing public interests or has been dictated by considerations on which Parliament could not have intended that the courts would substitute their views for the views of ministers or officials that the courts will hold that the issue is non-justiciable on the ground that the decision was made in the exercise of a statutory discretion. In Pamela's case there is no such ground for holding that her claim is non-justiciable and therefore the question to be determined is whether the damage relied on is foreseeable and proximate and whether it is just and reasonable to recognise a duty of care: *Caparo Industries plc v Dickman* [1990] 2 AC 605, 617–618. If a duty of care would exist where advice was given other than pursuant to the exercise of statutory powers, such duty of care is not excluded because the advice is given pursuant to the exercise of statutory powers. This is particularly important where other remedies laid down by the statute (e g an appeals review procedure) do not in themselves provide sufficient redress for loss which has already been caused.

Where, as in Pamela's case, a person is employed by a local education authority to carry out professional services as part of the fulfilment of the authority's statutory duty, it has to be asked whether there is any overriding reason in principle why (a) that person should not owe a duty of care (the first question) and (b) why, if the duty of care is broken by that person, the authority as employer or principal should not be vicariously liable (the second question).

I accept that, as was said in *X (Minors) v Bedfordshire County Council* [1995] 2 AC 633, there may be cases where to recognise such a vicarious liability on the part of the authority may so interfere with the performance of the local education authority's duties that it would be wrong to recognise any liability on the part of the authority. It must, however, be for the local authority to establish that: it is not to be presumed and I anticipate that the circumstances where it could be established would be exceptional.

As to the first question, it is long and well-established, now elementary, that persons exercising a particular skill or profession may owe a duty of care in the performance to people who it can be foreseen will be injured if due skill and care are not exercised, and if injury or damage can be shown to have been caused by the lack of care. Such duty does not depend on the existence of any contractual relationship between the person causing and the person suffering the damage. A doctor, an accountant and an engineer are plainly such a person. So in my view is an educational psychologist or psychiatrist and a teacher including a teacher in a specialised area, such as a teacher concerned with children having special educational needs. So may be an education officer performing the functions of a local education authority in regard to children with special educational needs. There is no more justification for a blanket immunity in their cases than there was in *Capital and Counties plc v Hampshire County Council* [1997] QB 1004.

I fully agree with what was said by Lord Browne-Wilkinson in the *X (Minors)* case [1995] 2 AC 633, 766 that a head teacher owes 'a duty of care to exercise the reasonable skills of a headmaster in relation to such [sc. a child's] educational needs' and a special advisory teacher brought in to advise on the educational needs of a specific pupil, particularly if he knows that his advice will be communicated to the pupil's parents, 'owes a duty to the child to exercise the skill and care of a reasonable advisory teacher.' A similar duty on specific facts may arise for others engaged in the educational process, eg an educational psychologist being part of the local authority's team to provide the necessary services. The fact that the educational psychologist owes a duty to the authority to exercise skill and care in the performance of his contract of employment does not mean that no duty of care can be or is owed to the child. Nor does the fact that the educational psychologist is called in in pursuance of the performance of the local authority's statutory duties mean that no duty of care is owed by him, if in exercising his profession he would otherwise have a duty of care.

That, however, is only the beginning of the inquiry. It must still be shown that the educational psychologist is acting in relation to a particular child in a situation where the law recognises a duty of care. A casual remark, an isolated act may occur in a situation where there is no sufficient nexus between the two persons for a duty of care to exist. But where an educational psychologist is specifically called in to advise in relation to the assessment and future provision for a specific child, and it is clear that the parents acting for the child and the teachers will follow that advice, prima facie a duty of care arises. It is sometimes said that there has to be an assumption of responsibility by the person concerned. That phrase can be misleading in that it can suggest that the professional person must knowingly and deliberately accept responsibility. It is, however, clear that the test is an objective one: *Henderson v Merrett Syndicates Ltd* [1995] 2 AC 145, 181. The phrase means simply that the law recognises that there is a duty of care. It is not so much that responsibility is assumed as that it is recognised or imposed by the law.

The question is thus whether in the particular circumstances the necessary nexus has been shown.

The result of a failure by an educational psychologist to take care may be that the child suffers emotional or psychological harm, perhaps even physical harm. There can be no doubt that if foreseeability and causation are established, psychological injury may constitute damage for the purpose of the common law. But so in my view can a failure to diagnose a congenital condition and to take appropriate action as a result of which failure a child's level of achievement is reduced, which leads to loss of employment and wages. Questions as to causation and as to the quantum of damage, particularly if actions are brought long after the event, may be very difficult, but there is no reason in principle to rule out such claims.

As to the second question, if a breach of the duty of care to the child by such an employee is established, prima facie a local education authority is vicariously liable for the negligence of its employee. If the educational psychologist does have a duty of care on the facts is it to be held that it is not just and reasonable that the local education authority should be vicariously liable if there is a breach of that duty? Are there reasons of public policy why the courts should not recognise such a liability? I am very conscious of the need to be cautious in recognising such a duty of care where so much is discretionary in these as in other areas of social policy. As has been said, it is obviously important that those engaged in the provision of educational services under the statutes should not be hampered by the imposition of such a vicarious liability. I do not, however, see that to recognise the existence of the duties necessarily leads or is likely to lead to that result. The recognition of the duty of care does not of itself impose unreasonably high standards. The courts have long recognised that there is no negligence if a doctor 'exercises the ordinary skill of an ordinary competent man exercising that particular art':

> '[A doctor] is not guilty of negligence if he has acted in accordance with a practice accepted as proper by a responsible body of medical men skilled in that particular art ... Putting it the other way round, a man is

> not negligent, if he is acting in accordance with such a practice, merely because there is a body of opinion who would take a contrary view': *Bolam v Friern Hospital Management Committee* [1957] 1 WLR 582, 586–587, per McNair J.

> The difficulties of the tasks involved and of the circumstances under which people have to work in this area must also be borne fully in mind. The professionalism, dedication and standards of those engaged in the provision of educational services are such that cases of liability for negligence will be exceptional. But though claims should not be encouraged and the courts should not find negligence too readily, the fact that some claims may be without foundation or exaggerated does not mean that valid claims should necessarily be excluded.

26.15 *S v Gloucestershire CC; L v Tower Hamlets LBC* (2000) 3 CCLR 294, CA

It was arguable that a decision by a social worker should be equated with the decisions of other professional persons, involving a duty of care, despite the statutory context

Facts: the claimants asserted that they had suffered personal injury as a result of sexual abuse perpetrated by their foster fathers, when in local authority care, and that this resulted from the local authorities' failure to exercise reasonable care and skill. The local authorities applied to strike out the claims for summary judgment.

Judgment: the Court of Appeal (Robert Walker, May and Tuckey LJJ) held that notwithstanding the statutory context, it was arguable that a duty of care in negligence existed: decisions of social workers in relation to individual children were capable of being equated with decisions of other professional people:

> In my view, a number of strands of the relevant law to be derived from *Barrett v Enfield* and the cases which preceded it may be summarised as follows:

> (a) depending on the particular facts of the case, a claim in common law negligence may be available to a person who claims to have been damaged by failings of a local authority who were responsible under statutory powers for his care and upbringing. In each of the cases before this court, the claims were sensibly limited to common law negligence claims.

> (b) the claim will not succeed if the failings alleged comprise actions or decisions by the local authority of a kind which are not justiciable. These may include, but will not necessarily be limited to, policy decisions and decisions about allocating public funds.

> (c) the borderline between what is justiciable and what is not may in a particular case be unclear. Its demarcation may require a more extensive investigation than is capable of being made from material in traditional pleadings alone.

> (d) there may be circumstances in which it will not be just and reasonable to impose a duty of care of the kind contended for. Here again, it may often be necessary to conduct a detailed investigation of the facts to determine this question.

> (e) in considering whether a discretionary decision was negligent, the court will not substitute its view for that of the local authority upon whom the

statute has placed the power to exercise the discretion, unless the discretionary decision was plainly wrong. But decisions of, for example, social workers are capable of being held to have been negligent by analogy with decisions of other professional people. Here again, it may well be necessary to conduct a detailed factual enquiry.

26.16 *Lister v Hesley Hall Ltd* [2001] UKHL 22, [2002] 1 AC 215

An employer is vicariously liable for the acts of an employee that were closely connected with his employment

Facts: the warden of a school boarding house sexually abused boys in his care, who then sued Hesley on the basis that Hesley was vicariously liable for the warden's tortious conduct, as the warden's employer.

Judgment: the House of Lords (Lords Steyn, Clyde, Hutton, Hobhouse and Millett) held that the warden's acts were so closely connected with his employment that it would be fair and just to hold Hesley vicariously liable:

> 28. Employing the traditional methodology of English law, I am satisfied that in the case of the appeals under consideration the evidence showed that the employers entrusted the care of the children in A House to the warden. The question is whether the warden's torts were so closely connected with his employment that it would be fair and just to hold the employers vicariously liable. On the facts of the case the answer is yes. After all, the sexual abuse was inextricably interwoven with the carrying out by the warden of his duties in A House. Matters of degree arise. But the present cases clearly fall on the side of vicarious liability.

26.17 *JD and others v East Berkshire CH and others* [2003] EWCA Civ 1151, (2004) 7 CCLR 63

Healthcare professionals owed a duty of care to children, when they were investigating possible abuse, but not parents

Facts: various protective steps had been taken in relation to children on the basis of assessments that their parents had perpetrated or exposed them to abuse. Those assessments were later shown to have been wrong. The children and the parents brought actions for damages in negligence.

Judgment: the Court of Appeal (Lord Phillips MR, Hale and Latham LJJ) held that, since the coming into force of the Human Rights Act 1998, it was no longer legitimate to rule that, as a matter of law, no duty of care was owed to a child in the investigation of suspected child abuse and the initiation and pursuit of care proceedings; but no duty of care arose in relation to the parents:

> 83. In so far as the position of a child is concerned, we have reached the firm conclusion that the decision in *Bedfordshire* cannot survive the Human Rights Act. Where child abuse is suspected the interests of the child are paramount – see S.1 Children Act 1989. Given the obligation of the local authority to respect a child's Convention rights, the recognition of a duty of care to the child on the part of those involved should not have a significantly adverse effect on the manner in which they perform their duties. In the context of suspected child abuse, breach of a duty of care in negligence will frequently also amount to a violation of Article 3 or Article 8. The difference,

of course, is that those asserting that wrongful acts or omissions occurred before October 2000 will have no claim under the Human Rights Act. This cannot, however, constitute a valid reason of policy for preserving a limitation of the common law duty of care which is not otherwise justified. On the contrary, the absence of an alternative remedy for children who were victims of abuse before October 2000 militates in favour of the recognition of a common law duty of care once the public policy reasons against this have lost their force.

84. It follows that it will no longer be legitimate to rule that, as a matter of law, no common law duty of care is owed to a child in relation to the investigation of suspected child abuse and the initiation and pursuit of care proceedings. It is possible that there will be factual situations where it is not fair, just or reasonable to impose a duty of care, but each case will fall to be determined on its individual facts.

85. In reaching this decision we do not suggest that the common law duty of care will replicate the duty not to violate Articles 3 and 8. Liability for breach of the latter duty and entitlement to compensation can arise in circumstances where the tort of negligence is not made out. The area of factual enquiry where breaches of the two duties are alleged are, however likely to be the same.

86. The position in relation to the parent is very different. Where the issue is whether a child should be removed from the parents, the best interests of the child may lead to the answer yes or no. The Strasbourg cases demonstrate that failure to remove a child from the parents can as readily give rise to a valid claim by the child as a decision to remove the child. The same is not true of the parents' position. It will always be in the parents' interests that the child should not be removed. Thus the child's interests are in potential conflict with the interests of the parents. In view of this, we consider that there are cogent reasons of public policy for concluding that, where child care decisions are being taken, no common law duty of care should be owed to the parents. Our reasoning in reaching this conclusion is supported by that of the Privy Council in *B v Attorney-General*.

87. For the above reasons, where consideration is being given to whether the suspicion of child abuse justifies taking proceedings to remove a child from the parents, while a duty of care can be owed to the child, no common law duty of care is owed to the parents.

Comment: the parents went to the House of Lords and lost (see para 26.19 below) but then went to the European Court of Human Rights and succeeded under Articles 8 and 13 ECHR: see *MAK and RK v United Kingdom* (para 26.26 below).[19]

26.18 *A and another v Essex CC* [2003] EWCA Civ 1848, (2004) 7 CCLR 98

Adoption agencies owed a duty of care to prospective adopters to give them information about the children that the agencies had decided ought to be communicated

Facts: Essex decided that it ought to inform foster carers and prospective adopters about the children's behaviour problems, but it failed to do so. The children were far more difficult than the carers would have agreed to look after had they known the full facts but, notwithstanding the personal injury and distress caused, they went on to adopt them in any event.

19 Application Nos 45901/05 and 40146/06, (2010) 13 CCLR 241, ECtHR.

Judgment: the Court of Appeal (Ward, Hale and Scott Baker LJJ) held that whilst adoption agencies did not owe a general duty to care to prospective adopters, they did owe a duty of care at least to pass on information that they had decided ought to be passed on (and information that it would be *Wednesbury* unreasonable not to pass on). Had the relevant information been passed on the adults would not have fostered and then adopted the children, so the local authority's breach of duty resulted in the injury and loss. Physical attacks were foreseeable, so that consequential psychiatric injury was also covered. However, there could not be any award of damages after the adoption proceeded because, by that time, the parents knew enough about the children to make a decision for themselves.

26.19 *JD v East Berkshire Community Health NHS Trust* [2005] UKHL 23, (2005) 8 CCLR 185

Healthcare professionals investigating the suspected of abuse of children did not owe a duty of care to the suspected perpetrators (the parents)

Facts: in a number of cases, children had been removed from their parents for a period of time, on the basis of doctors' opinions, that the parents had deliberately harmed them, or fabricated their symptoms. The parents sued the doctors in negligence. They established that the doctors owed the children a duty of care (*JD and others v East Berkshire CH and others*[20]) and the Trust did not appeal that. However, they appealed the conclusion of the Court of Appeal that the doctors did not owe the parents a duty of care.

Judgment: the House of Lords (Lords Bingham, Nicholls, Steyn, Rodger and Brown, Lord Bingham dissenting) held that for sound public policy reasons, doctors owed a duty of care to children undergoing medical tests for suspected child abuse, but not their parents/carers. The parents/carers might, however, have a claim under the ECHR.

Comment: the parents went to the European Court of Human Rights and succeeded under Articles 8 and 13 ECHR: see *MAK and RK v United Kingdom* (see para 26.26 below).[21]

26.20 *Lawrence v Pembrokeshire CC* [2007] EWCA Civ 446, (2007) 10 CCLR 367

Public authorities owe duties towards children not adults suspected of endangering them

Facts: thc Ombudsman found that Pembrokeshire had been guilty of maladministration in placing the names of L's children on the child protection register. L then brought a claim in negligence.

Judgment: the Court of Appeal (Auld, Scott Baker and Richards LJJ) held that the advent of the ECHR did not dilute the public policy that the need to protect children was the primary consideration, so that local authorities and other officials were not under a duty of care towards adults suspected of endangering children:

20 [2003] EWCA Civ 1151, (2004) 7 CCLR 63.
21 Application Nos 45901/05 and 40146/06, (2010) 13 CCLR 241, ECtHR.

55. In summary, my view, like that of Field J, is that Mr Weir's proposed 'small incremental step' in development of the common law would be a step too far. The public interest in effective and fair investigation and prevention of criminal behaviour has fashioned the common law to protect those suspected of it from malice or bad faith, but not from a well-intentioned but negligent mistake, as Lord Nicholls emphatically explained in *East Berkshire*, at paras 74, 77 and 78. The basis for that distinction is the need to provide protection to those who have a duty to enforce the law in good faith from the imposition of a duty in negligence that could or might tend to inhibit them in the effective fulfilment of that duty. The development proposed would fundamentally distort the law of negligence in this area, putting at risk the protection for children which it provides in its present form. Article 8, with its wholly different legal construct of engaging liability without reference to a duty of care, complements it in facilitating a similar protection through mechanism for justification. The provision of a discrete Convention remedy through the medium of the HRA, does not, on that account, necessitate change of the common law in the manner proposed. This Court and the House of Lords have recently clarified in *East Berkshire* the relevant principles of the common law, including the effect or lack of effect in relation to this issue of the impact of the HRA, concluding that they preclude the existence of such a duty to the parent. That reasoning, with respect, still stands, and is not, as Mr Weir would have it, 'consigned to history'.

26.21 *Sandford and Scherer v Waltham Forest LBC* [2008] EWHC 1106 QB, (2008) 11 CCLR 480

A local authority owed no duty of care to discharge its functions under section 2 of the Chronically Sick and Disabled Persons Act 1970 with reasonable care and skill

Facts: Wandsworth assessed Ms S as requiring cot sides for her bed but, before Wandsworth provided them, Ms S fell out of bed and sustained injuries, as a result of which she required nursing home care. After her death, her estate sued Wandsworth in negligence, for the injuries sustained by Ms S and also for the cost of nursing care.

Judgment: Deputy High Court Judge Richard Seymour QC dismissed the action on the ground that Wandsworth had not owed Ms S a common law duty of care in negligence: on analysis, the claim was simply that Wandsworth had been in breach of its statutory duty under section 2 of the Chronically Sick and Disabled Persons Act 1970.

26.22 *AK v Central and North West London Mental Health NHS Trust and another* [2008] EWHC 1217 QB, (2008) 11 CCLR 543

A duty of care was arguably owed to an extremely vulnerable man to whom an NHS Trust was providing services, on which the man was known to be reliant

Facts: after his discharge from the latest of many compulsory admissions, AK was placed in bed and breakfast accommodation but jumped from the window, suffering catastrophic injuries. He claimed damages from the Primary Care Trust and the local authority. The Master granted the defendants summary judgment and AK appealed.

Judgment: King J allowed the appeal on the basis that it was arguable that the defendants had owed AK a common law duty of care, based on their ongoing responsibility for the care of a highly vulnerable man they knew was reliant on them. Further, while the Article 2 ECHR claim was doomed to fail, in the absence of a plea of gross negligence, the same could not be said of the claims under Articles 3 or 8 ECHR.

26.23 *Connor v Surrey CC* [2010] EWCA Civ 286, (2010) 13 CCLR 491

A local authority owed a duty of care to a headteacher to take adequate steps to protect her from a campaign against her

Facts: new members of the governing body of a school engaged in a campaign to discredit and undermine the head teacher, as part of an attempt to change the school into a faith school. The local authority became aware of this but failed to take adequate steps to protect the head teacher, who ultimately retired permanently owing to psychiatric ill health.

Judgment: the Court of Appeal (Laws, Sedley and Thomas LJJ) held essentially that because the local authority owed the head teacher a pre-existing common law duty of care (arising out of the employment relationship), its gross failures to discharge its public law responsibilities reasonably amounted to a breach of that duty of care

26.24 *Jain v Trent Strategic Health Authority* [2009] UKHL 4, (2009) 12 CCLR 194

A health authority did not owe care home owners a duty of care when investigating suspected inadequate care provided to residents and securing an ex parte order cancelling the care home's registration

Facts: Nottingham Health Authority (Trent's predecessor's) applied ex parte without notice to the magistrates' court for an order under section 30 of the Registered Homes Act 1984, immediately cancelling the registration of Mr and Mrs Jain's care home. That resulted in the immediate closure of their care home business. Mr and Mrs Jain's only remedy was to appeal to the magistrates, which was a relatively lengthy process. By the time the appeal was heard, it was apparent that Nottingham's application under section 30 had been entirely misconceived and wholly unjustified. By that time, however, Mr and Mrs Jain had been financially ruined. They sued in negligence.

Judgment: the House of Lords (Lords Scott, Rodger, Baroness Hale, Lords Carswell and Neuberger) held that Nottingham had not owed Mr and Mrs Jain a common law duty of care because it had been acting under statutory powers conferred for the benefit of a separate class of persons and had obtained court authority for its actions. Lord Scott, Baroness Hale and Lords Carswell and Neuberger opined that had the relevant events occurred after the 2 October 2002, Mr and Mrs Jain might have had a remedy under the Human Rights Act 1998.

Comment: Mr and Mrs Jain brought proceedings in the European Court of Human rights and achieved a friendly settlement (£733,500 plus legal costs).[22]

26.25 *X and Y v Hounslow LBC* [2009] EWCA Civ 286, (2009) 12 CCLR 254

A local authority did not owe a duty of care to protect vulnerable adults from anti-social behaviour

Facts: X and Y, who were vulnerable adults requiring ongoing support in the community, were abused and victimised by a group of local youths as, meanwhile, Hounslow took ineffectual steps to transfer them elsewhere and protect them. The abuse then resulted in serious and sustained assaults. At first instance Maddison J held Hounslow liable in negligence but Hounslow then appealed.

Judgment: the Court of Appeal (Sir Anthony Clarke MR, Tuckey and Goldring LJJ) allowed Hounslow's appeal, on the ground that (i) it had not created the danger; (ii) it was not in control of or supervising the offenders, (iii) none of its officers had been in a conventional duty of care relationship with X and Y (such as doctor and patient); and (iv) it had simply exercised its statutory powers inadequately, without having assumed a special responsibility to protect X and Y from harm:

> 59. In *Mitchell* [2009] PTSR 778 it was common ground as it is here that the alleged duty was not part of the councils contractual duties as a landlord, which it was accepted did not extend to the exercise of discretionary powers under the relevant statute: *Hussain v Lancaster City Council* [2000] QB 1. As stated by Lord Hope, at [2009] PTSR 778, para 26, the question in the Mitchell case on the facts was whether, acknowledging that the council was the deceased's neighbours landlord, it was fair, just and reasonable that it should be held liable in damages for the omissions to warn relied upon. It was a matter of fairness and public policy. The House of Lords held that the answer was 'no'. Lord Hope said, at para 29, that the position would have been different if there had been a basis for saying that the council had assumed a responsibility to advise the deceased of the steps that they were taking or in some other way had induced the deceased to rely on them to do so.
>
> 60. In these circumstances, as we see it, the question is whether this case falls within Lord Hoffmann's category of cases in which public authorities have actually done acts or entered into relationships or undertaken responsibilities which give rise to a common law duty of care. Examples of such cases are given in the Mitchell case. Only in such a case would it be fair, just and reasonable to hold that a local authority such as the council on facts such as these owe a duty of care to the claimants. This is not a case of control like *Dorset Yacht* [1970] AC 1004. Nor is it a case where the defendant has created or increased the danger to the claimants. Moreover, it is not a case of assumption of responsibility unless it can properly be held that there was a voluntary assumption of responsibility: see *Rowley v Secretary of State for Work and Pensions* [2007] 1 WLR 2861, especially per Dyson LJ, at paras 51–54. This is because, as the cases cited above show, a public authority will not be held to have assumed a common law duty merely by doing what the statute requires or what it has power to do under a statute, at any

22 *Jain v United Kingdom* (2010) Application no 39598/09.

rate unless the duty arises out of the relationship created as a result, such as in Lord Hoffmann's example of the doctor patient relationship.

Comment: cf *Đorđević v Croatia* Application no 41526/10, (2012) 15 CCLR 657 (the authorities were in breach of Articles 3 and 8 ECHR by failing to protect a disabled man and his mother from harassment by local ragamuffins)(see also cases in chapter 25 'Human rights').

26.26 *MAK and RK v United Kingdom* Application nos 45901/05 and 40146/06, (2010) 13 CCLR 241

Disproportionate actions by a hospital doctor, resulting in his erroneously concluding that parents had abused their daughter, were incompatible with Article 8 ECHR

Facts: a hospital doctor negligently concluded that the daughter had been abused, resulting in the parents' access to their doctor being blocked, then impeded, for about a week. The English Court of Appeal struck out the parents' action in negligence (*JD v East Berkshire Community Health NHS Trust* [2005] 2 AC 373, (2005) 8 CCLR 185).

Judgment: the European Court of Human Rights held that whilst mistaken judgments or assessments by professionals do not in themselves render protection measures incompatible with Article 8 ECHR, in this case, the doctor's actions had been disproportionate: there had been a breach of Article 8 ECHR and, because the Human Rights Act 1998 had not been in force at the relevant time, of Article 13 ECHR.

26.27 *NA v Nottinghamshire CC* [2015] EWCA Civ 1139, [2016] QB 739

In the absence of negligence, a local authority is not liable for abuse perpetrated by foster carers

Facts: Nottinghamshire had placed NA with two foster families between 1985 and 1988. The first family abused NA physically, the second family abused her sexually. Nottinghamshire had not discharged its functions negligently.

Judgment: the Court of Appeal (Black, Tomlinson and Burnett LJJ) held that Nottinghamshire was not vicariously liable for the abuse and did not have a non-delegable duty of care that made it responsible.

26.28 *Cox v Ministry of Justice* [2016] UKSC 10, [2016] AC 660

A is vicariously liable for the torts of B who, whilst not being an employee, is undertaking activities as an integral part of A's undertaking and for A's benefit, rather than for an independent business, and where the risk arises out of A assigning B the activity that led to the tortious act

Facts: C, a catering manager employed at a prison, had been injured by the negligent act of a prisoner undertaking nominally paid prison work. C sued the Ministry of Justice for damages. The issue was, whether the Ministry of Justice was vicariously liable for the actions of the prisoner, given that the prisoner was not the Ministry of Justice's employee.

Judgment: the Supreme Court (Neuberger, Hale, Dyson, Reed and Toulson JJSC) held that the Ministry of Justice was vicariously liable because the prisoner had been undertaking activities in furtherance of the Ministry of Justice's aims, in the sense described in *Various Claimants v Catholic Child Welfare Society* [2012] UKSC 56, [2013] 2 AC 1 ('the *Christian Brothers* case'):

> 24. Lord Phillips's analysis in the *Christian Brothers* case wove together these related ideas so as to develop a modern theory of vicarious liability. The result of this approach is that a relationship other than one of employment is in principle capable of giving rise to vicarious liability where harm is wrongfully done by an individual who carries on activities as an integral part of the business activities carried on by a defendant and for its benefit (rather than his activities being entirely attributable to the conduct of a recognisably independent business of his own or of a third party), and where the commission of the wrongful act is a risk created by the defendant by assigning those activities to the individual in question.

26.29 *A M Mohamud v WM Morrison Supermarkets PLC* [2016] UKSC 11, [2016] AC 677

An employer is vicariously liable for the tortious action of an employee when there is a sufficiently close connection between the tortious action and what the employee had been employed to do, as when an employee abuses the position entrusted to him

Facts: Mr Mohamud, a customer, approached a member of staff of Morrison's ('K') with an enquiry but K responded with foul-mouthed abuse and a violent assault. The customer sued for damages but lost in the High Court and Court of Appeal on the basis that, although K's employment involved interaction with customers, that was insufficient to fix Morrison's with vicarious liability because there was an insufficiently close connection with the assault and what K had been employed to do. Mr Mohamud submitted there should be a new test of vicarious liability in which the courts applied a '*representative capacity*' test, rather than a '*close connection*' test.

Judgment: the Supreme Court (Neuberger, Hale, Dyson, Reed and Toulson JJSC) held that the '*close connection*' test in *Lister v Hesley Hall*[23] and *Dubai Aluminium Co Ltd v Salaam*[24] was to be applied although a simplification of the essence of the test was desirable:

> 44. In the simplest terms, the court has to consider two matters. The first question is what functions or 'field of activities' have been entrusted by the employer to the employee, or, in everyday language, what was the nature of his job. As has been emphasised in several cases, this question must be addressed broadly; see in particular the passage in Diplock LJ's judgment in *Ilkiw v Samuels* included in the citation from *Rose v Plenty* [1963] 1 WLR 991, 1004 at para 38 above, and cited also in *Lister* by Lord Steyn at para 20, Lord Clyde at para 42, Lord Hobhouse at para 58 and Lord Millett at para 77.

23 [2011] UKHL 22, [2002] 1 AC 215.

24 [2002] UKHL 2 AC, [2003] 2 AC 366.

45. Secondly, the court must decide whether there was sufficient connection between the position in which he was employed and his wrongful conduct to make it right for the employer to be held liable under the principle of social justice which goes back to Holt. To try to measure the closeness of connection, as it were, on a scale of 1 to 10, would be a forlorn exercise and, what is more, it would miss the point. The cases in which the necessary connection has been found for Holt's principle to be applied are cases in which the employee used or misused the position entrusted to him in a way which injured the third party. *Lloyd v Grace, Smith & Co, Peterson* and *Lister* were all cases in which the employee misused his position in a way which injured the claimant, and that is the reason why it was just that the employer who selected him and put him in that position should be held responsible. By contrast, in *Warren v Henlys Ltd* any misbehaviour by the petrol pump attendant, qua petrol pump attendant, was past history by the time that he assaulted the claimant. The claimant had in the meantime left the scene, and the context in which the assault occurred was that he had returned with the police officer to pursue a complaint against the attendant.

It had been K's job to attend to customers and respond to their enquiries and his conduct in answering Mr Mohamud's request in a foul-mouthed way was inexcusable but within the field of activities assigned to him and, when K followed Mr Mohamud outside and ordered him to leave, reinforcing that order with violence, he was forcing Mr Mohamud to leave Morrison's business premises and he was purporting to act in furtherance of his employer's business: since Morrison's had entrusted K with serving customers it was just that Morrison's should be held responsible for his abuse of that position.

26.30 *JR v Secretary of State for Justice* [2016] EW Misc B8 (CC)

The Probation Service was not liable for physical and emotional abuse suffered by a woman who had begun a relationship with a prisoner on licence without knowing that he had murdered his partner

Facts: JR entered into an intimate relationship with a man who had been convicted of murdering his partner and was released on licence. Information had been provided to the Probation Service that might have alerted them to this state of affairs. The man then assaulted JR and threatened to kill her. She sued the Probation Service in negligence.

Judgment: HHJ Saffman held that the Probation Service had not owed JR any duty of care because they had been discharging their statutory functions and there had not been any specific reliance on the Probation Service, in that the Probation Service had not told JR that it would investigate with a view to protecting her. In any event, on the facts, even if a duty of care had existed, the Probation Service would not have breached it because the information provided to it, about the relationship, had not been at all clear.

26.31 ## *London v Southampton CC* [2016] EWHC 2021 (QB)

There had been a breach of the duty of care towards an elderly man by failing to supervise him, as a result of which he had died

Facts: Mr London had been a 65-year-old man who suffered from a number of health conditions. He had been waiting for a minibus at a day centre run by the local authority. The driver, employed by the local authority, had briefly left Mr London unattended to adjust the tail lift at the back of the minibus. At that moment, Mr London stepped forward, tripped and fell. He needed a total hip replacement but never recovered fully and died 10 weeks later from deep vein thrombosis.

Judgment: May J held that the local authority had been in breach of its duty of care towards Mr London as the risk of him falling was known and that, on the facts, his death had been in consequence because his fall had increased his liability to deep vein thrombosis and his fall, operation and consequent immobility had caused it.

CHAPTER 27

Judicial review

continued

27.23 *R (Cowl) v Plymouth CC* [2001] EWCA Civ 1935, (2002) 2 CCLR 42
Alternative dispute resolution can be an alternative remedy to judicial review even in a case raising some issues of law and should always be seriously considered

27.24 *R (B) v Lambeth LBC* [2006] EWHC 639 (Admin), (2006) 9 CCLR 239
The function of judicial review is to pronounce upon the lawfulness or otherwise of public decision-making, not to investigate its merits

27.25 *R (F, J, S, R) v Wirral BC* [2009] EWHC 1626 (Admin), (2009) 12 CCLR 452
Minor criticisms of assessments, not likely to result in changed services, should be brought through a complaints procedure

27.26 *R (Bhatti) v Bury MBC* [2013] EWHC 3093 (Admin), (2014) 17 CCLR 64
A wholly new decision-making process in general required a fresh application for judicial review

27.27 *Re MN (An Adult)* [2015] EWCA Civ 411, (2015) 18 CCLR 521
The Court of Protection has no power to require a public authority to provide different services, only to consider whether services on offer are in P's best interests, so any legal challenge to the sufficiency of services offered must be brought by way of judicial review

27.28 *R (DAT) v West Berkshire Council* [2016] EWHC 1876 (Admin), (2016) 19 CCLR 362
Section 66 of the Local Government Finance Act 1992 did not prevent the court from quashing one component of the overall budget calculation where any increased expenditure could be met from reserves

27.29 Breaches of duty

27.30 *R v Islington LBC ex p Rixon* (1997–8) 1 CCLR 119, QBD
Where a resource is not available to meet needs that should not be the end of the matter; the local authority should consider acquiring a suitable resource

27.31 *R v Lambeth LBC ex p A1 and A2* (1997–8) 1 CCLR 336, CA
Where a necessary resource to meet a need is not available, a local authority must undertake a since and determined effort to find a solution but, if it does so, is not acting unlawfully in failing to meet the need

27.32 *R v Wigan MBC ex p Tammadge* (1997–8) 1 CCLR 581, QBD
Local authorities are required to meet needs that they have accepted as being eligible and a mandatory order may be granted ordering them to do so

27.33 *R (KM) v Cambridgeshire CC* [2012] UKSC 23, (2012) 15 CCLR 374
It is lawful to use a resource allocation system to guide assessment as to what level of personal budget to provide

Costs in judicial review

27.34 *R (Boxall) v Waltham Forest LBC* (2001) 4 CCLR 258, QBD
Guidance (now largely superseded) as to how costs liability will be determined when cases settle

27.35 *R (A, B, X and Y) v East Sussex CC* [2005] EWHC 585 (Admin), (2005) 8 CCLR 228
Legal costs incurred in general monitoring of the local authority's efforts would be disallowed but on the facts it was unrealistic to have expected the claimants to agree to mediation or that mediation would have resulted in settlement and, exceptionally, two sets of costs were awarded to separately represented claimants.

27.36 *R (B) v Lambeth LBC* [2006] EWHC 639 (Admin), (2006) 9 CCLR 239

Adverse costs orders would be made against lawyers who failed adequately to identify proper errors of law in their pleadings

27.37 *R (M) v Croydon LBC* [2012] EWCA Civ 595, [2012] 1 WLR 2607

In general, a claimant would recover costs when the order settling judicial review proceedings accorded them the relief sought in the pre-action protocol letter and judicial review grounds: this leading case sets out the principles of general application

27.38 *R (Hunt) v North Somerset Council* [2015] UKSC 51

If a party to judicial review proceedings establishes after a contested hearing that a public authority acted unlawfully, some good reason would have to be shown why he should not recover his reasonable costs

27.39 *R (MVN) v Greenwich LBC* [2015] EWHC 2663 (Admin), (2015) 18 CCLR 645

A Part 36 offer will not result in indemnity costs being awarded to the successful offeror unless the offer is a genuine attempt to negotiate involving 'give and take'

27.40 *R (Baxter) v Lincolnshire CC* [2015] EWCA Civ 1290, (2016) 19 CCLR 160

To recover costs, a claimant had to establish a sufficiently clear link between the consent order and the relief he had sought in his claim form

Other

27.41 *R (C) v Secretary of State for Justice* [2016] UKSC 2, (2016) 19 CCLR 5

There was no presumption of anonymity for mental patients challenging aspects of their treatment and care in the High Court but anonymity will be granted where that is necessary in the interests of the patient

27.42 *Wasif and Hossain v Secretary of State for the Home Department* [2016] EWCA Civ 82

An application for permission to apply for judicial review was totally without merit if it was so unarguable that it was bound to fail, such that neither oral advocacy nor a revised presentation of the case, at an oral renewal hearing, could render it arguable

Introduction

27.1 Judicial review is the power that the High Court derives from common law to supervise public functions, so as to ensure that they remains lawful. As Civil Procedure Rules 54.1(2)(a) provides, 'a "claim for judicial review" means a claim to review the lawfulness of – (i) an enactment; or (ii) a decision, action or failure to act in relation to the exercise of a public function'.

27.2 Judicial review is a supervisory jurisdiction, different from both ordinary adversarial litigation between private parties and an appeal on the merits. The question is not whether the judge considers that an enactment or what a public body has done is right, but whether the lawfulness of either is undermined by some recognisable public law wrong. In *Reid v Secretary of State for Scotland*,[1] Lord Clyde explained judicial review in this way in the context of applications for 'judicial review' of decisions:

> Judicial review involves a challenge to the legal validity of the decision. It does not allow the court of review to examine the evidence with a view to forming its own view about the substantial merits of the case. It may be that the tribunal whose decision is being challenged has done something which it had no lawful authority to do. It may have abused or misused the authority which it had. It may have departed from the procedures which either by statute or at common law as a matter of fairness it ought to have observed. As regards the decision itself it may be found to be perverse, or irrational, or grossly disproportionate to what was required. Or the decision may be found to be erroneous in respect of a legal deficiency, as for example, through the absence of evidence, or of sufficient evidence, to support it, or through account being taken of irrelevant matter, or through a failure for any reason to take account of a relevant matter, or through some misconstruction of the terms of the statutory provision which the decision-maker is required to apply. But while the evidence may have to be explored in order to see if the decision is vitiated by such legal deficiencies it is perfectly clear that in a case of review, as distinct from an ordinary appeal, the court may not set about forming its own preferred view of the evidence.

27.3 The main uses to which judicial review is put, in order to safeguard and promote the welfare of vulnerable adults, is (i) to supervise the lawfulness of decisions by public authorities about what services to offer, (ii) to ensure that human rights have not been violated.

Judicial review of service provision decisions

27.4 Insofar as judicial review is used to supervise the lawfulness of decisions by public authorities about what services to offer, there is often a fundamental tension between what the claimant actually wants (better or different services) and what the Administrative Court can deliver (a review as to whether a particular decision was lawful). This can result in the claimant pushing the court to review the merits of service provision decisions and the public authority urging the court to resist such pressure. Several of the cases below illustrate this creative tension.

1 [1999] 2 AC 512 at 541F–542A.

27.5 It is trite to observe that the function of judicial review is limited to supervising the lawfulness of public conduct so that, consequently, it is no part of the function of the court to review the merits of public decisions or, even when unlawfulness has been established, to require a public authority to reconsider its decision in any particular way (unless, very exceptionally there is plainly only one conclusion that the public authority could possibly reach).[2] Consistently with that, the court will almost never engage with factual disputes (in cases that do not involve EU or ECHR rights).[3]

27.6 Having said that, many judges do have regard to the underlying substantive merits of judicial review applications and may subject the lawfulness of public decision-making to more intense scrutiny, in cases where the decision seems aberrant, in particular the more that fundamental rights are involved.[4] There are, however, no hard and fast rules: sometimes, the right approach is to apply the law in favour of a claimant no matter how unappealing the underlying merits; other times, the right course is to maintain the law as it is and resist deflecting it so as to remedy a hard case.

27.7 The assumption of judicial review is that a public authority that has erred in public law has failed to see the question it has to decide clearly and in full and that, should it do so, there is a real possibility that it may reach a different decision. Judicial review has been used, very often successfully, to:

- require a local authority that has failed to complete a community care assessment to carry one out;[5]
- secure emergency provision pending the completion of an assessment;[6]
- quash an unlawful assessment or re-assessment and require a local authority to undertake the process again;[7]
- challenge decisions about service provision, and changes to service provision;[8]
- challenge budgetary and other policy changes;[9]

2 *R (S) v Secretary of State for the Home Department* [2007] EWCA Civ 546 at [46]; *R v Ealing LBC ex p Parkinson* (1996) 8 Admin LR 281 at 287F; see also the statutory bar on substitutionary remedies, at section 31(5) of the Senior Courts Act 1981.

3 *R (Ireneschild) v Lambeth LBC* [2007] EWCA Civ 234, [2007] HLR 34; *R v Board of Visitors of Hull Prison ex p St Germain (No 2)* [1979] 1 WLR 1401 at 1410H; cf *R (Al-Sweady) v Secretary of State for Defence* [2009] EWHC 2387 (Admin); *R (A) v Croydon LBC* [2009] UKSC 8, [2009] 1 WLR 2557.

4 *R (KM) v Cambridgeshire CC* [2012] UKSC 23, (2012) 15 CCLR 374 at para 36.

5 See, for example, *R (Patrick) v Newham LBC* (2001) 4 CCLR 48.

6 *R (AA) v Lambeth LBC* [2001] EWHC 741 (Admin), (2002) 5 CCLR 36; *R (Alloway) v Bromley LBC* [2004] EWHC 2108 (Admin), (2005) 8 CCLR 61.

7 See, for example, *R v Bristol CC ex p Penfold* (1997–8) 1 CCLR 315.

8 See, for example, *R v Gloucestershire CC ex p Barry* [1997] AC 584, (1997–8) 1 CCLR 7; *R (McDonald) v Kensington & Chelsea RLBC* [2011] UKSC 33, (2011) 14 CCLR 341; *R (KM) v Cambridgeshire CC* [2012] UKSC 23, [2012] 15 CCLR 374.

9 See, for example, *R (Hunt) v North Somerset Council* [2013] EWCA Civ 1320, (2013) 16 CCLR 502 and then at [2015] UKSC 51.

- achieve accommodation and support for persons subject to immigration control excluded from mainstream benefits;[10]
- contest local authority charges for service provision.[11]

27.8 One key feature of judicial review, which may become more important in cases under the Care Act 2014, is that it is a remedy of last resort and cannot be used where there is an adequate alternative remedy. A complaints/ADR (alternative dispute resolution) process will usually be an adequate alternative remedy where the complaint raises matters of fact and judgment.[12] A complaints/ADR process can even be an adequate alternative remedy when a case raises some issues of pure law – since the public authority might change its mind about the law in the course of the complaints/ADR process or, nonetheless, change its underlying decision.[13]

27.9 The government has created a power in section 72 of the Care Act 2014 to introduce an appeals procedure by way of regulations, in relation to all or many decisions made under Part 1 of the Care Act 2014. The government is currently undertaking a consultation about this.[14] If an appeals system is introduced then, depending of course on its scope, it is likely that judicial review will only be appropriate after the appeals process has been completed except, possibly, in some types of case where urgent relief is needed or the challenge includes a challenge to a macro policy. In other words, in future, judicial review challenges are likely usually to be focussing on the outcome of an appeal under a new appeals process.

27.10 In addition, the Senior Courts Act 1981 now provides, at section 31(2A), that the High Court must refuse to grant relief 'if it appears to the court to be highly likely that the outcome for the applicant would not have been substantially different if the conduct complained of had not occurred', unless there is an 'exceptional public interest' in granting relief.[15]

10 See, for example, *R (M) v Slough BC* [2008] UKHL 52, (2008) 11 CCLR 733; *R (Clue) v Birmingham CC* [2010] EWCA Civ 460, (2010) 13 CCLR 276; *R (SL) v Westminster CC* [2013] UKSC 27, (2013) 16 CCLR 161.

11 See, for example, in relation to residential accommodation, *R (Beeson) v Dorset CC* [2002] EWCA Civ 1812, (2003) 6 CCLR 5.

12 *R (F, J, S, R) v Wirral BC* [2009] EWHC 1626 (Admin), (2009) 12 CCLR 452.

13 *R (Cowl) v Plymouth CC* [2001] EWCA Civ 1935, (2002) 2 CCLR 42.

14 www.gov.uk/government/uploads/system/uploads/attachment_data/file/400757/2903104_Care_Act_Consultation_Accessible_All.pdf.

15 The Bingham Centre for the Rule of Law, the Public Law Project and Justice have suggested that this duty will only arise exceptionally: *Judicial Review and the Rule of Law: An Introduction to the Criminal Justice and Courts Act 2015, Part 4* at www.biicl.org/documents/767_judicial_review_and_the_rule_of_law_-_final_for_web_19_oct_2015.pdf. However, in *R (Hawke) v Secretary of State for Justice* [2015] EWHC 3599 (Admin), as a result of section 31(2A) of the Senior Courts Act 1981 Holman J declined to grant a declaration that the Secretary of State for Justice was in breach of the PSED (under section 149 of the Equality Act 2010); instead, he indicated that his judgment was a 'declaratory judgment', following the example of Blake J in *Logan v Havering LBC* [2015] EWHC 3193 (Admin). See also *R (Enfield LBC) v Secretary of State for Transport* [2015] EWHC 3758 (Admin) at para 106 (sometimes a witness statement is required from the public authority to establish that the outcome would not have been substantially different) and *R (HA) v The Governing Body of Hampstead School* [2016] EWHC 278 (Admin) at para 33 (these provisions may relate simply to 'technical flaws'). In *R (DAT) v West Berkshire Council* [2016] EWHC 1876 (Admin), Laing J found it hard to be satisfied that there was no chance of the council reaching a different decision on a reconsideration in case involving highly vulnerable children

Judicial review and human rights

27.11 Insofar as judicial review is used to ensure that human rights have not been violated:

- on the one hand, when it comes to the allocation of social welfare resources, public authorities are accorded a wide margin of judgment, so it is very difficult to use the ECHR to secure better or different services;[16]
- on the other hand, where resource allocation is not the real issue, the court may scrupulously review the facts so as to satisfy itself that human rights have not been violated, providing a highly effective safeguard: see chapter 25.[17]

Materials

27.12 The common law power of judicial review is supplemented by a statutory scheme:

- Sections 31 and 31A of the Senior Courts Act 1981;[18]
- Civil Procedure Rules Part 54;[19]
- CPR Practice Directions 54A[20] and 54D;[21]
- the Administrative Court judicial review guide 2016;[22]
- Judicial Review Pre-action Protocol.[23]

27.13 The main court forms are:[24]

- Judicial review claim form N461;
- Judicial review application for urgent consideration N463;
- Judicial review acknowledgement of service N462.

and, in any event, considered that in such a case there was an exceptional public interest in granting relief.

16 *McDonald v United Kingdom* Application no 4241/12, (2014) 17 CCLR 187.

17 *The Commissioner of Police for the Metropolis v ZH* [2013] EWCA Civ 69, (2013) 16 CCLR 109.

18 The Senior Courts Act 1981 has been recently amended by Criminal Justice and Courts Act 2015 the to add a section 31(2A), which prevents the court from granting relief where 'it appears to the court to be highly likely that the outcome for the applicant would not have been substantially different if the conduct complained of had not occurred' unless 'it considers that it is appropriate to do so for reasons of exceptional public interest' and a section 31, which prevents the court granting permission to apply for judicial review, on a similar basis.

19 www.justice.gov.uk/courts/procedure-rules/civil/rules/part54.

20 www.justice.gov.uk/courts/procedure-rules/civil/rules/part54/pd_part54a.

21 www.justice.gov.uk/courts/procedure-rules/civil/rules/part54/pd_part54d.

22 www.gov.uk/government/uploads/system/uploads/attachment_data/file/540607/administrative-court-judicial-review-guide.pdf.

23 www.justice.gov.uk/courts/procedure-rules/civil/pdf/preview/pre-action-protocol-amendments–6-april.pdf.

24 www.justice.gov.uk/courts/procedure-rules/civil/forms.

Cases

Human Rights Act cases

27.14 For cases in which the courts have exercised their public law jurisdiction under the Human Rights Act 1998, see chapter 25.

Alternative remedies and the limits of judicial review

27.15 *R v Avon CC ex p M* (1999) 2 CCLR 185, [1994] 2 FLR 1006, QBD

A local authority had to have a very good reason for departing from the cogently-reasoned conclusion of a complaints panel

Facts: a social services complaints review panel concluded that, as a result of his Down's Syndrome, M had developed the entrenched view that it was necessary for him to live in residential accommodation at a place called Milton Heights, such that to place him elsewhere would cause serious damage to his health; thus, he had a strong psychological need to live there. The panel recommended a placement at Milton Heights for three years, to allow for M to develop his living skills and be prepared to move elsewhere. In response, Avon concluded that whilst M had a strong personal preference to live at Milton Heights, his needs could be met at Berwick Lodge, which was substantial cheaper.

Judgment: Henry J held that Avon was under a duty to meet needs, including psychological needs of the kind that the panel held existed in this case and that Avon had not had *Wednesbury* rational reasons for disagreeing with the panel's assessment:

> Examining their reasons in detail, the following comments can be made:
>
> - The panel correctly found that in law the assessment must be based on current needs.
> - The panel correctly found that in law need is clearly capable of including psychological need. In particular, that must be so when (as it was on the evidence before them) that psychological need was contributed to by the congenital Down's Syndrome condition itself. I have recited the evidence that the panel had had as to that. That evidence was all one way once Mr Passfield had agreed that he was not an expert on Down's Syndrome.
> - Next, the panel had found that M's entrenched position was part of his psychological need. This is the crucial finding of fact. It is arrived at against the background, recited in these reasons, that M would not be forced to live anywhere against his will; that the only place he would presently consider would be Milton Heights, that that entrenched position was contributed to by the Down's Syndrome, and that his present needs included a need for a period of stability.
>
> ...
>
> But the making of the final decision did not lie with the review panel. It lay with the social services committee. I would be reluctant to hold (and do not) that in no circumstances whatsoever could the social services committee have overruled the review panel's recommendation in the exercise of their legal right and duty to consider it. Caution normally requires the court not to say 'never' in any obiter dictum pronouncement. But I have

no hesitation in finding that they could not overrule that decision without a substantial reason and without having given that recommendation the weight it required. It was a decision taken by a body entrusted with the basic fact-finding exercise under the complaints procedure. It was arrived at after a convincing examination of the evidence, particularly the expert evidence. The evidence before them had, as to the practicalities, been largely one way. The panel had directed themselves properly in law, and had arrived at a decision in line with the strength of the evidence before them. They had given clear reasons and they had raised the crucial factual question with the parties before arriving at their conclusion.

The strength, coherence, and apparent persuasiveness of that decision had to be addressed head on if it were to be set aside and not followed. These difficulties were not faced either by the respondents' officers in their paper to the social services committee, or by the social services committee themselves. Not to face them was either unintentional perversity on their part, or showed a wrong appreciation of the legal standing of that decision. It seems to me that you do not properly reconsider a decision when, on the evidence, it does not seem that that decision was given the weight it deserved. That is, in my judgment, what the social services committee failed to do here. To neglect to do that is not a question which merely, as is suggested in one of the papers, impugns the credibility of the review panel, but instead ignores the weight to which it is prima facie entitled because of its place in the statutory procedure, and further, pays no attention to the scope of its hearing and clear reasons that it had given.

It seems to me that anybody required, at law, to give their reasons for reconsidering and changing such a decision must have good reasons for doing so, and must show that they gave that decision sufficient weight and, in my judgment, it is that that the social services committee have here failed to do. Their decision must be quashed. As is often the case in Wednesbury quashings, it can be put in a number of ways: either unintentional perversity, or failure to take the review panel's recommendation properly into account, or an implicit error of law in not giving it sufficient weight.

27.16 *R v North Yorkshire CC ex p William Hargreaves* (1997–8) 1 CCLR 104, QBD

It can be rational to diverge from the conclusions of a complaints panel

Facts: a dispute arose between Mr Hargreaves and North Yorkshire as to what form suitable respite care ought to take, for Mr Hargreaves' intellectually impaired sister, Beryl Hargreaves. A complaints review panel had essentially upheld North Yorkshire's approach as to the provision of respite care, but recommended certain transitional arrangements. North Yorkshire accepted the principle of transitional arrangements, but modified them in a number of minor respects.

Judgment: Dyson J held that North Yorkshire had been entitled to depart from the recommendations of the complaints review panel: it was a question of rationality. He said:

The decision letter of 29 December 1993 accepted the principle of transitional arrangements and modified them in a number of respects. It is unnecessary to examine the modifications. I am satisfied that they were ones which the Respondent was entitled to put forward. Since the modifications were relatively minor I do not consider that the Respondent was obliged to give reasons for them. In fact it did give a reason for reducing

> the period in 1994/95 from ten weeks to six. Mr Gordon relies on *R v Avon County Council ex p M* to support his argument. In my judgment, that decision does not establish any general principle of universal application in relation to the rejection by local authorities of Review Panel recommendations. That case was decided on *Wednesbury* principles. It was, on its facts, very different from the present case. The Review Panel had recommended that the Applicant should go to a certain accommodation at Milton Keynes. The issue between the Applicant and the local authority was whether he should be placed in Milton Keynes, as the Applicant wished, or in other accommodation. The Panel reached its decision after conducting a fact-finding exercise, hearing expert evidence and so on. As the Judge said, the evidence had been largely one way, that is in favour of Milton Keynes, and yet the local authority rejected the Panel's recommendations without giving any, or any adequate reasons, for doing so. In the present case, the Review Panel had endorsed the Respondent on the subject of complaint, namely the offer of 2nd November 1993. In the *ex p M* case the Panel had decided the complaint in favour of the Applicant. All that Henry J was saying was that where a Panel has given a carefully reasoned decision adverse to the local authority on the subject of complaint, and the local authority rejects the Panel's recommendation without itself giving a rational reason for doing so, then there is a strong prima facie case for quashing the local authority's decision as unlawful. That is, as I say, no more that an application of the *Wednesbury* principle. In my judgment, it would be quite wrong to apply that approach to the mere refusal by the local authority to accept in full recommendations made by the Panel not on the subject of complaint but on a collateral matter, namely the proposed transitional arrangements put forward by the Panel in order to mitigate the consequences for the Applicant and Miss Hargreaves of the essential decision of the Panel to endorse the Respondent's position on the subject matter of complaint.

For the reasons given in relation to the first issue, however, the decision communicated by the Respondent's letter of 29 December 1993 must be quashed.

27.17 *R v Haringey LBC ex p Norton* (1997–8) 1 CCLR 168, QBD

Judicial review will not usually address factual disputes

Facts: Mr Norton was severely disabled as a result of Multiple Sclerosis. Haringey reduced his care provision from 24 hours/day live-in care, to five hours a day practical assistance for budgetary reasons. There was no suggestion that Mr Norton's needs had changed. However, on re-assessment, Haringey concluded that Mr Norton had not, in reality, needed his earlier care package and that five hours a day was sufficient to meet his needs.

Judgment: Mr Henderson QC (sitting as a Deputy High Court Judge) held:

> The 1994 decision is not under challenge in these proceedings. While it is a necessary part of the background properly to be taken into account, its lawfulness or unlawfulness and its substance or lack of substance could not determine the 1997 reassessment. The 1997 reassessment had to be decided on its own merits and although it was necessary to give appropriate weight to the 1994 decision there could have been no estoppel or fetter upon the Respondent in coming in 1997 to what it considered to be the correct evaluation of the Applicant's present needs consistent with the resources required to meet those needs.

...

The reasonableness or rationality of a decision can only be judged in the context of the statutory framework and of the particular facts of the case. Before turning to the statutory framework it is necessary to emphasise that it is only in extreme circumstances that a court will conclude that a decision is 'so unreasonable that no reasonable authority could ever have come to it'. (per Lord Greene MR at page 234). Warrington LJ in *Short v Poole Corporation* [1926] Ch 66 at 90/ 91 gave the example of the red-haired teacher dismissed because she had red hair. More apt to the present circumstances I have this week encountered a case in which a local authority applying its medical points system to housing need on a scale of 0–250 awarded 0 points to a lady with possibly recurrent cancer and gross breathing difficulty, of whom two consultants at London Teaching Hospitals said in categorical terms that were she to have to climb stairs this would endanger her life. In such circumstances a court can properly but most exceptionally conclude that the authority must have taken leave of its senses. I am reminded of Lord Brightman's caution in *R v Hillingdon Borough Council ex p Puhlhofer* [1986] AC 484 at page 518d, where he says:

> 'Where the existence or non-existence of a fact is left to the judgment and discretion of a public body and that fact involves a broad spectrum ranging from the obvious to the debatable to the just conceivable, it is the duty of the court to leave the decision of that fact to the public body to whom Parliament has entrusted the decision-making power save in a case where it is obvious that the public body, consciously or unconsciously, are acting perversely.'

In a case such as this, where the relevant facts include qualitative judgments of an individual's needs and the availability of resources to meet those needs and the needs of others, it must be especially difficult to establish perversity. We can now see from the recent speeches of the House of Lords in *R v Gloucester County Council ex p Barry* (1997–8) 1 CCLR 40; [1997] 2 WLR 459 that not only do the needs of particular applicants have to be considered under the statutory framework, but also a local authority's resources are to be taken into account when assessing or re-assessing the applicant's needs. The burden upon an applicant seeking to establish the irrationality or unreasonableness in law of a decision in that context is to persuade the court to step into the arena and to conclude that it is sufficiently informed of all relevant information such that no reasonable authority could have come to the conclusion that was in fact reached. Despite Mr Beloff's formidable advocacy, I am not persuaded that he has surmounted those obstacles.

...

It is not permissible to adduce, either by way of expert evidence or at all, evidence which purports to answer the question which it is for the Court to answer. Whether or not the Respondent's decision was within the realms of reasonableness in point of law is for the court and the court alone to decide. True it is that the court may in certain rare circumstances be assisted by knowing ex post facto how an expert in the field would have assessed the needs of a particular Applicant (eg a case where deficient enquiry led to ignorance of material facts or opinion and the evidence being proffered goes to the issue of what would have been discovered had due enquiry been made) but it can never be permissible for an expert either to express an opinion that a local authority's decision was or was not reasonable, nor to say whether such a decision fell within or outwith the spectrum of decisions of a local authority properly carrying out its community care duties.

> The opinion is the more objectionable in this case because an occupational therapist cannot claim to know as much as the Respondent about its available resources and competing needs, nor perhaps about Haringey's local standards. Furthermore, it is very doubtful whether, even if the opinion were appropriately limited so that it did not purport to usurp the court's function, it would be admissible consistent with *R v The Secretary of State for Environment ex p Powis*.

Comment: this decision illustrates a recurring theme in judicial review: the court will be astute to correct clear errors of law but highly circumspect in the arena of factual and evaluative judgments, notwithstanding evidence from the applicant, family, carers and experts.

27.18 *R v Sutton LBC ex p Tucker* (1997–8) 1 CCLR 251, QBD

In this case, issues of law meant that the complaints procedure was not an alternative remedy

Facts: the applicant's daughter, who was severely disabled and experienced substantial communication difficulties, had remained in hospital for two years after she was ready to be discharged, because of Sutton's failure to complete an assessment and care plan that addressed its long-term obligations so as to enable her discharge.

Judgment: Hidden J accepted the applicant's submission that Sutton had acted unlawfully by failing to 'act under' statutory guidance. He also held that the complaints procedure would not have been an adequate alternative remedy, so as to trigger the court's discretion to refuse judicial review relief because issues of law arose:

> As to whether I should in my discretion refuse relief on the basis of any alternate remedy, I find there is here a discrete point of law to be decided as to whether or not the respondent has acted unlawfully in failing to make a service provision decision under section 47(1)(b) of the National Health Service and Community Care Act 1990. That decision involves consideration of the statutory guidance issued under section 7 of the Local Authority Social Services Act 1970 and the non-statutory guidance as well. In particular it requires consideration of paragraphs 3.24 and 3.41 of the statutory policy guidance. In that situation I hold that the applicant is not precluded from making this application for judicial review by the availability of any other remedy such as the complaints procedure under section 7B of LASSA or the default powers under section 7D. I have to consider in relation to available remedies or avenues of redress, as they were referred to by Simon Brown LJ in *R v Devon County Council ex p Baker*, the question of which avenue is the more convenient, expeditious and effective. I am quite satisfied that judicial review is here the avenue to be preferred on those bases. I do not consider the default powers to be an alternative remedy where there is a discrete point of law (see *ex p S*). If the matter were to go by the complaints procedure under section 7A Mrs Tucker as a non-legally aided person would be forced to argue points of law before a non-qualified body. That could not be convenient, expeditious or effective. There is, in fact, no true alternative remedy. The position might be otherwise if the case were founded simply on *Wednesbury* irrationality or if it were a Children Act case (see *ex p T* at pages 814F and 815C). I am further satisfied that there is here a clear failure to follow the guidance given in paragraphs 3.24 and 3.41 of the policy guidance which is clearly binding on local authorities and the

respondent in particular. The respondent had discharged its duty under section 47(1)(a) of the 1990 Act to carry out an assessment of the applicant's needs by 13th April 1994. I find that the respondent is in clear breach of its duty under section 47(1)(b) in that it has still not made the decision which is called for by that section. There is still no service provision decision. Equally there is no care plan, as Mr Eccles accepts, in that there is still no provision for Therese's long term placement and therefore for her discharge from National Health Service care.

I accept the criticisms made by Mr Gordon of what is said to be the care plan in this case, those criticisms I have just referred to. I accept Mr Gordon's submissions that the care plan sought to be put forward in this case is as far from the policy guidelines as was that in the *Rixon* case. I find the respondent has acted unlawfully and departed without good reason from the policy guidance issued by the Secretary of State. I find that the respondent has used its undoubted discretion to make short term and interim decisions in relation to the care of the applicant.

The use of such discretion cannot in my view replace the duty to make a service provision decision as to the long term future of the applicant. I therefore find the respondent has acted unlawfully in the matters and in the manner I have indicated. I would also be prepared to find that such actions were *Wednesbury* unreasonable if that were necessary. As to the relief to be granted by the court I shall listen to any submissions from counsel.

27.19 *R v Gloucestershire CC ex p RADAR* (1997–8) 1 CCLR 476, QBD

A general issue of principle meant that the complaints procedure was not an alternative remedy

Facts: after the decision in *R v Islington LBC ex p Rixon* (below at para 27.30), Gloucestershire circulated 1,000 individuals facing removal or reduction of their services, inviting them to take up the offer of a re-assessment.

Judgment: Carnwath J held this did not satisfy the duty to re-assess community care needs before removing or reducing services: where there is an 'appearance of need' the duty to assess/re-assess arises without any explicit request having been made. Also, given that the case gave rise to a general issue of principle, the complaints procedure was not a reasonable alternative remedy:

> Next, Mr Eccles suggests that there is an alternative remedy by way of complaint, under the procedure set up pursuant to section 7B of the Local Authority Social Services Act 1970 (inserted by the 1990 Act s50). This may be relevant in particular cases, especially where individual relief is being sought. However, in relation to a general issue of principle as to the authority's obligations in law, such as I have been discussing here, I do not think that can be regarded as a suitable or alternative remedy to the procedure of judicial review.

27.20 *R v Wigan MBC ex p Tammadge* (1997–8) 1 CCLR 581, QBD

Once a local authority has assessed a need as existing, it is under a duty to meet that need and a mandatory order would be granted ordering it to do so

Facts: the social services complaints review panel concluded that the applicant and her family were in urgent need of re-housing for health and care reasons. Wigan accepted that and ascertained that the most cost-effective solution was knock together two adjacent houses in its area. However, Wigan then decided not to undertake that course because 'the potential benefits..... do not justify the significant costs'.

Judgment: Forbes J held that whilst resources were relevant to a limited extent, when determining whether and if so what needs existed for residential accommodation under section 21 of the National Assistance Act 1948, once a need has been assessed as existing, the local authority was under a duty to make provision for that need. That applied in this case and Wigan was ordered to undertake the work that it had itself determined as being the most cost-effective solution. At 597D-J, Forbes J said:

> In my view, SSCRP's finding as to Mrs Tammadge's need for larger accommodation is perfectly clear from the wording in which that particular conclusion is expressed. Moreover, that conclusion is entirely in keeping with views of Wigan's own professionally qualified staff and advisers, as expressed both before and after the hearing before the SSCRP. I am therefore satisfied that, by a date no later than 22 October 1996 (when it was acknowledged that Wigan had accepted the SSCRP finding ...), Mrs Tammadge's need for larger accommodation had been established.... As a result, from that date Wigan have been obliged to make provision of such accommodation to Mrs Tammadge and her family.....Once the duty had arisen in this way, it was not lawful of Wigan to refuse to perform that duty because of a shortage of or limits upon its financial resources or for any of the other reasons expressed ...'.

Comment: this is a relatively uncommon example of a judicial review directly resulting in enhanced service provision. The essential principle in the case should still apply under section 18 of the Care Act 2014 and, in relation to carers, under section 20. Also, this case arose after a decision by Wigan's complaints panel and so is an illustration of the type of case that might arise after a decision under any new appeals procedure under the Care Act 2014.

27.21 *R (Barker) v Barking, Havering and Brentwood Community Healthcare NHS Trust* (1999) 2 CCLR 5, CA

Detention should be challenged by way of judicial review, not habeas corpus, when the issue was whether administrative decision-making had been lawful

Facts: Ms Barker had a history of personality disorder and repeated admissions to hospital in a psychotic state. She was detained under section 3 of the Mental Health Act 1983 and then, later, allowed section 17 leave under which Ms Barker spent five days a week living at home, under conditions. Her psychiatrist renewed Ms Barker's section 3 detention, under section 20 of the Mental Health Act 1983. Ms Barker submitted that section 20 was inapplicable because she was no longer 'detained' or in receipt of/needing 'medical treatment in a hospital'.

Judgment: the Court of Appeal (Lord Woolf MR, Hobhouse and Thorpe LJJ) explained that, in detention cases, judicial review was the appropriate remedy, rather than habeas corpus, where 'what is in issue is the propriety of some prior administrative act', rather than where 'what is in issue is whether some precedent fact going to jurisdiction is in issue' (15D–H).

27.22 ## *R v Barking and Dagenham LBC ex p Lloyd* (2001) 4 CCLR 196, CA

In general, a complaint that an assessment or care plan was inadequate should be pursued through the complaints procedure

Facts: residents of care home accommodation submitted that the temporary closure and redevelopment of their home breached their legitimate expectations in a number of respects, including in relation to 'home for life' promises.

Judgment: the Court of Appeal (Schiemann, Sedley and Arden LJJ) dismissed the appeal, holding that, on the facts, the redevelopment plans would not necessarily involve a breach of any promises and that the assessments and care plans were adequate as provisional documents. Further, in general, a complaint that an assessment or care plan was inadequate should be pursued by way of a complaints procedure:

> 27. It seems to us however that, leaving aside for the moment any undertakings to the court, the court is not the appropriate organ to be prescriptive as to the degree of detail which should go into a care plan or as to the amount of consultation to be carried out with Ms Lloyd's advisers. In practice these are matters for the Council, and if necessary its complaints procedure. If the Council has failed to follow the Secretary of State's guidance and is arguably in breach of its statutory duties in relation to the way it carries out its assessment and what it puts into its care plans then aggrieved persons should in an appropriate case turn first to the Secretary of State. Where there is room for differences of judgment the Secretary of State and his advisers may have a useful input. The court is here as a last resort where there is illegality. Here there is not – It is right to say these matters have not been fully canvassed in argument.

27.23 ## *R (Cowl) v Plymouth CC* [2001] EWCA Civ 1935, (2002) 2 CCLR 42

Alternative dispute resolution can be an alternative remedy to judicial review even in a case raising some issues of law and should always be seriously considered

Facts: the claimants challenged the proposed closure of their care home on the basis of inadequate consultation, lack of proper assessments and breaches of 'home for life' promises; they rejected the offer of the complaints procedure, with Plymouth's assurance that it would pay very careful regard to the views of the social services complaints panel.

Judgment: the Court of Appeal (Woolf LCJ, Mummery and Buxton LJJ) dismissed the claimants appeal on the basis that the parties could have, and should still, engage in alternative dispute resolution, notwithstanding the fact that the claimants' case involved submissions that errors of law had been made. Handing down the judgment of the court, Lord Woolf LCJ said this:

> 25. We do not single out either side's lawyers for particular criticism. What followed was due to the unfortunate culture in litigation of this nature of over-judicialising the processes which are involved. It is indeed unfortunate that, that process having started, instead of the parties focusing on the future they insisted on arguing about what had occurred in the past. So far as the claimants were concerned, that was of no value since Plymouth were prepared, as they ultimately made clear was their position, to reconsider the whole issue. Without the need for the vast costs which

must have been incurred in this case already being incurred, the parties should have been able to come to a sensible conclusion as to how to dispose the issues which divided them. If they could not do this without help, then an independent mediator should have been recruited to assist. That would have been a far cheaper course to adopt. Today sufficient should be known about alternative dispute resolution to make the failure to adopt it, in particular when public money is involved, indefensible.

26. The disadvantages of what happened instead were apparent to the trial judge. They were also apparent to this court. At the opening of the hearing we therefore insisted on the parties focusing on what mattered, which was the future well-being of the claimants. Having made clear our views, building on the proposal which had been made in the 23 May letter, the parties had no difficulty in coming to a sensible agreement in the terms which are annexed to this judgment and will form part of the order of the court. The terms go beyond what Plymouth was required to do under the statutory complaint procedure. This does not however, matter because it is always open to the parties to agree to go beyond their statutory obligations. For example, sensibly the claimants are to have the benefit of representatives to appear on their behalf, who may well be non-lawyers who can be extremely experienced in handling issues of the nature of those which are involved. We trust that the parties will now draw a line under what has happened in the past and focus instead on what should happen in the future.

27.24 *R (B) v Lambeth LBC* [2006] EWHC 639 (Admin), (2006) 9 CCLR 239

The function of judicial review is to pronounce upon the lawfulness or otherwise of public decision-making, not to investigate its merits

Facts: the claimant, a 15-year-old girl, brought judicial review proceedings against Lambeth after she became homeless, alleging that Lambeth had failed adequately to assess her needs or make suitable provision. After a number of hearings, she withdrew those proceedings without permission to apply for judicial review having been granted. Lambeth applied for costs on the grounds that the judicial review grounds had failed to identify clearly any error of law and that, despite repeated requests, that had not been done until the last moment.

Judgment: Munby J held that there would no order for costs, but practitioners should be aware that cost and/or wasted costs might well be awarded in future when a judicial review application failed properly to identify any alleged errors of law: the whole of paragraphs 26–36 of the judgment contain salutary advice to practitioners. These passages commence thus:

1. This is yet another case exemplifying problems about which I have had to complain on too many occasions already. As I said in *R (P, W, F and G) v Essex County Council* [2004] EWHC 2027 (Admin) at paragraphs [30]–[31]:

'[30] The present litigation exemplifies a certain type of judicial review case which experience suggests can too often end up following a less than desirable course: I have in mind community care, housing and other cases involving either children or vulnerable adults, especially those where, as here, the first task of the local or other public authority is the preparation of an assessment.

[31] This is not the first time that I have felt impelled to express my unease about this particular type of litigation: see *R (A, B, X and Y) v*

> *East Sussex CC (No 2)* [2003] EWHC 167 (Admin), (2003) 6 CCLR 194, at paras [156]–[166], and *CF v Secretary of State for the Home Department* [2004] EWHC 111 (Fam), [2004] 1 FCR 577, at paras [217]–[219]. There is, I think, a problem here that needs to be addressed. Too often in my experience inadequate thought is given to what precisely the court is being asked or can properly be asked to do.'

2. I then went on to set out what I referred to as a few basic principles, starting with some observations on the proper function of the court in a case such as this:

> '[32] What the claimants here seek to challenge are decisions taken by the County Council in pursuance of the statutory powers and duties conferred on it by Part III of the Act. So I am here concerned with an area of decision-making where Parliament has chosen to confer the relevant power on the County Council: not on the court or anyone else. It follows that we are here within the realm of public law, not private law. It likewise follows that the primary decision maker is the County Council and not the court. The court's function in this type of dispute is essentially one of review – review of the County Council's decision, whatever it may be – rather than of primary decision making. It is not the function of the court itself to come to a decision on the merits. The court is not concerned to come to its own assessment of what is in these children's best interests. The court is concerned only to review the County Council's decisions, and that is not a review of the merits of the County Council's decisions but a review by reference to public law criteria: see *A v A Health Authority, in re J (A Child), R (S) v Secretary of State for the Home Department* [2002] EWHC 18 (Fam/Admin), [2002] Fam 213, and *CF v Secretary of State for the Home Department* [2004] EWHC 111 (Fam), [2004] 1 FCR 577, at paras [20]–[32]. Just as I pointed out in *R (A, B, X and Y) v East Sussex CC* (No 2) [2003] EWHC 167 (Admin), (2003) 6 CCLR 194, at para [161], that it was the function of the local authority and not the court to make and draw up the assessments that were there in issue, so too in the present case it is for the County Council and not the court to make the initial and core assessments of these children.
>
> [33] Now this has two important corollaries. Although I am, in a sense, concerned with the future welfare of very vulnerable children, I am not exercising a 'best interests' or 'welfare' jurisdiction, nor is it any part of my functions to monitor, regulate or police the performance by the County Council of its statutory functions on a continuing basis. A judge of the Family Division exercising the wardship jurisdiction has a continuing responsibility for the day to day life and welfare of the ward, exemplified by the principle that no important or major step in the life of a ward of court can be taken without the prior consent of the court: see *Kelly v British Broadcasting Corpn* [2001] Fam 59 at p 75. The function of the Administrative Court is quite different: it is, as it is put in CPR Part 54.1(2)(a), to review the lawfulness of a decision, action or failure to act in relation to the exercise of a public function. In other words, the Administrative Court exists to adjudicate upon specific challenges to discrete decisions. It does not exist to monitor and regulate the performance of public authorities: see in the context of community care *R v Mayor and Burgesses of the London Borough of Hackney ex p S* (unreported, 13 October 2000) at paras [8] and [11] and *R v Mayor and Burgesses of the London Borough of Hackney ex p S (No 2)* [2001] EWHC 228 (Admin) at para [4].

Comment: this really speaks for itself. Not only is it illegitimate to use the judicial review process to persuade the court to micro-manage a public authority's decision-making process, or to interfere with substantive decisions that are lawfully made, blatant attempts to do so may result in adverse or wasted costs orders.

27.25 *R (F, J, S, R) v Wirral BC* [2009] EWHC 1626 (Admin), (2009) 12 CCLR 452

Minor criticisms of assessments, not likely to result in changed services, should be brought through a complaints procedure

Facts: a supported living provider, Salisbury Independent Living, funded litigation brought by residents living in accommodation it provided, essentially claiming that due to inadequate assessments, Wirral had not provided the residents with funds that would in turn reimburse Salisbury Independent Living for the assistance it provided.

Judgment: McCombe J held that, leaving aside one potentially major point that had been raised at the hearing for the first time and which the claimants would not be permitted to rely on, the criticisms of the assessments were relatively minor and ought to be have been raised in a complaints procedure, in particular because no case had emerged where it was likely that there had been a failure to meet eligible needs; accordingly, he dismissed the application for judicial review as an abuse of process.

27.26 *R (Bhatti) v Bury MBC* [2013] EWHC 3093 (Admin), (2014) 17 CCLR 64

A wholly new decision-making process in general required a fresh application for judicial review

Facts: Ms Bhatti brought an application for a judicial review of a financial assessment undertaken by Bury, which was settled by a consent order, whereby Bury undertook a fresh community care assessment and consequent financial assessment. Ms Bhatti sought to amend her judicial review grounds to challenge those new decisions. Bury objected to that procedure.

Judgment: Deputy High Court Judge Pelling QC held that where, as here, a public authority went beyond reconsidering a decision but embarked on a new decision-making process leading to a wholly different decision, the correct approach in general was to issue fresh proceedings. Further, the proposed new grounds raised factual disputes which ought first to be addressed within the statutory complaints procedure.

27.27 *Re MN (An Adult)* [2015] EWCA Civ 411, (2015) 18 CCLR 521

The Court of Protection has no power to require a public authority to provide different services, only to consider whether services on offer are in P's best interests, so any legal challenge to the sufficiency of services offered must be brought by way of judicial review

Facts: MN was a severely disabled young adult. It was reluctantly conceded by his parents that it was in his best interests to live in a residential placement but they disputed that the package of care on offer was in MN's best interests and asked the Court of Protection (COP) to investigate and make a declaration on that issue. The COP declined to take that course on the basis that its role was limited to determining whether care packages actually on offer were in P's best interests. MN's parents appealed.

Judgment: the Court of Appeal (Sir James Munby, President of the COP, Treacey and Gloster LJJ) dismissed the appeal, holding that that the COP had no power to require a public authority to provide a different care package, only to consider whether what was on offer was in the best interests of P; if P or some other person wanted to secure change in the care package, then they had to bring judicial review proceedings. Accordingly, it was pointless and inappropriate for the COP to embark upon an investigation on whether a different care plan would be in P's best interests:

> 11. The starting point, in my judgment, is the fundamentally important principle identified by the House of Lords in *A v Liverpool City Council* [1982] AC 363 and re-stated by the House in *In re W (A Minor) (Wardship: Jurisdiction)* [1985] AC 791. For present purposes I can go straight to the speech of Lord Scarman in the latter case. Referring to *A v Liverpool City Council*, Lord Scarman said (page 795):
>
> > 'Authoritative speeches were delivered by Lord Wilberforce and Lord Roskill which it was reasonable to hope would put an end to attempts to use the wardship jurisdiction so as to secure a review by the High Court upon the merits of decisions taken by local authorities pursuant to the duties and powers imposed and conferred upon them by the statutory code.'
>
> He continued (page 797):
>
> > 'The High Court cannot exercise its powers, however wide they may be, so as to intervene on the merits in an area of concern entrusted by Parliament to another public authority. It matters not that the chosen public authority is one which acts administratively whereas the court, if seized by the same matter, would act judicially. If Parliament in an area of concern defined by statute (the area in this case being the care of children in need or trouble) prefers power to be exercised administratively instead of judicially, so be it. The courts must be careful in that area to avoid assuming a supervisory role or reviewing power over the merits of decisions taken administratively by the selected public authority.'
>
> 12. Lord Scarman was not of course disputing the High Court's power of judicial review under RSC Ord 53 (now CPR Pt 54) when exercised by what is now the Administrative Court: he was disputing the High Court's powers when exercising in the Family Division the parens patriae or wardship jurisdictions. This is made clear by what he said (page 795):
>
> > 'The ground of decision in *A v Liverpool City Council* [1982] AC 363 was nothing to do with judicial discretion but was an application in this field of the profoundly important rule that where Parliament has by statute entrusted to a public authority an administrative power subject to safeguards which, however, contain no provision that the High Court is to be required to review the merits of decisions taken pursuant to the power, the High Court has no right to intervene. If there is abuse of the power, there can of course be judicial review pursuant to RSC Ord 53: but no abuse of power has been, or could be, suggested in this case.'

It is important to appreciate that Lord Scarman was not referring to a rule going to the exercise of discretion; it is a rule going to jurisdiction.

...

80. The function of the Court of Protection is to take, on behalf of adults who lack capacity, the decisions which, if they had capacity, they would take themselves. The Court of Protection has no more power, just because it is acting on behalf of an adult who lacks capacity, to obtain resources or facilities from a third party, whether a private individual or a public authority, than the adult if he had capacity would be able to obtain himself. The *A v Liverpool* principle applies as much to the Court of Protection as it applies to the family court or the Family Division. The analyses in *A v A Health Authority* and in *Holmes-Moorhouse* likewise apply as much in the Court of Protection as in the family court or the Family Division. The Court of Protection is thus confined to choosing between available options, including those which there is good reason to believe will be forthcoming in the foreseeable future.

81. The Court of Protection, like the family court and the Family Division, can explore the care plan being put forward by a public authority and, where appropriate, require the authority to go away and think again. Rigorous probing, searching questions and persuasion are permissible; pressure is not. And in the final analysis the Court of Protection cannot compel a public authority to agree to a care plan which the authority is unwilling to implement. ...

Comment: the author cannot see any reason why a complaints process, or judicial review proceedings challenging a service provision decision, cannot be run in tandem with COP proceedings or, even, why a High Court judge entitled to sit in the Administrative Court and COP should not determine both the public law and best interests issues, providing that they carefully separated the different functions being exercised. All that this case decides, reflecting earlier case-law, is that one cannot use the best interests' jurisdiction to 'get around' the limits of judicial review.

27.28 *R (DAT) v West Berkshire Council* [2016] EWHC 1876 (Admin), (2016) 19 CCLR 362

Section 66 of the Local Government Finance Act 1992 did not prevent the court from quashing one component of the overall budget calculation where any increased expenditure could be met from reserves

Facts: West Berkshire reduced its funding of children's short breaks services in its annual budgetary decision.

Judgment: Laing J held that the decision was unlawful and that the prohibition in section 66 of the Local Government Finance Act 1992, the effect of which was to require all challenges to budget calculations to be brought by way of judicial review and to limit the grant of relief to a quashing order, did not prevent the court from quashing just one component of the budget where the council had financial reserves that could be utilised to furnish any consequential additional expenditure that might be required.

Breaches of duty

27.29 A clear breach of a clear duty to meet needs does not always result in a mandatory order to meet needs, for example, where the local authority establishes that the physical (cf. financial) resources to do so are simply not available. However, in such cases the court does not let the local authority off the hook completely; they are placed under a duty to do all they can to meet needs by pro-actively securing the necessary physical resources. However, where there is a clear breach of duty that can be remedied, the court can grant appropriately compelling orders.

27.30 *R v Islington LBC ex p Rixon* (1997–8) 1 CCLR 119, QBD

Where a resource is not available to meet needs that should not be the end of the matter; the local authority should consider acquiring a suitable resource

Facts: the applicant was a severely mentally and physically disabled 24-year-old man, whose mother considered that inadequate provision had resulted in him losing skills acquired at his special needs school and failing to develop his full potential. It was common ground that Islington's assessment and care plan failed to address comprehensively the applicant's needs and failed to comply with relevant central government guidance.

Judgment: Sedley J held that Islington had acted unlawfully in failing to 'act under' statutory guidance and properly to take into account non-statutory guidance (see above). He also held that Islington had acted unlawfully by providing an inadequate service because insufficient 'physical resources' were available: it should have considered increasing such resources:

> There are two points at which, in my judgment, the respondent local authority has fallen below the requirements of the law. The first concerns the relationship of need to availability. The duty owed to the applicant personally by virtue of section 2(1) of the Chronically Sick and Disabled Persons Act 1970 includes the provision of recreational facilities outside the home to an extent which Islington accepts is greater than the care plan provides for. But the local authority has, it appears, simply taken the existing unavailability of further facilities as an insuperable obstacle to any further attempt to make provision. The lack of a day care centre has been treated, however reluctantly, as a complete answer to the question of provision for Jonathan's recreational needs. As McCowan LJ explained in the *Gloucestershire* case, the section 2(1) exercise is needs-led and not resources-led. To say this is not to ignore the existing resources either in terms of regular voluntary care in the home or in budgetary terms. These, however, are balancing and not blocking factors. In the considerable volume of evidence which the local authority has provided, there is no indication that in reaching its decision on provision for Jonathan the local authority undertook anything resembling the exercise described in the *Gloucestershire* case of adjusting provision to need.

27.31 *R v Lambeth LBC ex p A1 and A2* (1997–8) 1 CCLR 336, CA

Where a necessary resource to meet a need is not available, a local authority must undertake a since and determined effort to find a solution but, if it does so, is not acting unlawfully in failing to meet the need

Facts: Lambeth had undertaken a number of assessments under various enactments; they were all flawed to a greater or lesser extent but the fact remained that Lambeth was aware and accepted that this family were in dire need of urgent rehousing because of adult care and children's welfare issues.

Judgment: The Court of Appeal (Hirst and Robert Walker LJJ, Harman) held that Owen J had been right to refuse relief, notwithstanding legal flaws in the assessments, because the heart of the matter was not Lambeth's failure to assess the problem but its failure to solve it:

> As I have said, what this court has to do is determine the appeal from Owen J. There are nine grounds of appeal in the notice of appeal against the rejection of Mrs A's application. The first is that the judge was wrong to defer questions under the Children Act, the 1970 Act and the 1995 Act until the issue of rehousing is resolved. Miss Maxwell has urged on us that comprehensive assessments were needed. She has said that only comprehensive assessments can meet the answer. I have to say that I do not accept that at all. There have been numerous assessments in this case, to some but not all of which I have referred. It may be that some are better than others. It may be that some do not explicitly state under what statute or statutes they have been made, but judicial review is a discretionary remedy. The judge exercised his discretion properly and, if I may say so, with eminent good sense, when he said that 'What this lad needs and what his parents need is a new home.' Everyone knows the problem. What is needed is a sincere and determined resumption of the search for a solution.
>
> The second ground of appeal is connected with the first. It seems to me that any correction of a lack of formal assessment in the past would simply be a bit of tidy minded putting the files in order and would not assist the resolution of the real problem.

Comment: notwithstanding the more pragmatically focussed language, this decision appears consistent with *Rixon* (see para 27.30 above): when a need is identified, but physical resources are not immediately available to meet it, the local authority must make 'a sincere and determined' effort to find a solution.

27.32 *R v Wigan MBC ex p Tammadge* (1997–8) 1 CCLR 581, QBD

Local authorities are required to meet needs that they have accepted as being eligible and a mandatory order may be granted ordering them to do so

Facts: the social services complaints review panel concluded that the applicant and her family were in urgent need of re-housing for health and care reasons. Wigan accepted that and ascertained that the most cost-effective solution was knock together two adjacent houses in its area. However, Wigan then decided not to undertake that course because 'the potential benefits ... do not justify the significant costs'.

Judgment: Forbes J held that while resources were relevant to a limited extent when determining whether and if so what needs existed for residential accommodation under section 21 of the National Assistance Act 1948, once a need has been assessed as existing, the authority is under a duty to make provision for that need. That applied in this case and Wigan was ordered to undertake the work that it had itself determined as being the most cost-effective solution:

I have come to the firm conclusion that Mr Gordon's submissions are correct. In my view, SSCRP's finding as to Mrs Tammadge's need for larger accommodation is perfectly clear from the wording in which that particular conclusion is expressed. Moreover, that conclusion is entirely in keeping with views of Wigan's own professionally qualified staff and advisers, as expressed both before and after the hearing before the SSCRP. I am therefore satisfied that, by a date no later than 22 October 1996 (when it was acknowledged that Wigan had accepted the SSCRP finding: see above), Mrs Tammadge's need for larger accommodation was established. I reject Miss Patterson's submissions to the contrary. As a result, from that date Wigan have been obliged to make provision of such accommodation to Mrs Tammadge and her family: see *ex p M* at pages 1009–1010. Once the duty had arisen in this way, it was not lawful of Wigan to refuse to perform that duty because of a shortage of or limits upon its financial resources or for any of the other reasons expressed in Mr Walker's letters of 30 July and 28 August 1997: see *ex p Sefton* at page 58 and also at page 67I–J, where Lord Woolf said this:

> 'However, in this case it is clear from the evidence that Sefton accepted that Mrs Blanchard met its own threshold as a person in need of care and attention. What it was seeking to do was to say that because of its lack of resources notwithstanding this it was not prepared to meet the duty which was placed upon it by the section. This it was not entitled to do.'

Accordingly, for those reasons, I have come to the firm conclusion that Wigan's decision not to provide Mrs Tammadge with larger accommodation is unlawful and must be quashed. Having regard to my conclusion on the central issue in this case and to the present length of this judgment, I do not propose to say anything further about Mrs Gordon's submissions on his core propositions four and five, except to acknowledge the compelling nature of his submissions with regard to core proposition four, which submissions are fully set out in his helpful written skeleton argument.

Comment: the principle should still apply under section 18 of the Care Act 2014 and, in relation to carers, under section 20.

27.33 *R (KM) v Cambridgeshire CC* [2012] UKSC 23, (2012) 15 CCLR 374

It is lawful to use a resource allocation system to guide assessment as to what level of personal budget to provide

Facts: Cambridgeshire assessed KM as having a range of critical needs for community care services and, using a resource allocation system (RAS), and an upper banding calculator (UBC) assessed his personal budget as £84,678.00. KM brought a judicial review, on the basis that this figure was too low.

Judgment: the Supreme Court (Justices Phillips, Walker, Hale, Brown, Kerr, Dyson and Wilson) held that:

1) when a local authority was required to decide whether it was necessary to make arrangements to meet the needs of a disabled person, for the purposes of section 2 of the Chronically Sick and Disabled Persons Act 1970 it was required to ask itself (i) what the needs of the disabled person were, (ii) whether in order to meet those needs it was necessary for the local authority to make arrangements to provide any services, and (iii) if

so, what the nature and extent of those services were. At stage (ii), the local authority was required to consider whether the needs of the disabled person could reasonably be met by family, friends, other state bodies, or charities, or out of the person's own resources. At stage (ii) the availability of resources was relevant and a local authority was entitled to have regard to the scale of its resources and the weight of other demands upon it;

2) where, as here, a disabled person qualified for a direct payment the local authority was required to ask a further question, (iv) what the reasonable cost was of securing provision of the services identified at stage (iii);

3) once stage (ii) had been passed, as in this case, the duty of the local authority to make provision for needs in accordance with stages (iii) and (iv);

4) it was lawful for a local authority to use a resource allocation scheme and an upper banding calculator, as Cambridgeshire had done, to ascertain a starting point or indicative figure, provided that the requisite services are then costed in reasonable detail to arrive a realistic direct payment figure;

5) in this case, Cambridgeshire had erred in not expressly stating that it did not accept the mother's assertion that KM would receive no family support and that it regarded the social worker's estimate of the cost of the claimant's needs as manifestly excessive, and it should have made a more detailed presentation to the claimant of how in its opinion he might reasonably choose to deploy the sum offered, and of its own assessment of the reasonable cost of the necessary services;

6) however, Cambridgeshire's reasoning had subsequently been amplified during the course of the litigation, the result of which left no real doubt about the lawfulness of the award; and that, accordingly, it would be a pointless exercise of the court's discretion to quash the determination so that the claimant's entitlement could be reconsidered.

In addition, Lord Wilson made these interesting observations, on behalf of the majority:

> 5. It is true that constraints upon its resources are a relevant consideration during one of the stages through which a local authority must pass in computing the size of a direct payment owed under section 2 of the 1970 Act. In paras 15 and 23 below I will identify four such stages; and constraints upon an authority's resources are undoubtedly relevant to the second stage. But the leading exposition of the law in this respect is to be found in the speeches of the majority of the appellate committee of the House of Lords in *R v Gloucestershire County Council ex p Barry* [1997] AC 584; and, if and in so far as it was there held that constraints upon resources were also relevant to what I will describe as the first stage, there are arguable grounds for fearing that the committee fell into error: see the concerns expressed by Baroness Hale of Richmond JSC in *R (McDonald) v Kensington and Chelsea Royal London Borough Council (Age UK intervening)* (2011) CCLR 341, paras 69–73.
>
> ...
>
> 36. ... I agree with Langstaff J in *R (L) v Leeds City Council* [2010] EWHC 3324 (Admin) at [59] that in community care cases the intensity of review will depend on the profundity of the impact of the determination. By reference to that yardstick, the necessary intensity of review in a case of this sort

> is high. Mr Wise also validly suggests that a local authority's failure to meet eligible needs may prove to be far less visible in circumstances in which it has provided the service-user with a global sum of money than in those in which it has provided him with services in kind. That point fortifies the need for close scrutiny of the lawfulness of a monetary offer. On the other hand respect must be afforded to the distance between the functions of the decision-maker and of the reviewing court; and some regard must be had to the court's ignorance of the effect upon the ability of an authority to perform its other functions of any exacting demands made in relation to the manner of its presentation of its determination in a particular type of case. So the court has to strike a difficult, judicious, balance.

Comment: the Supreme Court has not formally decided the point, but seems to have made it clear that a lack of resources is probably irrelevant when deciding whether or not a person has a particular 'need'. There may be a tension, however, been this position and the Supreme Court's position in *R (McDonald) v Kensington & Chelsea RLBC*,[25] in which the Supreme Court upheld Kensington & Chelsea's decision to re-describe Ms McDonald's needs in radically different terms, in order to save resources. *KM* would then mean, at least, that although a local authority can redefine a need, for resources reasons, to its cheapest possible description, it cannot pretend that it does not exist at all.

Costs in judicial review

27.34 *R (Boxall) v Waltham Forest LBC* (2001) 4 CCLR 258, QBD

Guidance (now largely superseded) as to how costs liability will be determined when cases settle

Facts: the claimant sought a judicial review of the lawfulness of Waltham Forest's failure to re-house her under community care provisions. After the issue of proceedings and the grant of permission to apply for judicial review Waltham Forest completed assessments and a care plan. The lawfulness of those documents remained in dispute but Waltham Forest then offered the claimant suitable re-housing, which she accepted. The issue was what order for costs should be made, given that the proceedings had become academic.

Judgment: Scott Baker J ordered Waltham Forest to pay the claimant's costs because there was little doubt that Waltham Forest would have been found, at a final hearing, to have acted unlawfully by failing to produce an assessment earlier:

> 22. Having considered the authorities, the principles I deduced to be applicable are as follows:
>
> (i) The court has power to make a costs order when the substantive proceedings have been resolved without a trial but the parties have not agreed about costs.
>
> (ii) It will ordinarily be irrelevant that the claimant is legally aided.
>
> (iii) The overriding objective is to do justice between the parties without incurring unnecessary court time and consequently additional cost.

25 [2011] UKSC 33, (2011) 14 CCLR 341.

(iv) At each end of the spectrum there will be cases where it is obvious which side would have won had the substantive issues been fought to a conclusion. In between, the position will, in differing degrees, be less clear. How far the court will be prepared to look into the previously unresolved substantive issues will depend on the circumstances of the particular case, not least the amount of costs at stake and the conduct of the parties.

(v) In the absence of a good reason to make any other order the fall back is to make no order as to costs.

(vi) The court should take care to ensure that it does not discourage parties from settling judicial review proceedings for example by a local authority making a concession at an early stage.

23. Applying these principles to the present case I think the following factors are relevant.

1. Prior to the commencement of proceedings a number of requests were made for an assessment but to no avail.

2. The first permission hearing was adjourned by consent on the defendant's agreement to carry out assessments.

3. The adjourned permission hearing was contested by the defendant unsuccessfully over a year later and this was followed shortly after by a carer's assessment that had been promised long before.

4. Costs are only claimed until 23 December 1999 when the further care plan was produced. It matters not whether it was a lawful plan, as the defendant contended, or not as the claimants contended. At the heart of this case lies the continued failure until December 1999 to assess the second claimant's need for accommodation under section 17(3) of the Children Act 1989. I reject the defendant's contention, which really comes to this. The second claimant's needs, including his accommodation needs, had been lawfully assessed well before December 1999 and the ultimate decision on housing was something that should be viewed as having occurred quite separately. It is true that housing lay at the heart of what the claimants were seeking, but the unlawfulness that is in my view relevant to the present application is not the failure to provide housing but the failure to carry out a proper assessment and to do so timeously.

5. The defendant's conduct in delaying to implement the terms of the consent order of 11 September 1998.

Comment: the *Boxall* principles have now been substantially modified.

27.35 *R (A, B, X and Y) v East Sussex CC* [2005] EWHC 585 (Admin), (2005) 8 CCLR 228

Legal costs incurred in general monitoring of the local authority's efforts would be disallowed but on the facts it was unrealistic to have expected the claimants to agree to mediation or that mediation would have resulted in settlement and, exceptionally, two sets of costs were awarded to separately represented claimants.

Facts: long-running and convoluted litigation was eventually compromised by way of a consent order, subject to judicial determination of costs liability.

Judgment: Munby J ordered East Sussex to pay a proportion of the claimants' costs, applying *Boxall*. He drew attention to some points of principle:

28. The second is the principle identified by Newman J in *R v The Mayor and Burgesses of the London Borough of Hackney ex p S* (unreported, 13 October 2000) at paras [8], [11]:

> 'I regard it as undesirable that a substantial bill of 'legal costs' should be incurred by a process of monitoring and regulating the performance of the public authority. In the situation which presented itself once LBH had been ordered to provide services and accommodation, it being the authority entrusted with the obligations and the resources, should have been able to decide upon a care plan and provide accommodation without the intervention of lawyers.
>
> The occasions when it will be appropriate for costly participation by a user's solicitor in the process of preparing a plan and the provision of accommodation by a local authority will be rare. The starting point must be that it is for the authority to act and produce its proposals.'

...

42. Ms Richards submits that this is a case in which the claimants could and should have agreed to [East Sussex County Council's] ESCC's offers of mediation. In particular, she says that the user independent trust issue cried out for mediation. She goes so far as to assert that if there had been mediation at the outset it is 'probable' that a huge amount of costs would have been avoided. She points to the comments and the actual order made by the Court of Appeal in *R (Cowl) v Plymouth CC (Practice Note)* [2001] EWCA Civ 1935, [2002] 1 WLR 803.

43. I have to say that I simply cannot accept this. In the first place, bearing in mind the vigour with which, seemingly, every conceivable point of law and every possible factual issue was canvassed in court, and the enthusiasm with which the forensic battle was apparently waged by all parties, the idea that mediation would have been successful at any earlier stage than in the event proved to be the case seems to me to verge on the fanciful. Moreover, the user independent trust issue raised questions of ESCC's *vires* which in the nature of things would have been difficult to resolve in the absence of a judicial determination – something which even ESCC appears to have recognised. Secondly, and as the claimants point out, ESCC's offers of mediation were for most of the time unrealistic. ESCC's attitude is, perhaps, best exemplified by the offer it made (without prejudice save as to costs) on 18 October 2002. True it offered to concede the user independent trust issue (but how could it?), but this was tied to a requirement that the claimants abandon their challenge to ESCC's manual handling policy and withdraw the judicial review proceedings. In my judgment the claimants were justified in the particular circumstances of this 'almost uniquely difficult case' (see paragraph [25] above) in taking the view that, however appropriate it might otherwise have been, mediation on the only terms being proposed by ESCC was inappropriate and likely to be futile. Of course parties should mediate wherever possible, but a party who reasonably rejects an unreasonable or unrealistic proposal for mediation may still recover his costs.

...

46. Ms Richards vigorously resists any order that allows both A and B and X and Y to recover their costs. She has particular submissions in relation to the user independent trust issue but more generally she submits that there was no justification for separate representation continuing – and certainly no reason why ESCC should have to pay for it – after the point in June 2002 when ESCC in effect abandoned the best interests claim.

47. Down to that point it hardly lies in ESCC's mouth to complain, for it was its own act in commencing the best interests proceedings which created the conflict between A and B on the one hand and X and Y on the other and the consequent necessity for their separate representation. Moreover, it is not unimportant that Wilson J in his order of 14 June 2002 awarded costs – very substantial costs – to *both* sets of claimants. Thereafter, I readily concede, matters are not so straight-forward. And Ms Richards can marshal powerful arguments – most helpfully set out in paragraphs 93–95 of her 'Submissions ... in response to the costs application made by X and Y' – as to why there should from then on be only one set of costs. As against that there are the points made by the claimants, in particular by Ms Mountfield in paragraphs 23 and 29 of her 'Written submissions on costs on behalf of the third and fourth claimants' and paragraph 17 of her 'Submissions ... in response'. Those submissions persuade me, I have to say without much enthusiasm, that it would not be right to limit the claimants to only one set of costs for the period down to 25 November 2002. They have persuaded me, essentially for the reasons they give, that it would in the circumstances be appropriate – fair, just and appropriate – to depart from what I accept is the typical starting point and to award the claimants two sets of costs. The facts of the present case are very different indeed, but in coming to this conclusion I have adopted the principles to be found in *Bolton MDC v Secretary of State for the Environment (Practice Note)* [1995] 1 WLR 1176 at 1178E and *R (Smeaton) v Secretary of State for Health and others (No 2)* [2002] EWHC 886 (Admin), [2002] 2 FLR 146, at paras [431]–[440], principles which, I believe, justify my coming to this conclusion.

27.36 *R (B) v Lambeth LBC* [2006] EWHC 639 (Admin), (2006) 9 CCLR 239

Adverse costs orders would be made against lawyers who failed adequately to identify proper errors of law in their pleadings

Facts: the claimant, a 15-year-old girl, brought judicial review proceedings against Lambeth after she became homeless, alleging that Lambeth had failed adequately to assess her needs or make suitable provision. After a number of hearings, she withdrew those proceedings without permission to apply for judicial review having been granted. Lambeth applied for costs on the grounds that the judicial review grounds had failed to identify clearly any error of law and that, despite repeated requests, that had not been done until the last moment.

Judgment: Munby J held that there would no order for costs, but practitioners should be aware that cost and/or wasted costs might well be awarded in future when a judicial review application failed properly to identify any alleged errors of law: paragraphs 26–36 of the judgment, in particular, contain salutary advice to practitioners.

27.37 *R (M) v Croydon LBC* [2012] EWCA Civ 595, [2012] 1 WLR 2607

In general, a claimant would recover costs when the order settling judicial review proceedings accorded them the relief sought in the pre-action protocol letter and judicial review grounds: this leading case sets out the principles of general application

Facts: after M had been granted permission to apply for judicial review, Croydon reconsidered and conceded his application for judicial review, leaving the issue of cost to be litigated.

Judgment: the Court of Appeal (Lord Neuberger MR, Hallett and Stanley Burnton LJJ) held that Croydon would be ordered to pay 50 per cent of the claimant's costs up to the grant of permission to apply for judicial review only (because of all the circumstances including that the Supreme Court had radically changed the perceived law) and 100 per cent of his costs thereafter. More importantly, in this leading case on costs in judicial review proceedings the court set the correct approach in principle:

> *The position where cases settle in the Administrative Court*
> 52. [Per Lord Neuberger MR] The question which then arises is whether the principles discussed in the preceding section of this judgment should apply in the Administrative Court, just as much as to other parts of the civil justice system: in particular, where the defendants accept that the claimant is entitled to all, or substantially all, the relief which he claims, should the defendants pay his costs unless they can show good reason to the contrary? At least on the face of it the fact that a claim is a public law claim should make no difference. Such claims are subject to the CPR, and a successful claimant who has brought such a claim is just as much entitled to his costs as he would be if it had been a private law claim. The court's duty to protect individuals from being wronged by the state, whether national or local government, is every bit as vital as its duty to enable them to vindicate their private law rights. And the fact that the defendants are public bodies should make no difference, as Pill LJ explained in the *Bahta* case [2011] 5 Costs LR 857, para 60. However, a number of points could be raised as to why defendants who concede claims in the Administrative Court should be less at risk on costs than those who concede in ordinary civil actions.
>
> 53. First, it may be said that government and public bodies should be encouraged to settle, and should not therefore be penalised in costs if they do so after proceedings have been issued. There are four answers to that. First, if it is a good point it should apply to any litigation, whether in private law or public law, and in very few if any private law cases would such an argument carry any weight. The implication that public authority defendants should be in a more privileged position than other defendants in this connection is not, in my view, maintainable. Secondly, it is simply unfair on the claimant or his lawyers if, at least in the absence of special factors, he does not recover his costs of bringing wholly successful proceedings, provided that they have been properly brought and conducted. Thirdly, while defendants may be more ready to concede a claim rather than fight it if they know that they will not thereby be liable for the claimant's costs, it can forcefully be said that the fact that, if defendants know they will have to pay the claimant's costs, it would be a powerful incentive to concede the claim sooner rather than later. Fourthly, if the defendants wish to settle, the time to do so is before proceedings are issued: that is one of the main reasons for the introduction of the Protocol.
>
> 54. Secondly, it may be said that because of the three-month time limit there will often be less time available for defendants in a public law claim to consider the merits of the claimant's case than in a private law claim, where the more generous time limits in the limitation normally apply. In my opinion, in some cases that factor might justify making a more generous order for costs from the defendants' perspective than the analysis in the previous section of this judgment might otherwise suggest. It would not be

good enough for defendants to say that they had not got round to dealing with the claimant's claim because of their 'heavy workload' or 'constraints upon [their] resources' (see the *Bahta* case, para 60). However, where the claim is one which reasonably requires more time to investigate than is available before the three-month period runs out, there may be a powerful case for defendants who thereafter concede the claim not being liable for any or some of the claimant's costs. However, that does not seem to me to give rise to a difference in principle between Administrative Court litigation and other civil litigation-for instance, where the letter before action is written very shortly before the expiry of the limitation period.

55. A third argument is that defendants sometimes concede claims in the Administrative Court simply because it is not worth the candle fighting the case, or because the claim is justified only on a relatively technical ground such as a procedural defect. In the first type of case it is said to be unfair to penalise the defendants in costs for taking a view which, while not necessarily reflecting the legal merits, is realistic and proportionate. In the second type of case the court normally then remits the decision to the defendants, who then go on to reconsider and often arrive at the same substantive conclusion as before. In the main it seems to me that the answer to this is that the defendants should make up their mind to concede the claim for such reasons before proceedings are issued. That is one of the main purposes of the Protocol, and if defendants delay considering whether they should concede a claim, that should not be a reason for depriving the claimant of his costs. If in fact the only reason the defendants did not take that course was that they had insufficient time to consider the claimant's claim, one is back to the point discussed in the preceding paragraph. In some cases Pill LJ's scepticism about this argument, as expressed at para 63 of the *Bahta* case, will apply; in others the defendants may be short of resources but, as mentioned, that is not a good reason for depriving the claimant of his costs.

56. A fourth argument is that in some public law cases the law (or what is understood to be the law) changes after the issue of proceedings, so that what appears to be a weak claim becomes transformed into a strong claim. An obvious example is where the Supreme Court overrules previous Court of Appeal authority, so that the defendants who (justifiably) thought they had a very strong case suddenly realise that they are very much on the back foot. In the *Bahta* case [2011] 5 Costs LR 857 Pill LJ was unimpressed with the UKBA's argument that they were entitled to refuse to agree the claimants' cases on the ground that, although Court of Appeal authority was against the UKBA, they were entitled to act on the assumption that the Supreme Court might take a different view, which in the event they did not. By parity of reasoning, it may seem rather harsh to visit defendants with liability for all the claimant's costs, because they assumed that the law was as the Court of Appeal had decided, until the Supreme Court took a different view. In such a case, however, while the defendants have a real argument for saying that they should not pay all the claimant's costs, the claimant can none the less raise all the normal reasons for receiving his costs. This argument would apply equally to ordinary civil cases.

57. A fifth argument, which also applies to ordinary civil cases, is based on a number of miscellaneous possible factual situations which arise in Administrative Court cases. They involve various failings on the part of the claimant, such as not having set out his case clearly in his letter before action, adding to his evidence well after the issue of proceedings, including a claim which does not succeed, or pursuing the claim in an unreasonable manner. In cases where such an argument is raised by the defendants, the

court may well be persuaded either that it would be wrong to award the claimant any costs for the reasons canvassed by Chadwick LJ in the *BCT Software Solutions* case [2004] FSR 150, para 24, or that the claimant should only receive a proportion of his costs. As in any civil litigation, a claimant who succeeds is only entitled to his costs in the absence of good reason to the contrary. Thus where the claim has been conceded in a consent order which does not deal with costs, the court will not award the claimant all or any of his costs save to the extent that it is satisfied, without looking at matters in detail, that the claimant is so entitled.

58. Accordingly, I conclude that the position should be no different for litigation in the Administrative Court from what it is in general civil litigation. In that connection, at any rate at first sight, there may appear to be a degree of tension between this conclusion, which applies the 'general rule' in CPR r 44.3(2)(a), and the fifth guideline in the *Boxall* case (2001) 4 CCLR 258, at least in a case where the settlement involves the defendants effectively conceding that the claimant is entitled to the relief which he seeks. In such a case the claimant is almost always the successful party, and should therefore, at least prima facie, be entitled to his costs, whereas the fifth guideline seems to suggest that the default position is that there should be no order for costs. Similarly, there could be said to be a degree of tension between what was said in paras 63 –65, and the view expressed in para 66 of the *Bahta* case [2011] 5 Costs LR 857.

59. In my view, however, on closer analysis there is no inconsistency in either case, essentially for reasons already discussed. Where, as happened in the *Bahta* case, a claimant obtains all the relief which he seeks, whether by consent or after a contested hearing, he is undoubtedly the successful party who is entitled to all his costs, unless there is a good reason to the contrary. However, where the claimant obtains only some of the relief which he is seeking (either by consent or after a contested trial), as in the *Boxall* case and the *Scott* case [2009] EWCA Civ 217, the position on costs is obviously more nuanced. Thus as in those two cases there may be an argument as to which party was more 'successful' (in the light of the relief which was sought and not obtained) or, even if the claimant is accepted to be the successful party, there may be an argument as to the importance of the issue, or costs relating to the issue, on which he failed.

60. Thus in Administrative Court cases just as in other civil litigation, particularly where a claim has been settled, there is, in my view, a sharp difference between (i) a case where a claimant has been wholly successful whether following a contested hearing or pursuant to a settlement, and (ii) a case where he has only succeeded in part following a contested hearing, or pursuant to a settlement, and (iii) a case where there has been some compromise which does not actually reflect the claimant's claims. While in every case the allocation of costs will depend on the specific facts, there are some points which can be made about these different types of case.

61. In case (i), it is hard to see why the claimant should not recover all his costs, unless there is some good reason to the contrary. Whether pursuant to judgment following a contested hearing, or by virtue of a settlement, the claimant can, at least absent special circumstances, say that he has been vindicated, and as the successful party that he should recover his costs. In the latter case the defendants can no doubt say that they were realistic in settling and should not be penalised in costs, but the answer to that point is that the defendants should on that basis have settled before the proceedings were issued: that is one of the main points of the pre-action protocols.

Ultimately it seems to me that the *Bahta* case [2011] 5 Costs LR 857 was decided on this basis.

62. In case (ii), when deciding how to allocate liability for costs after a trial, the court will normally determine questions such as how reasonable the claimant was in pursuing the unsuccessful claim, how important it was compared with the successful claim, and how much the costs were increased as a result of the claimant pursuing the unsuccessful claim. Given that there will have been a hearing, the court will be in a reasonably good position to make findings on such questions. However, where there has been a settlement, the court will, at least normally, be in a significantly worse position to make findings on such issues than where the case has been fought out. In many such cases the court will be able to form a view as to the appropriate costs order based on such issues; in other cases it will be much more difficult. I would accept the argument that, where the parties have settled the claimant's substantive claims on the basis that he succeeds in part, but only in part, there is often much to be said for concluding that there is no order for costs. That I think was the approach adopted in the *Scott* case [2009] EWCA Civ 217. However, where there is not a clear winner, so much would depend on the particular facts. In some such cases it may help to consider who would have won if the matter had proceeded to trial as, if it is tolerably clear, it may for instance support or undermine the contention that one of the two claims was stronger than the other. The *Boxall* case (2001) 4 CCLR 258 appears to have been such case.

63. In case (iii), the court is often unable to gauge whether there is a successful party in any respect and, if so, who it is. In such cases, therefore, there is an even more powerful argument that the default position should be no order for costs. However, in some such cases it may well be sensible to look at the underlying claims and inquire whether it was tolerably clear who would have won if the matter had not settled. If it is, then that may well strongly support the contention that the party who would have won did better out of the settlement, and therefore did win.

64. Having said that, I should add that I have read what Stanley Burnton LJ says in his judgment, and I agree with it.

65. Having given such general guidance on costs issues in relation to Administrative Court cases which settle on all issues save costs, it is right to emphasise that, as in most cases involving judicial guidance on costs, each case turns on its own facts. A particular case may have an unusual feature which would, or at least could, justify departing from what would otherwise be the appropriate costs order

...

Per Stanley Burnton LJ:

77. [Per Stanley Burnton LJ] Where the parties are unable to agree costs, and they are left to be determined by the court, it is important that both the work and costs involved in preparing the parties' submissions on costs, and the material the judge is asked to consider, are proportionate to the amount at stake. No order for costs will be the default order when the judge cannot without disproportionate expenditure of judicial time, if at all, fairly and sensibly make an order in favour of either party. This is not to say that there are not cases where the merits can be determined and no order for costs can be seen to be the appropriate order; but in such cases that order is not a default order, but an order made on the merits.

27.38 *R (Hunt) v North Somerset Council* [2015] UKSC 51

If a party to judicial review proceedings establishes after a contested hearing that a public authority acted unlawfully, some good reason would have to be shown why he should not recover his reasonable costs

Facts: the claimant sought judicial review of the local authority's decision to approve its budget for the year 2012/13 by way of an order quashing its reduction in the funding of youth services. He did not seek declaratory relief. In the Court of Appeal the claimant was ordered to pay half the local authority's costs, on the basis that although the claimant had established unlawful decision-making he had not obtained the quashing order he sought (it was refused because the budgetary year had already passed) and had not sought (or therefore obtained) any further relief.

Judgment: the Supreme Court (Hale, Wilson, Reed, Hughes and Toulson JJSC) held that Mr Hunt was entitled to two-thirds of his costs at first instance, in the Court of Appeal and in the Supreme Court. Notwithstanding the fact that Mr Hunt had lost on a number of issues he had succeeded on two points of principle of general public importance:

> 13. The appellant is on much stronger ground in relation to costs. The submissions to the Court of Appeal on his behalf made no reference to the costs at first instance, and it was remiss to agree to an order that the appeal should be dismissed, when there were obvious grounds for arguing that in relation to costs the judge's order should be set aside and replaced by an order in the appellant's favour. However, in relation to the costs in the Court of Appeal, the points were properly made that the appellant had succeeded on both the issues as to the respondent's statutory duty; that there were wider lessons for local authorities to learn from the case about their duties under each of the relevant sections; that the lapse of time, as a result of which the relevant financial year had now passed, was not the fault of the appellant; and that to deny the appellant his costs would be likely in practice to dissuade claimants from pursuing legitimate public law challenges. The respondent submitted that the appellant had not in substance been successful; that he had not obtained any result of any practical utility; and that he had known about the practical problems which would be involved in attempting to unwind the budget from evidence submitted by the respondent before the original hearing
>
> …
>
> 15. The discretion of a court in a matter of costs is wide and it is highly unusual for this court to entertain an appeal on an issue of costs alone. But the Court of Appeal said that it reached its decision as a matter of principle, treating the respondent as the 'successful party'. In adopting that approach, I consider that the court fell into error. The rejection of the respondent's case on the two issues on which the appellant was given leave to appeal was of greater significance than merely that the respondent had increased the costs of the appeal by its unsuccessful resistance. The respondent was 'successful' only in the limited sense that the findings of failure came too late to do anything about what had happened in the past, not because the appellant had been slow to raise them but because the respondent had resisted them successfully until the Court of Appeal gave its judgment. The respondent was unsuccessful on the substantive issues regarding its statutory responsibilities.

16. There are also wider public factors to consider. Public law is not about private rights but about public wrongs, as Sedley J said in *R v Somerset County Council ex p Dixon* [1998] Env LR 111 when considering a question of standing. A court may refuse permission to bring a judicial review claim if it considers the claimant to be a mere meddler or if it considers that the proceedings are unlikely to be of sufficient significance to merit the time and costs involved. But in this case the court considered that the issues were of sufficient significance to give permission. And the ruling of the court, particularly under section 149, contained a lesson of general application for local authorities regarding the discharge by committee members of the council's equality duty. If a party who has been given leave to bring a judicial review claim succeeds in establishing after fully contested proceedings that the defendant acted unlawfully, some good reason would have to be shown why he should not recover his reasonable costs.

17. I cannot see that the fact that in this case the determination of illegality came after it was too late to consider reopening the 2012/13 budget provided a principled reason for making the appellant pay any part of the respondent's costs. On the contrary, for the reasons stated the appellant was in principle entitled to some form of costs order in his favour.

27.39 *R (MVN) v Greenwich LBC* [2015] EWHC 2663 (Admin), (2015) 18 CCLR 645

A Part 36 offer will not result in indemnity costs being awarded to the successful offeror unless the offer is a genuine attempt to negotiate involving 'give and take'

Facts: in disputed age assessment proceedings, the claimant sought to obtain indemnity costs by dint of making a Part 36 offer, requiring the Greenwich to accept that the claimant was the age that he purported to be, without the need for a trial. Greenwich refused that offer, the claimant succeeded at trial and claimed indemnity costs.

Judgment: Picken J refused to award indemnity costs on the basis that the claimant's offer had not been a genuine offer to settle, involving real 'give and take', but rather a tactical ploy.

Comment: understandable: but can Part 36 offers ever be used in judicial review proceedings? Logic says 'why not' and yet the dearth of authority on this topic may suggest an underlying unease amongst practitioners about the application of a quintessentially private law weapon, in the public context. Having said that, there undoubtedly are occasions when a litigant in public law proceedings may richly deserve to pay costs on an indemnity basis and not just in those cases involving commercial litigation by another route.

27.40 *R (Baxter) v Lincolnshire CC* [2015] EWCA Civ 1290, (2016) 19 CCLR 160

To recover costs, a claimant had to establish a sufficiently clear link between the consent order and the relief he had sought in his claim form

Facts: Lincolnshire completed a community care assessment in relation to Mr Baxter, on the basis of which Lincolnshire proposed to move Mr Baxter from a residential placement to a supported living facility. Mr Baxter sought a judicial review of the assessment. After the issue of proceedings, Lincolnshire and Mr Baxter entered into a consent order whereby Lincolnshire undertook to hold a best interests meeting to determine the best type of placement for Mr Baxter, taking into account the views of an independent expert instructed by Lincolnshire. Mr Baxter then sought to recover his legal costs.

Judgment: the Court of Appeal (Floyd and Simon LJJ) held that Mr Baxter had not sent a pre-action letter, as required by the Pre-action Protocol, and could not show that it had been necessary to issue proceedings in order to achieve the settlement and that, also, Lincolnshire had neither conceded that its assessment had been unlawful, nor agreed to undertake a further assessment, so that there was an insufficiently clear link between the relief sought in the claim, and the consent order, for Mr Baxter to demonstrate that he had been the successful party, whose claim had been vindicated by the consent order. Accordingly, Mr Baxter was not entitled to his legal costs.

Other

27.41 *R (C) v Secretary of State for Justice* [2016] UKSC 2, (2016) 19 CCLR 5

There was no presumption of anonymity for mental patients challenging aspects of their treatment and care in the High Court but anonymity will be granted where that is necessary in the interests of the patient

Facts: C had been convicted of murder, then transferred to hospital as a mental patient. After many years in detention, the First-tier Tribunal recommended that he was suitable for conditional discharge but the Secretary of State for Justice refused to allow C trial periods of unescorted leave in the community. C sought a judicial review of that decision. His application was refused and the High Court judge revoked C's anonymity order. The Court of Appeal upheld that revocation.

Judgment: the Supreme Court (Hale, Clarke, Wilson, Carnwath and Hughes JJSC) held that there was no presumption of anonymity in the High Court and above, in relation to mental patients challenging aspects of their care and treatment under the Mental Health Act 1983, but that an anonymity order should be made in this case otherwise the patient's integration into the community would be jeopardised.

Comment: although this is a judgment on particular facts, the analysis of the Supreme Court, allowing the appeal from decisions by the High Court and Court of Appeal, suggests that there will be very few cases indeed, if any, where anonymity may be refused in this type of case – perhaps where there is no real prospect of the mental patient being discharged into the community, at all, or in the foreseeable future.

27.42 *Wasif and Hossain v Secretary of State for the Home Department* [2016] EWCA Civ 82

An application for permission to apply for judicial review was totally without merit if it was so unarguable that it was bound to fail, such that neither oral advocacy nor a revised presentation of the case, at an oral renewal hearing, could render it arguable

Facts: Mr Wasif and Mr Hossain appealed against decisions refusing their applications for permission to apply for judicial review and certifying them as being totally without merit ('TWM'), the effect of which was that they were not entitled to ask that their applications be reconsidered at an oral hearing.

Judgment: the Court of Appeal (Lord Dyson MR, Underhill and Floyd LJJ) held that permission to apply for judicial review was generally refused when the court considered that the claim was not 'arguable'; a case that is TWM is something beyond 'unarguable' – it is a case that is truly bound to fail, such that the power of oral advocacy at a renewal hearing, and the opportunity for the claimant to address perceived weaknesses in his claim at such a hearing, would serve no useful purpose. Claimants refused permission to apply for judicial review, whose claim was certified as being TWM, could appeal the refusal of permission to apply for judicial review.

CHAPTER 28

Ombudsman

continued

28.13 *Special Report – NHS Funding for long term care – investigations into Complaints Nos E 208/99-00 Dorset Health Authority and Dorset Health Care Trust and others* (2003) 6 CCLR 397

Health authorities were required to review their NHS Continuing Healthcare policies and provide redress to those wrongly charged for healthcare

28.14 *Report of an Investigation into Complaint No 07/A/01436 against London Borough of Hillingdon* (2008) 11 CCLR 675

There had been maladministration in that the social worker had failed to keep proper notes, to enquire carefully into the family's wish to care for the service user at home, to provide proper financial advice in writing, to complete a proper assessment and to investigate complaints of inadequate care

28.15 *Report on an investigation into Complaint No 12 001 464 against Kent County Council* (2013) 16 CCLR 465

There had been maladministration resulting in X not becoming a looked after child, to remedy which the Council ought to treat him as being such

28.16 *R (ER) v Local Government Ombudsman and Hillingdon LBC* [2014] EWCA Civ 1407, (2015) 18 CCLR 290

The LGO had no jurisdiction to investigate a complaint about the naming of a school in a Statement of Special Educational Needs

28.17 *Report on a joint PHSO and LGO investigation into complaint numbers JW–1999678 and 14006021 about Sheffield Health and Social Care Foundation Trust and Sheffield City Council*

The Council was directed to reimburse Ms D £14,000.00 being the sum she had spent on care, pay £12,000.00 compensation on account of Ms D's lack of social care and pay her a further £1,000.00 for distress

28.18 *R (Miller) v Parliamentary and Health Service Ombudsman* [2015] EWHC 2981 (Admin), (2015) 18 CCLR 697

It had been fair for the Ombudsman to have treated a complaint about one doctor as being implicitly a complaint about two doctors and he had given both doctors a fair opportunity to respond

Jurisdiction

28.1 The office of Local Government Ombudsman (LGO) is set up by Part 3 of the Local Government Act 1974 and Schedules 4 and 5 thereto, as amended.

28.2 The essential machinery is as follows:

- a complaint may be made by or on behalf of a member of the public (or their personal representative/some other suitable person, if they have died) if they claim to have 'sustained injustice' (section 26A);
- complaints can be referred to the LGO by various authorities (section 26C);
- a complaint must be made in writing and within 12 months of the day on which the person affected (or his or her personal representative) first had notice of the matter, although the LGO may extend time (section 26B);
- the LGO will not generally undertake an investigation unless the authority has been afforded a reasonable opportunity to investigate and respond (section 26(5));
- the LGO may or may not investigate a matter where the person has a right of appeal, reference or review to a tribunal and will not do so after such a right has been exercised (section 26(6) and (7));
- provision is made for investigations to be conducted in private, for the LGO to exercise a number of procedural powers and for him or her to issue reports on investigations (sections 28–30, 31B);
- the local authority has an opportunity of deciding what action to take to remedy any injustice, otherwise, the LGO will issue recommendations (section 31).

28.3 The critical provisions, relating to matters subject to investigation, are as follows:

> **Matters subject to investigation.**
>
> **26**(1) For the purposes of section 24A(1)(b), in relation to an authority to which this Part of this Act applies, the following matters are subject to investigation by a Local Commissioner under this Part of this Act–
>
> (a) alleged or apparent maladministration in connection with the exercise of the authority's administrative functions;
>
> (b) an alleged or apparent failure in a service which it was the authority's function to provide;
>
> (c) an alleged or apparent failure to provide such a service.
>
> (d) an alleged or apparent failure in a service provided by the authority in pursuance of arrangements under section 7A of the National Health Service Act 2006;
>
> (e) an alleged or apparent failure to provide a service in pursuance of such arrangements.

28.4 The Local Government Ombudsman has a useful and accessible website, www.lgo.org.uk, with information on adult social care complaints,[1]

1 www.lgo.org.uk/adult-social-care.

a searchable database of decisions[2] and an information centre with news, reports and complaints data.[3]

28.5 Of all the publications, the 'Guidance on Remedies', is particularly useful.[4]

28.6 It may also be useful to note that the Local Government Ombudsman has a policy of only investigating relatively serious complaints, in accordance with their policy.[5]

Maladministration

28.7 The term 'maladministration' is not defined in the statute. Its meaning was considered in *R v Local Commissioner for Administration for the North and East Area of England ex p Bradford MCC*,[6] where Lord Denning MR said as follows:

> *The meaning of maladministration*
>
> This brings me to the substantial point in this case. Has there been a sufficient claim of maladministration such as to justify investigation by the commissioner? The governing words of each statute are the same. There must be a written complaint made by or on behalf of a member of the public 'who claims to have suffered injustice in consequence of maladministration.'
>
> But Parliament did not define 'maladministration.' It deliberately left it to the ombudsman himself to interpret the word as best he could: and to do it by building up a body of case law on the subject. Now the Parliamentary ombudsman, Sir Edward Compton, has acknowledged openly that he himself gained assistance by looking at the debates in Parliament on the subject. He looked at *Hansard* and, in particular, at a list of instances of maladministration given by Mr. Crossman, the Lord President of the Council. It is called the 'Crossman Catalogue': and is used by the ombudsman and his advisers as a guide to the interpretation of the word. Now the question at once arises: Are we the judges to look at *Hansard* when we have the selfsame task? When we have ourselves to interpret the word 'maladministration.' The construction of that word is beyond doubt a question of law. According to the recent pronouncement of the House of Lords in *Davis v Johnson* [1978] 2 WLR 553, we ought to regard *Hansard* as a closed book to which we as judges must not refer at all, not even as an aid to the construction of statutes.
>
> By good fortune, however, we have been given a way of overcoming that obstacle. For the ombudsman himself in a public address to the Society of Public Teachers of Law quoted the relevant passages of *Hansard* (734 HC Deb, col. 51 (October 18, 1966)) as part of his address: and Professor Wade has quoted the very words in his latest book on *Administrative Law,* 4th edn (1977), p82 and we have not yet been told that we may not look at the writings of the teachers of law. Lord Simonds was as strict upon these matters as any judge ever has been but he confessed his indebtedness to their writings, even very recent ones: see *Jacobs v London County Council* [1950] AC

2 www.lgo.org.uk/decisions.

3 www.lgo.org.uk/information-centre.

4 PDF of 'Guidance on Remedies' available at www.lgo.org.uk/information-centre/advice-and-guidance/guidance-notes.

5 www.lgo.org.uk/information-centre/staff-guidance/assessment-code.

6 [1979] QB 287.

361, 374. So have other great judges. I hope therefore that our teachers will go on quoting *Hansard* so that a judge may in this way have the same help as others have in interpreting a statute.

So this is the guide suggested to the meaning of the word 'maladministration.' It will cover 'bias, neglect, inattention, delay, incompetence, ineptitude, perversity, turpitude, arbitrariness and so on.' It 'would be a long and interesting list,' clearly open-ended, covering the *manner* in which a decision is reached or discretion is exercised; but excluding the *merits* of the decision itself or of the discretion itself. It follows that 'discretionary decision, properly exercised, which the complainant dislikes but cannot fault the manner in which it was taken, is excluded': see *Hansard*, 734 HC Deb, col 51.

In other words, if there is no maladministration, the ombudsman may not question any decision taken by the authorities. He must not go into the merits of it or intimate any view as to whether it was right or wrong. This is explicitly declared in section 34 (3) of the Act of 1974. He can inquire whether there was maladministration or not. If he finds none, he must go no further. If he finds it, he can go on and inquire whether any person has suffered injustice thereby.

Cases

28.8 *Investigation into Complaint Nos 97/0177 and 97/0755 against the former Clwyd CC and Conwy County BC* (1997–8) 1 CCLR 546

A social services authority is required to provide after-care services under Mental Health Act 1983 s117 free of charge, from hospital discharge until it as a social services authority is satisfied that there is no longer any need of such services

28.9 *Investigation into Complaint No 97/A/2959 against Hackney LBC* (1999) 2 CCLR 67

About 22 months' delay in re-assessing the needs of person with learning difficulties remaining in a day centre that had been re-designated for persons with physical difficulties was maladministration, as was a failure to carry out risk assessments, complete a care plan, follow a Social Services Complaints Review Panel recommendation to review meal charges and to communicate effectively with the persons' parents: compensation of £1,500 was recommended

28.10 *Investigation into Complaint No 96/C/4315 against Liverpool CC* (1999) 2 CCLR 129

It is maladministration to set a limit of £100 per week (equivalent to the cost of residential care) on the cost of domiciliary services, when such services replace nursing home care costing about £190 per week

28.11 *Investigation into Complaint No 97/A/2870 against Newham LBC* (2000) 3 CCLR 47

In the case of a mentally disordered person particularly vulnerable to noise nuisance it was maladministration when the council failed to take adequate steps to ensure that the accommodation to which he was transferred was suitable for him and then failed to take timeous steps to remedy the deficiency

28.12 ***Investigation into Complaint No 97/A/2870 against Wiltshire CC*** **(2000) 3 CCLR 60**

It was maladministration to continue to charge service users for two years after receipt of legal advice that the charges were unlawful. It was maladministration to fail to adequately consider whether people who paid such charges should be reimbursed

28.13 ***Special Report – NHS Funding for long term care – investigations into Complaints Nos E 208/99-00 Dorset Health Authority and Dorset Health Care Trust and others*** **(2003) 6 CCLR 397**

Health authorities were required to review their NHS Continuing Healthcare policies and provide redress to those wrongly charged for healthcare

Strategic Health Authorities should review the criteria used by their predecessor bodies, and the way those criteria were applied, since 1996 taking into account the *Coughlan* judgment, guidance issued by the Department of Health and the Ombudsman's findings; and make efforts to remedy any consequent financial injustice to patients, where the criteria, or the way they were applied, were not clearly appropriate or fair. This includes attempting to identify any patients in their area who may wrongly have been made to pay for their care in a home and making appropriate recompense to them or their estates. The Department of Health should consider how they can support and monitor the performance of authorities and primary care trusts in this work. That might involve the Department assessing whether, from 1996 to date, criteria being used were in line with the law and guidance. Where they were not, the Department might need to co-ordinate effort to remedy any financial injustice to patients affected; review the national guidance on eligibility for NHS Continuing Healthcare, making it much clearer in new guidance the situations when the NHS must provide funding and those where it is left to the discretion of NHS bodies locally; consider being more proactive in checking that criteria used in the future follow that guidance; consider how to link assessment of eligibility for NHS Continuing Healthcare into the single assessment process and whether the Department should provide further support to the development of reliable assessment methods.

28.14 ***Report of an Investigation into Complaint No 07/A/01436 against London Borough of Hillingdon*** **(2008) 11 CCLR 675**

There had been maladministration in that the social worker had failed to keep proper notes, to enquire carefully into the family's wish to care for the service user at home, to provide proper financial advice in writing, to complete a proper assessment and to investigate complaints of inadequate care

Facts: following concerns about the quality of his home care package, 'Mr Davey' was admitted to hospital. Afterwards, Hillingdon placed him in residential accommodation despite his family's desire to have Mr Davey (properly) cared for at home, by carers and family members. The family agreed on the basis that the residential placement would be temporary only, but Hillingdon failed to resolve the issue of how Mr Davey was not be cared for long-term and placed a charge over his dwelling in relation to the accommodation fees. The family complained, ultimately to the ombudsman.

Conclusions: the Ombudsman held that there had been maladministration as follows:

1) There was maladministration by the Council in failing to follow up serious allegations as to the quality of care. Although it was not possible to conclude that Mr Davey's hospitalisation had been caused by the poor care, there would have been some adverse effect on him and increased anxiety for the family.

2) The council's view that Mr Davey needed a residential placement was reached without proper enquiry in the family's stated wish to care for him in his own home. The principle of promoting independence should not be lightly disregarded. There should have been an assessment which examined more carefully his level of need and how this could be met. In order to avoid delay in discharge, the council could have arranged a temporary admission to a care home pending assessment and consideration of the family's request for home care. There was no consideration of Mr Davey's wishes and feelings. The lack of a proper discharge assessment and the failure to carry out a further assessment after discharge was maladministration and this, along with the council's dismissive attitude to the family, had caused unnecessary and avoidable distress.

3) There was further maladministration by the social worker in failing to keep proper notes of relevant events.

4) The council did not set out in writing to the family the precise financial implications of Mr Davey's move to residential care.

5) As there was no proper assessment when Mr Davey was placed in residential care, the initial decision that he needed residential care was flawed. As there was no reassessment after his move, the council's decision to treat Mr Davey as a permanent resident of the home was maladministration. In any event, in this case the stay turned out to be temporary and Mr Davey should have been charged on that basis.

6) The council agreed a settlement of the complaint, including improvements to its monitoring of home care packages and assessment of residents on discharge from hospital, agreed to refund the excessive residential care charges levied on the basis that Mr Davey was a permanent resident, and paid compensation to Mr Davey and his family.

28.15 *Report on an investigation into Complaint No 12 001 464 against Kent County Council* (2013) 16 CCLR 465

There had been maladministration resulting in X not becoming a looked after child, to remedy which the Council ought to treat him as being such

Report summary

Subject: In early 2011, Mr X aged 16, became homeless because his parents abandoned him. Mr X approached Kent County Council's social services for help with both his housing and welfare needs. The council offered Mr X a foster placement. Mr X did not want this. The council offered no other alternatives. It did not help him with his welfare needs. Mr X moved between friends' houses. He remained with one friend between February and May 2012 and the council agreed to pay the friend's mother L30 per week. The friend's mother was unwilling to provide accommodation to Mr X when he became 18. Mr X became homeless again. Council A could not provide him with accommodation because Mr X was not considered in priority need.

Finding: Maladministration causing injustice.

Recommended remedy: Mr X should have been assessed as a looked after child. To remedy that the council should now confirm Mr X as a leaving care child and inform Council A. The council has agreed to this and it has written to Council A.

In addition, the council should:

- Assess Mr X's entitlement to services as a leaving care child and now provide those services;
- Set aside £3,000 for Mr X for the injustice caused to him by the loss of welfare benefits over a two-year period. This should be used, in consultation with the leaving care team, to promote Mr X's independent living and is in *addition* to the services Mr X is entitled to as a leaving care child;
- Review the implementation of its joint protocol to ensure it is meeting the council's responsibilities to all homeless young people; In bringing this report to the attention of the council's Committee, it should ensure the lead member of children's services is made aware of it.

28.16 *R (ER) v Local Government Ombudsman and Hillingdon LBC* [2014] EWCA Civ 1407, (2015) 18 CCLR 290

The LGO had no jurisdiction to investigate a complaint about the naming of a school in a Statement of Special Educational Needs

Facts: Hillingdon named a school on ER's son's Statement of Special Educational Needs, which was not ER's preferred choice. Her appeal to the SENDIST succeeded. She complained to the LGO about Hillingdon's failure to make educational provision for her son, in consequence of its naming decision. The LGO declined jurisdiction.

Judgment: the Court of Appeal (Moore-Bick, Aikens and Bean LJJ) held that the LGO had been right to decline jurisdiction, in that the naming decision fell within and was excluded by section 26(6)(a) of the Local Government Act 1974, as an appealable decision. The LGO's jurisdiction had been expanded by the Local Government and Public Involvement in Health Act 2007 to investigate service failures but that did not assist ER because the failure to provide ER's son with education was inextricably linked with the naming decision, which the LGO was barred from investigating.

28.17 *Report on a joint PHSO and LGO investigation into complaint numbers JW–1999678 and 14006021 about Sheffield Health and Social Care Foundation Trust and Sheffield City Council*[7]

The Council was directed to reimburse Ms D £14,000.00 being the sum she had spent on care, pay £12,000.00 compensation on account of Ms D's lack of social care and pay her a further £1,000.00 for distress

The Ombudsmen's decision

Summary: The Trust and the Council did not work quickly to provide a remedy to Ms D after her complaint was upheld in March 2014. So Ms D, a double amputee with significant mental health needs, has not had access to appropriate social care support for over 12 months, and had the stress of continuing to pursue a complaint which should have been resolved much sooner. The Trust and the Council should apologise, pay Ms D £12,000 to acknowledge the impact on her of their faults, reimburse the additional expenses she incurred, and take steps to avoid such a situation happening again.

...

Recommendations

64. In accordance with the Principles for Remedy, we make our recommendations on the basis that, where possible, the complainant should be returned to the position they would have been in if there had been no fault. If that is not possible, the complainant should receive a payment that acknowledges the impact of the fault. We therefore recommend the Trust and Council:

- Write to Ms D to apologise for the faults identified in this decision, and the distress these faults caused, within one month
- Reimburse Ms D £14,000 for the costs she incurred in buying support that should properly have come from her SDS budget, covering the period January 2014 to February 2015 inclusive
- Agree Ms D's monthly SDS budget as a matter of urgency and ensure that payments are made **within three months** at the latest and backdated appropriately
- Pay Ms D **£12,000** to acknowledge the impact on her of not having an adequate SDS budget in place. We have arrived at this figure by considering Ms D's vulnerability, the impact on her daily life, and the length of time she has been affected
- Pay Ms D a further **£1,000** to acknowledge the avoidable stress and frustration, and her justifiable outrage, from having to continue to pursue her complaint
- Disregard these payments when assessing Ms D's financial contribution to her SDS budget
- Produce an Action Plan **within three months** addressing the faults listed under paragraph 57 in this report, and setting out what action has and will be taken to address them.

28.18 *R (Miller) v Parliamentary and Health Service Ombudsman* [2015] EWHC 2981 (Admin), (2015) 18 CCLR 697

It had been fair for the Ombudsman to have treated a complaint about one doctor as being implicitly a complaint about two doctors and he had given both doctors a fair opportunity to respond

7 www.lgo.org.uk/decisions/adult-care-services/direct-payments/14-006-021.

Facts: Two doctors applied for a judicial review of the Ombudsman's decision that they had provided unacceptable care to a 76-year-old patient.

Judgment: Lewis J held that, whilst the patient's wife had explicitly complained only about the care provided by the second doctor, it had been reasonable for the Ombudsman to read her complaint as intending to encompass all the care her husband had received, including care from the first doctor, whom the wife's correspondence did refer to. The Ombudsman had provided both doctors with written notice of the complaint and both had been given a fair opportunity to respond; in addition, they had both had the opportunity of responding to the Ombudsman's draft report. The process had been fair and the Ombudsman had been entitled to assess financial redress having regard to damages awards in negligence actions.

CHAPTER 29

Regulation of adult social and health care

continued

29.35 *Bicknell v HM Coroner for Birmingham and Solihull* [2007] EWHC 2547 (Admin), (2008) 11 CCLR 431

An inquest should be held where the evidence suggested a possible connection between inadequate care and death in a care home

29.36 *Jain v Trent Strategic Health Authority* [2009] UKHL 4, (2009) 12 CCLR 194

A health authority did not owe care home owners a duty of care when investigating suspected inadequate care provided to residents and securing an ex parte cancelling the care home's registration

29.37 *R (Broadway Care Centre Ltd) v Caerphilly CBC* [2012] EWHC 37 (Admin), (2012) 15 CCLR 82

Termination of a framework contract with a care home was a private law, not a public law, decision and the care home did not have standing to complain about potential breaches of the residents' ECHR rights

29.37A *Old Co-operative Day Nursery Ltd v H M Chief Inspector of Education, Children's Services & Skills* [2016] EWHC 1126 Admin

The Chief Inspector of Education, Children's Services & Skills had no jurisdiction to investigate a complaint made by a member of the public and his investigation had in any event been irrational

Professional cases

29.38 *R (Raines) v Orange Grove* [2006] EWHC 1887 (Admin), (2006) 9 CCLR 541

A decision to deregister a foster carer had been taken in a procedurally unfair manner and was Wednesbury unreasonable

29.39 *Joyce v Secretary of State for Health* [2008] EWHC 1891 (Admin), (2008) 11 CCLR 761

The tribunal may consider allegations not included in the initial reference to the Secretary of State

29.40 *Wright and others v Secretary of State for Health* [2009] UKHL 3, (2009) 12 CCLR 181

The absence of any opportunity to make representations before being included in the POVA list breached the ECHR

29.41 *Southall v General Medical Council* [2010] EWCA Civ 407, [2010] 2 FCR 77

In simple cases the GMC need only set out what facts it had found proven but in more complex cases, it had to give sufficient reasons why it accepted some evidence but rejected other evidence

29.42 *Bonhoeffer v General Medical Council* [2011] EWHC 1585 (Admin), [2011] ACD 104

In disciplinary proceedings raising serious charges amounting to criminal offences likely if proven to have grave consequences for the accused, there would need to be compelling reasons to prevent him from cross-examining a witness whose evidence was critical to establishing the charges, if there were no problems associated with securing the attendance of that witness

29.43 *Perry v Nursing and Midwifery Council* [2013] EWCA Civ 145, [2013] 1 WLR 3423

The NMC was entitled to make an interim order against a nurse without hearing evidence from the nurse as to whether the allegations against them were well-founded; its role at that stage was not to decide the credibility or merit of allegations but to decide whether they justified making an interim order

29.44 *Obukofe v General Medical Council* [2014] EWHC 408 (Admin)
In appeals relating to fitness to practise and any sanction imposed, the court will accord considerable weight to the conclusions of the professional regulatory body and will bear in mind that its primary function is the protection of the public

29.44A *R (SPP Health Ltd) v Care Quality Commission* [2016] EWHC 2086 (Admin)
Fairness required the CQC to provide an independent review where a provider claimed that factual findings in a draft report were demonstrably wrong or misleading but the inspection team refused to vary the draft report

Confidential information cases

29.45 *R v Somerset CC ex p Prospects Care Services* (1999) 2 CCLR 161, QBD
It was lawful for a local authority to provide information about a fostering agency casting doubt on its competence where it adopted a fair and rational procedure and where the information was fair and rational

29.46 *R v Chief Constable of Wales ex p AB* (2000) 3 CCLR 25, DC
Providing they act fairly, by giving those affected the opportunity of comment, the police are entitled to disclose information about individuals to third parties where that is justified in the public interest

29.47 *R v Secretary of State for Health ex p C* (2000) 3 CCLR 412, CA
It had been lawful to maintain the Consultancy Service index

29.48 *R (S) v Plymouth CC* [2002] EWCA Civ 388, (2002) 5 CCLR 251
Fairness and the ECHR required disclosure of the son's mental health records to his mother, in nearest relative displacement proceedings

29.49 *MG v United Kingdom* (2002) 5 CCLR 525, ECtHR
Adults who were in local authority care as children are entitled to at least some level of access to their social services records

29.50 *R (A) v National Probation Service* [2003] EWHC 2910 (Admin), (2004) 7 CCLR 336
The disclosure of confidential information was unlawful when there had not been consideration of the need for a pressing justification or a balancing exercise

29.51 *A Local Authority v A Health Authority and Mrs A* [2004] EWHC 2746 Fam, (2004) 7 CCLR 426
Publication of a report into poor foster care would be too harmful to the children and vulnerable adults concerned

29.52 *Brent LBC v N and P* [2005] EWHC 1676 (Fam), (2006) 9 CCLR 14
Disclosure of a foster-carer's HIV status to the children's father was unjustified where the risks to the children were negligible and the disclosure opposed

29.53 *Roberts v Nottinghamshire Healthcare NHS Trust* [2008] EWHC 1934 (Admin), (2009) 12 CCLR 110
Disclosure of health records and reports could be refused where it might well cause damage to health

29.54 *R (L) v Metropolitan Police Commissioner* [2009] UKSC 3, (2009) 12 CCLR 573
The police may disclose personal information to an employer about a person who proposes to work with children or vulnerable adults when it is proportionate to do so

continued

29.55 *Chief Constable of Humberside Police v Information Commissioner* [2009] EWCA Civ 1079, [2010] 1 WLR 1136
It was lawful for chief constables indefinitely to retain information about convictions and cautions (spent or not)

29.56 *R (F (A child)) v Secretary of State for Justice* [2010] UKSC 17, [2011] 1 AC 331
It was incompatible with Article 8 ECHR to impose indefinite requirements on sexual offenders that did not include any possibility of review

29.57 *H and L v A City Council* [2011] EWCA Civ 403, (2011) 14 CCLR 381
It had been disproportionate to disclosure child sexual offences to organisations where the persons worked which were not involved with children and to personal assistants who were not allowed to bring children with them and the process had been unfair

29.58 *MM v United Kingdom* Application no 24029/07, [2012] ECHR 1096
A disclosure regime that did not include sufficient safeguards to protect private life would be incompatible with Article 8 ECHR

29.59 *R (A) v Chief Constable of Kent* [2013] EWCA Civ 1706, (2014) 135 BMLR 22
Court review of the proportionality of disclosure of sensitive personal information was intense but it was not a merits review and should ordinarily disregard new material

29.60 *R (L) v Chief Constable of Kent* [2014] EWHC 463 (Admin)
It was disproportionate to include in an ECRC allegations that had been rejected at a criminal trial as being manifestly unrealiable

29.61 *R (P) v Chief Constable of Thames Valley Police* [2014] EWHC 1436 (Admin), (2014) 17 CCLR 250
In this case, it had been disproportionate to disclose inappropriate remarks made to persons who were not vulnerable adults or children

29.62 *R (T) v Chief Constable of Greater Manchester Police* [2013] EWCA Civ 25, [2013] 1 WLR 2515
A disclosure scheme had to contain adequate safeguards against arbitrariness, designed to prevent disproportionate disclosures

29.63 *R (AB) v Chief Constable of Hampshire* [2015] EWHC 1238 (Admin)
A disclosure based on inadequate investigation and incorrect information was unlawful

29.64 *R (Catt) v Association of Chief Police Officers of England, Wales and Northern Ireland and others* [2015] UKSC 9, [2015] AC 1065
It was proportionate for the police to retain certain personal information for crime enforcement purposes

29.65 *R (W) v Secretary of State for Justice* [2015] EWHC 1952 (Admin)
It was primarily for the legislature to determine the length of time which different types of offences were disclosable

29.66 *R (SD) v Chief Constable of North Yorkshire and the Disclosure and Barring Service* [2015] EWHC 2085 (Admin)
Disclosure in an ECRC was proportionate

29.67 *Re C (A Child)* [2015] EWFC 79
Psychiatrists were not entitled to disclosure of confidential medical records to help them rebut defamatory comments

29.68 *R (P) v Secretary of State for Justice* [2016] EWHC 89 (Admin), [2016] 1 WLR 2009

Article 8 required there to be a mechanism for testing the proportionality of disclosure in individual cases

29.69 *R (MS) v Independent Monitor of the Home Office* [2016] EWHC 655 (Admin), [2016] 4 WLR 88

The Independent Monitor was required to scrutinise with a high degree of forensic care the credibility of allegations before assessing its weight and conducting the necessary disclosure balancing exercise

29.70 *R (C) v Secretary of State for Work and Pensions* [2016] EWCA Civ 47

It was lawful for the Secretary of State for Work and Pensions to retain records that showed that a person had changed their gender, where there was good reason for so doing and every effort had been made to minimise the distress caused

29.71 *R (LK) v Independent Monitor* [2016] EWHC 1629 (Admin)

It had been unreasonable to approve inclusion on the ECRC of information about an individual's acquittal of sexual offences when the decision was unsupported by the evidence at the trial and the judge's summing up

29.72 *R (G) v Chief Constable of Surrey Police* [2016] EWHC 295 (Admin), [2016] 4 WLR 94

The Police Act 1997 still contained inadequate safeguards against disproportionate disclosure

29.73 *A v B Local Authority* [2016] EWCA Civ 766

A head teacher had been fairly dismissed for gross misconduct for failing to disclose her relationship with a person convicted of making indecent images of children

Procedural and other cases

29.74 *Sarfraz v Disclosure and Barring Service* [2015] EWCA Civ 544, [2015] 1 WLR 4441

The Court of Appeal had no jurisdiction to give permission to appeal to itself, from a decision by the Upper Tribunal not to grant permission to appeal to itself

29.75 *MR v Disclosure and Barring Service (Safeguarding vulnerable groups: Adults' barred list)* [2015] UKUT 5 (AAC), 5 January 2015

The DBS reasons for including MR on the adult's barred list were wrong but the case would be remitted to the DBS for further consideration

29.76 *R (C) v Secretary of State for Justice* [2016] UKSC 2, (2016) 19 CCLR 5

There was no presumption of anonymity for mental patients challenging aspects of their treatment and care in the High Court but anonymity will be granted where that is necessary in the interests of the patient

29.1 A key distinction is between the regulation of services and the regulation of professionals.

Regulation of services

29.2 Adult health and social care services in England are, in the main, regulated by the Care Quality Commission (CQC),[1] an executive non-departmental public body of the Department of Health, set up by the Health and Social Care Act 2008, supplemented by Part 2 of the Care Act 2014. It replaces the Healthcare Commission, the Commission for Social Care Inspection and the Mental Health Act Commission and regulates hospitals, care homes, dental and general practices, domiciliary care providers and other mental health and care services.

29.3 Most children's services in England are regulated by Her Majesty's Chief Inspector of Education, Children's Services and Skills, backed up by Ofsted[2] (the Office for Standards in Education, Children's Services and Skills (a non-ministerial government department)) – including state and independent schools, children's homes, residential family centres, child-minding, child day care, children's social care, CAFCASS, teacher training providers, colleges and learning and skills providers and fostering and adoption agencies. The primary legislation is sections 1–5 of the Care Standards Act 2000, the Children Act 1989 and the Adoption and Children Act 2002.

29.4 In Wales, the Care and Social Services Inspectorate Wales regulates most adults' and children's services, including care homes, domiciliary care agencies, adult placement schemes, nurses' agencies, children's homes, child minders, day care services for under 8s, fostering agencies, adoption agencies, boarding schools, residential family centres, residential special schools and further education colleges which accommodate students under 18. It also reviews social services departments in Wales and conducts national reviews to monitor how well services are performing, under the Health and Social Care (Community Health and Standards Act) 2003, the Care Standards Act 2000, the Children Act 1989, the Adoption and Children Act 2002 and the Children and Families (Wales) Measure 2010.

29.5 There are numerous regulatory bodies concerned with health care provision:

- the Care Quality Commission[3] oversees the provision of safe, effective, compassionate and high quality care in hospitals, care homes, dental and GP surgeries and all other care services in England;
- NHS Improvement[4] brings together Monitor, the NHS Trust Development Agency and the Patient Safety elements operated by NHS England and aims to protect and promote the interests of patients by ensuring that the whole health sector works for their benefit – in effect

1 www.cqc.org.uk.
2 www.gov.uk/government/organisations/ofsted.
3 www.cqc.org.uk/.
4 https://improvement.nhs.uk/.

it regulates competition within the NHS and manages performance generally;

- NHS England[5] licenses and regulates Clinical Commissioning Groups;
- Healthwatch England and Local Healthwatch organisations[6] are founded by Chapter 1 of Part 5 of the Health and Social Care Act 2012 and are designed to feed the voice of the patient into the NHS and to champion their interests (there are now 152 Local Healthwatch groups);
- Health Overview and Scrutiny Committees, set up by Chapter 3 of Part 12 of the National Health Service Act 2006, are comprised of members of the local social services authority. They may review and scrutinise any matter relating to the planning, provision and operation of the health services in their area and are entitled to be consulted about any substantial development of the health service in their area and to refer any objection on their part to the Secretary of State for Health (see Part 4 of the Local Authority (Public Health, Health and Wellbeing Boards and Health Scrutiny) Regulations 2013;
- Health and Wellbeing Boards[7] were established by Chapter 1 of Part 5 of the Health and Social Care Act 2012, as committees of the local authority, as a forum where key leaders from the health and social care system work together to improve the health and wellbeing of their local population, in particular by promoting better joint working.

29.6 Throughout Great Britain, the Health and Safety Executive[8] operates as an independent regulator for health and safety in the workplace, which includes all private and publicly owned health and social care settings.

Regulation of professionals

29.7 A major function of professional regulatory bodies is to maintain a register of professionals who meet their standards and/or statutory standards to practise in that area and to exercise disciplinary functions over such members, including by removing them from the register, making it unlawful for them to continue to practice in the field.

29.8 Vulnerable adults who are concerned about the conduct of a professional in the health or social care field may raise their concern directly with the relevant regulatory body for investigation (as well, of course, as with the police or other relevant public agencies).

29.9 A complaint may result in the professional undergoing a 'fitness to practice' hearing, which is usually a public hearing, of a judicial nature, before the professional body's 'fitness to practice' panel.

29.10 In England, the regulation of health and social care professionals is, in the main, undertaken by the Health and Care Professions Council:

5 www.england.nhs.uk/.

6 www.healthwatch.co.uk/.

7 See the views of the LGA and the King's Fund at www.local.gov.uk/health/-/journal_content/56/10180/3510973/ARTICLE and www.kingsfund.org.uk/projects/new-nhs/health-and-wellbeing-boards.

8 www.hse.gov.uk/healthservices/arrangements.htm#a1.

they currently regulate arts therapists, biomedical scientists, chiropodists/podiatrists, clinical scientists, dietitians, hearing aid dispensers, occupational therapists, operating department practitioners, orthoptists, paramedics, physiotherapists, practitioner psychologists, prosthetists/orthotists, radiographers, social workers in England[9] and speech and language therapists.

29.11 The Health and Care Professions Council (HCPC)[10] operates under the Health and Social Work Professions Order 2001[11] (made under section 60 of the Health Act 1999) and the Health Professions Council (Constitution Order) 2009. The 2001 Order contains detailed provision about, inter alia, registration and 'fitness to practice' hearings.

29.12 There are a number of other regulatory bodies for particular categories of health and social care professionals (see below): all of which, including the HCPC, are themselves overseen by the Professional Standards Authority.[12] The other professional regulatory bodies are as follows:

- General Medical Council (GMC) which regulates doctors in the UK;[13]
- Nursing and Midwifery Council (NMC) which regulates nurses and midwives in the UK;[14]
- General Dental Council (GDC), which regulates dentists and professions complementary to dentistry in the UK;
- General Optical Council (GOC) which regulates optometrists, dispensing opticians, student opticians and optical businesses in the UK;[15]
- General Osteopathic Council (GOsC) which regulates osteopaths in the UK;[16]
- General Chiropractic Council (GCC) which regulates chiropractors in the UK;[17]
- General Pharmaceutical Council (GPhC) which regulates pharmacists and pharmacy technicians and regulates pharmacies in England, Wales and Scotland;[18]
- Pharmaceutical Society of Northern Ireland (PSNI) which regulates pharmacists in Northern Ireland.[19]

29.13 The regulatory body for social workers in Wales is the Care Council for Wales.[20] In Scotland, the regulatory body for social workers is the Scottish Social Services Council.[21]

9 In Wales, social care professionals are regulated by the Care Council for Wales, whose website is here: http://www.ccwales.org.uk/?force=1.
10 www.hcpc-uk.org.
11 http://www.hcpc-uk.org/Assets/documents/10004784HCPC-ConsolidatedHealthandSocialWorkProfessionsOrder(July2014).pdf.
12 www.professionalstandards.org.uk/about-us.
13 www.gmc-uk.org/.
14 www.nmc.org.uk/.
15 www.gdc-uk.org/.
16 www.optical.org/.
17 www.gcc-uk.org/.
18 www.pharmacyregulation.org/.
19 www.psni.org.uk/.
20 www.ccwales.org.uk.
21 www.sssc.uk.com.

29.14 While the regulation of health and care professionals is not devolved in Wales, regulation of health and care professionals is a devolved matter in Northern Ireland, and in Scotland it is devolved for health professionals brought into regulation since Scottish devolution (these are: operating department practitioners and practitioner psychologists regulated by the HCPC; dental nurses, dental technicians, clinical dental technicians and orthodontic therapists regulated by the GDC and pharmacy technicians regulated by the GPhC). The general position is that the jurisdiction of the regulatory bodies in respect of health professionals is UK-wide. The exception to this is the GPhC which covers Great Britain and the PSNI which covers Northern Ireland. The regulation of social care professionals falls within the legislative competence of each country.

29.15 It is estimated there are approximately 200 pieces of secondary legislation, which specifically address the regulatory bodies or professional regulation in general. This has led to the current legal framework becoming complex, inflexible, inconsistent and expensive to maintain. Accordingly, there is a need for reform, which has been recognised by the regulatory bodies as well as the Government. There has been a tripartite project between the Law Commission, the Scottish Law Commission and the Northern Ireland Law Commission resulting in the publication, in April 2014, of *Regulation of Health Care Professionals, Regulations of Social Care Professionals in England: a Joint Report*[22] and the government's response in January 2015.[23] There is, also, a very useful paper by Tim Spencer-Lane of the Law Commission, entitled *Safeguarding the Public by Regulating Health and Social Care Professionals.*[24] This has resulted in the Regulation of Health and Social Care Professions etc Bill 2016-17 which, at the time of writing has had its first reading in the House of Lords but does not have a second reading scheduled. The Bill if enacted commits the government to enacting legislation that gives effect to the Law Commissions' recommendations, most notably, that there should be a single statute which provides the framework for all regulatory bodies and the Professional Standards Authority.[25]

29.16 Onward appeals from decisions made by professional regulatory bodies, such as the HCPC and the GMC are in general to the High Court in England and Wales, the Court of Session in Scotland and the High Court of Northern Ireland.[26]

22 www.lawcom.gov.uk/document/regulation-of-health-care-professionals-regulation-of-social-care-professionals-in-england/.

23 www.gov.uk/government/uploads/system/uploads/attachment_data/file/420119/46547_Cm_8995_print_ready.pdf.

24 www.emeraldinsight.com/doi/abs/10.1108/JAP-06–2013-0024.

25 http://services.parliament.uk/bills/2016-17/regulationofhealthandsocialcareprofessionsetc.html.

26 In relation to the HCPC see www.hpc-uk.org/complaints/hearings/afterthehearing/ and see in relation to GMC www.gmc-uk.org/Appeals___Registration_appeals_factsheet___DC2861.pdf_49293478.pdf.

Disclosure and barring

29.17 In addition, all persons, including professionally registered persons, who work or seek to work with children or vulnerable adults are:

- liable to be barred from such work (this is in addition to the possibility that professionals may have their professional registration cancelled), subject to an appeal to the Upper Tribunal;
- subject to machinery which prohibits them from such work unless they disclose their full criminal history as well as information held by local police forces that it is reasonably considered might be relevant to the post applied for (eg complaints about the person's conduct that did not result in criminal proceedings and may never have been fully investigated let alone judicially determined).

29.18 The legislation that provides most of the relevant machinery is the Safeguarding Vulnerable Groups Act (SVGA) 2006, together with delegated legislation, the most important of which is:

- the Safeguarding Vulnerable Groups Act 2006 (Barring Procedure) Regulations 2008 (which prescribes the process to be undertaken before a person is included in one of the barred lists, or removed from a list);
- the Safeguarding Vulnerable Groups Act 2006 (Barred List Prescribed Information) Regulations 2008 (which prescribes the information that must be maintained about barred individuals).

29.19 The lynchpin of this statutory machinery is the Disclosure and Barring Service (DBS).[27] The DBS:

- maintains separate barred lists for regulated work with children and adults in accordance with Schedule 3 to the SVGA 2006 (which sets out the criteria for inclusion in the lists),
- provides three different levels of DBS checks for the benefit of employers in the field of child and adult care:
  - *Standard* (this checks for spent and unspent convictions, cautions, reprimands and final warnings);
  - *Enhanced* (this includes the standard check plus any additional information held by local police that is reasonably considered relevant to the workforce being applied for); and
  - *Enhanced with list checks* (this includes and enhanced check and a check of the DBS barred lists).

Barring

29.20 As far as concerns barring, a great deal of information provided to the DBS comes from the police and criminal justice system, but employers in regulated activities involving children or adults must report to the DBS any individual whom they dismissed because they harmed someone, whom they dismissed or removed from working in a regulated activity because they might have harmed someone or whom they were planning to

27 www.gov.uk/disclosure-barring-service-check/overview.

dismiss for either of these reasons, before they resigned; and it is a criminal offence to employ a barred person in a regulated activity from which they are barred: see sections 30–51 of the SVGA 2006.

29.21 By virtue of paragraphs 1 and 7 of Schedule 3 to the SVGA 2006, the DBS must automatically include on the children's or adult's barred list persons who have been convicted of prescribed offences.[28] Otherwise, by virtue of paragraphs 2 and 8 of Schedule 3, and the consequential provisions in Schedule 3, the DBS may include a person on one of the barred lists if (having considered the person's representations) it is satisfied that they have been or might be engaged in a regulated activity relating to children or vulnerable adults, if they have engaged in 'relevant conduct' and it is 'appropriate to include the person in the list'. The 'relevant conduct' is defined as follows (for the purposes of the adult's barred list) in SVGA 2006 Sch 3 para 10:

> **10**(1) For the purposes of paragraph 9 relevant conduct is–
> (a) conduct which endangers a vulnerable adult or is likely to endanger a vulnerable adult;
> (b) conduct which, if repeated against or in relation to a vulnerable adult, would endanger that adult or would be likely to endanger him;
> (c) conduct involving sexual material relating to children (including possession of such material);
> (d) conduct involving sexually explicit images depicting violence against human beings (including possession of such images), if it appears to DBS that the conduct is inappropriate;
> (e) conduct of a sexual nature involving a vulnerable adult, if it appears to DBS that the conduct is inappropriate.
> (2) A person's conduct endangers a vulnerable adult if he–
> (a) harms a vulnerable adult,
> (b) causes a vulnerable adult to be harmed,
> (c) puts a vulnerable adult at risk of harm,
> (d) attempts to harm a vulnerable adult, or
> (e) incites another to harm a vulnerable adult.
> (3) 'Sexual material relating to children' means–
> (a) indecent images of children, or
> (b) material (in whatever form) which portrays children involved in sexual activity and which is produced for the purposes of giving sexual gratification.
> (4) 'Image' means an image produced by any means, whether of a real or imaginary subject.
> (5) A person does not engage in relevant conduct merely by committing an offence prescribed for the purposes of this sub-paragraph.
> (6) For the purposes of sub-paragraph (1)(d) and (e), DBS must have regard to guidance issued by the Secretary of State as to conduct which is inappropriate.

29.22 A decision to include a person in either the adult's or children's barred list may be appealed to the Upper Tribunal, providing the Upper Tribunal grants permission to appeal, by virtue of section 4 of the SGVA 2006:

28 See the guide to prescribed offences at www.gov.uk/government/uploads/system/uploads/attachment_data/file/384712/DBS_referrals_guide_-_relevant_offences_v2.4.pdf.

Appeals

4(1) An individual who is included in a barred list may appeal to the Upper Tribunal against–
(a) ...
(b) a decision under paragraph 2, 3, 5, 8, 9 or 11 of Schedule 3 to include him in the list;
(c) a decision under paragraph 17, 18 or 18A of that Schedule not to remove him from the list.

(2) An appeal under subsection (1) may be made only on the grounds that DBS has made a mistake–
(a) on any point of law;
(b) in any finding of fact which it has made and on which the decision mentioned in that subsection was based.

(3) For the purposes of subsection (2), the decision whether or not it is appropriate for an individual to be included in a barred list is not a question of law or fact.

(4) An appeal under subsection (1) may be made only with the permission of the Upper Tribunal.

(5) Unless the Upper Tribunal finds that DBS has made a mistake of law or fact, it must confirm the decision of [DBS].

(6) If the Upper Tribunal finds that DBS has made such a mistake it must–
(a) direct DBS to remove the person from the list, or
(b) remit the matter to DBS for a new decision.

(7) If the Upper Tribunal remits a matter to DBS under subsection (6)(b)–
(a) the Upper Tribunal may set out any findings of fact which it has made (on which DBS must base its new decision); and
(b) the person must be removed from the list until DBS makes its new decision, unless the Upper Tribunal directs otherwise.

Disclosure

29.23 An Enhanced DBS certificate is required when, inter alia, a person will provide a 'regulated activity' to children or vulnerable adults, within the meaning of Schedule 4 to the SVGA 2006. The DBS publishes a range of guides as to 'eligibility' for different kinds of DBS certificates.[29]

29.24 The procedure is that (i) the registered body provides the candidate with a DBS application form for completion; (ii) the registered body checks that the information provided is accurate and completes its part of the form, which requires it to verify the candidate's identity; (iii) the form is sent to the DBS which checks it and may need to return it; (iv) the DBS searches the Police National Computer for any matches which reveal convictions (etc.), as well as the children and adult's barred lists; (v) the DBS then asks the police for any information held by them they consider to be relevant and ought to be included in the certificate; (vi) the DBS certificate is then printed securely and sent to the candidate; (vii) the registered body is able to track the process electronically; (viii) it is up to the candidate whether to disclose their DBS certificate to the registered body, although they must not be employed if they do not do so; (ix) the DBS has published guidance to assist registered bodies detect any fraudulent alteration of a DBS certificate and of course it is a criminal offence to alter such certificates.

29 www.gov.uk/government/publications/dbs-check-eligible-positions-guidance.

29.25 As will be apparent from the above, a major function of the DBS is to secure information from the police, for inclusion on the DBS certificate. The most contentious aspect of this arises out of section 113B of the Police Act 1997, which promotes the communication of information by the police to the DBS about the individual which may never have been judicially assessed for accuracy and which could range from gossip (although information '*unlikely to be true*'[30] ought not to be included) to highly evidenced allegations that are certainly true:

113B(4) Before issuing an enhanced criminal record certificate DBS must request any relevant chief officer force to provide any information which ....

(a) the chief officer reasonably believes to be relevant for the purpose described in the statement under subsection (2), and

(b) in the chief officer's opinion ought to be included in the certificate.

(4A) In exercising functions under subsection (4) a relevant chief officer must have regard to any guidance for the time being published by the Secretary of State.

29.26 The relevant statutory guidance is *Statutory Disclosure Guidance* (2nd edition, August 2015).[31] At paragraph 26 onwards, chief police officers are advised to consider affording applicants the opportunity to make representations about whether information should be included in an enhanced criminal record certificate.

29.27 This process can result in the applicant exercising their right to apply to the 'independent monitor' under sections 117A and 119B and/or applying for a judicial review of the chief police officer's decision, either before or after the issue of the DBS certificate.[32]

29.28 It may be surprising that legislation does not provide an appeal in relation to the content of DBS certificates. However, in judicial review proceedings, because ECHR rights are engaged, the court will intensely review the factors considered by the decision-maker and decide for itself whether the content of the DBS certificate is proportionate; though it will not consider evidence post-dating the relevant decision.[33]

Cases

Care homes

29.29 *Bettercare Group Ltd v The Director-General of Fair Trading* [2002] CAT 7

The North and West Belfast Health and Social Services Trust was an undertaking for the purposes of the Competition Act 1998

30 See paragraph 18 of the *Statutory Disclosure Guidance* (2nd edition, August 2015).

31 www.gov.uk/government/uploads/system/uploads/attachment_data/file/452321/6_1155_HO_LW_Stat_Dis_Guide-v3.pdf.

32 And see www.gov.uk/guidance/disclosure-and-barring-service-criminal-record-checks-referrals-and-complaints.

33 See *H and L v A City Council* [2011] EWCA Civ 403, (2011) 14 CCLR 381 at para 29.57 below.

Facts: Bettercare complained that The North and West Belfast Health and Social Services Trust was abusing its dominant position as the sole purchaser of care services from Bettercare, by offering unreasonably low prices and unfair terms, contrary to Chapter III of the Competition Act 1998. The Office of Fair Trading declined to investigate, on the ground that the Trust was not acting as an 'undertaking' within the meaning of section 18(1) of the Act.

Judgment: The Competition Commission Appeal Panel (Sir Christopher Bellamy, President, Mr Michael Davey and Mr David Summers) held that the Trust's activities in running its statutory residential homes and engaging in contracting out social care to independent providers were economic activities for the purposes of the Competition Act 1998, so that the Trust was an undertaking, subject to the Act.

29.30 *Alternative Futures Ltd v National Care Standards Commission* (2002) 101–111 NC, (2004) 7 CCLR 171, Care Standards Tribunals

A registered care home was unable unilaterally to change its status

Facts: Alternative Futures provided accommodation, board and care in a number of homes registered under the Registered Homes Act 1984. It then created a second company to deal with its property, which granted tenancies to the residents, with the original company continuing to provide care. The local authority refused to cancel the registration of the homes or pay housing benefit, on the basis that the homes remained registered and registrable.

Judgment: the Care Standards Tribunal held that a home could not unilaterally cease to be registered; it only ceased to be registered when the registration authority made a considered decision to remove it. If the home disagreed, with that or the housing benefits decision, it should invoke the appeals machinery that applied in both those types of case.

Comment: see the decision of the Court of Appeal under *Moore v Care Standards Tribunal* at para 29.32 below.

29.31 *Bettercare Group Ltd v North and West Belfast Health and Social Services Trust* Decision No CA98/09/2003 (2004) 7 CCLR 194, OFT

A commissioner was not in breach of Chapter II of the Competition Act 1998 because it did not set the prices paid

Facts: Bettercare complained that the North and West Belfast Health and Social Services Trust was abusing its dominant position as the sole purchaser of care services from Bettercare, contrary to Chapter III of the Competition Act 1998, by (i) paying excessively low prices for residential and nursing home services; (ii) paying significantly higher prices to its own statutory homes and (iii) requiring families placed in Bettercare homes to pay 'top ups', which acted as a disincentive. On the facts, however, it emerged that the prices were set by another body, the Eastern Health and Social Services Board, set up by the Department of Health, Social Services and Public Safety.

Judgment: since prices were set by the Eastern Health and Social Services Board, the North and West Belfast Health and Social Services Trust could not have been committing an abuse under Chapter II of the Competition Act 1998. In any event, there was insufficient evidence of excessively low prices (which was only unlawful, in any event, in exceptional circumstances) or of any form of discrimination. Since the setting of rates by the Eastern Health and Social Services Board was governmental, and not that of an undertaking, that activity fell outside the Competition Act 1998.

29.32 *Moore v Care Standards Tribunal* [2005] EWCA Civ 627, (2005) 8 CCLR 354

A home could in substance be a care home notwithstanding that occupiers had been granted assured tenancies, where in truth the establishment provided accommodation together with nursing or personal care

Facts: Alternative Futures provided accommodation, board and care in a number of homes registered under the Registered Homes Act 1984. It then created a second company to deal with its property, which granted tenancies to the residents, with the original company continuing to provide care. The local authority refused to cancel the registration of the homes or pay housing benefit, on the basis that the registered status of the homes precluded such payments.

Judgment: the Court of Appeal (Waller and Mance LJJ, Sir William Aldous) held that a home could in substance be a care home notwithstanding that occupiers had been granted assured tenancies, where in truth the establishment provided accommodation together with nursing or personal care and, in this case, Housing and Futures, together with each house, had operated as one establishment: it was a question of act, ultimately.

29.33 *Brooklyn House Ltd v CSCI* [2006] EWHC 1165 (Admin), (2006) 9 CCLR 394

Offences relating to the administration and availability of medication were offences of strict liability and it was a question of fact and degree whether an offence had been committed, in the light of the standards imposed by the Care Homes for Older People Minimum Standards

Facts: the judge at first instance found that on the occasion of one inspection visit, there were failures in the record-keeping in relation to the administration of medication, including an occasion where medication appeared not to have been administered with no explanation provided; and that on the occasion of a second visit, there were a number of failures in record-keeping and several instances of prescribed medication not being available. Brooklyn alleged that its prosecution had not been validly authorised and that it was not guilty of offences under section 25 of the Care Standards Act 2000 because it had instituted proper procedures but had been hampered by an inability to secure medication from GPs.

Judgment: the Divisional Court (Maurice Kay LJ, Tugendhat J) held that the Commission for Social Care Inspection was entitled to bring the prosecution and was not required to give evidence about its internal procedures and that the offences in question were offences of strict liability: the duty had been a duty to make effective arrangements for the administration and availability of medication and whether an offence had been committed was a question of fact and degree, in the light of the standards imposed by the Care Homes for Older People Minimum Standards.

29.34 *Welsh Ministers v Care Standards Tribunal and H* [2008] EWHC 49 (Admin), (2008) 11 CCLR 234

An appeal against a refusal to register a person as a manager could be allowed to proceed even after it had become academic

Facts: The Welsh Ministers refused to register H as manager of a care home because of concerns about her ability and H appealed to the Care Standards Tribunal. The owners of the care home appointed another manager, so H could no longer manage that home. However, H had been approached to manage another home, but could not do so unless she achieved registration. The Tribunal refused the Welsh Ministers' application to strike out H's appeal, on the ground that it had no realistic prospect of success, given that in point of form, H could no longer be registered as manager of the original care home. The Welsh Ministers appealed.

Judgment: Davis J dismissed the Welsh Ministers' appeal holding that whilst the registration of an individual as manager of a care home related to a specific establishment or agency it did not follow that an appeal against a refusal to register had to be struck out when the establishment or agency in question was no longer available to be managed by the appellant and it was legitimate to refuse to strike out such an appeal in circumstances where, if the appellant succeeded, there was a reasonable prospect of them securing management of a different establishment or agency.

29.35 *Bicknell v HM Coroner for Birmingham and Solihull* [2007] EWHC 2547 (Admin), (2008) 11 CCLR 431

An inquest should be held where the evidence suggested a possible connection between inadequate care and death in a care home

Facts: Ms Bicknell's father died about two weeks after entering Maypole Nursing Home. Afterwards a number of regulators started investigations and the GMC suspended the two doctors running the home. Ms Bicknell asked the coroner to hold an inquest into her father's death, presenting the coroner with evidence as to her father's condition on arrival at Maypole and expert evidence casting doubt on aspects of management there. The coroner refused to hold an inquest on the basis that, the cause of death being '*unknown*', the death was not an '*unnatural death*'. Ms Bicknell sought a judicial review of that decision.

Judgment: McCombe J allowed the application for judicial review, holding that there was a reasonable suspicion that the death had been an '*unnatural*' one and the coroner had been wrong to require a possible causative link between the improper treatment and the death to be established, it was enough that the death was abnormal or unexpected and, in any event, in this case, the evidence gave reasonable cause to suspect that Mr Bicknell's death had been caused or contributed to by inadequate care.

29.36 ### *Jain v Trent Strategic Health Authority* [2009] UKHL 4, (2009) 12 CCLR 194

A health authority did not owe care home owners a duty of care when investigating suspected inadequate care provided to residents and securing an ex parte order cancelling the care home's registration

Facts: Nottingham Health Authority (Trent's predecessor's) applied ex parte without notice to the magistrates' court for an order under section 30 of the Registered Homes Act 1984, immediately cancelling the registration of Mr and Mrs Jain's care home. That resulted in the immediate closure of their care home business. Mr and Mrs Jain's only remedy was to appeal to the magistrates, which was a relatively lengthy process. By the time the appeal was heard, it was apparent that Nottingham's application under section 30 had been entirely misconceived and wholly unjustified. By that time, however, Mr and Mrs Jain had been financially ruined. They sued in negligence.

Judgment: the House of Lords (Lords Scott, Rodger, Baroness Hale, Lords Carswell and Neuberger) held that Nottingham had not owed Mr and Mrs Jain a common law duty of care because it had been acting under statutory powers conferred for the benefit of a separate class of persons and had obtained court authority for its actions. Lord Scott, Baroness Hale and Lords Carswell and Neuberger opined that had the relevant events occurred after the 2 October 2002, Mr and Mrs Jain might have had a remedy under the Human Rights Act 1998.

Comment: Mr and Mrs Jain brought proceedings in the European Court of Human rights and achieved a friendly settlement (£733,500 plus legal costs).[34]

29.37 ### *R (Broadway Care Centre Ltd) v Caerphilly CBC* [2012] EWHC 37 (Admin), (2012) 15 CCLR 82

Termination of a framework contract with a care home was a private law, not a public law, decision and the care home did not have standing to complain about potential breaches of the residents' ECHR rights

Facts: as a result of performance-related concerns, Caerphilly terminated its framework contract with Broadway for the provision of care home places. Broadway applied for a judicial review, on the ground that Caerphilly's decision amounted to a decision to close its care home, and so it was unlawful in public law because of a lack of prior consultation with residents and because Caerphilly failed to have regard to the welfare of residents and, also because it was in breach of the residents' rights under Article 8 ECHR and Broadway's rights under Article 1 of the 1st Protocol ECHR.

Judgment: Deputy High Court Judge Seys Llewellyn dismissed the application, holding that Caerphilly was not amenable to judicial review because it had exercised a contractual power, that Braodway did not have standing to complain about potential breaches of residents' ECHR rights, that

34 *Jain v United Kingdom* (2010) Application no 39598/09.

Article 1 of the 1st Protocol ECHR was not engaged because Caerphilly had not resolved to close Broadway's care home and that, in any event, Broadway's claims were not well-founded factually.

29.37A *Old Co-operative Day Nursery Ltd v H M Chief Inspector of Education, Children's Services & Skills* [2016] EWHC 1126 (Admin)

The Chief Inspector of Education, Children's Services & Skills had no jurisdiction to investigate a complaint made by a member of the public and his investigation had in any event been irrational

Facts: the HM Chief Inspector of Education, Children's Services and Skills had investigated a complaint by a member of the public about inadequate care provided by the Old Co-operative Day Nursery, had found that inadequate care had been provided and had published a report to that effect on its website, criticising the standards of care provided by Old Co-operative Day Nursery.

Judgment: Coulson J held that (i) the HM Chief Inspector of Education, Children's Services and Skills had not had any jurisdiction to enquire into a complaint by a member of the public; (ii) its investigation and report had been so flawed as to be irrational; (iii) it had also been unlawful to disregard earlier reports and take into account Old Co-operative Day Nursery's history of excellence; but (iv) there had been no evidence of damage or loss warranting an award of financial compensation.

Professional cases

29.38 *R (Raines) v Orange Grove* [2006] EWHC 1887 (Admin), (2006) 9 CCLR 541

A decision to deregister a foster carer had been taken in a procedurally unfair manner and was Wednesbury unreasonable

Facts: After a severely disabled boy sustained an injury after a foster placement with Mrs Raines, the fostering panel recommended that she and her husband undergo further training. However, the defendant's director wrote to the panel recommending that Mrs Raines be de-registered and informed Mrs Raines that that was his recommendation. The panel met again and following representations by Mrs Raines decided to de-register Mrs Raines, although some members considered that she was being scapegoated.

Judgment: the director and decision-maker had been required to communicate the original panel's decision to Mrs Raines with his reasons for diverging from it, which he had failed to do and, in fact, he had not had a good reason for his divergence. Further, both he and the subsequent panel had relied on matters which, unfairly, had not been put to Mrs Raines for comment. A decision of this sort was not simply that of a private company dispensing with an independent contractor but a decision that would have to be disclosed to any other foster agency and would amount to a serious blot on Mrs Raines' career as a foster carer. The decision to de-register Mrs Raines was procedurally unfair and, also, *Wednesbury* unreasonable.

29.39 ***Joyce v Secretary of State for Health*** **[2008] EWHC 1891 (Admin), (2008) 11 CCLR 761**

The tribunal may consider allegations not included in the initial reference to the Secretary of State

Facts: Ms Joyce was dismissed from her employment in a care home after having been found sleeping on duty and, on that basis, the Secretary of State included her on the Protection of Vulnerable Adults (POVA) list. Ms Joyce appealed to the Care Standards Tribunal and the Secretary of State sought to rely on additional matters before the Tribunal, as evidence of Ms Joyce's misconduct, gleaned from documents sent by Ms Joyce's former employer, when he had referred her to the Secretary of State for sleeping on duty. The Tribunal held that it could take such matters into account and Ms Joyce appealed that holding.

Judgment: Goldring J dismissed the appeal holding that the Secretary of State had no control over the reference to him by the provider and it was only when the Secretary of State prepared the appeal that further issues might become apparent. It was well within the statutory language for the Secretary of State to raise such further matters and for the Tribunal to determine them and a narrower approach would contradict the protective purpose of the machinery.

29.40 ***Wright and others v Secretary of State for Health*** **[2009] UKHL 3, (2009) 12 CCLR 181**

The absence of any opportunity to make representations before being included in the POVA list breached the ECHR

Facts: when the Secretary of State invited provisionally included a person on the Protection of Vulnerable Adults list, maintained under the Care Standards Act 2000, provisional inclusion on the list immediately disqualified such persons from being employed in any caring capacity. It then took a considerable period of time to be able to challenge inclusion on the list.

Judgment: the House of Lords (Lords Phillips, Hoffman, Hope, Baroness Hale and Lord Brown) held that the scheme was incompatible with Articles 6 and 8 ECHR in that it did not begin fairly by entitling the person concerned to make representations before his provisional inclusion on the POVA list. Lady Hale said this:

> 28. However, in my view, Dyson LJ was entirely correct in his conclusion that the scheme as enacted in the Care Standards Act 2000 does not comply with Article 6(1), for the reasons he gave. The process does not begin fairly, by offering the care worker an opportunity to answer the allegations made against her, before imposing upon her possibly irreparable damage to her employment or prospects of employment.
>
> ...
>
> 39. However, I would not make any attempt to suggest ways in which the scheme could be made compatible. There are two reasons for this. First, the incompatibility arises from the interaction between the three elements of the scheme – the procedure, the criterion and the consequences. It is not for us to attempt to rewrite the legislation. There is, as I have already said, a delicate balance to be struck between protecting the rights of the care

workers and protecting the welfare, as well as the rights, of the vulnerable people with whom they work. It is right that that balance be struck in the first instance by the legislature. Secondly, both the Care Standards Act 2000 and the Protection of Children Act 1999 will in due course be replaced by a completely different scheme laid down by and under the Safeguarding Vulnerable Groups Act 2006. While we have been informed of its existence, we have not heard argument upon whether or not that scheme is compatible with the Convention rights as the question does not arise on these appeals. Nothing which I have said in this opinion is intended to cast any light upon that question.

29.41 *Southall v General Medical Council* [2010] EWCA Civ 407, [2010] 2 FCR 77

In simple cases the GMC need only set out what facts it had found proven but in more complex cases, it had to give sufficient reasons why it accepted some evidence but rejected other evidence

Facts: the GMC found that Mr Southall, a consultant paediatrician, was guilty of serious professional misconduct where it was alleged, by a mother, that he had accused her during an interview of drugging and murdering one of her children. Mr Southall's case was that he understood why the mother had formed this impression, but that he had not in fact made this accusation. His case was supported by the evidence of a social worker, who was present at the time. It was not clear from its determination why the GMC accepted the mother's allegation and rejected Mr Southall's explanation and the social worker's evidence.

Judgment: the Court of Appeal (Waller, Dyson and Leveson LJJ) held that whilst, in straightforward cases, setting out the facts to be proved and finding them proved or not proved would generally be sufficient in that it would be obvious whose evidence had been rejected and why. However, when the case was not straightforward more detailed reasons were required. In this case, the issue was more complex than a simple issue of fact and whilst a lengthy judgment was not needed, a few sentences dealing with the salient issues were essential. The panel's reasons were inadequate, and did not address some key evidential issues, including Mr Southall's credibility, and the panel's rejection of the social worker's evidence. Moreover, the panel seemed to have been extremely concerned about Mr Southall's belief that the circumstances of the older boy's death needed to be investigated by him; that concern might have informed their approach to the factual dispute. Yet such an approach was not based on evidence and they were not entitled to form a view about it. Further, the panel had not been entitled to consider the extent to which the social worker could be said to be independent of Mr Southall.

29.42 *Bonhoeffer v General Medical Council* [2011] EWHC 1585 (Admin), [2011] ACD 104

In disciplinary proceedings raising serious charges amounting to criminal offences likely if proven to have grave consequences for the accused, there would need to be compelling reasons to prevent him from cross-examining a witness whose evidence was critical to establishing the charges, if there were no problems associated with securing the attendance of that witness

Facts: Mr Bonhoeffer applied for judicial review of a decision by the GMC to admit hearsay evidence in disciplinary proceedings against him, to prove that he sexually abused a number of boys while working in Kenya in the 1990s, a charge he denied. Most of the evidence against him came from one man, who lived in Kenya but was willing to travel to the United Kingdom to give evidence. However, the GMC decided not to call him, applying instead to adduce his hearsay evidence on the basis that were he to give oral evidence he would be exposed to a risk of harm, in the form of the threat of reprisals from homophobic elements and from those allegedly loyal to Mr Bonhoeffer.

Judgment: the Divisional Court (Laws LJ and Stadlen J) allowed the application for judicial review. There was no general rule, whether under Article 6 ECHR, or in common law, entitling a person facing disciplinary proceedings to cross-examine a witness. Whether fairness required a person in Mr Bonhoeffer's position to be permitted to cross-examine the witness depended on all the circumstances, in particular the nature of the subject-matter of the proceedings: see, inter alia, *Bushell v Secretary of State for the Environment.*[35] The ultimate question was what protections were required for a fair trial. The more serious the allegation, the more astute the courts had to be to ensure a fair trial. In disciplinary proceedings raising serious charges amounting to criminal offences which, if proved, were likely to have grave adverse effects for the accused, there would need to be compelling reasons to prevent him from cross-examining a witness whose evidence was critical to establishing the charges, if there were no problems associated with securing the attendance of that witness. In this case, the GMC had not found that it was satisfied that the threat to the witness would be greater if he gave oral testimony than if his statements were read and no reasonable panel could reasonably have concluded that there were factors outweighing the powerful factors pointing against the admission of the hearsay evidence.

29.43 *Perry v Nursing and Midwifery Council* [2013] EWCA Civ 145, [2013] 1 WLR 3423

The NMC was entitled to make an interim order against a nurse without hearing evidence from the nurse as to whether the allegations against them were well-founded; its role at that stage was not to decide the credibility or merit of allegations but to decide whether they justified making an interim order

Facts: Mr Perry was summarily dismissed when a client made allegations that he had had an inappropriate and sexualised relationship with her and the NMC then made an interim order suspending his registration for 18 months. At the hearing, the committee allowed Mr Perry to give evidence on what he admitted and denied, and indicated that it would hear evidence that suggested that the allegations were clearly unfounded or malicious, but prevented Mr Perry's legal representative from exploring the allegations with him in evidence. Mr Perry submitted that fairness dictated that he was given an opportunity to give evidence to address the substance of the allegations against him, and that the committee had, in preventing

35 [1981] AC 75.

him from doing so, breached his rights under Articles 6 and 8 ECHR, and that the hearing had failed to comply with the common law requirements of fairness.

Judgment: the Court of Appeal (Hughes and Davis LJJ and Sir Stanley Burnton) dismissed the appeal, holding that in deciding whether an interim order was necessary for protection of the public or otherwise in the public interest the NMC had to permit both parties to make submissions on the need for an interim order, which involved considering the nature of the evidence on which the allegation was based. It was entitled to discount evidence that was inconsistent with objective or undisputed evidence or which was unreliable. It could also receive evidence on the effect of an order on a registrant, and a registrant was entitled to give evidence on that. A registrant could also give evidence to establish that the allegation was unfounded or exaggerated, but the committee was not required to hear evidence as to whether a substantive allegation was well-founded. It could not decide the credibility or merit of a disputed allegation; that was a matter for the panel at the substantive hearing. Fairness did not require that a registrant subject to an allegation of unfitness to practice be given an opportunity to give evidence on the substance of that allegation before the committee considered whether to make an interim suspension order: *R (Wright) v Secretary of State for Health*.[36] The NMC's approach was compatible with the common law and the Convention rights of registrants.

29.44 *Obukofe v General Medical Council* [2014] EWHC 408 (Admin)

In appeals relating to fitness to practise and any sanction imposed, the court will accord considerable weight to the conclusions of the professional regulatory body and will bear in mind that its primary function is the protection of the public

Facts: Dr Obukofe appealed under section 40 of the Medical Act 1983 against a decision on 18 April 2013 that his fitness to practice was impaired, and a decision on 20 June 2013 to impose a sanction of 12 months' suspension with a review at the end of that period. The decisions were made by a Fitness to Practice Panel of the General Medical Council.

Judgment: Popplewell J dismissed the appeal, citing some of the leading relevant authorities, as follows:

> **Impairment**
>
> 40. The first argument I shall address under this heading is that set out in ground 3 of the grounds of appeal, which is that the 2013 Panel was wrong to make another finding of impairment because Dr Obukofe had complied with and evidenced the concerns raised by the 2012 Panel.
>
> ...
>
> 43 ... Although an appeal under section 40 is by way of re-hearing there are three reasons why the court may be slow to interfere with such a finding. Those reasons were identified by Auld LJ in *Meadow v GMC* [2006] EWCA Civ 1390 [2007] 1 QB 462:
>
> > '197. On an appeal from a determination by the GMC, acting formerly and in this case through the FPP, or now under the new statutory regime, whatever label is given to the section 40 test, it is plain from the

36 [2009] UKHL 3, [2009] 1 AC 739.

authorities that the court must have in mind and give such weight as is appropriate in the circumstances to the following factors:

I) The body from whom the appeal lies is a specialist tribunal whose understanding of what the medical profession expects of its members in matters of medical practice deserve respect;

II) The tribunal had the benefit, which the Court normally does not, of hearing and seeing the witnesses on both sides;

III) The questions of primary and secondary fact and the over-all value judgement to be made by tribunal, especially the last, are akin to jury questions to which there may reasonably be different answers.'

44. Each of those factors is relevant in the present case

...

Sanction

...

50. The next point taken is that the suspension imposed was a disproportionate sanction.

...

51. It is important to keep in mind for this purpose the two strands in the authorities which were emphasised by Laws LJ in *Rashid v General Medical Council, Fatani v GMC* [2007] 1 WLR 1460 at paragraphs 16 to 20. The first strand is to differentiate the function of a Panel imposing sanctions from that of a court imposing retributive punishment. In that respect, Laws LJ quoted from the judgment of Lord Roger in *Gupta v General Medical Council (GMC)* [2001] UKPC 61 the passage at paragraph 21, as follows:

> 'It has frequently been observed that, where professional discipline is at stake, the relevant committee is not concerned exclusively, or even primarily, with the punishment of the practitioner concerned. Their Lordships refer, for instance, to the judgment of Sir Thomas Bingham MR in *Bolton v Law Society* [1994] 1 WLR 512, 517H–519E where his Lordship set out the general approach that has to be adopted. In particular he pointed out that, since the professional body is not primarily concerned with matters of punishment, considerations which would normally weigh in mitigation of punishment have less effect on the exercise of this kind of jurisdiction. And he observed that it can never be an objection to an order for suspension that the practitioner may be unable to re-establish his practice when the period has passed. That consequence may be deeply unfortunate for the individual concerned but it does not make the order for suspension wrong if it is otherwise right.'

52. The second strand is to emphasise the special expertise of the Panel or the committee in making the required judgment. In that respect, Laws LJ in *Rashid* quoted from the speech of Lord Hope in *Marinovich v General Medical Council* [2002] UKPC 36, giving the judgment of the Board of the Privy Council, where he said at paragraphs 28:

> 'In the appellant's case, the effect of the committee's order is that erasure is for life but it has been said many times that the Professional Conduct Committee is the body which is best equipped to determine questions as to the sanction that should be opposed in the public interest for serious professional misconduct assessment.
>
> This is because the assessment of the seriousness of misconduct is essentially a matter for the committee in the light of its experience. It is the body which is best qualified to judge what measures are required to maintain the standards and reputation of the profession.'

53. In the light of those two strands Laws LJ continued at paragraph 24 of the judgment in *Rashid* to say at paragraph 20:

> 'These strands in the learning then as it seems to me constitute the essential approach to be applied by the High Court on a section 40 appeal. The approach they commend does not emasculate the High Court's role in section 40 appeals. The High Court will correct material errors of fact and of course of law and it will exercise a judgment, though distinctly and firmly a secondary judgment, as to the application of the principles to the facts of the case.'

54. Bearing in mind those two strands and applying a judgment which is distinctly and firmly a secondary judgment I see no basis for treating the sanction which was imposed by the 2013 Panel as being in any way unfair or disproportionate notwithstanding the effect which it has on the ability of Dr Obukofe to earn his living ...

29.44A *R (SPP Health Ltd) v Care Quality Commission* [2016] EWHC 2086 (Admin)

Fairness required the CQC to provide an independent review where a provider claimed that factual findings in a draft report were demonstrably wrong or misleading but the inspection team refused to vary the draft report

Facts: the CQC inspected one of the GP practices operated by the claimant and then declined to correct factual inaccuracies in its draft report or vary its overall rating of that GP practice as 'inadequate'. Under the CQC's published procedures, providers could challenge the proposed rating and the factual accuracy of the findings on which it was based before publication and, after publication, could request a review of the rating only on the basis that CQC had not followed the process set out in its 'provider handbook'.

Judgment: Andrews J held that, on the particular facts, it had been *Wednesbury* unreasonable for the CQC not to revise its draft report, given that the claimant had provided evidence that demonstrated that aspects of that draft report were factually inaccurate. More widely, Andrews J held that fairness required the CQC to revise its procedures so as to provide a swift, fair and effective process whereby a provider could challenge a refusal to vary a draft report, on the ground that one or more of its factual findings was demonstrably wrong or misleading, involving an independent review.

Confidential information cases

29.45 *R v Somerset CC ex p Prospects Care Services* (1999) 2 CCLR 161, QBD

It was lawful for a local authority to provide information about a fostering agency casting doubt on its competence where it adopted a fair and rational procedure and where the information was fair and rational

Facts: After consulting with it and taking into account its views, Somerset drew up a standard document about Prospects, a private fostering agency, to send to other local authorities that made enquiries about

Prospects. Prospects complained that Somerset had no power to publish such a document and that its contents were so unfair as to be *Wednesbury* unreasonable.

Judgment: Dyson J held that local authorities had power under section 27 of the Children Act 1989 to provide information to other local authorities about fostering agencies and, in this case, bearing in mind the public importance of a free flow of information relating to concerns about the care of children, the procedure had been fair and rational and the content of what had been communicated was neither unfair nor irrational.

29.46 *R v Chief Constable of Wales ex p AB* (2000) 3 CCLR 25, DC

Providing they act fairly, by giving those affected the opportunity of comment, the police are entitled to disclose information about individuals to third parties where that is justified in the public interest

Facts: the applicants had been convicted of serious sexual offences against children and, having been unable to find anywhere safe to live, bought a caravan and moved to a site in North Wales. The Chief Constable was concerned about the potential risk to children who might stay at the caravan site during the Easter holidays and disclosed press Articles to the site owner, who then required the applicants to leave, which they did. They then sought a judicial review of the Chief Constable's decision.

Judgment: The Divisional Court (Lord Bingham LCJ and Buxton J) held that the Chief Constable should have made his policy public, but it was a lawful policy that permitted disclosure only to responsible persons and where there was a cogent public interest justification although, unlawfully, the Chief Constable failed to act fairly by giving the applicants the opportunity to make representations about the level of risk they posed: however, in this case, that failure made no difference to the outcome.

29.47 *R v Secretary of State for Health ex p C* (2000) 3 CCLR 412, CA

It had been lawful to maintain the Consultancy Service index

Facts: C had been dismissed by Kent CC as a child care worker, on the basis of allegations of sexual abuse of children, which Kent CC found proven but which C continued to contest. Kent referred C to the Secretary of State, who included C's name on his Consultancy Service Index. The Index could be checked by prospective employers. The reason for a person's inclusion on the Index was not disclosed but it enabled a prospective employer to contact the previous employer (whose name was also included on the Index) for a reference.

Judgment: the Court of Appeal (Lord Woolf MR, Hale LJ and Lord Mustill) held that the Crown had the same liberties as an individual citizen and was entitled to maintain the Consultancy Service Index although, being a public authority, it had to act rationally, in good faith and on lawful and relevant grounds of public interest and it had to balance the competing interests of an individual's privacy and reputation and the need to protect children. In principle, the Index was lawful in public law and compatible with the ECHR.

29.48 ## *R (S) v Plymouth CC* [2002] EWCA Civ 388, (2002) 5 CCLR 251

Fairness and the ECHR required disclosure of the son's mental health records to his mother, in nearest relative displacement proceedings

Facts: C suffered from a mental disorder and mental impairment. His mother, who was his nearest relative, opposed his being made subject to a guardianship order but, despite requests by her, she had not been shown the material on which that proposed application would be based, on the ground that it was confidential and C lacked capacity to consent to its disclosure to his mother.

Judgment: the Court of Appeal (Kennedy (dissenting in part), Clarke and Hale LJJ) held that such material would have to be disclosed in any proceedings to displace the nearest relative and that such proceedings were likely if the mother continued to object. For that reason, and because of the importance under the ECHR of involving the mother, disclosure would be ordered – not just to the mother's lawyers and expert, but also (Kennedy LJ dissenting) to the mother personally. Hale LJ said this:

> 48. Hence both the common law and the Convention require that a balance be struck between the various interests involved. These are the confidentiality of the information sought; the proper administration of justice; the mother's right of access to legal advice to enable her to decide whether or not to exercise a right which is likely to lead to legal proceedings against her if she does so; the rights of both C and his mother to respect for their family life and adequate involvement in decision-making processes about it; C's right to respect for his private life; and the protection of C's health and welfare. In some cases there might also be an interest in the protection of other people, but that has not been seriously suggested here.
>
> 49. C's interest in protecting the confidentiality of personal information about himself must not be underestimated. It is all too easy for professionals and parents to regard children and incapacitated adults as having no independent interests of their own: as objects rather than subjects. But we are not concerned here with the publication of information to the whole wide world. There is a clear distinction between disclosure to the media with a view to publication to all and sundry and disclosure in confidence to those with a proper interest in having the information in question. We are concerned here only with the latter. The issue is only whether the circle should be widened from those professionals with whom this information has already been shared (possibly without much conscious thought being given to the balance of interests involved) to include the person who is probably closest to him in fact as well as in law and who has a statutory role in his future and to those professionally advising her. C also has an interest in having his own wishes and feelings respected. It would be different in this case if he had the capacity to give or withhold consent to the disclosure: any objection from him would have to be weighed in the balance against the other interests, although as *W v Egdell* [1990] Ch 359 shows, it would not be decisive. C also has an interest in being protected from a risk of harm to his health or welfare which would stem from disclosure; but it is important not to confuse a possible risk of harm to his health or welfare from being discharged from guardianship with a possible risk of harm from disclosing the information sought. As *In re D (Minors) (Adoption Reports: Confidentiality)* [1996] AC 593 shows, he also has an interest in decisions about his future being properly informed.

50. That balance would not lead in every case to the disclosure of all the information a relative might possibly want, still less to a fishing exercise amongst the local authority's files. But in most cases it would lead to the disclosure of the basic statutory guardianship documentation. In this case it must also lead to the particular disclosure sought. There is no suggestion that C has any objection to his mother and her advisers being properly informed about his health and welfare. There is no suggestion of any risk to his health and welfare arising from this. The mother and her advisers have sought access to the information which her own psychiatric and social work experts need in order properly to advise her. That limits both the context and the content of disclosure in a way which strikes a proper balance between the competing interests.

29.49 *MG v United Kingdom* (2002) 5 CCLR 525, ECtHR

Adults who were in local authority care as children are entitled to at least some level of access to their social services records

Facts: MG sought disclosure of his social services records, relating to his time in care as a child but the local authority refused disclosure.

Judgment: The absence of any right of access to his social services records, and no right of appeal to an independent body, during the period before the Data Protection Act 1995 came into force, was in breach of MG's rights to respect for his private life Article 8 ECHR.

Comment: there are now rights of access to social services records under the Data Protection Act 1998: for a useful guide, see the *Subject Access Code of Practice: Dealing with requests from individuals for personal information.*[37]

29.50 *R (A) v National Probation Service* [2003] EWHC 2910 (Admin), (2004) 7 CCLR 336

The disclosure of confidential information was unlawful when there had not been consideration of the need for a pressing justification or a balancing exercise

Facts: A, who was 70, had been convicted of the murder of his wife and, on release, purchased a dwelling in a sheltered housing scheme. At the time of his trial, a report prepared for the CPS indicated that A was unlikely to re-offend and the Parole Board recommended his release on the expiry of his tariff. The probation service took the view that A's prospective accommodation was only suitable if the fact of his conviction was made known to the accommodation manager.

Judgment: Beatson J quashed this decision: the probation service was entitled to reach its own assessment of risk and how to manage it and, despite the difficulties of making disclosure to a person who was not a public body, and constrained by public law duties, was able to disclose information on a confidential basis, in the knowledge that obligations of confidentiality were enforced by the courts. However, its risk assessment had failed to start from the correct starting point, under the MAPPA guidelines, that there had to be a pressing need for disclosure, and it had failed to balance the need for disclosure against the potential harm to the claimant.

37 https://ico.org.uk/media/for-organisations/documents/1065/subject-access-code-of-practice.pdf.

29.51 *A Local Authority v A Health Authority and Mrs A* [2004] EWHC 2746 Fam, (2004) 7 CCLR 426

Publication of a report into poor foster care would be too harmful to the children and vulnerable adults concerned

Facts: over a number of years, Mrs A had fostered a number of highly vulnerable children. Concerns about Mrs A resulted in the Area Child Protection Committee setting up a panel of inquiry which produced a report and, also, care proceedings which resulted in an anonymised but public judgment. The local authority sought the court's permission to publish the report.

Judgment: The President of the Family Division refused permission, on the basis of the court's inherent jurisdiction to protect children and vulnerable adults from harmful publicity. Although starting from the position that there was a right to publish, in the absence of good reason, the concern was that, in this case, publication would be so harmful to the children and vulnerable adults that publication should be restrained by the grant of an indefinite injunction.

29.52 *Brent LBC v N and P* [2005] EWHC 1676 Fam, (2006) 9 CCLR 14

Disclosure of a foster-carer's HIV status to the children's father was unjustified where the risks to the children were negligible and the disclosure opposed

Facts: Brent had placed P, who was two, with foster carers, Mr and Mrs N, but were about to place her with her father, Mr S. An issue arose, as to whether Brent could/should disclose to S that Mr N was HIV+. Mr N objected to the disclosure. Medical evidence was obtained that demonstrated that any risk to P was negligible.

Judgment: Sumner J held that serious reasons were required to justify the disclosure of a person's medical condition and such reasons did not exist in this case where the risk to the children was negligible and disclosure was opposed.

29.53 *Roberts v Nottinghamshire Healthcare NHS Trust* [2008] EWHC 1934 (Admin), (2009) 12 CCLR 110

Disclosure of health records and reports could be refused where it might well cause damage to health

Facts: the claimant was detained at Rampton Hospital under sections 37 and 41 of the Mental Health Act 1983 and sought disclosure of a psychologist's report. The Trust did not intend to rely on this report in any tribunal proceedings and refused to disclose it to the claimant, or to give reasons why not. The claimant applied for disclosure under section 7(9) of the Data Protection Act 1998. A special advocate was appointed to read the report and make submissions on the claimant's behalf.

Judgment: Cranston J delivered a closed and an open judgment, refusing disclosure of the report. Under the Data Protection (Subject Access Modification) (Health) Order 2000 disclosure could be refused where there might well be a risk of harm to health falling short of a probability, whether that was the subject's health, or that of others. In this case, that risk was well-established, for reasons given in the closed judgment.

29.54 *R (L) v Metropolitan Police Commissioner* [2009] UKSC 3, (2009) 12 CCLR 573

The police may disclose personal information to an employer about a person who proposes to work with children or vulnerable adults when it is proportionate to do so

Facts: L was a midday assistant at a school but when the school obtained an enhanced criminal record certificate (ECRC) it showed that earlier L's 13-year-old son had been placed on the at-risk register under the neglect category and that there were allegations that L had failed to exercise proper care and supervision and refused to co-operate with social services. Shortly after that, L lost her job. She sought a judicial review of the Commissioner's decision to disclose her ECRC and his refusal to remove this information from it.

Judgment: the Supreme Court (Justices Hope, Saville, Scott, Brown and Neuberger) held that the provision of information in an ECRC could interfere with a person's rights under Article 8 ECHR, but could be justified: the question was, whether the disclosure was proportionate in all the circumstances, weighing in particular the pressing social need for children and vulnerable adults to be protected against the risk of harm against an applicant's right to respect for their private life. Neither consideration took precedence over the other, there were no presumptions and in cases of doubt the chief police officer should permit the applicant to make representations. In this particular case, the information about L was undoubtedly true and bore directly on whether she could safely be entrusted with supervising children, so its disclosure was proportionate.

Lord Hope said this:

> 42. So the issue is essentially one of proportionality. On the one hand there is a pressing social need that children and vulnerable adults should be protected against the risk of harm. On the other there is the applicant's right to respect for her private life. It is of the greatest importance that the balance between these two considerations is struck in the right place ... Increasing use of this procedure, and the effects of the release of sensitive information of this kind on the applicants' opportunities for employment or engaging in unpaid work in the community and their ability to establish and develop relations with others, is a cause of very real public concern as the written intervention submitted by Liberty indicates.
>
> 44. In my opinion the effect of the approach that was taken to this issue in *R (X) v Chief Constable of the West Midlands Police* has been to tilt the balance against the applicant too far. It has encouraged the idea that priority must be given to the social need to protect the vulnerable as against the right to respect for private life of the applicant ...
>
> 45. The correct approach, as in other cases where competing Convention rights are in issue, is that neither consideration has precedence over the other: *Campbell v MGN Ltd* [2004] 2 AC 457, para 12, per Lord Nicholls of Birkenhead ... careful consideration is required in all cases where the disruption to the private life of anyone is judged to be as great, or more so, as the risk of non-disclosure to the vulnerable group. The advice that, where

careful consideration is required, the rationale for disclosure should make it very clear why the human rights infringement outweighs the risk posed to the vulnerable group also needs to be reworded. It should no longer be assumed that the presumption is for disclosure unless there is a good reason for not doing so.

46. In cases of doubt, especially where it is unclear whether the position for which the applicant is applying really does require the disclosure of sensitive information, where there is room for doubt as to whether an allegation of a sensitive kind could be substantiated or where the information may indicate a state of affairs that is out of date or no longer true, chief constables should offer the applicant an opportunity of making representations before the information is released. In *R (X) v Chief Constable of the West Midlands Police* [2005] 1 WLR 65, para 37 Lord Woolf CJ rejected Wall J's suggestion that this should be done on the ground that this would impose too heavy an obligation on the chief constable. Here too I think, with respect, that he got the balance wrong. But it will not be necessary for this procedure to be undertaken in every case. It should only be resorted to where there is room for doubt as to whether there should be disclosure of information that is considered to be relevant. The risks in such cases of causing disproportionate harm to the applicant outweigh the inconvenience to the chief constable.

Lord Neuberger said this:

81. Having decided that information might be relevant under section 115(7)(a), the chief officer then has to decide under section 115(7)(b) whether it ought to be included, and, in making that decision, there will often be a number of different, sometimes competing, factors to weigh up. Examples of factors which could often be relevant are the gravity of the material involved, the reliability of the information on which it is based, whether the applicant has had a chance to rebut the information, the relevance of the material to the particular job application, the period that has elapsed since the relevant events occurred, and the impact on the applicant of including the material in the ECRC, both in terms of her prospects of obtaining the post in question and more generally. In many cases, other factors may also come into play, and in other cases, it may be unnecessary or inappropriate to consider one or more of the factors I have mentioned. Thus, the material may be so obviously reliable, relevant and grave as to be disclosable however detrimental the consequential effect on the applicant.

29.55 *Chief Constable of Humberside Police v Information Commissioner* [2009] EWCA Civ 1079, [2010] 1 WLR 1136

It was lawful for chief constables indefinitely to retain information about convictions and cautions (spent or not)

Facts: five individuals complained about the retention on the police national computer of details of their minor convictions over 20 years old and in one case a reprimand over five years old. The police agreed to 'step down' these details, so that only the police had access to them, but did not agree to delete them.

Judgment: the Court of Appeal (Waller, Carnwath and Hughes LJJ) held that the police were required by statute to be able to inform the CPS, the courts and the CRB of all offences, spent and otherwise; accordingly it was lawful to maintain these records under the Data Protection Act 1998.

Comment: as a result of this decision, the police abandoned their practice of 'stepping down'.

29.56 *R (F (A child)) v Secretary of State for Justice* [2010] UKSC 17, [2011] 1 AC 331

It was incompatible with Article 8 ECHR to impose indefinite requirements on sexual offenders that did not include any possibility of review

Facts: two claimants complained that, as a result of their having committed serious sexual offences, there were required indefinitely to comply with certain notification requirements under the Sexual Offences Act 2003, without limit of time and without the possibility of review.

Judgment: the Supreme Court (Phillips, Hope, Rodger, Hale and Clarke JJSC) held that the indefinite notification requirements amounted to a disproportionate interference with Article 8 rights because they included no provision for individual review whereby an individual might demonstrate that they no longer posed any significant risk.

29.57 *H and L v A City Council* [2011] EWCA Civ 403, (2011) 14 CCLR 381

It had been disproportionate to disclosure child sexual offences to organisations where the persons worked which were not involved with children and to personal assistants who were not allowed to bring children with them and the process had been unfair

Facts: H was disabled, and active in the disability rights movement. He had also been convicted of a sexual assault on a child, and also for failing to disclose that conviction when applying for a job; additionally he faced trial for a further sexual assault. The Council was alerted to these facts and, after a meeting with H and his solicitors (i) informed nine organisations with which H had connections of his convictions and the potential for further convictions, (ii) decided that H's personal disability assistants should be informed and should agree not to allow H unsupervised contact with children and that although H received direct payments, the assistants should be paid through a managed account.

Judgment: the Court of Appeal (Pill, Hooper and Munby LJJ) held that the Council had acted unfairly and disproportionately, in that it had adopted a blanket approach rather than asking whether there had been a pressing need for disclosure. The court had to apply an intense scrutiny and form its own conclusion. In this case, H and L were not involved in groups working with children unlawfully so that disclosure to those groups was disproportionate and, since H and L's personal assistants were contractually prohibited from bringing children to work, disclosure to them was also unnecessary and disproportionate. In addition, the process had been unfair in that H and L had not been afforded the opportunity of comment before the disclosures had been made. Munby LJ said this:

> *Disclosure: the law*
>
> 36. The first has to do with the respective functions of the local authority and the court and, in particular, the legal tests each had to apply. In relation to this Judge Langan fell into what I have to say was serious error.

37. The task for the local authority was, putting the matter shortly, to apply the principles to be found in *R v Chief Constable of the North Wales Police ex p Thorpe* [1999] QB 396 as adjusted by the re-calibration of the 'balancing exercise' undertaken in *R (L) v Commissioner of Police of the Metropolis (Secretary of State for the Home Department intervening)* [2009] UHSC 3, [2010] 1 AC 410. The latter case, although decided in relation to the statutory scheme under section 115 of the Police Act 1997, is, in my judgment, equally applicable in the present non-statutory context. As the authorities show, each case must be judged on its own facts. The issue is essentially one of proportionality. Information such as that with which we are here concerned is to be disclosed only if there is a 'pressing need' for that disclosure. There is no difference in this context between the common law test and the approach mandated by Article 8. The outcome is the same under both.

38. In considering proportionality the general principles are, as Mr Cragg submits, those to be extracted from the well-known passage in the speech of Lord Bingham of Cornhill in *Huang v Secretary of State for the Home Department, Kashmiri v Same* [2007] UKHL 11, [2007] 2 AC 167, para [19]: (i) the legitimate aim in question must be sufficiently important to justify the interference, (ii) the measures taken to achieve the legitimate aim must be rationally connected to it, (iii) the means used to impair the right must be no more than is necessary to accomplish the objective, and (iv) a fair balance must be struck between the rights of the individual and the interests of the community; this requires a careful assessment of the severity and consequences of the interference.

39. Prior to the decision of the Supreme Court in *L*, the effect of the decision of this court in *R (X) v Chief Constable of the West Midlands Police* [2004] EWCA Civ 1068, [2005] 1 WLR 65, had been to tilt the balance in favour of disclosure. As Lord Hope of Craighead put it in *L* at para [38], the effect of the approach in *X* was to encourage disclosure of any information that might be relevant, and to give priority to the social need that favours disclosure over respect for the private life of those who may be affected by the disclosure. He said (para [44]) that the effect of this approach had been to tilt the balance too far against the person about whom disclosure was being made.

40. Explaining the proper approach, Lord Hope said (para [42]):

> 'the issue is essentially one of proportionality. On the one hand there is a pressing social need that children and vulnerable adults should be protected against the risk of harm. On the other there is the applicant's right to respect for her private life. It is of the greatest importance that the balance between these two considerations is struck in the right place.'

He continued (para [45]):

> 'The correct approach, as in other cases where competing Convention rights are in issue, is that neither consideration has precedence over the other ... The [approach] should be restructured so that the precedence that is given to the risk that failure to disclose would cause to the vulnerable group is removed. It should indicate that careful consideration is required in all cases where the disruption to the private life of anyone is judged to be as great, or more so, as the risk of non-disclosure to the vulnerable group. The advice that, where careful consideration is required, the rationale for disclosure should make it very clear why the human rights infringement outweighs the risk posed to the vulnerable group also needs to be reworded. It should no longer be assumed that

the presumption is for disclosure unless there is a good reason for not doing so.'

41. That was the task the local authority had to undertake here. What was the task for the judge? His task was one of review, not decision on the merits. Judge Langan seems to have thought that the appropriate standard of review here was the *Wednesbury* test of irrationality. It was not. As Mr Cragg submitted, and Mr Pitt-Payne correctly conceded, what was required in this sensitive area of human rights was the more intense standard of review described by Lord Steyn in *R (Daly) v Secretary of State for the Home Department* [2001] UKHL 26, [2001] 2 AC 532, para [27]. In a case such as this, proportionality will require the reviewing court to assess the balance which the decision maker has struck, not merely whether it is within the range of rational or reasonable decisions; this goes further than the traditional grounds of review inasmuch as it requires attention to be directed to the relative weight accorded to interests and considerations.

29.58 *MM v United Kingdom* Application no 24029/07, [2012] ECHR 1906

A disclosure regime that did not include sufficient safeguards to protect private life would be incompatible with Article 8 ECHR

Facts: MM had taken her grandson away from his parents, briefly and without harming him, in an attempt to force them to reconcile their differences. She was cautioned for child abduction. Six years later she was refused employment because the criminal records check disclosed that caution. At the time of the caution, the policy had been to weed out cautions after five years but that had changed to a policy of indefinite retention of the record.

Judgment: the European Court of Human Rights held that:

195. The court considers it essential, in the context of the recording and communication of criminal record data as in telephone tapping, secret surveillance and covert intelligence-gathering, to have clear, detailed rules governing the scope and application of measures; as well as minimum safeguards concerning, inter alia, duration, storage, usage, access of third parties, procedures for preserving the integrity and confidentiality of data and procedures for their destruction, thus providing sufficient guarantees against the risk of abuse and arbitrariness (see *S and Marper* [*v United Kingdom* [2008] ECHR 1581], and the references therein). There are various crucial stages at which data protection issues under Article 8 of the Convention may arise, including during collection, storage, use and communication of data. At each stage, appropriate and adequate safeguards which reflect the principles elaborated in applicable data protection instruments and prevent arbitrary and disproportionate interference with Article 8 rights must be in place.

...

206. In the present case, the court highlights the absence of a clear legislative framework for the collection and storage of data, and the lack of clarity as to the scope, extent and restrictions of the common law powers of the police to retain and disclose caution data. It further refers to the absence of any mechanism for independent review of a decision to retain or disclose data, either under common law police powers or pursuant to Part V of the 1997 Act. Finally, the court notes the limited filtering arrangements in respect of disclosures made under the provisions of the 1997 Act: as regards mandatory disclosure under section 113A, no distinction is made

on the basis of the nature of the offence, the disposal in the case, the time which has elapsed since the offence took place or the relevance of the data to the employment sought.

207. The cumulative effect of these shortcomings is that the court is not satisfied that there were, and are, sufficient safeguards in the system for retention and disclosure of criminal record data to ensure that data relating to the applicant's private life have not been, and will not be, disclosed in violation of her right to respect for her private life. The retention and disclosure of the applicant's caution data accordingly cannot be regarded as being in accordance with the law. There has therefore been a violation of Article 8 of the Convention in the present case. This conclusion obviates the need for the court to determine whether the interference was 'necessary in a democratic society' for one of the aims enumerated therein.

29.59 *R (A) v Chief Constable of Kent* [2013] EWCA Civ 1706, (2014) 135 BMLR 22

Court review of the proportionality of disclosure of sensitive personal information was intense but it was not a merits review and should ordinarily disregard new material

Facts: A complained that inclusion of allegations of ill-treatment and neglect of care home residents in her enhanced criminal record certificate had been disproportionate because the allegations were unreliable. The judge at first instance allowed A's application for judicial review, taking into account new material not before the police at the time.

Judgment: the Court of Appeal (Pitchford, Beatson and Gloster LJJ) held that whilst a court determining whether ECHR rights had been violated had to determine that question for itself, which included determining whether an interference with qualified rights was proportionate, that did not amount to a full-scale merits review. Accordingly, to preserve the distinction between the function of the statutory decision-maker, and that of the court, the court ought not to take into account new material, until that had been considered by the statutory decision-maker. However, even disregarding the new material in this case, the ECRC had been unlawful. Beatson LJ said this:

36. It was common ground between the parties that, where the question before a court concerns whether a decision interferes with a right under the ECHR and, if so, whether it is proportionate and therefore justified, it is necessary for the court to conduct a high-intensity review of the decision. The court must make its own assessment of the factors considered by the decision-maker. The need to do this involves considering the appropriate weight to give them and thus the relative weight accorded to the interests and considerations by the decision-maker. The scope of review thus goes further than the traditional grounds of judicial review: see eg *R (Daly) v Secretary of State for the Home Department* [2001] 2 AC 532 at [27].

37. There are also clear statements that it is the function of the court to determine whether or not a decision of a public authority is incompatible with ECHR rights. In *R (SB) v Governors of Denbigh High School* [2006] UKHL 15 at [30], Lord Bingham stated that 'proportionality must be judged objectively by the court'. See also Lord Hoffmann at [68], Lord Neuberger MR in *L's* case [2009] UKSC 3 at [74], and *Belfast City Council v Miss Behavin' Ltd* [2007] UKHL 19. In the last of these decisions Baroness Hale stated

(at [31]) that it is the court which must decide whether ECHR rights have been infringed. In *Huang v Secretary of State for the Home Department* [2007] UKHL 11 Lord Bingham also stated that the court must 'make a value judgment, an evaluation'. But he made it quite clear (at [13]) that, despite the fact that cases involving rights under the ECHR involve 'a more exacting standard of review', 'there is no shift to a merits review' and it remains the case that the judge is not the primary decision-maker. In *Axa General Insurance Ltd v HM Advocate* [2011] UKSC 46, Lord Reed (at [131]) stated that, 'although the courts must decide whether, in their judgment, the requirement of proportionality is satisfied, there is at the same time nothing in the Convention, or in the domestic legislation giving effect to Convention rights, which requires the courts to substitute their own views for those of other public authorities on all matters of policy, judgment and discretion'.

38. In *SB*'s case Lord Bingham stated (at [30]) that the evaluation of proportionality must be made by reference to the circumstances prevailing 'at the relevant time'. In these proceedings, possibly the issue between the parties with the widest implications is what his Lordship meant by 'the relevant time'. I deal with this at [67]–[92] below.

39. Much consideration has also been given to the weight it is 'appropriate' for the court to give to the judgment of the person who has been given primary responsibility for the decision. That person has, in the words of Lord Bingham in *Huang's* case at [16], been given 'responsibility for a subject-matter' and 'access to special sources of knowledge and advice'. If that person has addressed his or her mind at all to the existence of values or interests which, under the ECHR, are relevant to striking the balance, his or her views and conclusions carry some weight. But, if the primary decision-maker has not done so, or has not done so properly, his or her views are bound to carry less weight and the court has to strike the balance for itself, giving due weight to the judgments made by the primary decision-maker on such matters as he or she did consider: see *Belfast City Council v Miss Behavin' Ltd* [2007] UKHL 19 per Baroness Hale at [37] and Lord Mance at [47].

29.60 *R (L) v Chief Constable of Kent* [2014] EWHC 463 (Admin)

It was disproportionate to include in an ECRC allegations that had been rejected at a criminal trial as being manifestly unrealiable

Facts: L's sister had made serious allegations against him of sexual abuse, but the judge halted the criminal trial against L after the conclusion of the prosecution evidence, on the basis that the evidence against L had been manifestly unreliable.

Judgment: Andrews J held that it had been disproportionate of the police to include the same allegations on L's ECRC.

29.61 *R (P) v Chief Constable of Thames Valley Police* [2014] EWHC 1436 (Admin), (2014) 17 CCLR 250

In this case, it had been disproportionate to disclose inappropriate remarks made to persons who were not vulnerable adults or children

Facts: P wished to work with young adults with autism but that wish was threatened by the Chief Constable's decision to include in P's enhanced criminal record certificate information that the manager of a drugs treatment programme where P had earlier worked on an agency basis had been informed that P had made inappropriate and sexual comments about bringing alcohol to a barbecue, a particular sexual position, prostitutes and Viagra (denied by P).

Judgment: Foskett J held that including this information on the ECRC amounted to a disproportionate interference with P's rights, in that even if P had said what was alleged, he had not been talking to a child or to a vulnerable adult and there was no reason to believe that P would make similar comments to a child or a young adult with autism.

29.62 *R (T) v Chief Constable of Greater Manchester Police* [2013] EWCA Civ 25, [2013] 1 WLR 2515

A disclosure scheme had to contain adequate safeguards against arbitrariness, designed to prevent disproportionate disclosures

Facts: the claimants received warnings/cautions for minor offences of dishonesty that were, some years later, disclosed to prospective care employers.

Judgment: the Supreme Court (Neuberger, Hale, Clarke, Wilson and Reed JJSC) held that the scheme under the Police Act 1997 was unlawful because it failed to contain adequate safeguards against arbitrary interference with private life and that the disclosures in question had been disproportionate: the point at which a conviction recedes into the past and becomes part of a person's private life will usually be the point at which it becomes spent.

29.63 *R (AB) v Chief Constable of Hampshire* [2015] EWHC 1238 (Admin)

A disclosure based on inadequate investigation and incorrect information was unlawful

Facts: The teacher, AB, had been dismissed in September 2010 for gross misconduct, having made inappropriate sexual comments to female students, however, the teaching council found the incident to fall short of unacceptable professional conduct. A year later, the teacher obtained another position at a girls' school. He disclosed his previous dismissal, but explained that it had not been ratified by the teaching council. The police got to hear about the teacher's new post and, having contacted his previous school, informed the new school that he had been dismissed twice before, once for '*touching pupils and getting them to touch him*'. That was untrue. The information was communicated to the Local Authority Designated Officer, who notified the teacher's new employer, who dismissed him.

Judgment: Jeremy Baker J allowed AB's application, holding essentially that the police failed to have regard to AB's rights under Article 8 ECHR and undertake proportionate enquiries, in particular, as to what the Disclosure and Barring Service had disclosed. The police investigation into its own actions had, also, been inadequate.

29.64 *R (Catt) v Association of Chief Police Officers of England, Wales and Northern Ireland and others* [2015] UKSC 9, [2015] AC 1065

It was proportionate for the police to retain certain personal information for crime enforcement purposes

Facts: the police kept information on their database about persons who had been involved in demonstrations against a commercial arms manufacturer, although there was no evidence that such persons had acted in breach of the criminal law and the police also kept copies, for seven years, subject to review, of letters written to individuals warning them that their conduct might amount to criminal harassment.

Judgment: the Supreme Court (Neuberger, Hale, Mance, Sumption and Toulson JJSC) held that, on both cases, retention of the information was proportionate in the light of the policing objectives pursued.

29.65 *R (W) v Secretary of State for Justice* [2015] EWHC 1952 (Admin)

It was primarily for the legislature to determine the length of time which different types of offences were disclosable

Facts: W had been required to disclose a 31-year-old conviction for assault occasioning actual bodily harm committed whilst he was a juvenile for which he had received a two-year conditional discharge and been bound over to keep the peace.

Judgment: Simon J held that this offence was disclosable under the current statutory regime and that this was not disproportionate:

> 59. In the event Parliament decided to draw the line so as to exclude common assault from disclosure, despite the argument which could be made that it should be included, and to include those offences of violence which were characterised as specified violence offences in Schedule 15 for the purposes of Chapter 5 or Part 12 of the 2003 Act.
>
> 60. As the Court of Appeal in *R (SG and others) v Secretary of State for Work and Pensions* [2014] EWCA Civ 156, [2014] PTSR 619 noted at [28], it was relevant to the intensity of the court's review that the legislation in issue had been approved by affirmative resolutions of both Houses of Parliament and had been subject to vigorous debate in both Houses of Parliament; and that there are areas of governmental life in which the court should be very slow to substitute its own view for that of the legislature or executive, although this did not mean that the legislation fell outwith the court's consideration, see [27].
>
> ...
>
> 78. The assessment of the advantages and disadvantages of various legislative alternatives is primarily a matter for Parliament and the existence of alternative solutions 'does not in itself render the contested legislation unjustified'; this conclusion is appropriate only where 'it is apparent that the legislature has attached insufficient importance to a person's Convention right' (*Wilson v First County Trust Ltd (No 2)* [2004] 1 AC 816 at §70, accepted in *R (T)* in the Supreme Court at [48].

29.66 *R (SD) v Chief Constable of North Yorkshire and the Disclosure and Barring Service* [2015] EWHC 2085 (Admin)

Disclosure in an ECRC was proportionate

Facts: in 2010, SD supervised a student trip, when he was a lecturer at the college. It was alleged that he had made inappropriate comments of a sexual nature in the presence of students aged 17–24 and other adults. The college investigated at the time and members of staff and students corroborated the allegations. The matter was not however taken any further by the college (largely because SD entered into a compromise whereby his employment was terminated with a positive reference), or by the police (no criminal offence had been committed), and SD was told that he would not be on the barred list for either children or adults. In 2013, SD applied for a job that required an enhanced criminal records check. It transpired that the Chief Constable had retained references to this incident in his ECRC and that the Disclosure and Barring Service proposed to disclose its copy of the ECRC to SD's prospective employer. SD sought a judicial review.

Judgment: Deputy High Court Judge Behrens held that, although SD denied it, it was more likely than not that the events on the ECRC had occurred, that the remarks made had been seriously inappropriate, that SD had had the opportunity of making representations and that the disclosure was accurate, balanced and fair so that, overall, applying a high intensity review, the disclosure was proportionate to the legitimate aim of protecting children or vulnerable people with whom SD might work in future.

Comment: this case is summarised as an example of the straight-forward application of the principles.

29.67 *Re C (A Child)* [2015] EWFC 79

Psychiatrists were not entitled to disclosure of confidential medical records to help them rebut defamatory comments

Facts: psychiatrists, who had treated the mother, and who had provided evidence in relation to the mother and her child, in family court proceedings, had been the subject of a complaint to the GMC (not upheld) and adverse press comment, in both cases by the mother. The psychiatrists sought disclosure of documents from the family court and the GMC hearing, so that they could openly discuss their experience of the family court proceedings, and have material available should anyone question their veracity: although they would not show any documents to a third party, they did wish to be able to offer redacted quotations from the original source material.

Judgment: Sir James Munby, President of the Family Division, held that the proposed disclosure represented a massive, unjustifiable breach of confidentiality, impossible to justify by reference to any asserted public interest, even though the psychiatrists had been traduced and defamed by the mother. (Presumably, that last statement by the President would have, however, greatly assisted the psychiatrists restore any diminution of their reputation).

29.68 *R (P) v Secretary of State for Justice* [2016] EWHC 89 Admin, [2016] 1 WLR 2009

Article 8 required there to be a mechanism for testing the proportionality of disclosure in individual cases

Facts: the claimants had been convicted of two relatively minor offences some years before that stood to be disclosed to employers under the Police Act 1997.

Judgment: the Divisional Court held that even as amended the Police Act 1997 was incompatible with Article 8 ECHR insofar as it contained no machinery for testing the proportionality of disclosure in individual cases and that, in these cases, disclosure would be disproportionate.

29.69 *R (MS) v Independent Monitor of the Home Office* [2016] EWHC 655 (Admin), [2016] 4 WLR 88

The Independent Monitor was required to scrutinise with a high degree of forensic care the credibility of allegations before assessing its weight and conducting the necessary disclosure balancing exercise

Facts: MS sought to return to work as a taxi driver and was dissatisfied with the proposal of the police to disclose information concerning a number of historic and unsubstantiated allegations against him of indecency towards females. The Independent Monitor upheld the police's approach.

Judgment: HHJ Blair QC, sitting as a Deputy High Court Judge, held that where the credibility of the allegations was in issue the Independent Monitor was not automatically to give considerable weight to the police view. Whilst the Independent Monitor was not required to conduct a comprehensive investigation, he was obliged to scrutinise with a high degree of forensic care the material said to incriminate the claimant and for that purpose was entitled to require information from the police. The Independent Monitor was required to reach his own conclusion about the weight to be attached to the allegations before conducting the necessary disclosure balancing exercise between the need to protect the vulnerable group and the individual's right to privacy.

29.70 *R (C) v Secretary of State for Work and Pensions* [2016] EWCA Civ 47

It was lawful for the Secretary of State for Work and Pensions to retain records that showed that a person had changed their gender, where there was good reason for so doing and every effort had been made to minimise the distress caused

Facts: C, a transgender person, was distressed by the fact that Department for Work and Pensions records showed that her gender had changed from male to female, including to the front desk officials that she had to meet on a regular basis.

Judgment: the Court of Appeal (Elias, Patten and Black LJJ) held that Article 8 ECHR was engaged but that the interference with C's personal autonomy was proportionate and justified by the need properly to calculate pension entitlements and to combat fraud, given that the Secretary of State for Work and Pensions had taken numerous steps to modify the system so as to meet the concerns of transgender persons.

29.71 *R (LK) v Independent Monitor* [2016] EWHC 1629 (Admin)

It had been unreasonable to approve inclusion on the ECRC of information about an individual's acquittal of sexual offences when the decision was unsupported by the evidence at the trial and the judge's summing up

Facts: LK had been acquitted of charges of rape and sexual assault on a child under 14 following a trial and had then applied for employment as a part-time social worker in the children's sector. The police and the Independent Monitor felt that the allegations against the claimant ought to be included in the ECRC.

Judgment: William Davis J accepted that the allegations could in principle be included in the ECRC despite the acquittal, providing that the material was relevant and the decision proportionate. In the present case, the police and the Independent Monitor had misrepresented important features of the case, to the extent that the material in the ECRC failed the relevance test.

29.72 *R (G) v Chief Constable of Surrey Police* [2016] EWHC 295 (Admin), [2016] 4 WLR 94

The Police Act 1997 still contained inadequate safeguards against disproportionate disclosure

Facts: the claimant was asked to disclose two reprimands for two counts of sexual assault on a male under 13 which he had received in 2006 when he himself had been 13, pursuant to the disclosure provisions of the Rehabilitation of Offenders Act 1997 and the Police Act 1997. In substance, the sexual assault had been nothing more sinister than teenage experimentation.

Judgment: Blake J held that the regime still failed to contain sufficient safeguards against disproportionate disclosure and that G had at least a highly arguable submission that in his case disclosure would be disproportionate:

> 47. In my judgment, the claimant has at least a highly arguable case that despite the statutory scheme as amended, disclosure of the data to a third party is not relevant and proportionate: (i) Until 1998 it is unlikely that a 12-year-old would have been held to have criminal responsibility for an act of sexual exploration with his peers. The UK has one of the youngest ages of criminal responsibility in Europe. It is necessary to temper the long arm of the criminal law with other measures designed to ensure that children do not become stigmatised as criminals for engaging in activity that might be seen as an ordinary part of the process of growing up.
>
> (ii) Given the investigator and prosecutor's assessment of the nature of the offending and the CPS guidance on sexual offences, the public interest did not require a prosecution and it was arguably a borderline line case for a reprimand. In reaching the decision that he did, the prosecutor did not consider that it was in the public interest to give G a record and did not intend to give him one and thereby damage his welfare and prospects of rehabilitation.
>
> (iii) Until March 2006, any reprimand given to a juvenile would have been weeded out under the terms of earlier document retention policy and therefore not available for mandatory disclosure.

(iv) Until October 2009 such material would have been 'stepped down' after ten years because of the absence of any other conduct causing concern and thus, as the police understand the law, not available for automatic disclosure. This practice changed after the *Humberside* case [2010] 1 WLR 1136 but that case did not consider the justification of interference with Article 8 by disclosure to a private employer.

(v) If the material had been weeded out and stepped down from central records but not deleted altogether, it would still be available for disclosure in an enhanced certificate if the chief constable considered it relevant and proportionate. This is the very judgment that the claimant submits is needed before a spent caution administered to a juvenile is ever disclosed.

(vi) Here the chief constable's own experienced disclosure officer considered that provision of the statutory information to an employer would have had a disproportionate effect. He sought to mitigate this by adoption of some explanation of the surrounding circumstance that tended to show that the offending was not abusive or exploitative and thus not evidence that G was a potential risk to young people.

(vii) Since 1974 Parliament has maintained the Rehabilitation of Offenders Act scheme where offenders sentenced to less than four years imprisonment or detention can treat their sentences as spent. In 2008 Schedule 2 paragraph 1(1)(b) of the ROA provided that an unconditional caution as this reprimand is now considered to be lapses immediately that it is issued. The provisions of the ROA and the previous 'weeding out' and 'stepping down' practices all point to a starting point in the proportionality analysis that not all such matters should be automatically disclosed.

(viii) Filtering out of single minor convictions is one way of achieving proportionality. In that context, the policy choice of which classes of conviction should not be filtered out is a matter to which a margin of appreciation should be afforded to the executive and the legislature, for the reasons given in *W*. However, merely filtering out of single minor convictions is insufficiently sensitive a means of distinguishing between disclosures that are relevant, necessary and proportionate to the legitimate aim that would justify interference with significant aspects of private life (see *Gallagher* [2015] NIQB 63 and *R (P and A) v Secretary of State for Justice* [2016] EWHC 89 (Admin)).

(ix) In the present case, the issue is not multiple cautions, but an overall examination of relevance and proportionality. These considerations could be sufficiently addressed by treating spent convictions and cautions as intelligence data that should only be disclosed when relevant and proportionate to the purpose of the request rather than automatically.

(x) Further, even if different considerations should apply to adult offenders, who could be assumed to be mature enough to understand what they were doing at the time they offended and the need to make a persuasive case that they had changed, the case for procedural safeguards where reprimands have been administered to offenders under 14 is that much more compelling. An interference with Article 8 rights that does not comply with the requirements of the international law obligations of the United Kingdom is unlikely to be justified. The requirements of international law relating to the welfare of the child generally are well known and have been applied in the Article 8 context. They were reviewed by Baroness Hale of Richmond in Durham and Lord Reed JSC in *T* [2014] UKSC 35]. Disclosure of a child's reprimand has a deleterious effect on subsequent social life and there are strong pointers that this should only take place where strictly necessary and proportionate.

(xi) Contrary to the concerns of the Secretaries of State and Ms Foulds, there is no complexity or impracticality about devising a procedure that enables such a judgement to be made as the statutory mechanism already exists in section 113B cases.

(xii) It is unfair to require the employer to make that kind of judgement, with no legal remedy available to the claimant to supervise errors of approach and ensure proportionality of decision making.

48. Cumulatively, in my judgment, these reasons amount to a compelling case that a review mechanism is both needed and is practicable. The claimant, therefore, falls within a class of people within the criteria set out in *MM v United Kingdom*. The Strasbourg Court concluded that the nature of the offence, the disposal in the case, the time which has elapsed since the offence took place or the relevance of the data to the employment sought, might reasonably result in a decision by a public authority applying human rights principles that disclosure was not relevant or necessary.

49. The claimant has no means of seeking to persuade a public authority of this fact, just as in F the registered sex offender, with indefinite notification requirements had no means of demonstrating that the continuation of those requirements remained necessary and proportionate.

50. In the circumstances, the conclusion is the same as in *R (P)*. In my judgment there are insufficient safeguards and the interference with the claimant's Article 8 rights was not in accordance with the law.

29.73 *A v B Local Authority* [2016] EWCA Civ 766

A head teacher had been fairly dismissed for gross misconduct for failing to disclose her relationship with a person convicted of making indecent images of children

Facts: although the head teacher and Y were not cohabiting they had a close personal relationship and the head teacher failed to disclose to the school authorities that Y had been convicted of making indecent images of children and had been sentenced to a community order and a sexual offences prevention order forbidding him from having unsupervised access to children under 18.

Judgment: the Court of Appeal (Elias, Black and Floyd LJJ) dismissed the head teacher's appeal from the employment tribunal's decision upholding the school's dismissal of the head teacher as being fair: her relationship with Y had posed a risk to children at the school and she ought to have disclosed it.

Procedural and other cases

29.74 *Sarfraz v Disclosure and Barring Service* [2015] EWCA Civ 544

The Court of Appeal had no jurisdiction to give permission to appeal to itself, from a decision by the Upper Tribunal not to grant permission to appeal to itself

Facts: Mr Sarfraz was a GP who had been removed from the register by the General Medical Council. The Independent Safeguarding Authority includes him on its children's and its adults' barred lists and the Disclosure and Barring Service (which succeeded the ISA) maintained that decision.

Mr Sarfraz applied to the Upper Tribunal for permission to appeal the DBS decision. The tribunal refused the application and refused permission to appeal to the Court of Appeal against that decision. The appellant argued that the Tribunals, Courts and Enforcement Act 2007 s13 conferred a right of appeal to the Court of Appeal from the Upper Tribunal except in the cases mentioned in section 13(8), which included appeals against decisions of the Upper Tribunal on an application for permission or leave to appeal from the First-tier Tribunal; it followed by necessary implication that appeals against decisions of the Upper Tribunal to refuse permission to appeal to itself from a body other than the First-tier Tribunal could be appealed under section 13.

Judgment: the Court of Appeal (Lord Dyson MR, Kitchin LJ), dismissed the application: whilst there was force in the argument that the exceptions to the right of appeal provided by section 13(1) were set out exhaustively in section 13(8), the principle in *Lane v Esdaile*[38] required to be followed: in the absence of express statutory language to the contrary, a provision giving a court the power to grant or refuse permission to appeal should be construed as not extending to an appeal against a refusal of permission to appeal.

29.75 *MR v Disclosure and Barring Service (Safeguarding vulnerable groups: Adults' barred list)* [2015] UKUT 5 (AAC), 5 January 2015

The DBS reasons for including MR on the adult's barred list were wrong but the case would be remitted to the DBS for further consideration

Facts: the DBS included MR on the adults' barred list, largely on the basis that he had had a sexual relationship with patient B.

Judgment: the Upper Tribunal (UTJ Rowland, Ms M Tynan and Mr J Hutchinson) held that the oral evidence disclosed that MR had not had a sexual relationship with patient B. However, since there could still be grounds to include MR on the adult's barred list, the case was remitted to the DBS.

Comment: this case is included as an example of day-to-day decision-making in the Upper Tribunal in DBS cases.

29.76 *R (C) v Secretary of State for Justice* [2016] UKSC 2, (2016) 19 CCLR 5

There was no presumption of anonymity for mental patients challenging aspects of their treatment and care in the High Court but anonymity will be granted where that is necessary in the interests of the patient

Facts: C had been convicted of murder, then transferred to hospital as a mental patient. After many years in detention, the First-tier Tribunal recommended that he was suitable for conditional discharge but the Secretary of State for Justice refused to allow C trial periods of unescorted leave in the community. C sought a judicial review of that decision. His application was refused and the High Court judge revoked C's anonymity order. The Court of Appeal upheld that revocation.

38 [1891] AC 210.

Judgment: the Supreme Court (Hale, Clarke, Wilson, Carnwath and Hughes JJSC) held that there was no presumption of anonymity in the High Court and above, in relation to mental patients challenging aspects of their care and treatment under the Mental Health Act 1983, but that an anonymity order should be made in this case otherwise the patient's integration into the community would be jeopardised.

Comment: although this is a judgment on particular facts the analysis of the Supreme Court, allowing the appeal from decisions by the High Court and Court of Appeal, suggests that there will be very few cases indeed, if any, where anonymity may be refused in this type of case – perhaps where there is no real prospect of the mental patient being discharged into the community, at all, or in the foreseeable future.

Index